5 Update in Intensive Care and Emergency Medicine

Edited by J. L. Vincent

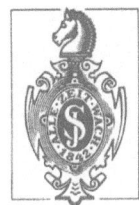

Update 1988

Edited by
J. L. Vincent

With 175 Figures and 77 Tables

Springer-Verlag
Berlin Heidelberg New York
London Paris Tokyo

Dr. Jean Louis Vincent   Assistant-Director, Department
of Intensive Care, Erasme Hospital
Free University of Brussels
Route de Lennik 808
B-1070 Brussels, Belgium

ISBN-13: 978-3-540-18981-7   e-ISBN-13: 978-3-642-83392-2
DOI: 10.1007/978-3-642-83392-2

© Springer-Verlag Berlin Heidelberg 1988

The use of registered names, trademarks, etc. in the publication does not imply, even in
the absence of a specific statement, that such names are exempt from the relevant protective laws and regulations and therefore free for general use.

Product Liability: The publisher can give no guarantee for information about drug dosage and application thereof contained in this book. In every individual case the respective user must check its accuracy by consulting other pharmaceutical literature.

2119/3140-543210

Contents

Acute Respiratory Failure

Severe Asthmatic Crisis

Right Ventricular Failure – Pulmonary Hypertension

Myocardial Ischemia and Necrosis

Management of Cardiac Crisis

Monitoring of the Critically Ill: Invasive and Non-Invasive

Cardiopulmonary Resuscitation

Emergency and Trauma

Outcome After Trauma

Cerebral Crisis – Psychological Support

List of Contributors

Abraham, E.
Emergency Medicine Center, University of California,
Los Angeles, CA 90024, USA

Adgey, A. A. J.
Cardiology, Royal Victoria Hospitale,
Grosvenor Road, Northern Belfast BT12 6BA, Ireland

Aloy, A.
Anästhesiologie, University of Vienna
Spitalgasse 23, 1090 Wien, Austria

Arfors, K. E.
Experimental Medicine,
10901 N. Torrey Pines Road, La Jolla, CA 92037, USA

Artigas, A.
Cuidados Intensivos, Hospital Santa Creu i Sant Pau,
Av San Antoni M. Claret 167, Barcelona 08025, Spain

Askenasi, R.
Service des Urgences, Hôpital Erasme,
Route de Lennik 808, 1070 Bruxelles, Belgium

Atwater, B. W.
Technical Center, BOC Group,
100 Mountain Avenue, New Providence, NJ 07974, USA

Baron, J. F.
Anesthésie-Réanimation, C. H. U. Pitié-Salpêtrière,
83 Bld de l'Hôpital, 75013 Paris Cédex 13, France

Barriot, P.
Service Médical d'Urgence, Sapeurs-Pompiers de Paris,
47 rue Saint Fargeau, 75020 Paris, France

Baum, M.
Klinik für Anaesthesiologie, University of Innsbruck,
Anichstrasse 35, 6020 Innsbruck, Austria

Beaufils, F.
Réanimation Pédiatrique, Hôpital Bretonneau,
2 rue Carpeaux, 75018 Paris, France

Beeley, J. M.
Director of Naval Medicine, Royal Naval Hospital,
Haslar, Gosport, Hampshire PO12 2AA, UK

Benito, S.
Servicio de Cuidados Intensivos, Hospital Santa Creu i Sant
Pau, Av San Antoni M. Claret 167, Barcelona 08025, Spain

Benzer, H.
Klinik für Anaesthesiologie, University of Innsbruck,
Anichstrasse 35, 6020 Innsbruck, Austria

Berkenboom, G.
Cardiologie, Hôpital Erasme,
Route de Lennik 808, 1070 Bruxelles, Belgium

Beutler, B.
Research Laboratories, Howard Hughes Medical Institute,
5323 Harry Hines Bld Y5-210, Dallas, TX 75235-9050, USA

Biagioli, B.
Cardiovascular Surgery, University of Siena,
Viale Bracci, 53100 Siena, Italy

Boldt, J.
Intensive Care Medicine, Justus Liebig University,
Klinikstrasse 29, 6300 Giessen, FRG

Bossaert, L. L.
Intensieve Zorgen, University Antwerp-UIA,
Universiteitsplein 1, 2610 Antwerpen, Belgium

Bradley, J. A.
Department of Surgery, University of Glasgow,
Western Infirmary, Glasgow G11 6NT, UK

Brandt, L.
Department of Neurosurgery, University Hospital,
22185 Lund, Sweden

Brimioulle, S.
Soins Intensifs, Hôpital Erasme
Route de Lennik 808, 1070 Bruxelles, Belgium

Brochard, L.
Réanimation Médicale, Hôpital Henri Mondor,
51 Av de Lattre de Tassigny, 94010 Créteil Cédex, France

Bruère, D.
Anesthésie-Réanimation, C. H. U. Pitié-Salpêtrière,
47 Bld de l'Hôpital, 75671 Paris Cédex 13, France

Brunet, F.
Réanimation Polyvalente, C. H. U. Cochin-Port Royal,
27 rue du Faubourg St Jacques, 75674 Paris Cédex 14, France

Busse, O.
Department of Neurology, Klinikum Minden,
Friedrichstrasse 17, 4950 Minden, FRG

Campbell, R. W. F.
Department of Cardiology, Freeman Hospital,
High Heaton, Newcastle/Tyne NE7 7DN, UK

Chatterjee, K.
Division of Cardiology, University of California,
1186 Moffit Long Hospital, San Francisco, CA 94143, USA

Chiara, O.
Emergency Surgery, Universita di Milan,
Via F. Sforza 33, 20122 Milan, Italy

Chilcoat, R. T.
Technical Center, BOC Group,
100 Mountain Avenue, New Providence, NJ 07974, USA

Clark, R. J.
Respiratory Division, Hammersmith Hospital,
London W12 OHS, UK

Cohen, R. D.
Department of Medicine, The London Hospital,
Mile End 275 Bancroft Road, London E1 1BB, UK

Coriat, P.
Anesthésie-Réanimation, C. H. U. Pitié-Salpêtrière,
83 Bld de l'Hôpital, 75651 Paris Cédex 13, France

Coutenye, M.
Department of Nephrology, AZ Stuyvenberg,
Lange Beeldekensstraat 267, 2008 Antwerpen, Belgium

Cunningham, S. R.
Cardiology, Royal Victoria Hospital,
Grosvenor Road, Northern Belfast BT12 6BA, Ireland

Dall'ava-Santucci, J.
Réanimation Médicale, C. H. U. Cochin-Port Royal,
27 Faubourg St Jacques, 75674 Paris Cédex 14, France

da Luz, P. L.
Faculdade de Medicina, Hospital des Clinicas,
CJTO 141-Rue Itapeva 366, Sao Paulo, CEP 01332, Brazil

Dalzell, G. W. N.
Cardiology, Royal Victoria Hospital,
Grosvenor Road, Northern Belfast BT12 6BA, Ireland

Dantzker, D. R.
Pulmonary Medicine, University of Texas Health Center,
6431 Fannin Suite 1274, Houston, TX 77030, USA

De Broe, M. E.
Department of Nephrology, AZ Stuyvenberg,
Lange Beeldekensstraat 267, 2008 Antwerpen, Belgium

Decaux, G.
Service de Médecine, Hôpital Erasme,
Route de Lennik 808, 1070 Bruxelles, Belgium

Dhainaut, J. F.
Réanimation Médicale, C. H. U. Cochin-Port Royal,
27 rue du Faubourg St Jacques, 75674 Paris Cédex 14, France

Downs, J. B.
Department of Anesthesiology, Ohio State University,
410 West Tenth Avenue, Colombus, Ohio 43210, USA

Ducas, J.
Department of Medicine, Health Science Center,
700 William Avenue, Winnipeg, Manitoba R3E OZ3, Canada

Duroux, P.
Service de Réanimation, Hôpital Antoine Beclère,
157 rue de la Porte de Trivaux, 92140 Clamart, France

Duvelleroy, M.
Laboratoire de Biophysique, Hôpital Fernand Widal,
200 rue du Faubourg St Denis, 75010 Paris, France

Edwards, J. D.
Intensive Care Unit, Withington Hospital,
West Didsbury, Manchester M20 8LR, UK

Estenne, M.
Service de Pneumologie, Hôpital Erasme,
Route de Lennik 808, 1070 Bruxelles, Belgium

Falke, K. J.
Anesthesiologie, Universitätskrankenhaus,
Moorenstrasse 5, 4000 Düsseldorf, FRG

Fanconi, S.
Intensivstation, Universitätskinderklinik,
Steinwiesstrasse 75, 8032 Zürich, Switzerland

Ghannad, E.
Réanimation Médicale, C. H. U. Cochin-Port Royal,
27 rue du Faubourg St Jacques, 75674 Paris Cédex 14, France

Giomarelli, P.
Cardiovascular Surgery, University of Siena,
Viale Bracci, 53100 Siena, Italy

Goldberg, L. I.
Department of Pharmacology, University of Chicago,
947 East 58th Street, Chicago, Illinois 60637, USA

Goldberg, P.
Meakins-Christie Laboratories, McGill University,
3775 University Street, Montreal, Quebec H3A 2B4, Canada

Goldstein, J. P.
Chirurgie Cardiaque, Hôpital Erasme,
Route de Lennik 808, 1070 Bruxelles, Belgium

Gouin, F.
Anesthésie-Réanimation, Hôpital Sainte Marguerite,
270 Bld de Sainte-Marguerite, 13277 Marseille Cédex 9, France

Hartenauer, U.
Klinik für Anästhesiologie, Westfälische Wilhelms-Universität,
Albert Schweitzer Strasse 33, 4400 Münster, FRG

Hartmann, J. F.
Réanimation Pédiatrique, Hôpital Bretonneau,
2 rue Carpeaux, 75018 Paris, France

Haupt, M. T.
Medical Intensive Care Unit, Wayne University,
540 East Canfield Avenue, Detroit, MI 48201, USA

Heidendal, G. A. K.
Nucleaire Geneeskunde, St Annadal Ziekenhuis,
St Annadal 1, 6201 BX Maastricht, The Netherlands

Heinrich, H.
Anästhesiologie, Universität Ulm,
Steinhövelstrasse 9, 7900 Ulm, FRG

Hemmer, M.
Anesthésiologie, Centre Hospitalier, Rue Barblé 4,
Luxembourg

Hempelmann, G.
Intensive Care Medicine, Justus Liebig University,
Klinikstrasse 29, 6300 Giessen, FRG

Hillman, K.
Intensive Care Unit, The Liverpool Hospital,
Box 103 Liverpool, Sydney, NSW 2170, Australia

Holbrook, P. R.
Department of Child Health, Children's Hospitale,
111 Michigan Avenue NW, Washington, DC 20010, USA

Kaste, M.
Department of Neurology, University of Helsinki,
00290 Helsinki, Finland

Kling, D.
Intensive Care Medicine, Justus Liebig University,
Klinikstrasse 29, 6300 Giessen, FRG

Kuch, K.
Department of Psychiatry, Toronto General Hospital,
200 Elizabeth Street, Toronto M5G IL7, Canada

Laborde, F.
Chirurgie Cardio-vasculaire, Clinique de la Porte de Choisy,
75018 Paris, France

Lazarus, G.
Institut für Anästhesiologie, Universität Würzburg,
Josef Schneider Strasse 2, 8700 Würzburg, FRG

Leal, J.
Intensive Care Unit, Hospital de Santo Antonio,
4200 Porto, Portugal

Lebert, M.
Intensivstation, Universitätskinderklinik,
Steinwiesstrasse 75, 8032 Zürich, Switzerland

Ledingham, I. McA.
Department of Surgery, University of Glasgow,
Western Infirmary, Glasgow G11 6NT, UK

Lemaire, F.
Réanimation Médicale, Hôpital Henri Mondor,
51 Av de Lattre de Tassigny, 94010 Créteil Cédex, France

Lenclud, C.
Service de Pneumologie, Hôpital Erasme,
Route de Lennik 808, 1070 Bruxelles, Belgium

Levene, M. I.
Department of Child Health, Leicester Royal Infirmary,
Infirmary Square, Leicester LE1 5WW, UK

Lheureux, P.
Service des Urgences, Hôpital Erasme,
Route de Lennik 808, 1070 Bruxelles, Belgium

Lins, R. L.
Department of Nephrology, AZ Stuyvenberg,
Lange Beeldekensstraat 267, 2008 Antwerpen, Belgium

Ljunggren, B.
Department of Neurosurgery, University Hospital,
22185 Lund, Sweden

Mancebo, J.
Servicio de Cuidados Intensivos, Hospital Santa Creu i Sant
Pau, Av Sant Antoni M. Claret 167, Barcelona 08025, Spain

Martin, C.
Anesthésie-Réanimation, Hôpital Sainte Marguerite,
270 Bld de Sainte-Marguerite, 13277 Marseille Cédex 9, France

Martinez, R.
Cuidados Intensivos, Hospital Santa Creu i Sant Pau,
Av Sant Antoni M. Claret 167, Barcelona 08025, Spain

Mayer, N.
Anästhesiologie, University of Vienna,
Spitalgasse 23, 1090 Wien, Austria

McNeill, A. J.
Cardiology, Royal Victoria Hospital,
Grosvenor Road, Northern Belfast BT12 6BA, Ireland

Mercier, J. C.
Réanimation Pédiatrique, Hôpital Bretonneau,
2 rue Carpeaux, 75018 Paris, France

Messmer, K.
Experimentelle Chirurgie, Ruprecht-Karls-Universität,
Im Neuenheimer Feld 347, 6900 Heidelberg 1, FRG

Montejo, L. S.
Anesthésie-Réanimation, C. H. U. Pitié-Salpêtrière,
83 Bld de l'Hôpital, 75013 Paris Cédex 13, France

Morel, D. R.
Department of Anesthesia, University Hospital,
1211 Geneva, Switzerland

Mutz, N.
Klinik für Anaesthesiologie, University of Innsbruck,
Anichstrasse 35, 6020 Innsbruck, Austria

Neild, G. H.
Department of Renal Medicine, St Philip's Hospital
Sheffield Street, London WC2A 2EX, UK

Nienaber, C.
Department of Radiological Sciences, UCLA School of Medicine,
Room CHS/045, Los Angeles, CA 90024, USA

Nikki, P.
Department of Neurology, University of Helsinki,
00290 Helsinki, Finland

Ohtomo, Y.
Critical Care Medicine, Nippon Medical School,
1-1-5 Sendagi/Bunkyo-Ku, Tokyo 113, Japan

Otsuka, T.
Critical Care Medicine, Nippon Medical School,
1-1-5 Sendagi/Bunlyo-Ku, Tokyo 113, Japan

Paes Cardoso, A.
Intensive Care Unit, Hospital de Santo Antonio,
4200 Porto, Portugal

Palandri Chagas, A. C.
Faculdade de Medicina, Hospital des Clinicas,
CJTO 141-Rue Itapeva 366, Sao Paulo, CEP 01332, Brazil

Parker, J. W.
Technical Center, BOC Group,
100 Mountain Avenue, New Providence, NJ 07974, USA

Parratt, J. R.
Department of Physiology, Royal College,
204 George Street, Glasgow G1 1XW, UK

Perret, C.
Service des Soins Intensifs, C. H. U. Vaudois,
1011 Lausanne, Switzerland

Peters, J.
Institut für Anästhesiologie, Universität Düsseldorf,
Moorenstrasse 5, 4000 Düsseldorf 1, FRG

Pileggi, F.
Faculdade de Medicina, Hospital des Clinicas,
CJTO 141-Rue Itapeva 366, Sao Paulo, CEP 01332, Brazil

Pinsky, M. R.
Critical Care Medicine, Presbyterian University Hospital,
1385 Scaife Hall, Pittsburgh, Pennsylvania 15261, USA

Prewitt, R. M.
Department of Medicine, Health Science Center,
700 William Avenue, Winnipeg, Manitoba R3E 0Z3, Canada

Priebe, H. J.
Anesthesiologie, Kantonsspital,
4031 Basel, Switzerland

Primo, G.
Chirurgie Cardiaque, Hôpital Erasme,
Route de Lennik 808, 1070 Bruxelles, Belgium

Räsänen, J.
Department of Anesthesiology, Central Hospital,
Haartmaninkatu 4, 00290 Helsinki 29, Finland

Reinhart, K.
Anästhesiologie, Universitätsklinikum Steglitz,
Hindenburgdamm 30, 1000 Berlin 45, FRG

Riou, B.
Anesthésie-Réanimation, C. H. U. Pitié-Salpêtrière,
83 Bld de l'Hôpital, 75013 Paris, France

Robertson, C. E.
Emergency Medicine, Western General Hospital,
Crewe Road South, Edinburgh EH4 2XU, UK

Roca, J.
Servicio di Pathologia Resp., Hospital Clinic i Provincial,
Via Villarroel 170, 08036 Barcelona, Spain

Rodriguez-Roisin, R.
Servicio di Pathologia Resp., Hospital Clinic i Provincial,
Via Villarroel 170, 08036 Barcelona, Spain

Rogerson, M. E.
Department of Renal Medicine, St Philip's Hospital,
Sheffield Street, London WC2A 2EX, UK

Roglan, A.
Cuidados Intensivos, Hospital Santa Creu i Sant Pau,
Av Sant Antoni M. Claret 167, Barcelona 08025, Spain

Roine, R. O.
Department of Neurology, University of Helsinki,
00290 Helsinki, Finland

Rosi, R.
Cardiovascular Surgery, University of Siena,
Viale Bracci, 53100 Siena, Italy

Rossignon, M. D.
Anesthésie-Réanimation, C. H. U. Pitié-Salpêtrière,
83 Bld de l'Hôpital, 75651 Paris Cédex 13, France

Roussos, C.
Meakins-Christie Laboratories, McGill University,
3775 University Street, Montreal, Quebec H3A 2B4, Canada

Rua, F.
Intensive Care Unit, Hospital de Santo Antonio,
4200 Porto, Portugal

Saux, P.
Anesthésie-Réanimation, Hôpital Sainte Marguerite,
270 Bld de Sainte-Marguerite, 13277 Marseille Cédex 9, France

Säveland, H.
Department of Neurosurgery, University Hospital,
22185 Lund, Sweden

Schäfer, M.
Anästhesiologie, Universitätsklinikum Steglitz,
Hindenburgdamm 30, 1000 Berlin 45, FRG

Scheidegger, D.
Anesthesiologie, Kantonsspital,
4031 Basel, Switzerland

Schelbert, H. R.
Department of Radiological Sciences, UCLA School of Medicine,
Room CHS/045, Los Angeles, CA 90024, USA

Schellekens, J. F. P.
Department of Clinical Microbiology, Academisch Ziekenhuis,
Catharijnesingel 101, 3511 GV Utrecht, The Netherlands

Scherer, R.
Klinik für Anästhesiologie, Clemens-Hospital,
Düesbergweg 124, 4400 Münster, FRG

Schwaiger, M.
Division of Nuclear Medicine, University of Michigan Hospitals
Ann Arbor, Michigan, USA

Scott, I.
Special Care Baby Unit, St. David's Hospital,
Cowbridge Road East, Cardiff CF2 1SZ, UK

Shortland, G. J.
Special Care Baby Unit, St. David's Hospital,
Cowbridge Road East, Cardiff CF2 1SZ, UK

Sinclair, M. E.
Nuffield Department of Anaesthetics, John Radcliffe Hospital,
Headington, Oxford 0X3 9DU, UK

Soeters, P. B.
Afdeling Chirurgie, St Annadal Ziekenhuis,
St Annadal 1, 6214 PA Maastricht, The Netherlands

Sold, M.
Institut für Anästhesiologie, Universität Würzburg,
Josef Schneider Strasse 2, 8700 Würzburg, FRG

Specht, M.
Anästhesiologie, Universitätsklinikum Steglitz,
Hindenburgdamm 30, 1000 Berlin 45, FRG

Steedman, D. J.
Emergency Medicine, Western General Hospital,
Crewe Road South, Edinburgh EH4 2XU, UK

Stoutenbeek, C. P.
Intensieve Zorgen, Onze Lieve Vrouw Gasthuis,
1e Oosterparkstraat 179, 1091 HA Amsterdam, The Netherlands

Swinson, R. P.
Department of Psychiatry, Toronto General Hospital,
200 Elizabeth Street, Toronto M5G IL7, Canada

Thijs, L. G.
Inwendige Geneeskunde, A.Z. Amsterdam,
De Boelelaan 1117, 1007 MB Amsterdam, The Netherlands

Turner, A. F.
Department of Radiology, Community Hospital of San Gabriel,
612 W Duarte Road, Arcadia, CA 91006, USA

Unger, P.
Cardiologie, Hôpital Erasme,
Route de Lennik 808, 1070 Bruxelles, Belgium

van der Merwe, C. J.
Emergency Department, HF Verwoerd Hospital,
P.O. Box 667, Pretoria 0001, South Africa

Van Gossum, A.
Gastro-Entérologie, Hôpital Erasme,
Route de Lennik 808, 1070 Bruxelles, Belgium

van Saene, H. K. F.
Medical Microbiology, Royal Liverpool Hospital,
P. O. Box 147, Liverpool L69 3BX, UK

Verhoef, J.
Department of Clinical Microbiology, Academisch Ziekenhuis,
Catharijnesingel 101, 3511 GV Utrecht, The Netherlands

Verrier Jones, E. R.
Special Care Baby Unit, St David's Hospital,
Cowbridge Road East, Cardiff CF2 1SZ, UK

Versprille, A.
Pulmonary Diseases, Erasmus Universiteit,
Postbus 1738, 3000 Rotterdam, The Netherlands

Viars, P.
Anesthésie-Réanimation, C. H. U. Pitié-Salpêtrière,
47 Bld de l'Hôpital, 75671 Paris Cédex 13, France

Vicaut, E.
Laboratoire de Biophysique, Hôpital Fernand Widal,
200 rue du Faubourg St Denis, 75010 Paris, France

von Meyenfeldt, M. P.
Afdeling Chirurgie, St Annadal Ziekenhuis,
St Annadal 1, 6214 PA Maastricht, The Netherlands

Wainwright, C. L.
Department of Physiology, Royal College,
204 George Street, Glasgow G1 1XW, UK

Yamamoto, Y.
Critical Care Medicine, Nippon Medical School,
1-1-5 Sendagi/Bunkyo-Ku, Tokyo 113, Japan

Yernault, J. C.
Service de Pneumologie, Hôpital Erasme,
Route de Lennik 808, 1070 Bruxelles, Belgium

Zandstra, D. F.
Intensieve Zorgen, Onze Lieve Vrouw Gasthuis,
1e Oosterparkstraat 179, 1091 HA Amsterdam, The Netherlands

Zimpfer, M.
Anästhesiologie, University of Vienna,
Spitalgasse 23, 1090 Wien, Austria

Circulatory Failure:
The Importance of Tissue Oxygen Supply

Cardiocirculatory Control Mechanisms in Health and Disease

N. Mayer and M. Zimpfer

Introduction

The cardiovascular system is regulated by different control principles including *local* metabolic control at tissue levels and the *overall* neural and humoral regulation. It remains a major concern as to whether these complicated mechanisms remain intact or get affected by various diseases and/or anesthetic drugs in the perioperative period. The present paper briefly reviews the above mentioned control mechanisms and focuses on some clinically relevant disturbances of these regulatory circuits as result of diseases or pharmacological manipulations.

Local Control Mechanisms

The major determinant of local blood flow is the rate of metabolism of the tissues and the availability of oxygen whereby an increase in the metabolic rate and a decrease of the availabilty of oxygen are directly linked to a local blood flow augmentation. However, in several tissues like in kidney and the brain a certain invariability of blood flow is of such importance that additional factors play a dominant role for the blood supply of these organs, thus uncoupling the blood flow rates from the instantaneous perfusion pressure, i.e. autoregulation.

Regulation of *cerebral blood flow* is mainly linked to changes of the carbon dioxide concentration, the hydrogen ion concentration and the oxygen tension whereas the autonomic nervous system is only of minor importance. Besides occlusive cerebral vascular disease, the integrity of the cerebral autoregulation is threatened by several pathophysiological conditions and pharmacological interventions with the common mechanisms of cerebral vasodilation.

Volatile anesthetics reduce the autoregulative capacity of the cerebral blood flow causing a more or less pressure-dependent brain perfusion at higher concentrations. It is a typical feature of the inhalation anesthetics that the slope of the autoregulation curve is altered both on the high and the low pressure range [1]. While the latter might have a beneficial effect because it augments cerebral perfusion at lower blood pressures [2], the shift of the upper limit of the autoregulation to the left leads to a direct transfer of high arterial pressures on the intracranial pressure. However, there exist also indirect influences besides the above mentioned direct effects. These include an altered carbon dioxide sensitivity [3] as well as alterations of the cerebral metabolism.

As both *nitroprusside and nitroglycerin* have direct vasodilator properties it is not surprising that they may reduce or even abolish the cerebral autoregulation. However, their impact on cerebral blood flow and intracranial pressure depends on the effect on systemic arterial pressure. When the latter is not reduced due to the action of nitroprusside or nitroglycerin on the peripheral vasculature, as might be the case in hypertensive individuals, one must face the possibility of deleterious intracranial pressure increases [4, 5].

While hypercapnia, hypoxia or volatile anesthetics impair the overall integrity of the cerebral autoregulation, in the surrounding of tumors or cerebral infarcts the autoregulation is terminated at a regional level. Cerebral vessels in the vicinity of these pathological structures are already maximally dilated due to accumulation of acidic metabolites. On the basis of these alterations cerebral steal might occur when carbon dioxide tension increases thereby inducing a dilation of normal vessels which might shunt blood away from the zone of permanent vasodilation. On the other hand, a salutary effect on ischemic zones can be accomplished by reduction of carbon dioxide tension and consequent constriction of normal vessels which leads to a blood shift in favour of hypoperfused brain structures (Robin Hood phenomenon).

Local regulation of blood flow is also of fundamental importance in the *lung* for the matching of ventilation and perfusion. Since blood flow trough the lung

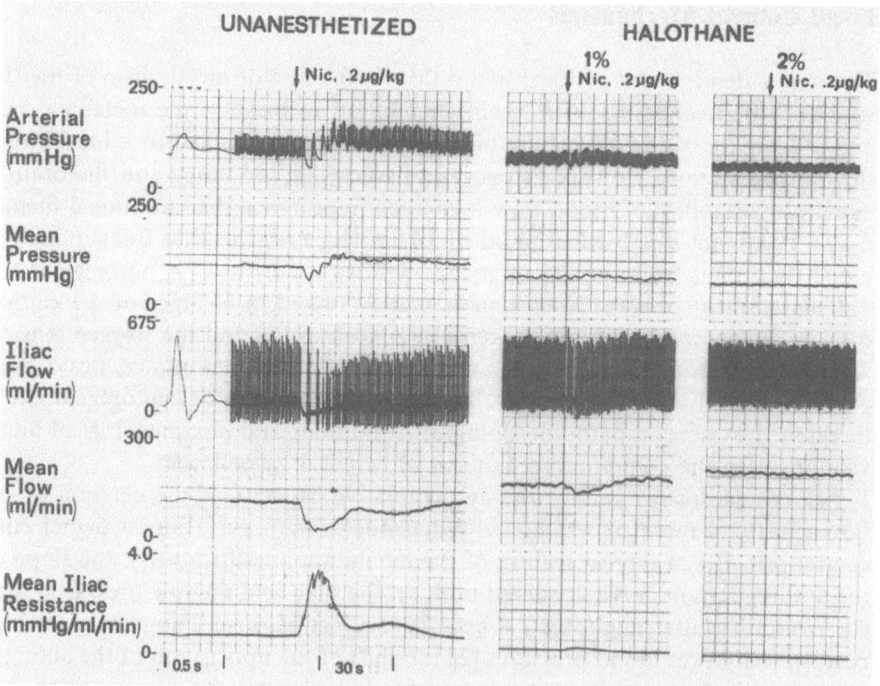

Fig. 1. Effects of a temporary occlusion of the left circumflex coronary artery in a conscious dog with intact coronary circulation. As a result of metabolic autoregulation, dramatic reactive hyperemia is observed after release of the occluder

is essentially equal to cardiac output, the factors that control cardiac output also determine pulmonary blood flow. However, as opposed to other tissues a low alveolar oxygen pressure increases pulmonary vascular resistance in order to adapt the regional lung perfusion to the instantaneous degree of ventilation, keeping the shunt fraction within physiological limits. This potent so called hypoxic pulmonary vasoconstriction is inhibited both by inhalation anesthetics and by systemic vasodilators. This feature has been ascribed to halothane [6, 7], enflurane [8], isoflurane [9], nitroprusside and nitroglycerin [10] and to the calcium antagonists nifedipine [11], verapamil [12] and nimodipine [13].

Although the *coronary circulation* has no autoregulatory properties in terms of blood flow maintenance over an array of blood pressure changes it will be discussed here because of certain other characteristics (Fig. 1). One of these features is the fact that the heart – even in the resting state – removes about 70% of oxygen from the arterial blood. Thus, an increased oxygen demand can only be met by an increase of coronary blood flow which closely parallels myocardial oxygen usage. It might be anticipated that overall coronary vasodilation protects against silent or overt myocardial ischemia. However, in contrast to the initial enthusiasm, small vessel coronary dilators, e.g., dipyridamole can actually aggravate myocardial ischemia as a result of blood flow redistribution away from ischemic areas i.e. "coronary steal". Similar mechanisms are currently under discussion of inducing myocardial ischemia during inhalation anesthesia [14–16]. In contrast to results obtained from acute animal preparations [17], which might be perturbated from baseline anesthesia and recent surgical trauma, both halothane [18] and isoflurane [19] fail to cause exaggerated or permanent ischemic myocardial dysfunction in the animals with a chronic coronary stenosis suggesting absence of regional flow redistribution.

Neural Control Mechanisms

The neural control of the cardiovascular system is not only accomplished by impulse transmission from the central nervous system to peripheral blood vessels (Fig. 2) but also includes special cardiovascular reflexes which mainly act within the scope of short-term arterial pressure regulation.

The baroreceptor reflex originates at spray type nerve endings situated in the aortic arch and the carotid sinus. When an increase in arterial pressure causes a stretch of these receptors, a number of nerve impulses travelling to the inhibitory area of the vasomotor center increases and in turn decreases sympathetic vasoconstrictor tone. This results in peripheral vasodilation, reduced myocardial contractility and heart rate. The opposite mechanism becomes operative when blood pressure declines. The maximum gain of this reflex is within the range of normal mean arterial pressures where only a small change causes strong baroreceptor-mediated cardiovascular responses. While the baroreceptor reflex system acts within seconds in response to a blood pressure change, with impulses increasing during systole and decreasing during diastole [20], it has no importance for the long-term arterial pressure regulation because adaptation occurs within 1–3 days irrespective of the actual pressure they are exposed to. The volatile anesthetics

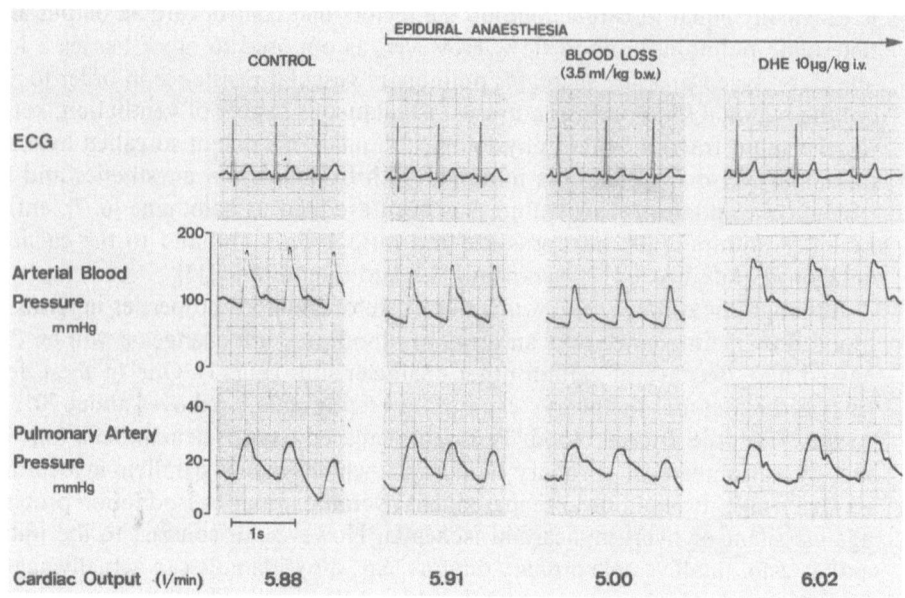

Fig. 2. Hemodynamic effects of dihydroergotamine during epidural anesthesia and mild blood loss. In spite of preinfusion of 1000 ml Ringer, cardiac output and arterial pressure are reduced after mild hemorrhage due to the disruptive effects on neural control principles. The circulatory depression is abolished by dihydroergotamine (DHE)

halothane, enflurane and, to a lesser extent, isoflurane [21] as well as the barbiturates [22] impair the integrity of the baroreceptor reflex whereas with morphine anesthesia the reflex remains intact [23]. It might also be of clinical relevance that the sensitivity of the baroreceptor reflex is reduced with volume loading [24] and in presence of heart disease [25].

The chemoreflex: It is often overlooked that the chemosensitive cells, located in the carotid bodies near the bifurcation of the common carotid artery, and the aortic bodies in the aortic arch triggers one of the most powerful cardiovascular reflexes, mediating bradycardia and an intense peripheral vasoconstriction (Fig. 3) with the teleological significance to preserve the supply of oxygen to the vital organs. The carotid chemoreceptor reflex is impaired by increasing concentrations of volatile anesthetics (Fig. 3), [26, 27], barbiturates [26] and also opioids [23] although the latter class of anesthetics is often held to be devoid of effects on cardiocirculatory control principles.

A failure in the afferent or efferent loop of the chemoreceptor reflex and/or its central integration is the pathophysiological basis of the central hypoventilation syndromes like the Pickwick syndrome [28].

The *low pressure receptors,* located in the walls of the atria and the pulmonary arteries, are sensitive to pressure changes in connection with alterations of the circulating blood volume. Stretching the atria induces 1) reflex vasodilation and reduction in peripheral vascular resistance, 2) dilation of the afferent arterioles in the kidneys thereby increasing renal blood flow and glomerular filtration rate, 3) inhibition of the release of antidiuretic hormone, and 4) increase of cardiac

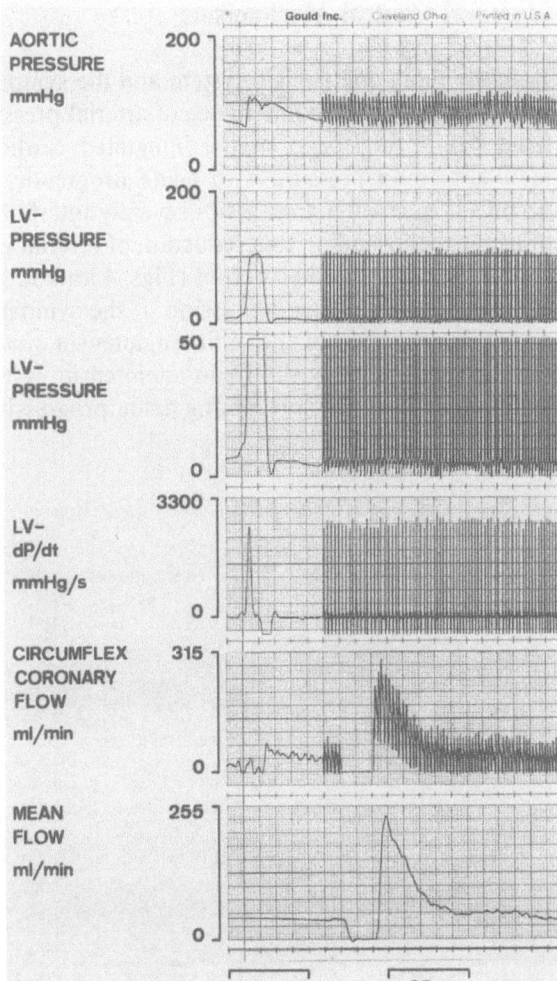

Fig. 3. Responses to coronary chemoreceptor stimulation with nicotine (0.2 μg/kg) are shown on measurements of phasic and mean arterial pressure, phasic and mean iliac blood flow, and computed mean iliac resistance in an unanesthetized dog with controlled ventilation in the left-hand panel and in the same dog after the addition of halothane 1 vol% and 2 vol% (right-hand panel). The iliac constriction and bradycardia induced by coronary chemoreflex stimulation was depressed considerably by 1 vol% halothane, whereas 2 vol% of halothane abolished these responses

rate and the strength of contraction. The documentation of the latter, known as the Bainbridge reflex, which has been challenged [29], depends on low physiological heart rates [30], and is of lesser importance in man than in the subhuman primate or in the dog [31]. However, although cardiovascular responses to volume loading in anesthetized animals are at variance to those observed in conscious animals, it remains uncertain whether the Bainbridge reflex is specifically affected by anesthetics or various diseases.

Humoral Control Mechanisms

Both the renin-angiotensin system and the sympathoadrenal system play an important role for the maintenance of arterial pressure during progressive hemorrhage. While the ability of the integrated cardiovascular control principles to maintain blood pressure with acute progressive hemorrhage is unaffected by opioids [32], volatile anesthetics severely interfere with hemodynamic responses to hemorrhage leading to a reduction of arterial pressure in spite of only moderate reductions in cardiac output (Figs. 4 and 5). These differences can partly be explained by a striking depression of the sympathoadrenal system in spite of a powerful activation of the renin-angiotensin system. Nonetheless, vasoconstriction accomplished by the renin-angiotensin system is not powerful enough to maintain arterial pressure during acute progressive hemorrhage [33].

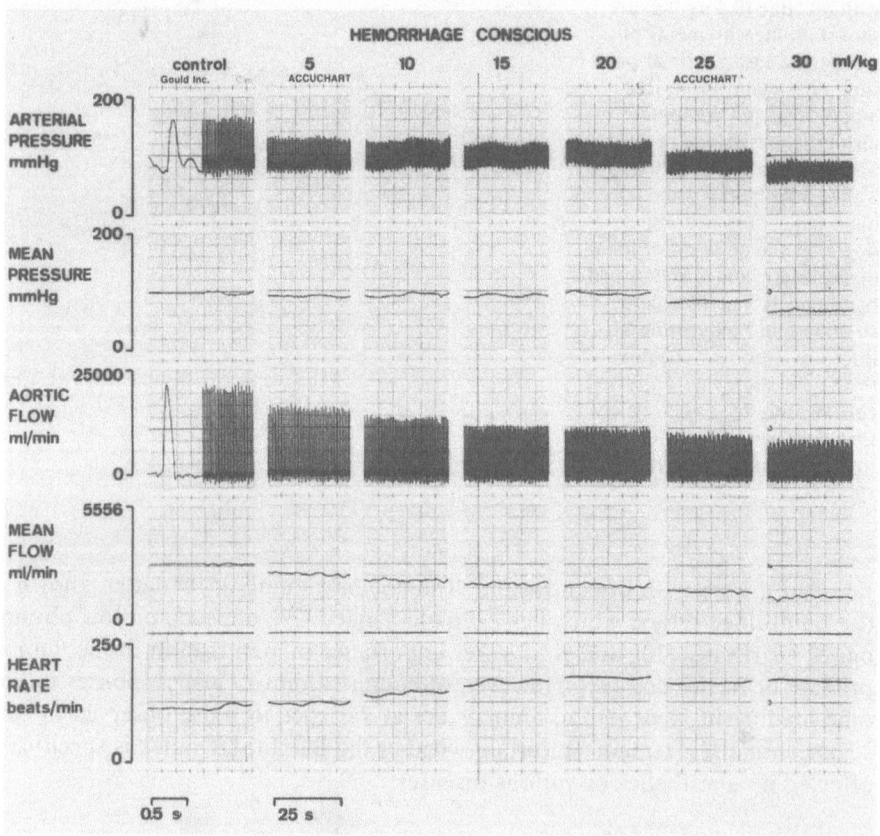

Fig. 4. Typical response showing the effects of hemorrhage in a conscious dog on phasic and mean arterial pressure, phasic and mean aortic blood flow and heart rate. Recordings are shown at control and at every 5 ml/kg of blood loss up to 30 ml/kg. While arterial pressure was well maintained throughout the entire experiment, aortic flow fell markedly

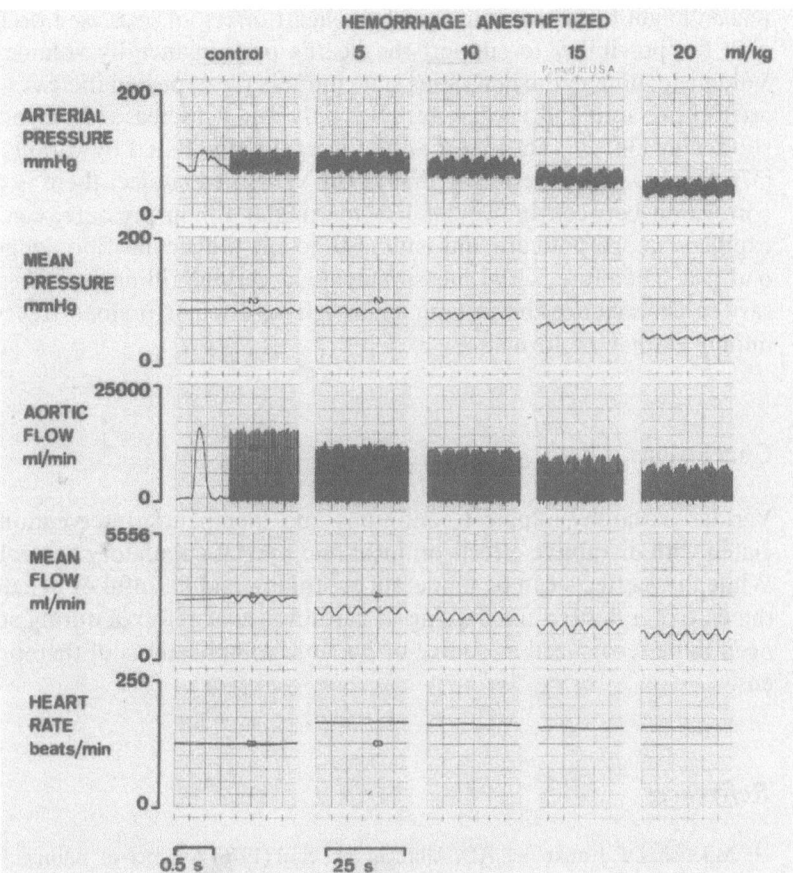

Fig. 5. In contrast to the conscious state, with 3% enflurane inspired, hemorrhage led to striking progressive decreases in arterial pressure, forcing the investigator to terminate the experimental protocol untimely

Intrinsic Regulation of Cardiac Output – The Frank-Starling Law of the Heart

The concept of the control of cardiac performance by the rate of venous return, i.e. preload, is one of the corner stones of cardiac physiology. More recent studies, however, looked at the efficacy of these important cardiovascular control principles in the conscious reclining state. In this situation the heart is working on the sharp upslope of the pressure-volume curve [34] and an increase in preload, i.e. myocardial fiber length, is followed by only trivial increases in stroke length while cardiac output is mainly augmented via chronotropic mechanisms. On the other hand, left ventricular preload decreases with a variety of common clinical situations, e.g. preexisting intrinsic plasma volume deficit [35], inhibition of venous return by intermittent positive pressure ventilation of pharmacologically induced vasodilation or along with tachycardia. However, whatever the reason might be, a reduced size of the heart offers an increased preload reserve with the possibility to support the heart's performance by volume expansion. Volume loading in the conscious state induces the expected increases in systemic arterial pressure and cardiac rate but only minor increases in myocardial fiber shortening [34, 36]. These responses are again modulated by various anesthetics [37]. Finally, it is noteworthy that in the ventilated subject there is only a poor correlation between indices of left ventricular filling pressure, e.g. pulmonary capillary wedge pressure and enddiastolic left ventricular fibre length, i.e. preload [38]. Therefore, serial measurements at various filling pressures are necessary to characterize the instantaneous left ventricular preload reserve in determining cardiac performance.

Conclusions

Various pathophysiological conditions and therapeutic interventions are associated with disruptive effects on local and overall circulatory control principles. While these effects can be moderate or striking and harmful or beneficial, e.g. in the case of a desired uncoupling of cardiovascular reflexes during surgery, they need to be recognized as source of possible complications of therapeutic regimens.

References

1. Miletich, DJ, Ivankovich AD, Albrecht RF, et al (1976) Absence of autoregulation of cerebral blood flow during halothane and enflurane anesthesia. Anesth Analg 55:100–109
2. Fitch W, MacKenzie ET, Harper AM (1975) Effects of decreasing arterial blood pressure on cerebral blood flow in the baboon; influence of sympathetic nervous system. Circ Res 37:550–557
3. Smith AL, Wollman H (1972) Cerebral blood flow and metabolism: effects of anesthetic drugs and techniques. Anesthesiology 36:378–395
4. Shapiro HM (1974) Intracranial hypertension. Anesthesiology 43:445–471
5. Marsh ML, Shapiro HM, Smith RW, et al (1979) Changes in neurologic status and intracranial pressure associated with sodium nitroprusside administration. Anesthesiology 51:336–338
6. Buckley MJ, NcLaughlen JS, Fort L III, et al (1964) Effects of anesthetic agents on pulmonary vascular resistance during hypoxia. Surg Forum 15:183–184
7. Lumb TD, Silvay G, Weinreich AI, et al (1979) A comparison of the effects of continuous ketamine infusion and halothane on oxygen during one lung anesthesia in dogs. Can Anaesth Soc J 26:394–401
8. Bjertnaes LJ, Mundal R, Hauge A, et al (1980) Vascular resistance in atelectatic lungs: Effect of inhalation anesthetics. Acta Anaesthesiol Scand 24:109–118
9. Mathers J, Benumof JL, Wahrenbrock EA (1977) General anesthetics and regional hypoxic pulmonary vasoconstriction, Anesthesiology 46:111–114
10. Benumof JL (1979) Hypoxic pulmonary vasoconstriction and sodium nitroprusside infusion. Anesthesiology 50:481–483
11. Bishop MJ, Cheney FW (1983) Minoxidil and nifedipine inhibit hypoxic pulmonary vasoconstriction. J Cardiovasc Pharmacol 5:184–189
12. Tucker A, McMurtry IF, Grover RF, et al (1976) Attenuation of hypoxic pulmonary vasoconstriction by verapamil in intact dogs. Proc Soc Exp Biol Med 151:611–614

13. Germann P, Aloy A, Zabloudil B, et al (1987) Treatment of subarachnoid hemorrhage with the calcium entry blocker nimodipine affects pulmonary gas exchange in patients requiring controlled mechanical ventilation. Anesthesiology 67:A115
14. Lowenstein E, Foex P, Francis M, et al (1981) Regional ischemic ventricular dysfunction in myocardium supplied by a narrowed coronary artery with increasing halothane concentration in the dog. Anesthesiology 55:349–359
15. Reiz S, Balfors E, Sorensen E, et al (1983) Isoflurane – a powerful coronary vasodilator in patients with coronary artery disease. Anesthesiology 59:91–97
16. Buffington CW, Romson JL, Levine A, et al (1987) Isoflurane induces coronary steal in a canine model of chronic coronary occlusion. Anesthesiology 66:280–292
17. Priebe HJ, Foëx P (1987) Isoflurane causes regional myocardial dysfunction in dogs with critical coronary artery stenoses. Anesthesiology 66:293–300
18. Mayer N, Steinbereithner K, Zimpfer M (1986) Effects of halothane on the contractile performance of myocardium supplied by a chronically narrowed coronary artery in the dog. Anesthesiology 65:A59
19. Zimpfer M, Mayer N, Steinbereithner K (1987) Dissimilar effects of isoflurane versus dipyridamole on myocardium supplied by a chronically narrowed coronary artery in the dog. Anesthesiology 67:A587
20. Stoelting RK, (ed) (1987) Pharmacology and physiology in anesthetic practice. JB Lippincott, Philadelphia London Mexico City New York St. Louis Sao Paulo Sydney
21. Kotrly KJ, Ebert TJ, Vucins E, et al (1984) Baroreceptor reflex control of heart rate during isoflurane anesthesia in humans. Anesthesiology 60:173–179
22. Cox RH, Bagshaw RJ (1979) Influence of anesthesia on the response to carotid hypotension in dogs. Am J Physiol 237:H424–H432
23. Zimpfer M, Beck A, Mayer N, et al (1983) Einfluß von Morphium auf die Kontrolle des kardiovaskulären Systems durch den Carotis-Sinus-Reflex und den Carotis-Chemoreflex. Anaesthesist 32:60–66
24. Vatner SF, Boettcher DH, Heyndrickx GR, et al (1975) Reduced baroreflex sensitivity with volume loading in conscious dogs. Circ Res 37:236–242
25. Eckberg DL, Drabinsky M, Braunwald E (1971) Defective cardiac parasympathetic control in patients with heart disease. N Engl J Med 285:877–883
26. Zimpfer M, Sit SP, Vatner SF (1981) Effects of anesthesia on the carotid chemoreceptor reflex. Circ Res 48:400–406
27. Beck A, Zimpfer M, Raberger G (1982) Inhibition of the carotid chemoreceptor reflex by enflurane in chronically instrumented dogs. Naunyn-Schmied. Arch Pharmacol 321:145–148
28. Peters UH, Rieger H (Hrsg) (1976) Das Pickwick-Syndrom. Urban & Schwarzenberg, München
29. Pathak CL (1966) The fallacy of the Bainbridge reflex. Am Heart J 72:577–581
30. Vatner SF, Zimpfer M (1981) Bainbridge reflex in conscious unrestrained, and tranquilized baboons. Am J Physiol 240:H164–H167
31. Boettcher DH, Zimpfer M, Vatner SF (1982) Phylogenesis of the Bainbridge reflex. Am J Physiol 242:R244–R246
32. Zimpfer M, Kotai E, Mayer N, et al (1983) Einfluß von Morphin auf die Kreislaufkontrolle bei akuter progressiver Hämorrhagie. Anaesthesist 32:259–264
33. Mayer N, Kotai E, Placheta P, et al (1985) Enflurane alters compensatory humoral and hemodynamic responses to hemorrhage. 7th Annual Meeting, Society of Cardiovascular Anesthesiologists, Phoenix, Arizona, p 111
34. Boettcher DH, Vatner SF, Heyndrickx GR, et al (1978) Extent of utilization of the Frank Starling mechanism in conscious dogs. Am J Physiol 234:H338–H345
35. Cohn LH, Klovekorn P, Moore FD, et al (1974) Intrinsic plasma volume deficits in patients with coronary artery disease. Arch Surg 108:57–60
36. Zimpfer M, Mayer N, Gilly H, et al (1987) Cardiodynamics during rapid volume expansion and fuction of chronically ischemic myocardium under isoflurane: A study in chronically instrumented dogs. In: Peter K, Brown BR, Martin E, Norlander O (eds) Inhalation Anesthetics. New Aspects. Anaesthesiology and Intensive Care Medicine Vol 185. Springer, Berlin Heidelberg New York London Paris Tokyo, p 133–148

37. Mayer N, Maurer E, Zimpfer M (1987) Untersuchungen zur Wertigkeit des Frank-Starling-Mechanismus im Verlauf akuter Volumsexpansion in Inhalationsanaesthesie. Anaesthesist 36 (Suppl):442, (V 30.1)
38. Zimpfer M, Blazek G (1983) Effects of prolonged inspiratory: expiratory ratio in critically ill patients – an echochardiographic evaluation. Crit Care Med 11:243

Can Primary Resuscitation Therapy Be Improved?

K. Messmer and K. E. Arfors

Introduction

Rapid restoration of blood volume after hemorrhage, trauma and shock is the goal of primary resuscitation. For about two decades the controversy whether colloids or crystalloids are preferable for resuscitation in hypovolemic shock has been entertained by researchers and clinicians. But until today agreement has not been achieved. There is, however, general agreement that the time during which the patient remains hypovolemic and in shock is decisive for the final outcome.

As result of improved primary care less patients suffering trauma, multiple injuries or other forms of shock will succumb within the first hours except those presenting with lethal injuries of the vital organs [1]. Independent upon the fluid regimen used for primary volume replacement patients do survive the initial critical hours and even days and appear under stable reconvalescent conditions when approximately 2-4 weeks after the injury the patients deteriorates, dysfunction of one or several of his organs becomes apparent and the patient will eventually die from late complications in sepsis and multiple systems organ failure [2]. Baker et al. [3] have demonstrated, that age, severity of the injury, shock with pressures below 80 mm Hg and the duration of the shock are the most important factors for the prognosis after multiple trauma.

The attempts to treat multiple systems organ failure (MOF) were particularly unsuccessful sofar [4, 5] so that measures to prevent development of MOF after trauma and shock are needed.

Hypotheses for Development of MOF

Four different hypotheses to explain the pathogenesis of MOF after shock have been forwarded:

1. Patients after severe injury or major surgery do suffer from reduced intestinal perfusion allowing microorganisms to enter the systemic circulation resulting in bacteremia, endotoxinemia and sepsis. In this hypothesis endotoxin is the most important factor.
2. Bacteria invade lung, liver and kidney where they activate macrophages and monocytes to release Interleukin I (IL1), a small peptide known to affect the function of most organs and tissues.

3. MOF results from general activation of the immune system [4].
4. Local ischemia and local reperfusion trigger leukocyte sticking, release of oxygen free radicals and generation of mediators e. g. IL1, which in turn activate the arachidonic acid pathway [6].

Ischemia and Reperfusion Injury

According to the last concept, the primary volume therapy does not abolish the shock-specific impairment of microcirculation even though central hemodynamic parameters might be normalized. It is known today that irreversible tissue damage is not entirely the result of lack of oxygen, but that much of the damage occurs after the ischemia-hypoxia during reperfusion and reoxygenation, e.g. when blood flow is restored.

Temporary lack of oxygen makes the affected cells more susceptible to the oxygen free radicals which are formed during non-enzymatic reduction of oxygen. This "oxygen paradox" results in lipid peroxidation and irreversible denaturation of cellular proteins and damage of tissue cells. Reperfusion injury can partially be prevented by means of scavenging the oxygen radicals being produced.

The implementation of scavenging substances into the resuscitation regimen is not particulary easy, though theoretically attractive. Therefore efficient reversal of the microcirculation defect and of local ischemia appears as promising alternative. This would need instantaneous restoration of nutritional flow and tissue drainage at the very time of primary treatment. It is therefore reasonable to ask the question whether the resuscitation in shock conditions today occurs fast and efficient enough to avoid local reperfusion injury and eventually MOF.

Efficiency of Primary Shock Treatment

Surprisingly, systematic studies addressing this important issue are scarce. However, the prospective randomized study of Modig [7, 8] provides most valuable information. Victims of severe traumatic shock received Dextran 70 versus Ringer's acetate to treat shock and to prevent trauma-induced ARDS. The hemodynamics improved significantly faster in the Dextran-treated group (mean blood pressure was restored within 110 ± 18 min ($M \pm SD$)). In contrast, in patients receiving Ringer's acetate mean blood pressure (MAP) of 65 mm Hg was reached only after 170 ± 40 min. Cardiac index of the Dextran-treated patients was significantly higher and rose significantly more upon challenge with 500 ml of Dextran 70 as compared to patients challenged with 2 liters of Ringer's acetate. During the 7–8 day posttrauma period none of the 14 patients receiving Dextran developed ARDS as compared to 5/17 patients presenting with ARDS after treatment with Ringer's acetate. Modig concludes that initial aggressive shock treatment with Dextran 70 followed by continued Dextran administration after trauma can prevent complications such as ARDS.

Without discussing the potential of either treatment modality to prevent initial pulmonary edema and consequently ARDS, the *differences in time* required for stabilization of arterial pressure and the *differences in total perfusion rate* (cardiac index) should be heralded. Nevertheless, with regard to ischemia and reperfusion injury a resuscitation time of 110 min is by far too long.

Hypertonic Saline Solution

In this context the observations of Velasco et al. [9] and de Filippe et al. [10] are of particular interest. These authors have demonstrated in dogs and humans that the infusion of hypertonic sodium chloride solution with an osmolarity of 2400 mOsml/l has the potential to restore the cardiovascular function within minutes when given in volumes of 4 ml/kg.

The response of animals in severe hemorrhagic shock and of patients in refractory hypovolemic shock to small volumes of hypertonic saline has attracted attention of research groups throughout the world. The original findings have unequivocally been confirmed in various species, namely instantaneous increase of cardiac output with release of vasoconstriction [11–14]. The most striking advantage of this concept is certainly the notion that only small infusion volumes are necessary. Hence, it would become feasible to restore cardiovascular function, already at the site of the accident, more rapidly as compared to present resuscitation techniques requiring much higher volumes of fluid, particularly when crystalloids are used.

Nutritional Blood Flow During Resuscitation with Hypertonic Saline

So far nutritional flow has neither been assessed in the earlier studies on the effect of hypertonic solutions [15] nor in the more recent studies with use of 7.5% saline mentioned above. Kreimeier et al. [16] have therefore compared the effect of 7.2% NaCl versus 7.2% NaCl and 10% Dextran 60, versus 0.9% NaCl and 10% Dextran 60. The protocol in anesthetized dogs included hemorrhagic hypotension with MAP 40 mm Hg for 45 min and infusion of the test fluids in volumes corresponding to 10% of the reservoir blood volume (approx. 3.8 ml/kg BW).

The infusion of both hypertonic solutions was most efficient and resulted in rapid restoration of cardiac output while MAP reached approx. 60% of control within 5 min after infusion (Fig. 1). Nutritional blood flow to the brain, heart and adrenals rose beyond control values, but flow to the other organs reached control values within 5 min after onset of infusion except blood flow to gastric mucosa and pancreas. Hence it has been demonstrated that hypertonic solutions do normalize nutritional blood flow upon infusion of small volumes already within 5 min. Prolongation of the hypotension did neither change the macronor the microhemodynamic response [16, 17].

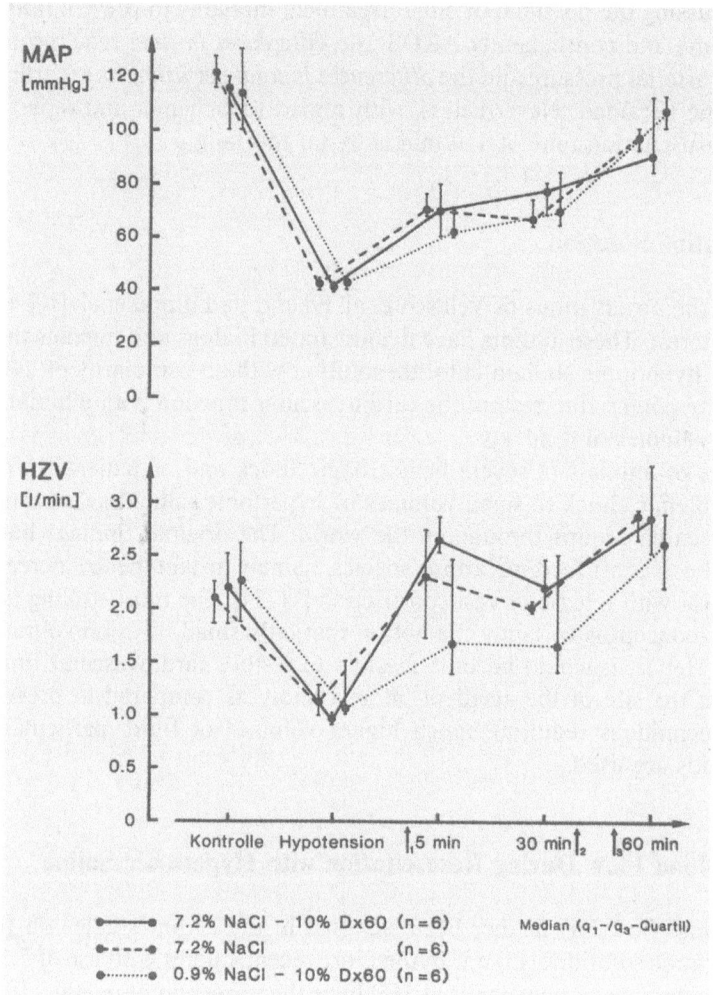

Fig. 1. Changes of mean arterial pressure (MAP) and cardiac output (HZV) during 45 min of hemorrhagic hypotension during primary resuscitation (arrow 1) as well as after intravenous infusion of 3.8 ml/kg BW 6% Dextran 60 (arrow 2 and 3). (From [17] with permission)

Resuscitation Fluids for the Future

Hypertonic solutions containing or notcontaining colloids offer new aspects in primary resuscitation and are explored in great detail today [14, 17]. Further improvement of their efficiency towards preventing focal ischemia and reperfusion injury is envisaged by the implementation of drugs affecting leukocyte sticking and/or scavenging of oxygen free radicals. In this context, the monoclonal antibodies directed against the membrane complex CDw18 responsible for leukocyte sticking are of particular interest [7].

References

1. Carmona R, Catalano R, Trunkey DD (1984) Septic shock. In: Shires GT (ed) Shock and related problems. Churchill Livingstone, Edinburg, pp 156–177
2. Baue AE (1975) Multiple, progressive or sequential systems failure – A syndrome of the "70"s. Arch Surg 110:779–781
3. Baker CC, DeSantis J, Degutis LD, Baue AE (1985) The impact of a trauma service on trauma care in a University Hospital. Am J Surg 149:453–548
4. Baue AE (1981) Multiple organ or systems failure: In: Haimovici FD (ed) Vascular emergencies. Chap 7. Appleton-Century-Crofts, New York, p 125
5. Fry EE, Pearlstein L, Fulton RL, et al (1980) Multiple systems organ failure. Arch Surg 115:136–140
6. Messmer K, Zeintl H, Kreimeier U, Schoenberg M (1986) Neue Trends in der Schockforschung. In: Eigler FW, Peiper HJ, Schildberg FW, Witte J, Zumtobel V (eds) Stand und Gegenstand chirurgischer Forschung. Springer, Berlin Heidelberg New York Tokyo, pp 58–65
7. Modig J (1986) Effectiveness of Dextran 70 versus Ringer's acetate in traumatic shock and adult respiratory distress syndrome. Crit Care Med 14:454–457
8. Modig J (1983) Advantages of Dextran 70 over Ringer's acetate solution in shock treatment and in prevention of adult respiratory distress syndrome. A randomized study in man after traumatic-hemorrhagic shock. Resuscitation 10:219–226
9. Velasco IT, Pontieri V, Rocha e Silva M, Lopes OU (1980) Hyperosmotic NaCl and severe hemorrhagic shock. Am J Physiol 239:H664–73
10. de Felippe J Jr, Gimoner J, Velasco IT, Lopes OU, Roche e Silva M Jr (1980) Treatment of refractory hypovolemic shock by 7.5% sodium chloride injections. Lancet 11:1002–4
11. Nakayama S, Sibley L, Gunther RA, Holcroft JW, Kramer GC (1984) Small volume resuscitation with hypertonic saline (2400 mOsm/liter) during hemorrhagic shock. Circ Shock 13:149–59
12. Peters R, Shackford S, Hogan J, Cologne J (1986) Comparison of isotonic and hypertonic fluids in resuscitation from hypovolemic shock. Surg Gyn ecol Obstetr 163:219–224
13. Kramer G, Perron P, Lindsey D, Ho H, Gunther RA, Boyle W, Holcroft JW (1986) Small-volume resuscitation with hypertonic saline dextran solution. Surgery 100:239–247
14. Luypaert P, Vincent JL, Domb M, Van der Linden P, Blecic S, Azimi G, Bernard A (1986) Fluid resuscitation with hypertonic saline in endotoxic shock. Circ Shock 20:311–320
15. Messmer K, Mokry G, Jesch F (1969) The protective effect of hypertonic solutions in shock. Br J Surg 56:626
16. Kreimeier U, Schmidt J, Brückner UB, Schoenberg M, Yang Zh, Messmer K (1987) Primary resuscitation using hypertonic saline/colloid solution. Langenbecks Arch Klin Chir, Suppl. Chir Forum 329–332
17. Kreimeier U, Messmer K (1987) New perspectives in resuscitation and prevention of multiple organ system failure. In: Baethmann A, Messmer K (eds) Surgical Research: Recent Concepts and Results. Springer, Berlin Heidelberg New York London Paris Tokyo, pp 39–50

Oxygen Transport and Utilization in Critically Ill Patients

M. T. Haupt

Introduction

Because of a high affinity for electrons, oxygen is uniquely suited to the "capturing" of foodstuff derived electrons, a process which releases energy. In turn, under normal conditions, about 42% of the energy released during oxidation is coupled to the synthesis of ATP, a compound responsible for providing energy to a large and diverse number of cellular processes; processes which include active transport, enzymatic reactions, and muscle contraction [1]. The viability of virtually all living mammalian tissues is thus dependent on a continuous supply of oxygen.

To maintain a continuous oxygen supply to the cell in humans, an elaborate system of adjustable processes has evolved. If, for example, the oxygen and energy demands of the cell increase, adjustments in pulmonary oxygen exchange, cardiac output, hemoglobin oxygen binding, and capillary resistance increase oxygen extraction and facilitate the availability of oxygen to the cell. Furthermore, when one component of the system fails, the remaining components adjust in an attempt to meet cellular oxygen demands.

Failure to maintain oxygen consumption consistant with cellular needs remains a fundamental problem in many patients who are critically ill. Patients with severe reductions in oxygen delivery, from cardiogenic shock for example, frequently fail to satisfy systemic energy requirements if compensatory mechanisms to increase oxygen extraction are overwhelmed. Although patients with septic shock may have increased systemic oxygen delivery and consumption, they may fail to meet systemic energy demands from increased metabolism, fever, tachypnea, and tachycardia associated with the septic process. When cellular energy demands are not satisfied, active transport fails, sodium enters the cell, and cellular swelling develops. Lysosomal membranes eventually rupture, and lytic enzymes are released and result in autodigestion and cell death. Progressive loss of vascular tone, circulatory failure, and multiple organ system failure are also characteristic of advanced sepsis. Lactic acidosis emerges, reflecting the use of inefficient anaerobic pathways to maintain ATP synthesis in the absence of oxygen.

Clinical Methods to Assess Oxygen Delivery and Consumption

The assessment of systemic oxygen delivery (DO_2) and consumption ($\dot{V}O_2$) is now possible in the clinical setting. In addition, clinicians may conveniently measure biochemical markers of anaerobic metabolism to determine whether DO_2 and $\dot{V}O_2$ are sufficient to meet systemic oxygen demands.

Several clinical methods are available to monitor DO_2 and $\dot{V}O_2$ in critically ill patients [2]. The most widely applied technique in intensive care units utilizes the Fick method. Following insertion of a pulmonary artery catheter, cardiac output (CO) is measured, simultaneous determinations of hemoglobin concentration (Hb-gm/dl), arterial and mixed venous oxygen saturations (SaO_2, $S\bar{v}O_2$) and oxygen tensions (PaO_2, $P\bar{v}O_2$) are made. The following formulas are utilized:

$$CaO_2 = (1.38 \cdot Hb \cdot SaO_2) + (.003 \cdot PaO_2)$$

$$C\bar{v}O_2 = (1.38 \cdot Hb \cdot S\bar{v}O_2) + (.003 \cdot P\bar{v}O_2)$$

$$DO_2 = CaO_2 \cdot (CO/BSA) \cdot 10 \text{ (normal 520–720 ml/min/m}^2)$$

$$\dot{V}O_2 = (CaO_2 - C\bar{v}O_2) \cdot (CO/BSA) \cdot 10 \text{ (normal 100–180 ml/min/m}^2)$$

Gas exchange methods (open and close circuit techniques) may also be utilized to measure $\dot{V}O_2$ through exhaled and/or inhaled gas analysis. These methods, as well as the Fick method, have important advantages and disadvantages in the clinical setting which have been discussed in excellent reviews [2, 3].

The ability to assess the activity of anaerobic metabolic pathways complements measurements of DO_2 and $\dot{V}O_2$. Lactic acidosis is one sequella of anaerobic metabolism and is conveniently determined in the clinical setting. Lactic acid elevations in critically ill patients suggest that $\dot{V}O_2$ is insufficient to meet metabolic demands. Drugs, poisons, liver disease, tumors, hypercapnea and hypocapnea, and congenital metabolic defects may cause elevations of lactate levels that are independent of anaerobic metabolic pathways [4]. When these conditions are present, clinicians should be aware that elevated lactate levels may not precisely reflect the presence of anaerobic metabolism or inadequate oxygen relative to demands. Fortunately, these conditions are usually easy to identify.

Accelerated glycolysis is characteristic of sepsis and other inflammatory disorders, and may also increase lactate levels independently of anaerobic mechanisms. Progressive lactic acidosis associated with clinical deterioration in these patients may nevertheless reflect the development of anaerobic metabolism. Laboratory models of endotoxemia and sepsis in which progressive reductions in ATP synthesis and increases in lactate to pyruvate ratios are observed support the development of anaerobic metabolism in these conditions [5, 6].

The presence of metabolic acidosis or an elevated anion gap may reflect the presence of lactic acidosis if other types of metabolic acidosis are absent. However, the use of these methods have serious limitations in the clinical setting. One clinical study demonstrated that up to 58% of patients with lactic acidosis ($>2:4$ mM) had no evidence of metabolic acidosis. In addition, only 8.5% of patients with metabolic acidosis (pH <7.36 and CO_2 content <22 mM) and elevated lactate levels had an increased anion gap (>16 mM). Frequently observed hypoal-

buminemia lowered the anion gap in these patients. Thus the absence of metabolic acidosis or an elevated anion gap does not rule out clinically significant
anaerobic metabolism [7].

Other methods to evaluate the presence of anaerobic metabolism may be more
precise than the measurement of lactate, but currently are not readily available
or convenient in the clinical setting. Enzymatic techniques are being evaluated to
assess levels of redox couplets, such as lactate and pyruvate, beta-hydroxybuty-
rate and acetoacetate [8]. ADP degradation products accumulate when ATP synthesis declines or its degradation increases. One product of ADP degradation,
hypoxanthine, correlates with tissue hypoxia [9]. Hypoxanthine, however, remains difficult to measure in the clinical setting. Phosphorus nuclear magnetic
spectroscopy and position emission tomography may also be used to assess the
presence of tissue oxygen debt, but these methods do not currently lend themselves to bedside care in the intensive care unit setting.

Patterns of Oxygen Delivery and Consumption in the Clinical Setting

The assessment of DO_2 and $\dot{V}O_2$ in the clinical setting has revealed important
patterns of oxygen utilization that have previously been defined in the laboratory. When DO_2 is decreased in laboratory animals, through progressive normovolemic anemia, hypoxic hypoxia, and hypovolemia, $\dot{V}O_2$ remains constant or independent of DO_2 until a critical DO_2 level is reached [10–12]. Below this critical
DO_2, further decreases in DO_2 will result in corresponding decreases in $\dot{V}O_2$;
$\dot{V}O_2$ then becomes supply dependent (Fig. 1). In this circumstance, normal adaptive mechanisms fail to maintain $\dot{V}O_2$ in the presence of decreasing DO_2. Clinical observations of patients with severe reductions in cardiac output [13], stable
pulmonary hypertension [14], and of patients under general anesthesia [15] are
consistant with a supply dependent pattern of oxygen utilization below critical
DO_2's.

Patients with ARDS, sepsis, and multiple trauma exhibit supply dependency
over a much wider range of DO_2's [16–18], a pattern that has been termed *pathologic supply dependency* [12] (See figure). Characteristics of the systemic inflammatory response may contribute to this abnormal pattern of oxygen utilization.
In sepsis and other inflammatory disorders, increased levels of circulating mediators produce changes in vascular tone, increase capillary permeability, and

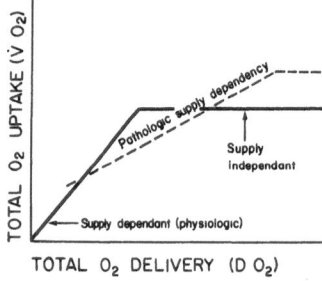

Fig. 1. Oxygen consumption, as a function of oxygen
delivery, is illustrated. (From Cain [12])

increase interstitial edema. Cellular aggregates and fibrin emboli may occlude microvascular beds. Experimental models of microembolism, endothelial swelling with tissue edema, and alpha-adrenergic blockage simulate characteristics of the inflammatory response and lead to changes characteristic of pathologic supply dependency [19–21]. One explanation for pathologic supply dependency based on these experiments is that these changes result in a maldistribution of blood flow such that oxygen diffusion distances from capillary to cell are increased. Since increased DO_2 is required to overcome these increased diffusion distances and maintain $\dot{V}O_2$ at levels that preceded the distributive defect the critical DO_2 will be shifted to the right. Supply dependency will thus be observed over a wider range of DO_2's.

Conditions which accelerate oxidative metabolism may increase the tendency for supply dependency and anaerobic metabolism to develop over a wider range of DO_2's. These conditions may include fever, tachycardia, tachypnea, and elevated endogenous or exogenous catecholamine levels, conditions frequently observed in critically ill patients.

Pathologic supply may also develop when extramitochondrial or non-ATP producing oxidase systems are activated by the inflammatory process. These systems include the cyclooxygenase, lipoxygenase and xanthine oxidase systems. The affinity of these extramitochondrial systems is less than the terminal oxidase of the mitochondrial electron transport chain (cytochrome aa_3) [22]. For this reason, if anaerobic conditions are present, delivered oxygen will preferentially be utilized by mitochondria. Thus, supply dependency may characterize early stages of sepsis, ARDS, trauma, and other inflammatory conditions when mitochondrial oxidative pathways are saturated and anaerobic metabolism is absent.

Therapeutic Guidelines

Critically ill patients with decreased DO_2, decreased $\dot{V}O_2$ and signs of anaerobic metabolism frequently respond to interventions which increase DO_2. Accordingly, patients with hypovolemia respond to fluid loading, hemorrhagic shock may be treated with blood transfusions, and patients with cardiogenic shock may respond to vasodilating agents and inotropic support.

The treatment of patients with conditions such as sepsis, ARDS and multiple trauma who show signs of inadequate $\dot{V}O_2$ relative to estimated demand and anaerobic metabolism is more difficult. Although it is rational to correct volume and hemoglobin, hemoglobin oxygen saturation, and cardiac output deficits, these measures frequently fail to correct the microvascular, cellular and subcellular abnormalities that characterize these conditions. In fact, conventional supportive measures have failed to significantly change the mortality of ARDS and sepsis over the past 10 years, a mortality which remains over 50% in most series.

Specific measures to minimize or reverse inflammatory conditions may be of benefit. Unfortunately, however, significant benefits from more specific, newer generation antibiotics have been realized in patients with bacterial sepsis. The anti-inflammatory effects of corticosteroids do not appear to benefit patients with established sepsis. A number of investigational agents may be promising in the reversal of detrimental inflammatory changes and include [23]:

Anti C5a Antibodies: The complement cascade is activated during severe inflammatory insults and results in the formation of C5a which attracts and aggregates neutrophils in areas such as the capillary beds of the lung. Neutrophils subsequently release toxic products such as oxygen-free radicals, proteases, prostaglandins, leukotrienes, and platelet activating factors. Anti C5a antibodies may prevent this activation of neutrophils.

Antibodies to neutrophil receptor sites: Monoclonal antibodies to Mo l, a granulocyte – adhesion – promoting surface glycoprotein may modulate granulocyte activity.

Tumor necrosis factor antibodies and endotoxin antibodies: These antibodies appear to protect laboratory animals from the lethal effects of endotoxin.

Oxygen-free radical scavengers: Many agents are toxic. Dimethyl sulfoxide (DMSO), N-acetylcysteine (Mucomyst), Vitamin E, superoxide dismutase, catalase and mannitol are effective scavengers in animal models.

Anti-arachidonic acid metabolic agents: These agents include cyclooxygenase inhibitors (e.g. ibuprofen) and lipoxygenase inhibitors.

Agents which increase red cell flexibility: These agents may be useful in conditions associated with mediator release and capillary microembolism. Increasing flexibility with agents such as *pentoxifylline,* for example, may enhance red cell flow through partially blocked capillary beds and improve systemic uptake of oxygen [24].

When progressive decreases in $\dot{V}O_2$ and signs of anaerobic metabolism are observed, interventions which decrease elevated systemic oxygen demand are also rational. A variety of interventions may be employed.

Sedation is an important fundamental measure. Drugs such as the benzodiazepines will decrease the secretion of catecholamines, agents which stimulate oxidative metabolism. Some reports have demonstrated reductions in $\dot{V}O_2$ after use of these agents [25]. Analgesia is an important mechanism for sedation when pain is present.

Decreasing heart rate is important if tachycardia is responsible for reductions in stroke volume, cardiac output, and DO_2. Calcium blocking agents and digitalis may be useful in supraventricular tachycardia, multifocal atrial tachycardias, and atrial fibrillation. Beta-blockade is useful in slowing heart rate in thyrotoxicosis and excessive agitation. One must avoid reductions in heart rate if elevations are a major mechanism for maintenance of cardiac output and DO_2.

Mechanical ventilation reduces the work of breathing and the oxygen demands of the respiratory muscles. Assisting a patient's ventilation may thus lead to a redistribution of cardiac output and oxygen delivery to systemic areas in greater need. A decrease in total body oxygen consumption has been demonstrated following the initiation of mechanical ventilation in the clinical setting [26].

Decreasing body temperature lowers metabolic rate and decreases oxygen consumption if shivering is prevented. Induced hypothermia appears to prolong survival time in animal models of cardiogenic shock [27]. Hypothermia has also been employed in near-drowning to improve CNS recovery. The efficacy of hypothermia has not been documented in the clinical setting. However, efforts to avoid extreme elevations of temperature in patients with circulatory shock are rational.

The clinician should also be aware of pharmacological agents which increase metabolism and oxygen consumption. This includes catechalomine type intravenous agents (e. g., dopamine, dobutamine, norephinephrine), inhalational beta-agonists (terbutuline, albuterol), aminophylline and thyroid hormone. These agents may unfavorably increase the oxygen demand relative to supply.

Conclusion

The understanding of patterns of abnormal utilization of oxygen may guide the clinician's choice of therapeutic and pharmacologic interventions in critically ill patients. Methods to optimize oxygen delivery and to minimize systemic oxygen demands seem rational in patients with progressive signs of anaerobic metabolism. One must be aware of the possibility, however, that increases in DO_2 may be unfavorable, especially in early sepsis and inflammatory conditions when activated extra-mitochondrial oxidase systems may utilize oxygen to produce toxic mediators. More precise management of patients with abnormal patterns of oxygen utilization awaits innovations in the control of the generalized inflammatory response.

References

1. Weibel ER (1984) The pathway for oxygen: Structure and function in the mammalian respiratory system. Cambridge, Harvard University Press
2. Weissman C (1987) Measuring oxygen uptake in the clinical setting. In: New Horizons: Oxygen Transport and Utilization. Bryan-Brown, Ayres (eds) Society of Critical Care Medicine, pp 25–64
3. Westenkow DR, Cutler CA, Wallace WD (1984) Instrumentation for monitoring gas exchange and metabolic rate in critically ill patients. Crit Care Med 12:183–187
4. Kruse JA, Carlson RW (1987) Lactate metabolism. Crit Care Clin 5:725–746
5. Tavakoli H, Mela L (1982) Alterations of mitochondrial metabolism and protein concentration in subacute septicemia. Infection and Immunity 38:536–541
6. Holtzman S, Schuler JJ, Earnest W, Erve PR, Schumer W (1974) Carbohydrate metabolism in endotoxemia. Circ Shock 1:99–105
7. Mehta K, Kruse JA, Carlson RW (1984) The relationship between the anion gap and elevated lactate. Crit Care Med 14:405
8. Davies AO, Samuelson WM (1986) Assessing redox status in human plasma: Experience in critically ill patients. Crit Care Med 14:942–946
9. Grum CM, Simon RH, Dantzker DR, Fox IH (1985) Evidence for adenosine triphosphate degradation in critically ill patients. Chest 88:763–767
10. Cain SM (1977) Oxygen delivery and uptake in dogs during anemic and hypoxic hypoxia. J Appl Physiol 42:228–234

11. Schwartz S, Frantz RA, Shoemaker WC (1981) Sequential hemodynamic and oxygen transport responses in hypovolemia, anemia, and hypoxia. Am J Physiol 241:H864–H871
12. Cain SM (1984) Review: Supply dependence of oxygen uptake in ARDS: Myth or reality? Am J Med Sci 288:119–124
13. Bauman DJ, Pierce MJ, Kuida H (1973) Decreased oxygen consumption in cardiac patients with severe reduction in cardiac output. Am J Med Sci 265:281–285
14. Chappell TR, Rubin LS, Makham RV Jr, Firth B (1983) Independence of oxygen consumption and systemic oxygen transport in patients with either stable pulmonary hypertension or refractory left ventricular failure. Am Rev Respir Dis 128:30–33
15. Shibutani K, Komatsutt, Kubal K, Sanchala V, Kumar V, Bizzari DV (1983) Critical level of oxygen delivery in anesthetized man. Crit Care Med 11:640–643
16. Danek SJ, Lynch JP, Weg JD, Dantzker DR (1980) The dependence of oxygen uptake on oxygen delivery in the adult respiratory distress syndrome. Am Rev Resp Dis 122:387–395
17. Haupt MT, Gilbert EM, Carlson RW (1985) Fluid loading increases oxygen consumption in septic patients with lactic acidosis. Am Rev Respir Dis 131:912–916
18. Powers SR Jr, Mannal R, Neclerio M et al. (1973) Physiologic consequences of positive end-expiratory pressure (PEEP) ventilation. Ann Surg 178:265–272
19. Landau SE, Alexander RS, Powers SR Jr, Stratton HH, Goldfarb RD (1982) Tissue oxygen exchange and reactive hyperemia following microembolism. J Surg Res 32:38–43
20. Shah GM, Powers SR Jr, Stratton HH, Newell JC (1981) Effects of hypertonic mannitol on oxygen utilization in canine hind limbs following shock. J Surg Res 30:593–601
21. Cain SM (1978) Effects of time and vasoconstrictor tone on oxygen extraction during hypoxic hypoxia. J Appl Physiol 45:219–224
22. Robin E (1980) Of men and mitochondria: coping with hypoxic dypoxia. Am Rev Respir Dis 122:517–531
23. Raffin TA (1986) Novel approaches to ARDS and sepsis. In Critical Care: State of the Art, Vol 7, 247–276
24. Baker CH, Wilmoth FR, Sutton ET (1986) Reduced RBC versus plasma microvascular flow due to endotoxin. Circ Shock 20:127–139
25. Cote P, Campeau L, Bourassa MG (1976) Therapeutic implications of diazepam in patients with elevated left ventricular filling pressure. Am Heart J 91:747–751
26. Field S, Kelly SM, Macklem PT (1982) The oxygen cost of breathing in patients with cardiorespiratory disease. Am Rev Respir Dis 126:9–13
27. Boyer NH, Gerstein MM (1977) Induced hypothermia in dogs with acute myocardial infarction and shock. J Thorac Cardiovasc Surg 74:286–294

Oxygen Transport Following Major Trauma

J. D. Edwards

Oxygen Transport – The System

The concepts of oxygen delivery (DO_2) are now well established and measurement of related variables are routinely made in critically ill patients [1], not least because measurement and manipulation of these variables has been shown to predict [2] and improve [3] outcome. Therefore the physiology of DO_2 will not be reviewed in detail in this chapter but the terms used will be defined at the onset:

CaO_2 = arterial O_2 content (ml/dl)

$C\bar{v}O_2$ = mixed venous O_2 content (ml/dl)

SaO_2 = arterial oxyhemoglobin saturation (%)

$S\bar{v}O_2$ = mixed venous oxyhemoglobin saturation (%)

CI = cardiac index (l/min/m²)

as will the relevant equations:

1. Oxygen consumption ($\dot{V}O_2$) = CI × (CaO_2 − $C\bar{v}O_2$) × 10 (ml/min/m²)

2. Oxygen delivery (DO_2) = CI × CaO_2 × 10 (ml/min/m²)

3. Oxygen extraction ratio (OER) = $\dfrac{CaO_2 - C\bar{v}O_2}{CaO_2}$ (%)

Pivotal to the management of any critically ill patient is the principle that maintenance of a normal or high $\dot{V}O_2$ in the face of low or inadequate DO_2 will mean an increase in OER and a fall in $S\bar{v}O_2$ [4]. If $S\bar{v}O_2$ is 60% or less there is reduced tissue oxygen availability and $S\bar{v}O_2$ levels approaching 40% are critical and not sustainable for long periods [5, 6]. Below a critical level of DO_2, shown to be 330 ml/min/m² in anesthetized subjects but possibly lower in some shock states, $S\bar{v}O_2$ does not fall further and lactic acidosis supervenes [7]. In sepsis and adult respiratory distress syndrome (ARDS), $\dot{V}O_2$ will fall at much higher levels of DO_2 [4, 8] and critically ill patients have optimal survival rates when CI ⩾ 4.5 l/min/m², DO_2 ⩾ 600 ml/min/m² and VO_2 ⩾ 170 ml/min/m² [2, 3, 9], (Fig. 1).

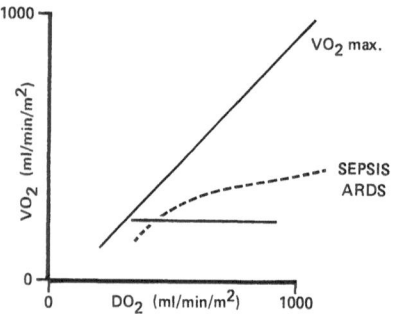

Fig. 1. Dependence of $\dot{V}O_2$ on DO_2

Assessment of the Size of the Injury

Outcome from major trauma can be audited by combining the initial trauma score (TS) with the injury severity score (ISS) calculated at discharge from hospital or death – the so-called TRISS methodology [10]. The classical TS depends on observations of respiratory effort, Glasgow Coma Scale, capillary refill and systolic blood pressure. The ISS is calculated from the three worse injuries to various bodily compartments. The details of TRISS are beyond the scope of this chapter but essentially TS decreases as the patients physiologic status deteriorates and the ISS increases as the number and severity of injuries increase [11]. A line separating expected survivors from non-survivors can be drawn by plotting ISS against TS based on a study of large numbers of trauma victims in North America – The Multiple Trauma Outcome Study [12]. TRISS can be used to quantify the severity of trauma in an individual patient, predict expected outcome and thereby identify anomalous outcome whether survival or non-survival, and to audit trauma care [13]. Any study on any aspect of trauma can be put into perspective by inclusion of TRISS data into the methodology and we shall include such data, wherever possible, in this account of DO_2 in relation to trauma. Studies of DO_2 in trauma would be of most interest and pertinence in trauma victims with a high risk of death – those with low TS and high ISS.

DO_2 Studies After Trauma

Early studies on $\dot{V}O_2$ following trauma such as those of Cuthbertson [14] were based on measurements of volume and O_2 content of inspired and expired gases. Cuthbertson divided the period following injury into two phases – an early 'ebb phase' of low $\dot{V}O_2$, lasting 48 hours, and a later period or 'flow phase' of high $\dot{V}O_2$ [15]. A vast amount of experimental work in small laboratory animals apparently lends support to this concept which has achieved the level of dogma [16–18]. However, the initial study was of a small number of patients [7], of which three were not injured but had elective orthopedic procedures performed under spinal or general anesthesia. The ISS of the injured patients can be calculated from the data provided to be low at 4,4,4 and 9, respectively. Analysis of the results shows that in five patients, $\dot{V}O_2$ measured on the first day was higher than on subsequent occasions. Incredibly, based almost entirely on this one study the concept of ebb and flow phases has dominated the surgical attitude and approach to management of the multiply injured patients. As far as the apparently corroborative laboratory work is concerned Stoner has recently extensively reviewed the available data and has pointed out the problems of extrapolating the results of work on small laboratory animals to the responses of large primates such as man [19].

As early as 1943 Cournand [20] published data which could allow DO_2 and $\dot{V}O_2$ to be calculated in patients with major injuries. He studied a group of 16 patients with a varying combinations of chest, abdominal and limb trauma, many of whom had ISS in the range of 16–40. He studied the patients before any resuscitation in order to determine the cause of post-traumatic shock – he showed conclusively that it was due to hemorrhage and fluid loss. He did not record serial values in individual patients but divided shock into mild and moderate categories based on measurements of mean arterial blood pressure (MAP) made from femoral arterial lines. DO_2 and $\dot{V}O_2$ calculated from his raw data are shown in Table 1.

In the patients who were most shocked – who would have been assessed today as having low TS and high ISS – $\dot{V}O_2$ was maintained in the face of falling DO_2 by increases in OER leading to critically low $S\bar{v}O_2$ levels in many patients. The reduced DO_2 in his patients was due to a combination of low CI and CaO_2 in the absence of any blood, fluids or supplemental inspired O_2 therapy.

Table 1. DO_2 and $\dot{V}O_2$ following major trauma. (From [20])

	MAP	DO_2	$\dot{V}O_2$	CI
No shock	94	556	184	3.57
Mild shock	54	303	174	2.46
Moderate shock	44	243	176	2.06

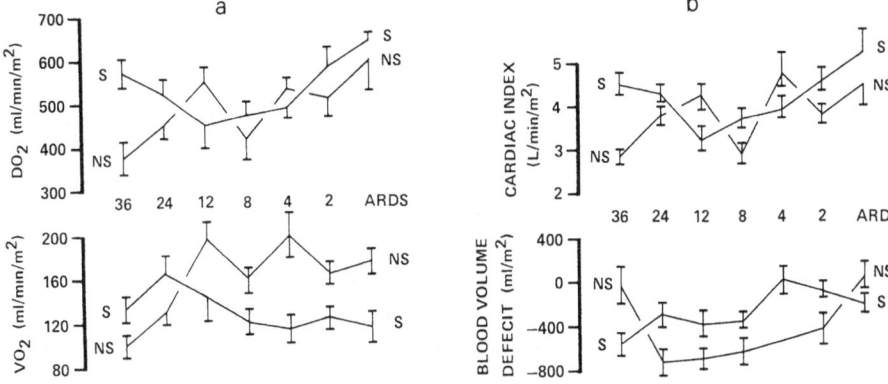

Fig. 2a, b. Pathogenesis of ARDS after trauma

Shoemaker et al. [21] studied DO_2 and $\dot{V}O_2$ in a group of 42 patients after trauma in an attempt to identify at an early stage variables which could identify those patients ultimately destined to survive or die from post-traumatic ARDS. From the limited amount of clinical data given ISS can be calculated to have been a minimum of 16 in all patients and in excess of 30 in many. He showed that $\dot{V}O_2$ measured at an early stage was higher in survivors than non-survivors but in many of the latter was still within the normal range (Fig. 2a).

Those non-survivors with reduced $\dot{V}O_2$ had DO_2 levels below the accepted critical value of 330 ml/min/m^2. These low DO_2 levels were not associated with greater blood volume deficits than in survivors (Fig. 2b) and were thus not due to greater blood loss but to poorer left ventricular function. The relatively normal $\dot{V}O_2$ in some non-survivors in the earlier stages was maintained by increases in OER. Although $S\bar{v}O_2$ levels are not recorded in the results mean values in the early stages can be calculated from the information given to 57% in survivors and 48% in non-survivors.

From the results of Cournand and Shoemaker in which DO_2 variables were measured in larger numbers of seriously injured patients no clear evidence of an ebb phase response in man emerges. On the contrary, analysis of the results of both studies shows an attempt to maintain normal or high $\dot{V}O_2$ by increases in OER in the face of inadequate DO_2 leading to low $S\bar{v}O_2$ levels and potential tissue hypoxia. In Cournand's study $S\bar{v}O_2$ was measured in blood samples taken from the right atrium. True mixed venous blood in the critically ill can only be sampled from the right ventricular outflow tract or pulmonary artery [23]. In Shoemaker's study the relationship between time of injury, resuscitation, anesthesia, definitive surgery, TS and ISS are not clear. It has been previously pointed out that DO_2 data from patients studied following surgery and anesthesia cannot be used to define the responses to trauma and basic resuscitation [25]. We therefore decided to study prospectively the DO_2 responses in victims of major blunt trauma transferred from the Accident & Emergency Department to the Intensive Care Unit within hours of receiving their trauma and before anesthesia or surgery, in whom invasive monitoring was indicated on routine clinical grounds.

The University Hospital of South Manchester Study of DO_2 Variables Following Major Trauma

We were able to study 16 patients in an 11 month period. The mean time from injury to DO_2 variables being measured was 1.6 hours (range 0.8 to 9 hours). The patients were vigorously resuscitated with modified fluid gelatin and/or blood before and during the initial period on the Intensive Care Unit before surgery. Mean TS was 9 ± 2 and ISS was 38 ± 10. All patients required mechanical ventilation and an FiO_2 ≥ .55 to maintain PAO_2 at a satisfactory level. The DO_2 varables of the 16 patients are shown in Table 2 and Fig. 3.

$\dot{V}O_2$ was higher than normal in ten patients, normal in four and reduced in only two, both of whom were hypothermic on admission to the Intensive Care Unit. In the face of low or inadequate DO_2 the $\dot{V}O_2$ was maintained by increases

Table 2. Oxygen transport variables in 16 major trauma victims in South Manchester

Case Number	CI	CaO_2	DO_2	$\dot{V}O_2$	OER	$S\bar{v}O_2$
1	5.8	14.5	841	145	17	92
2	2.7	13.0	351	119	34	71
3	3.5	18.2	637	155	24	79
4	4.4	14.8	651	105	16	87
5	5.5	18.5	1018	176	17	85
6	4.2	18.2	764	176	23	75
7	2.5	14.3	357	110	31	52
8	2.8	16.8	470	308	65	36
9	5.3	15.1	800	175	22	79
10	4.9	16.9	828	176	21	82
11	3.4	16.4	558	190	34	66
12	1.8	14.5	261	94	36	64
13	5.4	15.3	826	238	29	77
14	6.6	15.0	990	198	20	82
15	6.9	13.8	952	186	20	81
16	2.6	12.9	335	190	56	43

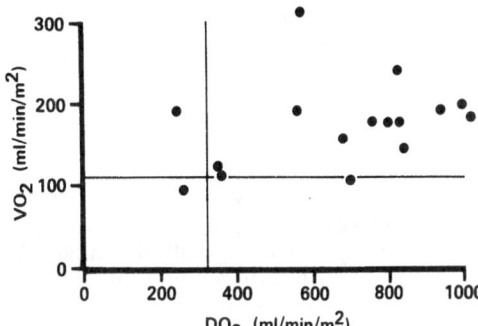

Fig. 3. Oxygen transport following trauma

in OER, seven patients leading to low $S\bar{v}O_2$ levels. Those patients with an inadequate DO_2 – defined as $DO_2 < 600$ ml/min/m^2, OER > 25% or $S\bar{v}O_2 < 75\%$ all had pulmonary artery occlusion pressure (PAOP) $\geqslant$ 18 mm Hg with adequate hemoglobin and CaO_2. The major cause of reduction in DO_2 was inadequate CI despite optimal levels of PAOP. We have found therefore, as did Shoemaker that left ventricular dysfunction can limit the CI response to fluid transfusion after trauma. Only one of these seven patients had evidence of underlying heart disease, the others were previously fit and well and we presume that the cause for the cardiac dysfunction was myocardial contusion. One of these young patients died and autopsy examination revealed extensive contusion of the myocardium effecting the right ventricle, anterior septum and left ventricle.

Adequate DO_2 was achieved in six of these seven patients by inotropic support in the form of dobutamine 7.5 to 55 µg/kg/min. There were four deaths and twelve survivors. Ten of the 12 survivors were above the LD_{50} line constructed by TRISS and therefore represent anomalous survivors. There was one anomalous death due to delay in transfer from the referring hospital. The initial resuscitation of these patients in the Emergency Room was supervised directly be senior staff members. The patients were transferred directly to the Intensive Care Unit where mechanical ventilation was instituted, monitoring lines inserted immediately and monitoring continued throughout the definitive surgical procedures that were required – laparotomy, external fixation of fractures, amputation of limbs etc. Following surgery they were supported through the lengthy recovery period by maintenance of $DO_2 \geqslant 600$ ml/min/m^2, again by inotropic support if necessary.

In conclusion, the evidence for an ebb phase of reduced $\dot{V}O_2$ following major trauma in man is poor. There is much more convincing evidence that $\dot{V}O_2$ is increased in those with the severest injuries, at the expense of increased OER and decreased $S\bar{v}O_2$ if DO_2 is not maintained at a supranormal level. Outcome can be improved if DO_2 is increased to adequate levels by inotropic support if required.

References

1. Buran JM (1987) Oxygen consumption. In: Snyder JV, Pinsky MR (eds) Oxygen transport in the critically ill. Chicago, Year Book Medical Publishing Inc: pp. 16–21
2. Bland RD, Shoemaker WC, Abraham E, Cobo JC (1985) Hemodynamic and oxygen transport patterns in surviving and non surviving postoperative patients. Crit Care Med 13:85–90
3. Shoemaker WC, Appel PL, Waxman K, et al (1982) Clinical trial of survivors cardiorespiratory patterns as therapeutic goals in critically ill postoperative patients. Crit Care Med 10:398–402
4. Snyder JV (1987) Patterns of hemodynamic response. In: Snyder JV, Pinsky MR (eds) Oxygen transport in the critically ill. Chicago, Year Book Medical Publishing Inc, pp 46–66
5. Kandel G, Aberman A (1983) Mixed venous saturation. Its role in the assessment of the critically ill patient. Arch Intern Med 143:1400–1402
6. Kasnitz P, Druger GL, Yorra F, et al (1976) Mixed venous oxygen tension and hyperlactemia. Survival in severe cardiopulmonary disease. JAMA 236:570–574
7. Shibutani K, Komatsu T, Kubal K (1983) Critical level of oxygen delivery in anesthetized man. Crit Care Med 11:640–643
8. Danek SJ, Lynch JP, Weg JG, Dantzker DR (1980) The dependence on oxygen uptake on oxygen delivery in the Adult Respiratory Distress Syndrome. Am Rev Respir Dis 122:387–395
9. Shoemaker WC (1987) Circulatory mechanisms of shock and their mediators. Crit Care Med 15:787–794
10. Champion HR, Sacco WJ (1986) Trauma severity scales. In: Maull KI, Cleveland HC, Strauch GO, Wolferth CC (eds) Advances in trauma, Vol 1, 1-20. Year Book Medical Publishers Inc Chicago
11. Campion H, Sacco WJ, Hurst J (1983) Trauma severity scoring to predict mortality. World J Surg 7:4–11
12. Lowe DK, Gately HL, Goss JR, Frey CL, Peterson CG (1983) Patterns of death, complications, and error in the management of motor vehicle accident victims: implications for a regional system of trauma care. J Trauma 23:503
13. Boyd CR, Tolson MA, Copes WS (1987) Evaluating trauma care: The TRISS method. J Trauma 27:370–378
14. Cuthbertson DP (1932) Observations on the disturbance of metabolism produced by injury to the limbs. Quart J Med 1:233–246

15. Wilmore DW (1986) The wound as an organ. In: Little RA, Frayn KN (eds) The scientific basis for the care of the critically ill. Manchester University Press, pp 45–59
16. Odling-Smee GW (1981) The metabolic response to injury. In: Odling-Smee GW, Crockard A (eds) Trauma care. London, Academic Press, pp 33–52
17. Cuthbertson DP (1942) Post-shock metabolic response. Lancet 1:433–437
18. Shoemaker WC (1987) Relationship of oxygen transport patterns to the pathophysiology and therapy of shock states. Intensive Care Med 13:230–243
19. Stoner HB (1987) Interpretation of the metabolic effects of trauma and sepsis. J Clin Pathol 40:1108–1117
20. Cournand A, Riley RL, Bradley SE, et al (1943) Studies of the circulation in clinical shock. Surgery 13:964–995
21. Shoemaker WC, Appel P, Czer LSC, et al (1980) Pathogenesis of respiratory failure (ARDS) after haemorrhage and trauma. Crit Care Med 8:504–512
22. Mayall RM, Edwards JD, Wilkins RG (1987) Importance of sampling site for measurement of mixed venous oxygen saturation. Crit Care Med 15:405 (Abstract)
23. Little RA (1985) Heat production after injury. Brit Med Bull 41:226–231
24. Shatney CH (1985) Management of traumatic shock. In: Vincent JL (ed) Update in intensive care and emergency medicine. Springer, Berlin Heidelberg New York Tokyo, pp 247–253

Limits of Hemodilution in Patients with Coronary Artery Disease

J. F. Baron, E. Vicaut, and M. Duvelleroy

Introduction

Preoperative intentional hemodilution is induced by an isovolemic exchange of whole blood with colloid or crystalloid solutions to gain autologous blood while maintaining normovolemia. Intentional hemodilution has been introduced into surgery because transfusion donor blood is associated with significant risks. The appearance of AIDS and its possible transmission by transfusion despite a selection of donors, is a very sensitive problem for patients and physicians [1]. However, it is probably not the major problem since the risk of non-A non-B hepatitis transmission is quantitatively more important. In addition, the evidence that transfusions of homologous blood can induce immunosuppression and thereby impair the host resistance of surgical patients is a cause of new concern [2]. These problems with homologous transfusion have promoted all techniques of autotransfusion. Among these, intentional hemodilution is the one which has probably known the greater development since it is the simplest and least expensive.

The pathophysiology of normovolemic hemodilution has been studied extensively in the past decade [3]. It has been established that a reduction in hematocrit and, as a result, in arterial oxygen content, is not deleterious since compensating mechanisms are involved to maintain systemic oxygen transport. However, it has been suggested by experimental studies that the cardiovascular adaptations involved by hemodilution may be either deleterious or limited in patients with coronary artery disease [4]. Nevertheless, some clinical studies have been conducted in patients with coronary artery disease and have brought some conflicting results. At present, it remains from all these experimental and clinical studies that rather than to speak about hemodilution as a contraindication in patients with coronary artery disease, it is probably more appropriate to call up its safe limits in this setting [5].

Cardiovascular Adaptations to Normovolemic Hemodilution

The decrease in hematocrit results in an improvement of rheologic properties of blood. In normovolemic conditions, the enhanced blood fluidity induces a large increase in cardiac output [6] as a result of an enhanced venous return [7]. Stroke volume increases while at the same time the emptying of the left ventricle is facilitated due to a reduced afterload [8]. It is generally admitted that the increase in cardiac output is not due to a change in heart rate as long as normovolemia is preserved. Heart rate increases as soon as hypovolemia occurs, due to either an insufficient infusion of the plasma substitute or to its rapid extravasation [3]. However, when considering control groups, clinical studies found a trend to a higher heart rate in patients with hemodilution [9]. In addition, an experimental study, comparing cardiac adaptations to normovolemic hemodilution in dogs with chronic cardiac denervation to those occurring in normal dogs, found a lower increase in cardiac output in former group than in the second [10]. In this study, this result was due to a decrease in the relative contribution of heart rate to the increase in cardiac output. These results suggest an involvement of the autonomic nervous system by hemodilution through an activation of chemoreceptors and baroreceptors [11]. The same mechanisms might explain the increase in myocardial contractility during normovolemic hemodilution [12].

Despite the decreased oxygen carrying capacity during normovolemic hemodilution, systemic oxygen transport is not compromised since cardiac output increases. Based on theoretical considerations, Hint first predicted that systemic oxygen transport may be at least maintained until hematocrit reaches 20% [13]. These results were fully corroborated by many experimental and clinical studies [14, 15]. Global oxygen consumption is maintained during normovolemic hemodilution for a large range of hematocrits (from 60 to 20%) [6]. This is associated with a decrease in venous oxygen content [6]. Continuous and simultaneous measurements of oxygen pressure distribution in various organs revealed that the local PO_2 in the liver, pancreas, intestine, kidney and skeletal muscle increased slightly as a result of normovolemic hemodilution [16]. The shift of the tissue PO_2 distribution profiles towards higher PO_2 values while the hematocrit was lowered was interpreted as a reflection of a more homogeneous flow distribution of capillary flows [17].

Coronary Circulation Adaptations to Normovolemic Hemodilution

The enhanced cardiac output is distributed to the vital organs in approximatively the same fraction during normovolemic hemodilution as at normal hematocrit with the exception of the coronary circulation. Coronary blood flow increases proportionately more than other local blood flows [18]. This finding indicates that the increase in coronary blood flow is not only due to the decrease in viscosity but that it also reflects a coronary vasodilation [19]. In addition, hemodilution may induce a decrease in the coronary perfusion pressure since the mean arterial pressure generally slightly decreases while the right atrial pressure increases.

Myocardial oxygen consumption is maintained for a large range of hematocrits (from 20 to 60%) as well as for the total body. However, no change in coronary sinus oxygen saturation is observed during hemodilution even at a very low hematocrit [19] while a decrease in mixed venous oxygen saturation is generally observed with hematocrits below 25%. Other studies found a slight decrease in coronary sinus oxygen saturation, but this decrease is more limited than for other local circulations. This particular adaptation of the myocardium to hemodilution is imposed by the nearly maximal oxygen extraction in basal conditions. These experimental findings have been confirmed in the human coronary circulation [20]. Thus, when compared to other tissues, a strict maintenance of myocardial oxygen supply is necessary during hemodilution.

Furthermore, the endocardial/epicardial distribution of coronary blood flow may also be modified by hemodilution. Brazier et al [21] demonstrated that oxygen delivery to both subepicardium and subendocardium is adequately maintained over a wide range of hemoglobin levels (down to 5 g/100 ml) in normal dogs with patent coronary arteries. This was achieved by a proportional increase in coronary blood flow to both areas. With a hemoglobin concentration lower than 5 g/100 ml a further increase in both total coronary and subendocardial blood flow was observed. However, there was a significant reduction in the proportion of that flow delivered to the subendocardium, leading to a decrease in endocardial/epicardial flow ratio. These changes were associated with myocardial ischemia detected with an intracavitary electrocardiogram. These results demonstrate that during hemodilution the subendocardium is more vulnerable to ischemia than other layers because it must receive most or all of its flow during diastole. Thus, for the subendocardium to receive the same amount of flow as other layers, it must have a lower vascular resistance. Since the capacity of subendocardial vessels to vasodilate is more limited, maximum coronary dilatation will occur first in this region. In addition, Geha [4] showed that the maximal coronary blood flow is not modified during normovolemic hemodilution. As a result, the coronary flow reserve, or the ratio of peak increase in flow after 10 second occlusion to preocclusion flow is decreased by 50% at a hematocrit of 30%. This decrease is only due to the increase in the resting flow with hemodilution. Thus, at half normal hematocrit, coronary reserve is severely compromised indicating cardiac vulnerability especially if a rise in oxygen requirements occurs.

Hemodilution and Experimental Coronary Stenosis or Occlusion

Experimental studies were conducted with models of acute myocardial ischemia to determine whether normovolemic hemodilution is deleterious or not. A study in open-chest dogs revealed that a decrease in arterial oxygen content obtained by hemodilution does not increase myocardial ischemia evaluated by summating S-T elevations from epicardial electrocardiographic mapping [22]. The same decrease in arterial oxygen content obtained by hypoxia at a normal hematocrit increases the severity of ischemia in the same experiments. Similar studies performed in isolated, isovolemic hearts under controlled hemodynamic conditions confirmed that hemodilution does not increase myocardial ischemia after coronary occlusion [22]. These last experiments suggested that an increased collateral flow during normovolemic hemodilution is the mechanism by which a decrease in arterial oxygen content is not further deleterious when obtained by hemodilution rather than by hypoxia. This increase in collateral flow is probably directly related to the decreased viscosity at the microcirculatory level. These experiments are in agreement with those of Stucker et al. [23] who compared the myocardial performances of isolated working hearts reperfused after a prolonged global myocardial ischemia according to the hematocrit of the perfusate. They found that after a global ischemia, coronary blood flow increased in the hemodiluted group in order to maintain the same myocardial oxygen transport than in the non hemodiluted group. In addition, myocardial performance evaluated by the aortic blood flow of this isolated working heart was better in the group with hemodilution after global ischemia. These results contrasted with the similarity in both groups of the myocardial oxygen consumption.

Few studies investigated the effects of hemodilution with experimental coronary artery stenosis. Hagl et al [24] demonstrated that after a partial occlusion of a coronary artery, the increase in coronary blood flow induced by hemodilution was extremely limited, while it was adapted in another normal coronary artery. As a result, oxygen transport was reduced in the region irrigated by the narrowed artery. However, these experimental preparations are probably not appropriate to simulate coronary adaptations in the setting of coronary artery disease. In addition, coronary adaptations probably depends on the degree of stenosis, as well as on the existence of a collateral circulation.

Hemodilution and Coronary Artery Disease

Based on these experimental data, acute normovolemic hemodilution has been considered to be contraindicated in patients with coronary artery disease. Nevertheless, such a technique is commonly used during cardiac surgery including coronary bypass procedures [5]. During vascular surgery, hemodilution is also commonly used despite the high incidence of coronary artery disease in such patients [25]. Although postoperative myocardial infarction is a frequent complication after these types of surgery, normovolemic hemodilution has not been identified as a determinant or as a contributing factor for this complication. In

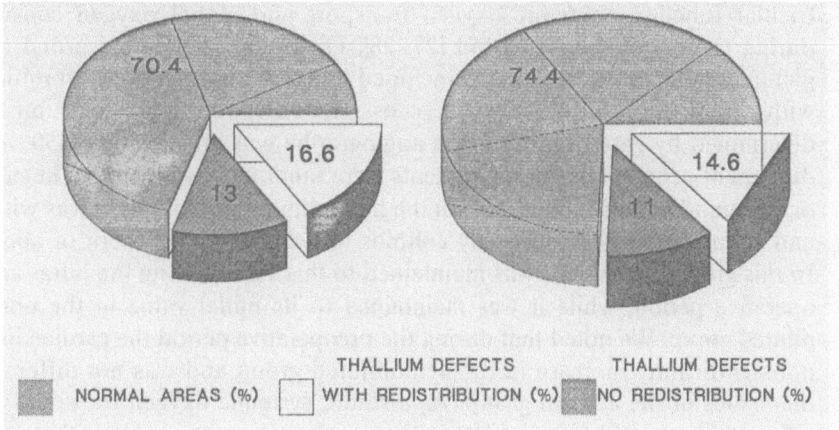

Fig. 1. Myocardial dipyridamole-thallium gammatomography before (*left*) and after (*right*) normovolemic hemodilution in patients with coronary artery disease. (From [26])

fact, to our knowledge, no randomized clinical study has been conducted to determine this.

One approach to investigate the effects of normovolemic hemodilution on coronary dynamics and on myocardial metabolism in patients with coronary artery disease is to study myocardial thallium uptake. Such a study conducted by Laxenaire et al [26] did not reveal any further impairment in basal thallium uptake after normovolemic hemodilution decreasing hematocrit to 30% (Fig. 1). Furthermore, basal thallium uptake was improved in three patients. In addition, when comparing dipyridamole-thallium scans before and after normovolemic hemodilution, no change in thallium uptake was observed in 7 of the 10 patients included in this study, an improvement was observed in two patients and an increase in thallium defects was observed in only one patient. This last patient had disabling angina with chest pain at rest. These results indicated that despite the hemodilution-induced decrease in coronary vascular resistance, resulting from both coronary vasodilation and decrease in blood viscosity, no coronary steal phenomenon was observed in these patients since no significant change in basal thallium uptake was observed. On the contrary, the increase in basal thallium uptake in three patients suggested that the collateral flow may be improved and/or that the flow downstream to the coronary artery stenosis was better distributed. However, the increase in dipyridamole-thallium scans defects in one patient with disabling angina suggested a dipyridamole-induced coronary steal and fixed a limit to the tolerance of hemodilution in patients with coronary artery disease. Furthermore, this study pointed out that left ventricular function at rest was not altered by hemodilution in these patients with coronary artery disease. However, one should wonder to what extent these results might be extrapolated to anesthetic situations in which both global and myocardial oxygen consumption may dramatically vary especially at recovery from general anesthesia. In this situation, myocardial oxygen imbalance may impair left ventricular function which in turn may limit systemic oxygen transport.

We conducted a randomized study in anesthetized patients with coronary artery disease to investigate the effects of normovolemic hemodilution on left ventricular function, systemic oxygen transport and global oxygen consumption during the perioperative period [27, 28[. On preoperative myocardial thallium gammatomography, all patients included had at least one defect on initial scans with a redistribution on delayed scans. Their left ventricular ejection fraction determined by gated radionuclide angiography was greater than 0.50. After induction of general anesthesia, patients were randomly assigned to a hemodiluted or to a non-hemodiluted group. In the hemodiluted group, blood was withdrawn and simultaneously replaced by colloids to achieve a hematocrit of about 25%. In this group, hematocrit was maintained to this value during the intra- and postoperative period, while it was maintained to its initial value in the non-hemodiluted group. We noted that during the preoperative period the cardiac index did not significantly increase in the hemodiluted group and was not different from the values of the control group. As a result, systemic oxygen transport was significantly lower after hemodilution than in the other group. Nevertheless, global oxygen consumption was not different between the two groups, this was achieved by a significant decrease in mixed venous oxygen content. The lack of increased cardiac index in these patients with coronary artery disease and normal left ventricular function could not be explained by an insufficient volume replacement since the same amount of colloids was infused. In addition, no significant changes in pulmonary capillary wedge pressure and in left ventricular end-diastolic area monitored by transesophageal echocardiography, were observed. Impairment in left ventricular function due to myocardial ischemia was also unlikely since no significant change in ejection fraction area was noted. An increased venous compliance due to fentanyl benzodiazepine anesthesia may not be excluded and would have interfered with the effects of hemodilution on venous return. During the postoperative period, after rewarming, global oxygen consumption significantly increased to the same extent in both groups. However, cardiac index was not significantly higher in the hemodiluted group. This situations does not appear to be deleterious since there is a trend to a lower lactate concentration in the hemodiluted group. In addition, myocardial ischemic episodes retrospectively evidenced by the analysis in Holter tapes were not more frequent in the hemodiluted than in the control group. This study illustrates that normal hemodynamic adaptations to hemodilution may not occur during the intra- and postoperative period in patients with coronary artery disease even with a normal preoperative left ventricular function. Several mechanisms may lead to these results : interference with general anesthesia, impairment in left ventricular function, myocardial ischemia, decreased autonomic nervous system tone by general anesthesia. Some of these mechanisms are not deleterious as illustrated in this study. Therefore, a cardiac monitoring included ECG monitoring with ST-T segment analysis, an hemodynamic monitoring to evaluate preload pressures associated or not to a $S\bar{v}O_2$ monitoring, and if possible a monitoring of left ventricular function by transesophageal echo, appears to be recommended in these patients to determine which is the predominant mechanism in the case of mismatching between systemic oxygen transport and global oxygen consumption.

Conclusions

Normovolemic hemodilution may be a well-suited method for blood management during surgery. Its pathophysiology has been extensively studied in the past decade evidencing that a reduction in hematocrit was perfectly well tolerated in patients without cardiac disease. It has been suggested by experimental studies that cardiovascular adaptations involved by hemodilution might be either deleterious or limited in patients with coronary artery disease. Nevertheless, normovolemic hemodilution is largely used during cardiac surgery even with coronary bypass procedures and during vascular surgery. It has not been shown in these high risk groups of patients that hemodilution may be causative of postoperative myocardial infarction. In addition, myocardial thallium scans performed after hemodilution in patients with coronary artery disease evidenced rather beneficial than deleterious effects on myocardial metabolism. However, some limitations must be re-emphasized : normovolemic hemodilution must not be performed either in patients with a recent myocardial infarction or with disabling angina or with an impairement in left ventricular function. Hematocrit must be kept greater than 30% especially during the recovery period. In addition, the absence of adequate cardiac monitoring is a real limit for the use of such a technique in patients with coronary artery disease.

References

1. Bove JR (1984) Transfusion associated AIDS – a cause for concern. N Engl J Med 310:115–116
2. Horsey PJ (1985) Blood transfusion and surgery. Br Med J 291:234
3. Messmer K, Kreimeier U, Intaglietta M (1986) Present state of intentional hemodilution. Eur Surg Res 18:254–263
4. Geha AS (1976) Coronary and cardiovascular dynamics and oxygen availability during acute normovolemic anemia. Surgery 80:47–53
5. Niinikoski J, Laaksonen V, Meretoja O, Jalonen J, Inberg MV (1981) Oxygen transport to tissue under normovolemic moderate and extreme hemodilution during coronary bypass operation. Ann Thorac Surg 31:134–143
6. Laks H, Pilon RN, Klovekorn WP, Anderson W, McCallum JR, O'Connor NE (1974) Acute hemodilution: its effect on hemodynamics and oxygen transport in anesthetized man. Ann Surg 180:103–109
7. Guyton AC, Richardson TQ (1961) Effect of hematocrit on venous return. Circ Res 9:157–161
8. Carey JS (1975) Determinants of cardiac output during experimental therapeutic hemodilution. Ann Surg 18:196–202
9. Rose D, Coussofides T (1981) Intraoperative normovolemic hemodilution. J Surg Res 31:375–381
10. Glick G, Plauth WH, Braunwald E (1964) Role of the autonomic nervous system in the circulatory response to acutely induced anemia in anesthetized dogs. J Clin Invest 43:2112–2124
11. Hatcher JD, Chiu KL, Jennings DB (1978) Anemia as a stimulus to aortic and carotid chemoreceptors in the cat. J Appl Physiol 44:696–702
12. Rodriguez JA, Chamorro GA, Rapaport E (1974) Effect of isovolumic anemia on ventricular performance at rest and during exercise. J Appl Physiol 36:28–33
13. Hint H (1968) The pharmacology of dextran and physiological background of the clinical use of Rheomacrodex. Acta Anaesth Belg 19:119–138
14. Sunder-Plassmann L, Klovekorn WP, Holper K, Hase U, Messmer K (1971) The physiological significance of acutely induced hemodilution. In: Ditzel J, Lewis DH (eds) 6th European Conference on Microcirculation. Karger, Basel, pp 23–28
15. Shah DM, Prichard MN, Newell JC, Karmody AM, Scovill WA, Powers SR (1980) Increased cardiac output and oxygen transport after intraoperative isovolumic hemodilution – A study in patients with peripheral vascular disease. Arch Surg 115:597–600
16. Messmer K, Sunder-Plassmann L, Jesch F, Gornandt L, Sinagowitz E, Kessler M (1973) Oxygen supply to the tissues during normovolemic hemodilution. Resp Exp Med 159:152–166
17. Vicaut E, Stucker O, Teisseire B, Duvelleroy M (1987) Changes in systemic hematocrit and red cell fluxes at capillary bifurcations in rat cremaster muscle. Int J Microcirc: Clin Exp 6:225–235
18. Race D, Dedichen H, Schenk WG (1967) Regional blood flow during dextran-induced normovolemic hemodilution in the dog. J Thorac Cardiovasc Surg 53:578–586
19. Jan KM, Chien S (1977) Effect of hematocrit variations on coronary hemodynamics and oxygen utilisation. Am J Physiol 233:H106–H113
20. Gisselsson L, Rosberg B, Ericsson M (1982) Myocardial blood flow, oxygen uptake and carbon dioxide release of the human heart during hemodilution. Acta Anaesth Scand 26:589–591

21. Brazier J, Cooper N, Maloney JV, Buckberg G (1974) The adequacy of myocardial oxygen delivery in acute normovolemic anemia. Surgery 75:508-516
22. Yoshikawa H, Powell J, Bland JHL, Lowenstein E (1973) Effect of acute anemia on experimental myocardial ischemia. Am J Cardiol 32:670-678
23. Stucker O, Trouve R, Vicaut E, et al (1983) Effects of differents hematocrits on the isolated working rabbit heart reperfused after ischemia. Int J Microcirc Clin Exp 2:325-335
24. Hagl S, Heimlich W, Meisner H, Erben R, Baum M, Mendler N (1977) The effect of hemodilution of regional function in the presence of coronary stenosis. Basic Res Cardiol 72:344-364
25. Davies MJ, Cronin KD, Domaingue C (1982) Haemodilution for major vascular surgery using 3.5% polygeline (Haemaccel). Anaesth Intens Care 10:265-270
26. Laxenaire MC, Aug F, Voisin C, Chevreaud C, Bauer P, Bertrand A (1986) Effects of haemodilution on ventricular function in coronary heart disease patients. Ann Fr Anesth Réanim 5:218-222
27. van der Linden P, Baron JF, Philip I, et al (1987) Normovolemic hemodilution in anesthetized patients with coronary artery disease: Effects on hemodynamic and left ventricular function. Anesthesiology 67 (suppl):A135
28. van der Linden P, Baron JF, Philipp I, et al (1987) Normovolemic hemodilution in anesthetized patients with coronary artery disease: Hemodynamic and metabolic responses to recovery. Anesthesiology 67 (suppl):A79

Pathophysiology of Lactic Acidosis

R. D. Cohen

By far the most common cause of clinical lactic acidosis is the circulatory insufficiency of shock (Type A lactic acidosis). There are a large number of other conditions in which lactic acidosis appears in the absence of clinical evidence of shock (Type B). The withdrawal from general use of the more toxic anti-diabetic biguanides has made significant inroads into the frequency of severe Type B lactic acidosis and this condition is often a relatively minor component of a more major illness – for example in diabetic ketoacidosis and alcoholic intoxication poisoning. Type A lactic acidosis is likely to be more relevant to intensive care medicine and is therefore the main subject of this paper.

The principal organs producing lactate in normal resting man are skeletal muscle, erythrocytes, brain, gut and skin (approximately 1300 mmol/day). An equimolar quantity of H^+ is produced with the lactate and titrates tissue and blood bicarbonate; the bicarbonate is restored when the lactate is converted to electroneutral products such as glucose, glycogen or CO_2 and water.

$$2H_2O \rightarrow 2H^+ + 2OH^-$$

$$2CH_3CHOHCOO^- + 2H^+ \rightarrow C_6H_{12}O_6$$

$$2OH^- + 2CO_2 \rightarrow 2HCO_3^-$$

Sum: $2CH_3CHOHCOO^- + 2CO_2 + 2H_2O \rightarrow C_6H_{12}O_6 + 2HCO_3^-$

This conversion takes place mainly in the liver (40–70%) but also in kidney, heart, and under some circumstances in resting skeletal muscle.

Type A lactic acidosis is traditionally ascribed to anaerobic glycolysis in ischemic tissues, which is undoubtedly true, but there is much evidence in animals, and a little in man, that the lactate and H^+ removal capacity of the liver is severely compromised by the ischemia of shock, resulting in further accumulation of blood and tissue lactate and H^+. There are two obvious factors in this effect. Firstly, the actual process of gluconeogenesis from lactate and H^+ requires 6 ATP per mole of glucose formed; the majority of this ATP is of course derived from aerobic respiration, which is markedly reduced in shock. Secondly, poor perfusion of lactate-removing organs, e.g. the liver, results in decreased presentation of lactate and H^+ for gluconeogenesis.

Fig. 1 summarizes the results of observations in isolated perfused rat livers which were made ischemic to different degrees [1]. The rate of decline of lactate uptake with flow is relatively gentle at first, but becomes increasingly precipitous as ischemia increases. From mathematical analysis it appears likely that the slowness of the initial decline is simply due to the effect of reduced delivery of lactate to the liver being partly offset by the increased residence time of each microvolume of blood in the liver, thereby allowing more lactate to be taken up. At lower flows (25% of normal) the liver becomes oxygen deficient and ATP synthesis [1] and lactate uptake fall more rapidly. Fig. 1 also shows that at about this stage of ischemia, intracellular pH (pH_i) begins to fall and hepatic venous PCO_2 to rise.

In these studies, perfusate pH and PCO_2 were normal. But in shock, systemic acidosis is present as well as ischemia. Although compensatory hypocapnia is frequently present in arterial blood in the lactic acidosis of shock, hepatic and mixed venous PCO_2 are usually elevated [2,3]; it may be assumed that PCO_2 within tissues is also elevated and that this effect and the production of H^+ during anaerobic glycolysis contribute to the fall in pH_i, which is reinforced by the low extracellular pH (pH_e). The raised PCO_2 is due to (a) poor wash out of PCO_2 from residual aerobic metabolism and (b) titration of tissue and blood bicarbonate by the H^+ produced with lactate.

Some of the important effects of the acidosis on the situation in shock are as follows:

1. A negative inotropic effect due to inhibition of the cardiac sarcolemmal slow calcium channels by low cardiac pH_i. Cardiac output in rats falls with increasing acidosis and so therefore does hepatic and renal blood flow and the perfusion of organs producing lactate and H^+ blood flow [4]. The acidosis itself therefore worsens the shock.
2. If the blood lactate is below 2 mM, hepatic lactate uptake and conversion to glucose and bicarbonate is stimulated by increasing pH_e relative to hepatic

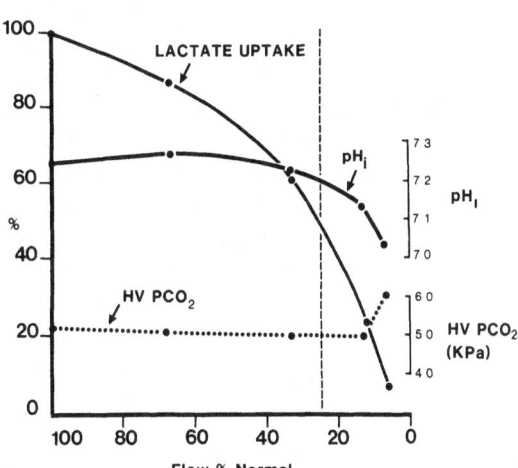

Fig. 1. Lactate uptake, intracellular pH and hepatic venous PCO_2 in isolated perfused rat liver as perfusion rate is progressively lowered from normal (100%). Portal venous lactate was 2 mM. (From [1])

pH$_i$ [5]. This is due to increased activity of a semi-specific lactate transporter in the plasma membrane of the hepatocyte, thereby improving the presentation of lactate to the reactions of gluconeogenesis [6,7]. This could be a homeostatic mechanism in mild circulatory insufficiency.

3. If, however, blood lactate is > 2 mM, as is the case in more advanced circulatory insufficiency, the main effect of acidosis is, via a low pH$_i$, to *inhibit* lactate conversion into glucose [8,9] and bicarbonate regeneration, by an effect on one of the intermediate steps of gluconeogenesis (conversion of pyruvate to oxaloacetate [10]). The development of lactic acidosis is therefore accelerated.

   It has been shown in isolated liver preparations that the inhibitory effects of acidosis and low perfusion on lactate uptake are additive [14]. The combined effects of moderate ischemia and acidosis can be largely overcome by the addition of epinephrine to the perfusion at concentrations similar to those observed during hemorrhagic shock in man [15].

4. Intracellular acidosis – whether it be generated in situ, or by the effects of low pH$_e$ or high PCO_2 – has a marked inhibitory effect on glycolysis. This phenomenon has been described in many tissues, including skeletal and cardiac muscle, brain, erythrocytes and liver, and is mediated by inhibition of phosphofructokinase, a rate-limiting enzyme of glycolysis. It serves as a brake on anaerobic glycolysis, without which lactic acidosis in shock or exercise might be even more severe.

The effect described in paragraph 3 above has further anti-homeostatic implications. It has been shown that hepatic pH$_i$ is directly related to the rate of lactate uptake and metabolism [11]. Increasing this rate alkalinizes the liver cell because of the bicarbonate generated. Conversely, a reduction of the rate of lactate uptake and metabolism, which may result in some circumstances - e.g. fructose infusion – in conversion of lactate uptake to output, results in a lowering of hepatic pH$_i$ [12]. This type of effect may, as indicated in paragraph 3, result in further inhibition of lactate uptake and metabolism.

   With this in mind we were intrigued by the relatively uncommon appearance of severe lactic acidosis during diabetic ketoacidosis, when extracellular acidosis may be very severe, and the site of generation of ketoacids, i.e. the liver, might lead one to expect severe inhibition of lactate uptake and metabolism. To examine this problem we have made measurements of hepatic pH$_i$ by ^{31}P-magnetic resonance spectroscopy in intact lightly anaesthetised rats [13], which have been made progressively acidotic by either (a) streptozotocin-induced diabetic ketoacidosis (b) oral administration of ammonium chloride or (c) slow intravenous infusion of hydrochloric acid. At milder degrees of extracellular acidosis there is little difference between hepatic pH$_i$ in the three groups, but at the more severe degrees of extracellular acidosis, pH$_i$ in the ketoacidotic rats falls much less than in the other two groups. This could explain why lactic acidosis is relatively infrequent in diabetic ketoacidosis; lactate uptake and conversion into glucose is maintained at a high level in diabetic ketoacidosis, perhaps by elevated mitochondrial concentration of acetyl CoA which stimulates gluconeogenesis from lactate at the pyruvate carboxylase step. Consistent with this explanation is the observation that it is much more difficult to demonstrate inhibition of gluconeo-genesis from lactate (at lactate levels > 2 mM) in perfused livers from diabetic as compared to normal rats [13].

Conclusions

The above discussion indicates the complexity of the influences on lactate meta-bolism during shock. Clearly there are some aspects of the scheme which are very much in unstable equilibrium and might help to account for the rapid and irreversible deterioration which is frequently seen clinically. Because of the inter-play of effects it is not surprizing that clear conclusions have not been reached about the success or failure of various direct therapeutic approaches to the lactic acidosis of shock.

References

1. Iles RA, Baron PG, Cohen RD (1979) The effect of reduction of perfusion rate on lactate and oxygen uptake, glucose output and energy supply in the isolated perfused liver of starved rats. Biochem J 184:635–642
2. Tung SH, Bettice J, Wang BC, Brown E (1976) Intracellular and extracellular acid-base changes in haemorrhagic shock. Respir Physiol 26:229–237
3. Weil MH, Rackow EC, Trevino R, Grundler W, Falk JL, Griffel MI (1986) Difference in acid-base state between venous and arterial blood during cardiopulmonary rescuscitation. N Engl J Med 315:153–156
4. Yudkin J, Cohen RD, Slack B (1976) The haemodynamic effects of metabolic acidosis in the rat. Clin Sci Mol Med 50:177–184
5. Sestoft L, Marshall MO (1986) Hepatic lactate uptake is enhanced by low pH at low lactate concentration in perfused rat liver. Clin Sci 70:19–22
6. Monson JP, Smith JA, Cohen RD, Iles RA (1982) Evidence for a lactate transporter in the plasma membranes of rat hepatocytes. Clin Sci 62:411–420
7. Fafournoux P, Demigné C, Rémésy C (1985) Carrier-mediated uptake of lactate in rat he-patocytes. J Biol Chem 260:292–299
8. Hems R, Ross BD, Berry MN, Krebs HA (1966) Gluconeogenesis in the perfused rat liver. Biochem J 101:284–292
9. Lloyd MH, Iles RA, Simpson BR, Strunin JM, Layton JM, Cohen RD (1973) The effect of simulated metabolic acidosis on intracellular pH and lactate metabolism in the isolated perfused liver. Clin Sci Mol Med 45:543–549
10. Iles RA, Cohen RD, Rist AH, Baron PG (1977) The mechanism of inhibition by acidosis of gluconeogenesis from lactate. Biochem J 164:185–191
11. Cohen RD, Iles RA, Barnett D, Howell MEO, Strunin J (1971) The effect of changes in lactate uptake in the intracellular pH of the perfused rat liver. Clin Sci 41:159–170
12. Cohen RD, Henderson RM, Iles RA, Smith JA (1982) Metabolic interrelationships of intra-cellular pH measured by double-barrelled microelectrodes in perfused rat liver. J Physiol (Lond) 330:69–80
13. Beech JS, Williams SR, Iles RA (1987) Models of metabolic acidosis investigated by ^{31}P-NMR. Proceedings of the Society of Magnetic Resonance in Medicine. 6th Annual Meet-ing, p 105
14. Iles RA, Cohen RD, Baron PG (1981a) The effect of combined ischemia and acidosis on lactate uptake and gluconeogenesis in the perfused rat liver. Clin Sci 60:537–42
15. Iles RA, Cohen RD, Baron PG, Smith JA, Henderson RM (1981b) The effect of adrenaline on hepatic lactate uptake in the acidotic partially ischaemic rat liver. Clin Sci 60:543–548

Transport and Consumption of Oxygen in Septic Shock

L. G. Thijs

The primary function of intensive care is in essence the maintenance or improvement of oxygen uptake in critically ill patients. Its immediate objective is to preserve life and prevent, minimize or reverse damage to vital organs. In order to achieve this, adequate supply of oxygen to the tissues is mandatory, a condition sine qua non for the organism to survive and to buy time for the underlying disease or injury to resolve.

In septic shock, as in all shock states, reduced oxygen consumption (relative to the metabolic demands) is presumably the earliest pathogenetic event which occurs at or even prior to the initial hypotensive crisis [1]. Throughout a septic episode the basic physiologic problem seems to be a disparity between the uptake of oxygen by the cells and the demand of oxygen. In patients with septic shock systemic oxygen consumption ($\dot{V}O_2$) is frequently normal or even decreased despite a hyperdynamic circulation, a response that seems highly inappropriate in the presence of fever, tissue inflammation increased protein catabolism, and increased circulating catecholamines [2, 3]. Recent clinical evidence indicates that inadequate $\dot{V}O_2$ is a major determinant of outcome and it is suggested that this is associated with the degree of $\dot{V}O_2$ deficit [1]. Limitations of $\dot{V}O_2$ may significantly contribute to morbidity and mortality by predisposing to multiple organ failure which is often the cause of death. A substantial oxygen debt has been found in critically ill, mostly septic patients with dysfunction of two or more organ systems who subsequently died [4]. This observation suggests that inadequate tissue oxygenation is a central mechanism mediating the widespread and irreversible tissue damage that is associated with multiple organ failure and fatal outcome [4].

With this in mind it will be worthwhile to analyze the various components of the oxygen transport chain and their alterations in septic shock. In this way we may find a sound basis for therapeutic interventions aimed at improvement of tissue oxygenation. Delivery of oxygen to tissues depends upon the functional capability of three organ systems. These are the ability of the lungs to restore venous oxygen tension to acceptable levels in arterial blood, the blood's ability to carry oxygen and the perfusion of tissues and lung capillaries by the circulatory system [5].

Therefore, the components of oxygen transport and consumption are: pulmonary gas exchange, total systemic blood flow (cardiac output), distribution of cardiac output (regional blood flow), arterial oxygen content and peripheral oxygen extraction. The main abnormality found in septic shock is a defect in peripheral oxygen extraction, but abnormalities in all other components may additionally impair adequate oxygenation and therefore contribute to an unfavorable outcome.

Pulmonary Gas Exchange

To ensure transfer of sufficient oxygen from the atmosphere to the blood adequate *alveolar ventilation, pulmonary perfusion, ventilation to perfusion ratio* and *diffusion capacity* of the lungs are necessary. In septic shock a large number of abnormalities may interfere with these mechanisms (e.g. pneumonia, COPD, atelectasis, ARDS) either pre-existent or associated with sepsis. Interventions aimed at improvement of pulmonary gas exchange such as oxygen therapy, physiotherapy, early intubation and mechanical ventilation (with PEEP) contribute significantly to overall oxygen transport. However, some interventions such as mechanical ventilation with PEEP may adversely interfere with circulation and oxygen transport: although PaO_2 increases cardiac output may decline. This stresses the necessity to consider all components of oxygen transport at the same time.

Cardiac Output

Since total oxygen delivery is determined by the product of cardiac output and arterial oxygen content ($DO_2 = CO \cdot CaO_2$) adequate total systemic flow is a prerequisite for tissue oxygenation. Whereas in most forms of shock oxygen supply is limited by a decrease in cardiac output, cardiac output in septic shock is usually elevated or in the upper limit of normal. Provided that arterial hypoxemia is prevented oxygen delivery is therefore usually well preserved. In view of the abnormal supply dependency of $\dot{V}O_2$ in septic shock (as will be discussed later) cardiac output is still a potential crucial variable even when total systemic flow is not lowered. Moreover, myocardial depression may occur and compromized myocardial function can ultimately result in a low cardiac output. In patients with pulmonary hypertension right heart failure may be an important mechanism contributing to a decline in cardiac output [6]. It has been estimated that about one-third of nonsurvivors of a septic insult develop a low cardiac output prior to demise [7]. A decline of cardiac output and therefore DO_2 forms a serious threat, additional to all other abnormalities that interfere with oxygen delivery and calls for vigorous treatment. The heart itself is also dependent upon adequate oxygen supply and interventions should maintain or improve the balance between myocardial oxygen supply and demand. Delivery of oxygen to the myocardium is determined by coronary perfusion (dependent upon *diastolic blood pressure, filling pressures of the heart, length of diastole* and *coronary vascular resistance*) and CaO_2. In two recent studies it has been shown that in early human septic shock oxygen supply to the heart is increased due to selective coronary vasodilation [8, 9]. Myocardial oxygen consumption was not significantly different from controls. In these studies blood pressure was maintained at acceptable levels and therefore significant reduction of myocardial oxygen supply may occur at lower blood pressures. Myocardial oxygen demand is influenced by *heart rate, contractility* and *wall tension* (related to ventricular diameters: Laplace law). Inotropic drugs that increase contractility and heart rate therefore significantly increase myocardial oxygen demand while an enlarged heart needs more oxygen than a normal heart. All these factors should be taken into consideration in the circulatory management of patients with septic shock.

Distribution of Cardiac Output

Results from a large number of experimental studies indicate that in endotoxin and septic shock models blood flow is redistributed and preferentially directed to heart, brain, liver and adrenals [10]. In general, redistribution of blood flow seems to subserve preservation of oxygen supply in vital organs such as heart and brain at the expense of most other organs. Our knowledge of blood flow redistribution in human septic shock is only fragmentary. As already mentioned, coronary vascular resistance is lowered relatively more than systemic vascular resistance in septic shock, favoring a proportionally higher coronary blood flow [8, 9]. In a recent study in hyperdynamic septic patients splanchnic blood flow was found to be elevated and higher than in a nonseptic trauma group. However, in both groups the proportion of cardiac output directed to the splanchnic area was essentially identical [11]. In contrast to the nonseptic group, a disproportionate increase in splanchnic oxygen consumption relative to total body oxygen consumption was found in patients with sepsis [11]. Capillary muscle flow also increases in patients with sepsis but in direct proportion to increases in cardiac output [12]. In these last mentioned studies patients did not meet the criteria of shock and therefore results may not necessarily apply when shock supervenes. However, it is highly likely that also in human septic shock a significant redistribution of blood flow occurs to preserve to a large extent oxygen supply to vital organs and probably also to direct oxygen to metabolically highly active organs.

Regulation of regional blood flow is likely due to a balance between local tissue regulation of arteriolar tone and the activity of central mechanisms such as the autonomous nervous system. In severe sepsis strong vasodilating mechanisms (e.g. vasodilating mediators) are operative that probably overrule normal autoregulation, while simultaneously sympathetic nervous activity is increased and levels of several vasoconstricting mediators may be elevated. The balance between these many, often opposing, vasoactive forces ultimately determines the arterial blood flow to organs.

From a clinical point of view no therapeutic measures other than supporting or improving DO_2 seem possible, although theoretically selective drugs are necessary that direct oxygen supply to those tissues most in need of oxygen. However, at present no bedside tools are available to detect such tissues nor do we have these magic drugs.

Arterial Oxygen Content

Oxygen is transported in the blood bound to hemoglobin and dissolved in plasma. The amount of oxygen combined with hemoglobin is determined by its oxygen capacity and its percentage saturation with oxygen (SaO_2), while the volume in solution depends upon the partial preserve of oxygen (PaO_2). Therefore, the factors determining CaO_2 are: hemoglobin concentration, SaO_2 and PaO_2. Hemoglobin concentration is a major determinant of CaO_2 but the hematocrit value is on the other hand the major determinant of blood viscosity. High hematocrit values may therefore adversely affect microcirculatory rheology and exacerbate microcirculatory derangements. The optimal hematocrit in septic shock is still not defined and may well be variable in individual cases.

The relation between SaO_2 and PaO_2 can be expressed as the sigmoid shaped oxygen dissociation curve. This curve shows how important it is to maintain PaO_2 above about 60 mm Hg as below this number saturation (and therefore CaO_2) rapidly falls. The curve may be shifted to the right thereby increasing the unloading capacity of oxygen at the cellular level by increases in temperature, acidosis and high levels of 2,3 DPG in red cells. A left shifted curve indicates higher affinity of hemoglobin for oxygen (and lower unloading capacity) which may be induced by decreases in temperature, alkalosis and low 2,3 DPG levels [13]. Hypophosphatemia and transfusion of stored blood are well recognized causes of low 2,3 DPG levels [13] but are usually preventable or correctable. In general, changes in the oxygen dissociation curve appear to represent a minor influence upon the availability of oxygen at the tissue level in septic shock [14] but some observations indicate that a left shifted curve may contribute to organ dysfunction [15].

Peripheral Oxygen Extraction

One of the most striking and puzzling features of human septic shock is the usually observed narrowed arterio-venous oxygen difference together with lactacidemia. Arterial blood lactate levels are assumed to reflect in some way the severity of anaerobic metabolism in tissues following an oxygen debt accumulated in the shock state [16]. Apparently, tissue hypoxia may occur despite a normal or elevated cardiac output and DO_2. Oxygen requirements appear to be elevated in sepsis to maintain a large number of processes and lactacidemia may thus be reflecting a disbalance between systemic oxygen utilization and demand that is not reflected in the extraction ratio [3]. This defect in peripheral oxygen uptake seems to be a fundamental tissue in septic shock. At present, so-called *functional shunting* appears to be the most likely explanation for this phenomenon. At least three mechanisms in the microcirculation seem to be involved: *vasodilation, microembolization* and *endothelial cell injury* [17]. The normally finely tuned autoregulation of tissues that adapts perfusion to oxygen demand may be blunted by vasodilation with resulting loss of precapillary regulating capacity [18]. Impairment of such adaptation may result in overperfusion of relatively low oxygen requiring tissues and hypoperfusion of tissues in need of high amounts of oxygen. In the latter areas cellular hypoxia may develop stimulating lactic acid production. In one study a positive correlation was found between systemic vascular resistance and oxygen extraction ratio: the lower the vascular resistance the lower the extraction ratio [16]. Also, a decrease in systemic vascular resistance during the course of a septic shock episode was associated with an increase in lactate levels and vice versa [16]. Therefore, strong vasodilation as such may presumably result in loss of autoregulation and maldistribution of flow with ineffective oxygen extraction.

Microembolization may result in loss of autoregulatory function, limitation of recruitable capillary surface, increase in variance of capillary transit times and inhomogeneity of flow [18, 19]. Impairment of capillary recruitment may increase functional diffusion pathways for oxygen and limit total capillary surface [19]. Increases in variance of transit times may limit local oxygen uptake because capillary PO_2 in some capillaries with a long transit time falls below a critical level needed to maintain sufficient diffusion of oxygen [18]. Also, other capillaries would have too short a transit time to allow effective unloading of O_2 from hemoglobin [18]. Following experimental microembolization using polysterene microspheres oxygen uptake at a given oxygen supply declined (i.e. extraction ratio fell) and venous PO_2 in the microembolized area was higher than in a corresponding normal area [20, 21]. In human septic shock microembolization may be induced by aggregation of granulocytes and platelets. It has been proposed that among others thromboxane A_2 is involved and amplifies the mechanical effects by intense vasoconstriction and additional platelet aggregation [17]. Markedly elevated levels of TXB_2 (a stable metabolite of TXA_2) have been demonstrated in patients dying with septic shock compared with survivors and normal controls [22]. In a recent study using administration of prostacyclin which antagonizes the effects of excessive release of TXA_2 and inhibits platelet aggregation and granulocyte adherence the majority of patients who increased their $\dot{V}O_2$ had increases in peripheral extraction ratio [4]. This suggests that prostacyclin improved distribution of microcirculatory flow. Endothelial cell injury may result in increased microvascular permeability and tissue edema which further impairs oxygen diffusion by increases in diffusion distances and may compress capillaries, thereby contributing to maldistribution of flow. This pathological increase in the normal heterogeneity of microcirculatory flow unrelated to oxygen demand of respiring tissues underlies functional shunting and presumably forms the basis of abnormal oxygen supply dependency of $\dot{V}O_2$ observed in septic shock. A number of studies have shown that $\dot{V}O_2$ may be dependent on DO_2 over a much wider range of DO_2 than normally found [2, 3, 16, 23, 24]. Although it may be argued that the observed relationship between DO_2 and $\dot{V}O_2$ would be spurious because of mathematical coupling a number of arguments are in favor of this concept of abnormal supply dependency [18]. Some studies have shown that septic patients who exhibited this phenomenon had elevated blood lactate levels while corresponding increases in $\dot{V}O_2$ to increases in DO_2 upon volume loading were not found in patients without lactacidemia [2, 3]. This suggests that elevated lactate levels may predict whether further increases in cardiac output and DO_2 by volume therapy will result in increases in $\dot{V}O_2$.

It is at present not known whether these microcirculatory derangements occur uniformly in all organs. In experimental studies increases in transvascular albumin flux (and presumably of microvascular permeability) show differences in various organs [25, 26]. In patients with septic shock abnormally high coronary sinus oxygen contents and low myocardial oxygen extraction have been demonstrated [8, 9]. These findings suggest similar microcirculatory abnormalities in the coronary circulation as in the systemic circulation. In contrast, the oxygen extraction fraction in the splanchnic area was higher than the systemic extraction ratio in one series of septic patients [11]. These scanty clinical data suggest that microcirculatory behavior might be different in the various organ systems.

Practical Consequences

There is a growing body of evidence that tissue hypoxia is a central mechanism mediating multiple organ failure and the immediate goal of treatment is to restore tissue oxygenation. Fluid loading is usually the first step to increase oxygen delivery. There is evidence that this will result in increases in $\dot{V}O_2$ especially in patients with elevated lactate levels [2, 3]. An important question is whether the increased $\dot{V}O_2$ associated with increased DO_2 represents a lessened degree of tissue hypoxia. An alternative possibility is that increased consumption of oxygen by extra-mitochondrial oxidase systems (and even for production of oxygen free radicals) may be responsible for the increased uptake [18]. This point remains to be clarified. However, Shoemaker et al. [27] have shown that it is important to maintain DO_2 and $\dot{V}O_2$ at supra-normal levels in order to reduce the incidence of multiple organ failure and overall mortality. For this purpose cardiovascular drugs are usually added when volume loading alone fails to restore adequate DO_2. It should be realized that catecholamines stimulate oxidative metabolism and even may be detrimental by increasing metabolic (and oxygen) demands in areas that are near or beyond the threshold for anaerobic metabolism [3]. Although optimal hematocrit levels are still not well defined a near normal hemoglobin value is presumably desirable [18] and a left shifted oxygen dissociation curve should be avoided. PaO_2 is best maintained above a minimum level of 60 mm Hg but should be considered in the context of the total chain of oxygen delivery.

Interventions aimed at improving microcirculatory flow are likely to be most beneficial. Prostacyclin and PGE_1 have possible beneficial effects and number of studies have indeed shown promising results. Further studies with these and other drugs with effects on the microcirculation will decide whether such an approach will really alter the outcome of patients with septic shock.

References

1. Shoemaker WC (1987) Relation of oxygen transport patterns to the pathophysiology and therapy of shock states. Intensive Care Med 13:230-243
2. Haupt MI, Gilbert EM, Carlson RW (1985) Fluid loading increases oxygen consumption in septic patients with lactic acidosis. Am Rev Respir Dis 131:912-916

3. Gilbert EM, Haupt MT, Mandanas RY, Huaringa AJ, Carlson RW (1986) The effect of fluid loading, blood transfusion, and catecholamine infusion on oxygen delivery and consumption in patients with sepsis. Am Rev Respir Dis 134:873-878

4. Bihari D, Smithers M, Gimson A, Tinker J (1987) The effects of vasodilation with prostacyclin on oxygen delivery and uptake in critically ill patients. N Engl J Med 317:397-403

5. Cain SM (1983) Peripheral oxygen uptake and delivery in health and disease. Clin Chest Med 4:139-148

6. Thijs LG, Groeneveld ABJ (1987) The circulatory defect of septic shock. In: Vincent JL, Thijs LG (eds) Septic shock - European view. Springer, Berlin Heidelberg New York London Paris Tokyo (Update in Intensive Care and Emergency Medicine vol 4, pp 161-178)

7. Parillo JE (1985) Cardiovascular dysfunction in septic shock: new insights into a deadly disease. Int J Cardiol 7:314-321

8. Cunnion RE, Schaer GL, Parker MM, Natanson C, Parillo JE (1986) The coronary circulation in human septic shock. Circulation 73:637-644

9. Dhainaut J-F, Huyghebaert M-F, Monsallier JF, et al (1987) Coronary hemodynamics and myocardial metabolism of lactate, free fatty acids, glucose, and ketones in patients with septic shock. Circulation 75:533-541

10. Thijs LG, Groeneveld ABJ. Peripheral circulation in septic shock. ACP (in press)

11. Dahn MS, Lange P, Lobdell K, Hans B, Jacobs LA, Mitchell RA (1987) Splanchnic and total body oxygen consumption differences in septic and injured patients. Surgery 101:69-80

12. Finley RJ, Duff JH, Holliday RL, Jones D, Marchuk JB (1975) Capillary muscle blood flow in human sepsis. Surgery 78:87-94

13. McConn R (1975) The oxyhemoglobin dissociation curve in acute disease. Surg Clin North Am 55:627-656

14. Houtchens BA, Westenkow DR (1984) Oxygen consumption in septic shock: collective review. Circ Shock 13:361-384

15. Weisel RD, Vito L, Dennis RC, Valeri CR, Hechtman HB (1977) Myocardial depression during sepsis. Am J Surg 133:512-521

16. Groeneveld ABJ, Kester ADM, Nauta JJP, Thijs LG (1987) Relation of arterial blood lactate to oxygen delivery and hemodynamic variables in human shock states. Circ Shock 22:35-53

17. Cain SM (1984) Supply dependency of oxygen uptake in ARDS: myth or reality? Am J Med Sci 288:119-124

18. Schumacher PT, Cain SM (1987) The concept of critical oxygen delivery. Intensive Care Med 13:223-229

19. Kreutzer F, Cain SM (1985) Regulation of the peripheral vasculature and tissue oxygenation in health and disease. Crit Care Clin 1:463-470

20. Ellsworth ML, Goldfarb RD, Alexander RS, Bell DR, Powers SR Jr (1981) Microembolization induced oxygen utilization impairment in the canine gracilis muscle. Adv Shock Res 5:89-99

21. Shah DM, Newell JC, Saba TM (1981) Defects in peripheral oxygen utilization following trauma and shock. Arch Surg 116:1277-1281

22. Reines H, Halushka P, Cook J, Wisc W, Rambo W (1982) Plasma thromboxane concentrations are raised in patients dying with septic shock. Lancet II:174-175

23. Astiz ME, Rackow EC, Falk JL, Kaufman BS, Weil MH (1987) Oxygen delivery and consumption in patients with hyperdynamic septic shock. Crit Care Med 15:26-28

24. Kaufman BS, Rackow EC, Falk JL (1984) The relationship between oxygen delivery and consumption during fluid resuscitation of hypovolemia and septic shock. Chest 85:336-340

25. Van Lambalgen AA, Van den Bos GC, Thijs LG (1987) Changes in regional plasma extravasation in rats following endotoxin infusion. Microvasc Res 34:116-132

26. Groeneveld ABJ, Heidendal GAK, Den Hollander W, Nauta JJP, Thijs LG. Noninvasive assessment of regional plasma extravasation in porcine septic shock. J Crit Care (in press)

27. Shoemaker WC, Appel P, Kram H, et al (1982) Clinical trial of an algorithm for outcome prediction in acute circulatory failure. Crit Care Med 10:390-393

New Aspects of Sepsis:
Relevance to Shock and MOF

The Molecular Basis of Shock:
The Role of Cachectin

B. Beutler

In its final stages, shock, regardless of the cause, evokes a picture familiar to all clinicians. Diffuse end-organ damage, a coagulopathic state, metabolic acidosis, hypotension, and sequestration of fluid are all elements of this picture. Yet, these common features reveal little about the molecular pathogenesis of shock, or about the events that lead to its development.

One type of shock, often seen in the context of gram-negative septicemia, is particularly common among hospitalized patients. So-called "endotoxic" shock is frequently fatal, and is perhaps the type of shock best studied so far as its pathogenic mechanisms are concerned.

For many years, it has been known than that a single class of molecules, present in the outer membrane of gram-negative bacteria, can induce a syndrome of physiologic decompensation that is strikingly similar to the shock produced by an actual infection. These molecules, the lipopolysaccharides (LPS; endotoxin), were once believed to possess toxic properties directly responsible for vascular collapse, aberrant coagulation, and widespread inflammatory lesions. However, the elegant studies of Michalek and her colleagues [1] revealed that LPS possess no profound toxicity of their own; rather, they evoke the production of highly toxic endogenously mediators, principally by cells of the host hematopoietic system. Michalek et al. observed that mice of the endotoxin-resistant strain C3H/HeJ become highly sensitive to endotoxin when irradiated and then injected with hematopoietic stem cells derived from an endotoxin-sensitive donor. Conversely, endotoxin-sensitive mice become endotoxin-resistant when irradiated and reconstituted with endotoxin-resistant marrow. Thus, it would seen that, whatever its effects on fixation of complement, coagulation, and tissue in culture, the lethal effect of endotoxin depends upon its ability to activate cells derived from hematopoietic precursors.

The nature of the mediators produced by these hematopoietic cells, and indeed, the identity of the cells involved, have only recently been determined. In a remarkably short period of time, the tools of molecular biology have been harnessed to reveal the primary structure of a protein that now seems central to the pathogenesis of shock, as well as wasting in chronic disease states.

This molecule is a macrophage-derived hormone as "cachectin", or "tumor necrosis factor (TNF)". Its dual name reflects the fact that it was discovered by two entirely separate lines of investigation. "Cachectin" was purified as a mediator of wasting and lipid catabolism, as observed in chronic neoplastic and parasitic disease processes. Rouzer and Cerami [2] noted that trypanosome-induced wasting in rabbits was often accompanied by a paradoxical hypertriglyceridemia, apparently caused by an endogenous mediator. Kawakami and Cerami [3] then showed that mice also became hypertriglyceridemic following LPS administration, and noted that endotoxin-induced macrophages produced a hormone capable of suppressing lipoprotein lipase (LPL) activity in fat and in adipocyte cultures. LPL is essential for the clearance of plasma triglyceride; thus, this hormone appeared to mediate at least one of the metabolic derangements (hypertriglyceridemia) observed both in wasting and endotoxemic states.

Beutler et al. purified cachectin to homogeneity [4], and observed that the murine hormone had a sequence strongly homologous to that reported for human TNF [5]. Subsequent immunologic studies, molecular cloning work, and reciprocal measurements of biological activity revealed that cachectin and TNF were identical proteins [5, 6].

"TNF", as such was purified as a macrophage product responsible for inducing the hemorrhagic necrosis of transplantable tumors in mice [7], and for eliciting lysis of certain transformed cell lines *in vitro* [8]. Since induction of tumor necrosis, like the induction of a hypertriglyceridemia state, are both aspects of the host response to LPS, Beutler and Cerami, reasoned that this hormone might, in fact, mediate many of the effects of LPS, including the lethal effect.

It was shown that mice passively immunized against cachectin became markedly resistant to the lethal effect of LPS [9]; moreover, it became apparent that cachectin is a highly toxic molecule, capable of provoking a shock state in mice, rats [10], and dogs [11], following its parenteral administration.

Perhaps the toxicity of cachectin has best been studied in rats. Intravenous infusion of cachectin causes a mild degree of hypotension, moderate tachypnea, and an abrupt respiratory arrest in this species. Profound metabolic acidosis, hemoconcentration, and hyperkalemia are also observed, together with biphasic changes in plasma glucose concentration. At necropsy, rats treated with lethal doses of cachectin show widespread end organ damage. Severe pathologic changes are observed in the lung, where leukostasis and thickening of the alveolar septa are generally found. The gastrointestinal tract is also affected, and shows varying degrees of ischemia and luminal hemorrhage. The kidney, too, is often injured by cachectin, which cause acute tubular necrosis and acute glomerulonephritis.

In dogs, a variety of similar changes are observed, together with a generalized stress response, characterized by marked elevation in plasma cathecholamines, insulin, and cortisol levels. One feature of shock that has never been fully explained involves changes in muscle cell transmembrane potential. Cachectin elicits a sharp fall in skeletal muscle cell transmembrane potential, whether administered systemically (with recording done *in vivo*) or applied to isolated muscle preparations [12]. This change may relate to the accumulation of fluid within the intracellular compartment.

Cachectin may evoke many of its effects directly; however, it is likely that at least some responses (and perhaps most of them) arise through its ability to induce the release of terminal mediators of inflammation. Among these, products of arachidonate metabolism (prostaglandins and leukotrienes) as well as platelet activating factor (PAF) are important candidates. Cachectin is known to induce the release of PGE_2 from human dermal fibroblasts and human synovial cells

[13], and acts to induce the accumulation of cysteinyl leukotrienes in bowel (Keppler, D., personal communication). It has also been reported that cyclooxygenase inhibitors (ibuprofen and indomethacin) markedly attenuate the toxic effect of cachectin [14]. The relative contributions of terminal inflammatory mediators (and the cells that produce them) to the pathogenesis of cachectin-induced shock, as compared with the direct effect of the hormone on target tissues, remains to be fully evaluated.

When chronically administered, cachectin leads to a severe wasting diathesis which is at least partly attributable to a decrease in food consumption. Oliff et al. have provided the clearest evidence of cachectin's "cachexia-inducing" potential [15]. These investigators transformed Chinese hamster ovary (CHO) cells with a vector that caused the continuous secretion of recombinant human cachectin. Nude mice inoculated with these genetically altered cells developed a small, non-metastatic tumor confined to the hind limb, as did control animals inoculated with cells that failed to produce cachectin. Animals exposed to cachectin suffered a dramatic weight lost over a period of several weeks, while animals bearing control tumors continued to gain weight at a normal rate.

Just as animals are sensitized to the lethal effect of LPS by such agents as galactosamine and lead, so they are also sensitized to the lethal effect of cachectin. Rats, for example can be killed by microgram quantities of cachectin if pretreated with D-galactosamine [16]. This finding would seem to offer a major clue as to the mechanism of cachectin's lethal effect; however, the precise biochemical action of such sensitizing agents remains to be elucidated.

Cachectin is but one of two closely related polypeptide hormones. The second member of the "family" is a protein produced not by macrophages, but by lymphocytes, termed "lymphotoxin". Cachectin, in its mature form, contains 156 amino acids in man; lymphotoxin contains 171 residues and exhibits approximately 30% sequence identity at the protein level.

While cachectin is produced in very large quantities by macrophages following exposure to LPS (and in somewhat smaller quantities in response to other invasive agents), lymphotoxin is produced in response to specific antigenic stimuli (to which the responder T-lymphocytes have previous been exposed) and in response to non-specific mitogenic stimuli. Both proteins appear to bind to the same plasma membrane receptor [17], and to evoke a highly concordant range of cellular responses. The need for production of both cachectin and lymphotoxin, by different immunocytes under different pathologic conditions, remains puzzling.

Cachectin and lymphotoxin are both produced as prohormones. Interestingly, when interspecific comparisons of propeptide sequence are made, a high degree of homology is observed (86% homology between the propeptide of human and murine cachectin, for example) suggesting that the propeptide may fulfill an important biological function. The cachectin propeptide (76 amino acids in length in man) is even more conserved among species than is the mature hormone. Yet, it appears to be extensively cleaved in processing to produce secreted cachectin [18].

Cachectin biosynthesis is controlled at several levels. In response to LPS, the cachectin gene is transcribed at an accelerated rate (at least 3-fold more rapidly than in resting cells) [19]. However, this comparatively modest increase in transcriptional activity is associated with a 50- to 100-fold increase in the intracellular content of cachectin mRNA, and with a greater than 1000-fold increase in the quantity of cachectin that is synthesized and released by the cell.

The 3'-untranslated region of mRNA molecules encoding cachectin, as well as a variety of other cytokines and protooncogenes contains a conserved AT-rich sequence consisting repeating and overlapping octameric units (UUAUUUAU) [6]. This sequence has been shown to confer instability to mRNA molecules that contain it, and presumably, it acts as a target for the action of a selective ribonuclease. The same sequence may also be involved in the control of translation.

Cachectin mRNA may apparently exist within cells in an untranslated form, since relatively high levels of the message may be detected within macrophages obtained from endotoxin-resistant mice, despite the fact that these cells are producing little or no cachectin. Similarly, dexamethasone treated macrophages derived from endotoxin-responsive mice may express cachectin mRNA in considerable abundance; yet, they fail to produce cachectin protein. Inhibition of cachectin biosynthesis by dexamethasone may, in part, account for the strong protective effect of this glucocorticoid when administered to animals before endotoxin challenge.

Considerable speculation has been devoted to the beneficial role fulfilled by cachectin: the role that has justified its conservation throughout mammalian evolution. It seems almost certain that, while the hormone has markedly detrimental effects when produced in excessive quantities, it must have protective effects when produced on a smaller scale in the course of a limited infectious process. Some evidence has now emerged to suggest that passive immunization against cachectin, while protective against endotoxin challenge, may have a negative impact on survival in the course of an actual infection (for example, murine malaria infection) [20]. In years to come our increased understanding of the role played by cachectin may enable us to grasp the essential benefits conferred by the inflammatory response as a whole, and our ability to manipulate the production of cachectin may allow us to modulate inflammatory response, in both its acute and chronic forms.

References

1. Michalek SM, Moore RN, McGhee JR, et al (1980) The primary role of lymphoreticular cells in the mediation of host responses to bacterial endotoxin. J Inf Dis 141:55–63
2. Rouzer CA, Cerami A (1980) Hypertriglyceridemia associated with Trypanosoma brucei infection in rabbits: role of defective triglyceride removal. Molec Biochem Parasitol 2:31–38
3. Kawakami M, Cerami A (1981) Studies of endotoxin-induced decrease in lipoprotein lipase activity. J Exp Med 154:631–639
4. Beutler B, Mahoney J, Le Trang N, et al (1985) Purification of cachectin, a lipoprotein lipase-suppressing hormone secreted by endotoxin-induced RAW 264.7 cells. J Exp Med 161:984–995
5. Beutler B, Greenwald D, Hulmes JD, et al (1985) Identity of tumour necrosis factor and the macrophage-secreted factor cachectin. Nature 316:552–554

6. Caput D, Beutler B, Hartog K, et al (1986) Identification of a common nucleotide sequence in the 3'-untranslated region of mRNA molecules specifying inflammatory mediators. Proc Natl Acad Sci 83:1670–1674

7. Carswell EA, Old LJ, Kassel RL, et al (1975) An endotoxin-induced serum factor that causes necrosis of tumors. Proc Natl Acad Sci 72:3666–3670

8. Aggarwal BB, Kohr WJ, Hass PE, et al (1985) Human tumor necrosis factor. Production, purification, and characterization. J Biol Chem 260:2345–2354

9. Beutler B, Milsark IW, Cerami A (1985) Passive immunization against cachectin/tumor necorsis factor (TNF) protects mice from the lethal effect of endotoxin. Science 229:869–871

10. Tracey KJ, Beutler B, Lowry SF, et al (1986) Shock and tissue injury induced by recombinant human cachectin. Science 234:470–474

11. Tracey KJ, Lowry SF, Fahey III TJ, et al (1987) Cachectin/tumor necrosis factor induces lethal shock and stress hormone responses in the dog. Surg Gynecol Obstet 164:415–422

12. Tracey K, Lowry S, Beutler B, et al (1986) Cachectin/tumor necrosis factor mediates changes in skeletal muscle transmembrane potential. J Exp Med 164:1368–1373

13. Dayer JM, Beutler B, Cerami A (1985) Cachectin/tumor necrosis factor (TNF) stimulates collagenase and PGE$_2$ production by human synovial cells and dermal fibroblasts. J Exp Med 162:2163–2168

14. Kettelhut IC, Fiers W, Goldberg AL (1987) The toxic effects of tumor necrosis factor in vivo and their prevention by cyclooxygenase inhibitors. Proc Natl Acad Sci 84:4273–4277

15. Oliff A, Defeo-Jones D, Boyer M, et al (1987) Tumors secreting human TNF/cachectin induce cachexia in mice. Cell 50:555–563

16. Lehmann V, Freudenberg MA, Galanos C (1987) Lethal toxicity of lipopolysaccharide and tumor necrosis factor in normal and d-galactosamine-treated mice. J Exp Med 165:657–663

17. Aggarwal BB, Eessalu TE, Hass PE (1985) Characterization of receptors for human tumor necrosis factor and their regulation by gamma-interferon. Nature 318:665–667

18. Beutler B, Cerami A (1986) Cachectin and tumor necrosis factor as two sides of the same biological coin. Nature 320:584–588

19. Beutler B, Krochin N, Milsark IW, et al (1986) Control of cachectin (tumor necrosis factor) synthesis: mechanisms of endotoxin resistance. Science 232:977–980

20. Grau GE, Fajardo LF, Piguet PF, et al (1987) Tumor necrosis factor (cachectin) as an essential mediator in murine cerebral malaria. Science 237:1210–1212

Immunologic Abnormalities Following Hemorrhage and Trauma

E. Abraham

Despite rigorous prophylactic therapy and the availability of a variety of increasingly powerful antimicrobial agents, infections are the major cause of mortality and morbidity after traumatic injury and burns [1, 2]. It has been estimated in different studies [3, 4] that from 60 to 88% of deaths occurring more than 7 days after blunt trauma or thermal injury were caused by sepsis. These infectious episodes following injury generally are characterized by multiple organ system failure (MOSF). Pulmonary processes either directly related to infection, such as *Pseudomonas aeruginosa* pneumonia, or secondarily caused by infection, such as the adult respiratory distress syndrome (ARDS), are invariably a major aspect of the post-injury MOSF.

The initial host defense mechanism preventing entrance of bacteria through skin and mucosal barriers is the localized inflammatory response. Bacteria entering the organism through cutaneous or endothelial sites induce the formation of a polymorphonuclear and then mononuclear infiltrate that usually is capable of preventing systemic bacterial invasion. Utilizing a standard laparotomy procedure in rats, Kinnaert et al. [5] demonstrated that surgery inhibits the inflammatory response. Inflammation also is reduced during hypovolemic shock. The inflammatory response remains suppressed for more than 24 hours after hemorrhage, even if the blood volume is restored by blood transfusion [6]. The post hemorrhage depression in inflammatory response is related directly to the severity of the hemorrhagic insult and the time elapsed before retransfusion.

Deterioration of fixed reticuloendothelial phagocytic activity is present within hours after surgery, burns, accidental trauma, hemorrhage, ischemic intestinal injury, cardiopulmonary bypass, transfusion reaction, and myocardial injury in proportion to the severity of the physiologic insult [7]. Pretreatment of animals with substances that stimulate reticuloendothelial cell phagocytic function is associated with increased tolerance to the above forms of systemic stress. Similarly, materials that block or depress the phagocytic capacity of the reticuloendothelial system increase mortality.

Fibronectin is a major opsonic protein, capable of enhancing the phagocytic capacity of reticuloendothelial cells, that has been purified and well-characterized. Purified fibronectin stimulates reticuloendothelial phagocytosis of test particles and antibody to fibronectin inhibits phagocytic function [8]. Decreases in the serum levels of fibronectin parallel depression of reticuloendothelial phagocytosis after burns, trauma, surgery, and other major physiological insults. Replacement of fibronectin by intravenous opsonin therapy with either cryoprecipitate or purified fibronectin can prevent the depression of phagocytic function observed postoperatively in experimental animals [9]. Several clinical series have examined the effects of therapy with cryoprecipitate or purified fibronectin in critically ill surgical patients with low serum fibronectin levels [10]. No improvement in the incidence of infections or in outcome was found in these studies [11].

Skin test reactivity to recall antigens such as mumps, Candida, streptokinase-streptodornase (SKSD), purified protein derivative (PPD) and dinitrochloroben-zene (DNCB) frequently is depressed after significant surgical or accidental trauma. For example, approximately 40% of patients undergoing major cardio-vascular procedures, such as abdominal aortic aneurysm resection, coronary artery bypass grafting, aortic or mitral valve replacement, became anergic to a battery of four recall antigens by postoperative day 3 [12].

The presence of complete anergy to a battery of at least four recall antigens on skin testing after operative or accidental trauma defines a patient population that may have as high as a 60% probability of developing a clinically important septic episode [13]. Sequential skin testing has been advocated in critically ill patients; a change from a reactive to an anergic state may be predictive of a septic episode and should instigate a search for a septic focus.

Despite the apparent clinical utility of skin testing in identifying patients at risk for sepsis, several factors confuse interpretation of skin testing results. The major problem is simply quantitative; most patients in a critical care unit are anergic. In Bradley's study [14] for example, 73% of patients were nonreactive to skin testing on admission to the critical care unit. Possible factors contributing to this elevated incidence of anergy, aside from surgery and trauma, include increased age, immunosuppressive drugs (such as corticosteroids, chemotherapeutic agents, cimetidine, coumadin, heparin, and anti-inflammatory agents), the presence of pre-existing disease (such as uremia, cirrhosis, and malignancy), and undernutrition.

Directed movement of neutrophils (chemotaxis) toward a site of bacterial infiltration is a prerequisite for the effective elimination of the organisms. There have been conflicting reports on the existence of abnormalities in neutrophil chemotaxis after surgical and accidental trauma, with several studies showing decreased chemotaxis after severe trauma, probably related to production of complement fragments with relative suppressive actions on granulocyte locomotion [15]. Hemorrhage alone seems to have little effect on neutrophil chemotaxis [16].

Intracellular bacterial killing by neutrophils is markedly decreased after major thermal injury [17]. In contrast, hemorrhage and trauma do not seem to affect either phagocytosis or intracellular bacterial killing [18].

There is a striking association between abnormalities in cell-mediated immunity and life-threatening infection after major trauma. The parameter that has been measured most frequently is the proliferation of lymphocytes in response to a mitogen such as phytohemagglutinin (PHA). Both Keane et al. [19] and O'Mahony et al. [20] found that multitrauma patients who subsequently became infected had lower lymphocyte proliferative responses to PHA than that in patients who did not become infected.

There is no common agreement as to the mechanisms responsible for the diminished cell-mediated immunity after hemorrhage and trauma. In different systems T-suppressor-cells, B-lymphocytes, monocytes/macrophages and serum polypeptide factors have been blamed for the observed suppression in immune response. Despite the varying evidence implicating different cell types as being the initiators of the suppressed state of cell-mediated immunity, the major expression of this immunosuppressed state is abnormal T-cell-function. As mentioned previously, both accidental and surgical trauma produce significant depression in the polyclonal cellular proliferative response induced by mitogens that primarily act on T-cells. In addition, proliferative response of T-cells to cell surface (MHC type I) antigens in cultures duplicating a transplantation rejection (mixed lymphocyte reactions [MLR]) is diminished when the responding and proliferating T-cells are obtained from a burned or injured animal or human. Finally, production of several lymphokines, the polypeptide products of activated T-lymphocytes that participate in a variety of cellular responses regulating the immune system, are diminished after injury and hemorrhage.

Several studies have suggested that functionally active suppressor cells are generated after tissue injury, such as that associated with trauma or burns. Surgical trauma produced suppressor cells which inhibited the proliferative response of normal lymphocytes when added to cultures of these cells (MLR) [21]. These trauma induced suppressive cells appeared to be macrophages since they were insensitive to treatment with antibodies that react to T- and B-cells, and their activity could be blocked by antibodies directed towards antigens (Ia) usually associated with macrophages. In experimental models for surgical trauma, these functionally active suppressor macrophages were detected as soon as 2 hours after injury.

Thermal injury, in contrast to surgical trauma, has been shown to produce two populations of suppressor T-cells, capable of inhibiting proliferation of normal T-lymphocytes [22]. One population, with cell surface markers consistent with T-helper/inducer-lymphocytes, appeared 5 to 7 days after experimental burns. This population was then supplanted by activation of another set of T-lymphocytes with markers consistent with suppressor/cytotoxic cells. This second group of post-burn suppressor cells was detectible 7 to 15 days after the burn injury. No suppressive activity could be demonstrated in macrophages obtained after burns.

Burn induced suppressor cells appear to be capable of affecting host defenses against bacterial infection [23]. Suppressor/cytotoxic T-cells (Lyt-2$^+$) obtained form the spleens of mice 7 days post burn increased the mortality rate from 15% to 100% when injected into normal mice with a well-characterized experimental model of intra-abdominal infection. No increase in mortality was found when similar T-cells from normal, unburned mice were injected into infected animals.

We and others have shown that hemorrhage alone, without any tissue injury, brings about abnormalities in cell-mediated immune response [24]. In particular, T-cell-proliferation in both mitogen-stimulated and mixed lymphocyte cultures is markedly depressed starting within 2 hours of hemorrhage and continuing for as long as 9 days post-hemorrhage. This decrease in T-cell-proliferation after hemorrhage is due, at least in part, to the appearance of activated T-suppressor-cells as early as 2 hours after loss of 30% of blood volume [25]. As few as $1 \cdot 10^4$ of the hemorrhage induced T-suppressor-cells can reduce proliferation of $5 \cdot 10^5$

normal peripheral blood mononuclear cells (lymphocytes and monocytes) by more than 50%. Like thermal injury, hemorrhage did not bring about the appearance of suppressor macrophages.

Although a subset of activated T-suppressor-cells appears after hemorrhage, we were unable to find any changes in cell numbers in lymphoid organs, such as the spleen, thymus, bone marrow or lymph nodes. Similarly, the numbers and percentages of T-helper- and suppressor-cells in these organs was the same after hemorrhage as in normal mice. These results indicated that hemorrhage induced important functional changes in immune function, produced in part by activated suppressor cells, and which were not simply due to relative changes in the numbers of T-cell subpopulations.

Lymphokines are important in modulating the immune response to antigens. Interleukin 1 (IL 1) is produced by macrophages, as well as various other cell types including skin keratocytes, mesangial cells, vascular endothelial cells and microglia. In addition to activating resting T-cells, so that these lymphocytes can induce an expanded immune response to the recognized antigen, IL-1 is a primary mediator of the acute-phase response. IL-1 induces fever, the synthesis of hepatic acute-phase proteins, release of neutrophils, and prostaglandin synthesis.

Experiments have shown a five-fold increase in IL-1 release within 2 hours of the loss of 30% of blood volume [26]. By 24 hours post-hemorrhage, IL-1 production has returned to normal levels. However, this marked increase in IL-1 release immediately following the hemorrhagic insult may be the initiating event that produces the acute phase reaction that follows injury.

Interleukin 2 (IL 2) is produced primarily by activated T-cells and has the ability to further induce the proliferation of these activated cells. High-affinity receptors for IL-2 are absent on resting T-cells but appear within hours of activation. The binding of IL-2 to these receptors gives rise to the clonal expansion of T-cells activated by a specific antigen. Withdrawal or elimination of the antigen leads to the involution of the IL-2 receptor and the cessation of T-cell proliferation even in the presence of IL-2, thus limiting the extent of clonal expansion.

Accidental injury and burns in previously healthy individuals cause marked decreases in IL-2 production [27, 28]. Within less than an hour of severe injury (injury severity score [ISS] > 30), IL-2 production is reduced to approximately 10% of normal levels. In experimental settings, after a single episode of hemorrhage, with no further physiologic insults, IL-2 release returns to normal after 48 hours [29]. However, injured patients usually are exposed to surgical procedures and medications which often have significant effects on immune function. In these cases, IL-2 production and host defense mechanisms may be depressed for prolonged periods. For example, in a group of patients after burn injury, who required repeated operations for debridement and skin grafting, IL-2 generation was demonstrated to be diminished for more than 50 days [27].

Because of the central role that IL-2 occupies directly in T-lymphocyte activation, and secondarily in modulation of both T- and B-cell response to antigen presentation, such as occurs with bacterial invasion, this substantial and prolonged suppression of IL-2 production induced by injury may contribute significantly to the high incidence of infections after trauma. Unfortunately, the abnormalities in lymphocyte proliferative response after injury are not directly produced by the decrease in IL-2 release. Addition of highly purified, recombinant IL-2 to lymphocyte cultures obtained from injured patients resulted in only minimal improvement in lymphocyte function which did not approach normal levels [30]. These results suggested that IL-2 independent steps in lymphocyte activation were affected by hemorrhage and trauma. Such steps could include inhibition of T-lymphocyte activation by suppressor cells, such as have been demonstrated to exist after hemorrhage, or inhibition of expression of IL-2 receptors on T-cells.

T-cells produce other lymphokines that have important effects on multiple cellular responses. We recently have found hemorrhage-induced depression in interleukin-3, which supports the growth of pluripotent (multilineage) bone marrow stem cells, and in release of interleukin-5, which maintains B-cell proliferation, maturation and differentiation to antibody producing cells after activation through antigen presentation.

The rapidity with which lymphocyte proliferation and production of lymphokines is suppressed after hemorrhage and trauma is unusual in terms of cellular activation mechanisms, and is more suggestive of exogenous factors inhibiting cellular function. We and other have found serum factors after hemorrhage and injury that are capable of depressing lymphocyte proliferation and function. In particular, we have described a polypeptide with molecular weight of approximately 15000 daltons which appears in the serum of rats within 2 hours of removal of 30% of the blood volume [31]. Addition of this hemorrhage-induced factor to normal lymphocytes is capable of depressing proliferation and IL-2 release to the same low levels found with lymphocytes obtained from hemorrhaged animals. In addition, washing lymphocytes obtained from normal animals with serum from hemorrhaged animals activates the same population of T-suppressor-cells that are found in hemorrhaged animals. It therefore seems that all of the suppressive effects of hemorrhage on lymphocyte function could be mediated through the effects of this hemorrhage-induced serum suppressive factor.

Serum factors, less well characterized than the hemorrhage-induced polypeptide but also capable of inhibiting lymphocyte proliferation, have been demonstrated to be present after accidental and operative trauma, as well as after severe burns. At least in thermal injury, immunosuppressive activity of postburn serum does not appear to correlate with serum cortisol levels, serum endotoxin levels, serum prostaglandin E_e (PGE_2) levels, blood transfusion, protein-calorie malnutrition, or anesthesia [32].

In summary, hemorrhage, accidental injury, operative trauma and burns have significant and widespread effects on the immune system that are associated with an unexpectedly high incidence of infection in these patient groups. Further characterization of these abnormalities in immune function and development of methods to reverse their effects may result in significant improvement in outcome for critically injured patients.

References

1. Baker CC, Oppenheimer L, Stephens B, Lewis FR, Trunkey DD (1980) Epidemiology of trauma deaths. Am J Surg 140:144–150
2. Polk HC (1979) Consensus summary on infections. J Trauma 19 (suppl):894–896
3. Sturm JA, Lewis FR, Trentz, et al (1979) Cardiopulmonary parameters and prognosis after severe multiple injury. J Trauma 19:305–318
4. Goris RJA, Draaisma J (1982) Causes of death after blunt trauma. J Trauma 22:141–146
5. Kinnaert P, Geertryden NV, Mahieu A, et al (1984) Effects of surgical trauma on various aspects of the immune response in rats. Eur J Surg Res 16:99–105
6. Abraham E, Chang Y-H (1984) The effects of hemorrhage on inflammatory response. Arch Surg 119:1154–1157
7. Altura BM (1983) Endothelium, reticuloendothelial cells, and microvascular integrity: roles in host defense. In: Altura BM, Lefer AM, Schumer W (eds) Handbook of shock and trauma. Raven Press, New York, pp 51–95
8. Saba TM, Lanser ME, Dillon BC (1983) Opsonic fibronectin and phagocytic defense after trauma. In: Altura BM, Lefer AM, Schumer W (eds) Handbook of shock and trauma. Raven Press, New York, pp 167–181
9. Saba TM (1978) Prevention of liver reticuloendothelial systemic host defense failure after surgery by opsonic glycoprotein therapy. Ann Surg 188:142–150
10. Scovill WA, Saba TM, Blumenstock FA, et al (1978) Opsonic 2 surface binding glycoprotein therapy during sepsis. Ann Surg 188:142–151
11. Hesselvek S, Brodin B, Carlsson C, Cedergren B, Gorfeldt L, Lieden J (1987) Cryoprecipitate infusion fails to improve organ function in septic shock. Crit Care Med 15:473–483
12. McLoughlin GA, Wu AV, Saporoschetz I, et al (1979) Correlation between anergy and a circulating immunosuppressive factor following major surgical trauma. Ann Surg 190:297–303
13. Meakins JL, McLean APH, Kelly R, et al (1982) Delayed hypersensitivity and neutrophil chemotaxis: effect of trauma. J Trauma 20:833–839
14. Bradley JA, Hamilton DNH, Brown MW, et al (1984) Cellular defense in critically ill patients. Crit Care Med 12:565–570
15. Maderazo EG, Albano SD, Woronick CL, Drezner ADF, Quercia R (1983) Polymorphonuclear leukocyte migration abnormalities and their significance in seriously traumatized patients. Ann Surg 198:736–742
16. Esrig BC, Frazee L, Stephenson SF, Fulton RL, Jones CE (1976) Predisposition to infection and neutrophil function following hemorrhagic shock. Rev Surg 33:431–433
17. Alexander JW, Wixson D (1970) Neutrophil dysfunction and sepsis in burn injury. Surg Gynecol Obstet 130:431–439
18. Palder SB, O'Mahony JB, Rodrick M, Demling RH, Mannick JA (1984) Alteration of polymorphonuclear leukocyte function in the trauma patient. J Trauma 23:655
19. Keane RM, Birmingham W, Shatney CM, Winchurch RA, Munster AM (1983) Prediction of sepsis in the multitraumatic patient by assays of lymphocyte responsiveness. Surg Gynecol Obstet 156:163–167
20. O'Mahony JB, Palder SB, Wood JJ, et al (1984) Depression of cellular immunity after multiple trauma in the absence of sepsis. J Trauma 24:869–875
21. Wang BS, Heacock EH, Wu AVO, Mannick JA (1980) Generation of suppressor cells in mice after surgical trauma. J Clin Invest 66:200–209
22. Kupper TS, Green DR (1984) Immunoregulation after thermal injury: sequential appearance of I-J$^+$, LY-1 T suppressor inducer cells and LY-2 T suppressor effector cells following thermal trauma in mice. J Immunol 136:3047–3053
23. Kupper TS, Baker CC, Ferguson TA, Green DR (1985) A burn induced LY-2 suppressor T cell lowers resistance to bacterial infection. J Surg Res 38:606–613
24. Abraham E. Chang Y-H (1985) The effects of hemorrhage on lymphocyte proliferation. Circ Shock 15:141–149
25. Abraham E, Chang Y-H (1987) Effects of hemorrhage and hemorrhagic serum on macrophage and T cell function. Clin Res 35:383A

26. Richmond NJ, Abraham E, Chang Y-H (1987) The effects of hemorrhage on macrophage function and interleukin 1 production. Crit Care Med 15:429
27. Abraham E, Regan RF (1985) The effects of hemorrhage and trauma on interleukin 2 production. Arch Surg 120:1341–1344
28. Wood JJ, Rodrick ML, O'Mahoney JB, et al (1984) Inadequate interleukin 2 production: a fundamental immunological deficiency in patients with major burns. Ann Surg 200:311–320
29. Abraham E, Lee RJ, Chang Y-H (1986) The role of interleukin 2 in hemorrhage induced abnormalities of lymphocyte proliferation. Circ Shock 18:205–214
30. Abraham E, Regan RF, Chang Y-H (1986) The lack of effect of exogenous recombinant interleukin-2 on trauma-induced abnormalities in lymphocyte proliferation. Crit Care Med 14:847–851
31. Abraham E, Chang Y-H (1986) Cellular and humoral bases of hemorrhage-induced depression of lymphocyte function. Crit Care Med 14:81–86
32. Wolfe JHN, Wu AVO, O'Conner Ne, Saporoschetz I, Mannick JA (1982) Anergy, immunosuppressive serum, and impaired lymphocyte blastogenesis in burn patients. Arch Surg 117:1266–1271

Update in Host Defence Mechanisms

I. McA. Ledingham and J. A. Bradley

Introduction

Infection is a major problem in general and some specialized Intensive Therapy Units (ITU). A number of patients are admitted to ITU suffering from life-threatening infection while others become infected during the course of treatment of unrelated conditions. Irrespective of the reason for admission, the majority of patients whose stay in the ITU exceeds a few days, become infected to a greater or lesser extent. In the case of multiple trauma, more than 80% of late mortality in one series [1] was associated with, if not caused by, infection.

It is now increasingly accepted that most infection acquired in the ITU is ednogenous in origin and follows colonisation of the alimentary tract by organisms not usually present in significant numbers in healthy individuals e.g. aerobic gram-negative bacteria such as E.coli, Klebsiella, Proteus and Ps. aeruginosa. Exogenous infection without previous alimentary tract colonization may occur but is unusual.

The mechanisms leading to infection amongst these patients are complex and multifactorial; bacteriological, immunological and environmental factors are all involved. The resulting morbidity and mortality have proved resistant to a wide range of therapeutic procedures; in particular, conventional environmental control and a steady stream of new and powerful antibiotics appear to have made little difference to outcome. These observations have led to an increasing interest in the role of host defence mechanisms in the critically ill and in the possibility of correcting at least some of the immunological disturbances.

Host Defence Mechanisms

Resistance to colonization of the alimentary tract by aerobic bacteria depends on a variety of complex factors. These include mucosal integrity, normal gastrointestinal motility, desquamation of mucosal cells, mucus and immunoglobulin A secretion as well as the indigenous intestinal anaerobic flora which inhibit proliferation of aerobic organisms. Following major surgery or trauma these factors are often altered with a resultant decrease in resistance to colonization, to which is added the invariable breaching of local defences by the presence of many invasive devices necessary for treatment. Consequently it falls on the generalized cellular and humoral defences to prevent or contain infection.

Possible mechanisms involved in suppression of cellular immunity in such patients include hormonal effects (e.g. steroids, "stress"), durgs (e.g. antibiotics, chemotherapeutic agents, H_2 receptor blockers, anti-inflammatory agents), anesthesia (including prolonged low levels) and nutritional status.

Assessment of Host Defence

Although tests of inflammatory and immune function have often indicated alterations in many different aspects of host defence it is apparent that these defences are extremely complex. No single defect has been found which would in isolation account for the problem of infection in these patients and indeed it is unclear whether many of the observed alterations are harmful or protective to the host.

A range of the currently available tests is listed below:

Humoral response (B-cell response)
1. Estimation of B-lymphocytes (both absolute numbers and percentage).
2. Estimation of serum immunoglobulin (IgG, IgM and IgA) levels.
3. Lymphocyte transformation.
4. Specific antibody response.

Cell mediated immune response (T-cell response)
1. Estimation of T-lymphocytes and subpopulations (absolute numbers and percentage) using monoclonal antibodies.
2. Lymphocyte transformation.
3. Delayed hypersensitivity skin testing.
4. Measurement of lymphokine production.

Phagocyte function
1. Estimation of neutrophils and monocytes (absolute numbers and percentage).
2. Nitroblue tetrazolium (NBT) test.
3. Ingestion and killing of S.aureus or C.albicans.
4. In vivo leukocyte migration (Rebuck skin window).

Complement
1. Measurement of total hemolytic complement activity (CH_{50})
2. Measurement of specific complement components.

Since most of these investigations only assess a particular aspect of the immune system, it is common practice to include a selection of such tests to obtain an overall assessment of immune profile. A limitation of most of the measurements of immune function is that they are made from only one anatomical compartment viz. peripheral blood.

Treatment strategies: A wide variety of strategies are presently under investigation including:
1. Prevention of penetration
2. Promotion of killing (via complement, antibodies and phagocytes)
   - opsonisation (specific and non-specific antibodies)
   - transfusion of phagocytic cells

    – stimulation of phagocytic funtion
    – stimulation of antidoby-dependent cell mediated or T cell cytotoxicity
    – stimulation of antibody production
3. Inactivation of toxic bacterial products
    – exotoxins
    – endotoxin (cell wall)
    – enzymes
    – adherence/recognition products
4. Removal of toxic products (apheresis)
5. Inactivation of host-cell binding sites
6. Blockage of host-cell metabolic responses
7. Killing by
    – antibiotics
    – targeted or "assisted" antibiotics

The earlier treatment is started the greater the prospect of success. The most practically significant observation to date has been that prevention of colonization via the alimentary tract reduces the incidence of secondary infection in critically ill patients [2, 3].

Nutrition and immunity are closely related and the role of nutritional support in improving host defence in patients who are anergic is considered important. Intravenous infusion of fibronectin-rich cryoprecipitate can restore deficient fibronectin levels and reverse the opsonic defect in critically ill patients; some evidence of improved physiological function is emerging from current studies of septic shock but increased survival has yet to be demonstrated [4]. Other suggestions for improving opsonic activity have included the administration of fresh frozen plasma in patients with depressed C3 levels. Of more limited clinical success is the present range of immunostimulatory agents but new developments are awaited.

The possible role of endotoxin in producing the cardiovascular complications of severe infection has prompted attempts to administer serum containing antibodies to the toxic part of lipopolysaccharide. A parallel approach lies in the vaccination of critically ill patients against specific organisms when these are known to be a common threat. Plasmapheresis and plasma exchange combine a number of potential advantages in the management of septicemia [5] but further clinical experience is required.

References

1. Goris RJA, Draaisma J (1982) Causes of death after trauma. J Trauma 22:141
2. Stoutenbeek CJ, van Saene HKF, Miranda DR, van der Waaÿ, Zandstra DF (1984) The effect of selective decontamination of the digestive tract on colonisation and infection rate in multiple trauma patients. Intens Care Med 10:185
3. Ledingham I McA, Mc Donald JC, Alcock SR (1988) Adult Respiratory Distress Syndrome and Selective Decontamination of the digestive tract (in press)
4. Ramsay G, Newman P, Ledingham I McA (1986) Cryoprecipitate replacement of fibronectin in septic shock. 3rd European Congress on Intensive Care Medicine, Hamburg
5. Bjorratn B, Bjertnes L, Fadnes HO, et al (1984) Meningococcal septicaemia treated with combined plasmapheresis and leucopheresis or with blood exchange. Br Med J 288:439

Selective Elimination of Oropharyngeal and Gastro-Intestinal Flora: A Step Forward in the Control of Infection in ICU?

H. K. F. van Saene, C. P. Stoutenbeek, and D. F. Zandstra

Introduction

Selective flora elimination is a technique for prevention/treatment of colonization/infection in high risk patients. This is achieved by elimination of aerobic, potentially pathogenic microorganisms from throat and gastro-intestine whilst preserving the indigenous, mostly anaerobic flora [1]. This method is based on *three fundamentals* in clinical bacteriology, as follows.

Potentially Pathogenic Microorganisms

Practically all infections in the compromised host are caused by about fourteen aerobic potentially pathogenic microorganisms (i.e. microorganisms only able to cause infections in hosts with impaired defence mechanisms) [2, 3]. *Streptococcus pneumoniae, Hemophilus influenzae, Branhamella catarrhalis, Escherichia coli, Staphylococcus aureus* and *Candida albicans* are six 'community' acquired microorganisms. Varying percentages of healthy people carry these 'community' acquired microorganisms in throat and/or gastro-intestinal tract. Oropharyngeal and/or intestinal carriage of *Klebsiella, Proteus, Morganella, Enterobacter, Citrobacter, Serratia* and *Acinetobacter* species as well as *Pseudomonadaceae* are uncommon in healthy people. These eight microorganisms only colonize people with impaired defence following underlying disease, medical interventions and advanced age. As this type of host is hospitalised frequently, these eight bacteria are called 'hospital'/'nosocomial'/'ICU' associated flora. The flora which man carries in throat and intestine is mostly anaerobic (99.9%). This indigenous flora lives in symbiotic relationship with the host and has low pathogenic potential. The indigenous flora is rarely involved in infections and has important physiological functions [4] contributing to defence against colonization by the fourteen aerobic microorganisms (0.1% of human flora) [5]. An inverse relation is seen between microbial carriage and intrinsic pathogenicity (and infection frequency).

Defence (Fig. 1)

Man is exposed daily to the above-mentioned fourteen aerobic potentially pathogenic microorganisms often present in food (e.g. vegetable salads) and beverages (e.g. milk shakes). The human host is able to cope with the daily supply of high bacterial concentrations ($> 10^9$ colony forming units per ml or g) by two defence mechanisms, as follows:

Colonization defence: The first line of defence is formed by the defence of oropharyngeal cavity and gastro-intestinal canal, respiratory tract, urinary tract and skin against *colonization* [6]. The aim of that line of defence is the clearing of microorganisms attempting to colonize the mucosae and skin. This first line depends on a complex of similar factors (Tables 1 and 2). The only difference between the factors building up colonization defence of throat and intestine and the factors forming the first line of defence of respiratory tract, urinary tract and skin is the fact that in oropharynx and gut indigenous flora is normally present in large

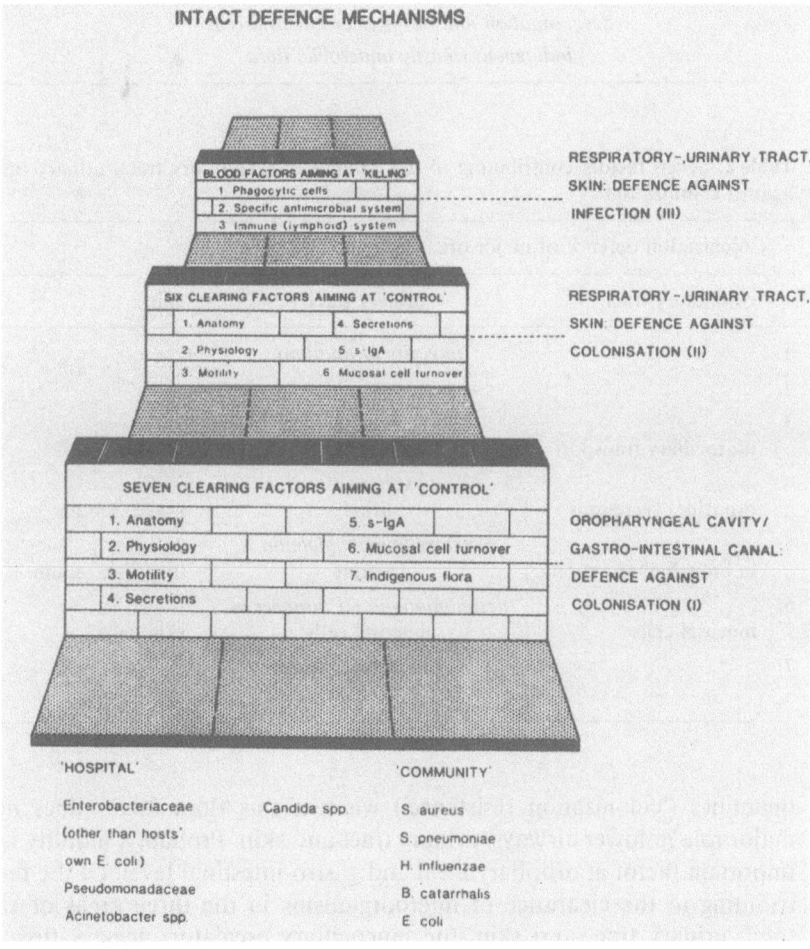

Fig. 1. Schematic representation of three barriers constituting the defence against the aerobic potentially pathogenic microorganisms, and the factors contributing to each of these barriers

Table 1. Seven factors contributing to the defence of oropharyngeal cavity and gastrointestinal canal against colonization

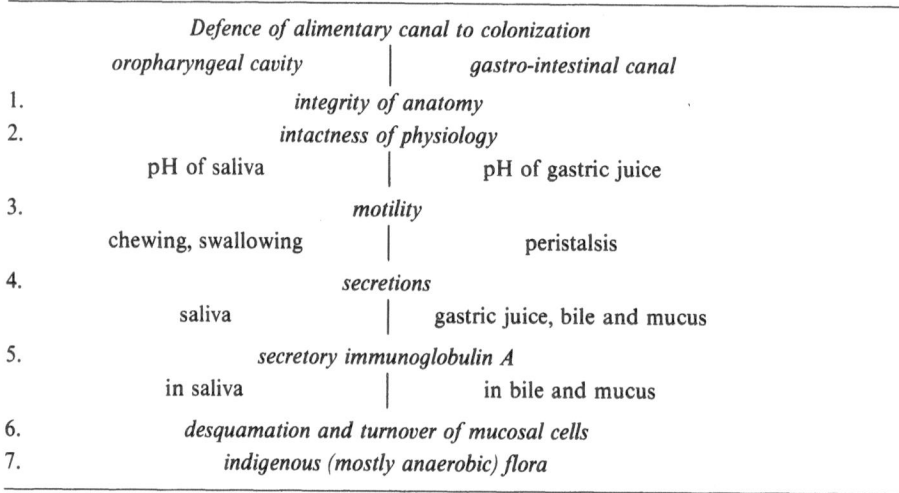

	Defence of alimentary canal to colonization	
	oropharyngeal cavity	*gastro-intestinal canal*
1.	*integrity of anatomy*	
2.	*intactness of physiology*	
	pH of saliva	pH of gastric juice
3.	*motility*	
	chewing, swallowing	peristalsis
4.	*secretions*	
	saliva	gastric juice, bile and mucus
5.	*secretory immunoglobulin A*	
	in saliva	in bile and mucus
6.	*desquamation and turnover of mucosal cells*	
7.	*indigenous (mostly anaerobic) flora*	

Table 2. Seven factors contributing to the defence of respiratory tract, urinary tract and skin against colonization

	Colonization defence of major organ systems		
	respiratory tract	urinary tract	skin
1.	*integrity of anatomy*		
2.	*intactness of physiology*		
3.	*motility*		
	mucociliary transport	urinary flow	−
4.	*secretions*		
	bronchial secretions	urine	sweat, sebum
5.	*secretory immunoglobulin A*		
	in bronchial secretions	in urine	in sweat, sebum
6.	*desquamation and turnover of*		
	mucosal cells	mucosal cells	skin cells
7.	*indigenousflora*		
	−	−	+

quantities ('colonization resistance') whereas this flora factor does not play a major role in lower airways, urinary tract and skin. Probably, motility is the most important factor at oropharyngeal and gastro-intestinal level. Of the factors contributing to the clearance of microorganisms in the three areas of respiratory tract, urinary tract and skin, the mucociliary escalator, urinary flow and skin integrity are the most important. From the microbiological point of view, intactness of colonization defence of throat and gut is associated with the virtual absence of the eight 'hospital' bacteria, while integrity of defence of respiratory and urinary tracts and skin results in sterile bronchial secretions and urine, and skin only colonized with low grade pathogens (e.g. *Staphylococcus epidermidis*).

Infection defence: The second line of defence is formed by the defence against infection [7]. This system is situated behind skin and mucous membranes and is based on cells (macrophages) and proteins (IgM, IgG and complement). The host mobilizes these infection defence mechanisms only in the presence of impaired colonization defence followed by adherence, overgrowth and invasion. The aim of this 'reactive' system is the 'killing' of the aerobic invader. Colonization defence is a mucous membrane and skin associated 'preventive' system based on 'neutralizing' and not on killing aerobic microorganisms.

Pathogenesis of Infection : Endogenous

An infection can only develop in hosts suffering impairment of defence against both colonization and infection (of respiratory tract, urinary tract and skin). As long as the defence of throat and gut against colonization is intact, microorganisms involved in infection belong to the group of six 'community' microorganisms. If this important line of defence is also impaired (Fig. 2) the patient may acquire microorganisms from the hospital environment via highly colonized patients or contaminated sinks and food, i.e., the 'hospital', 'nosocomial' or 'ICU' flora. Acquisition may then be followed by oral and/or gastro-intestinal colonization or carriage. This carrier state is crucial, occurring before colonization and infection of the respiratory tract, urinary tract and wounds. This sequence of events describes the genesis of an *endogenous* infection [8]. An infection is called endogenous when the infection is caused by microorganisms that are part of the patient's oropharyngeal and/or gastro-intestinal flora. *Primary endogenous* infection is distinguishable from *secondary endogenous* infection. The admission flora is involved in primary endogenous infections, while microorganisms acquired during hospital stay are associated with secondary endogenous infections. Although the microorganisms involved in 'secondary endogenous' infections are acquired in the hospital ('exogenous' microorganisms), the infection is called endogenous, because oral and gastro-intestinal carriage forms an essential stage in the development of infection. An exogenous infection is defined as an infection caused by microorganisms not present in the patient's oral and gastro-intestinal flora, e.g. lower airway infections associated with ventilatory equipment and humidifiers. Modern hygienic measures have virtually eliminated this type of infection.

ICU-Patient

Careful microbiological monitoring of throat, gut, lower airways, urinary tract and wounds only allows description of the magnitude of the problem of colonization/infection in the ICU patient (Fig. 3) [9]. More than 90% of ICU patients are colonized in throat and/or intestine with 'ICU' associated bacteria within

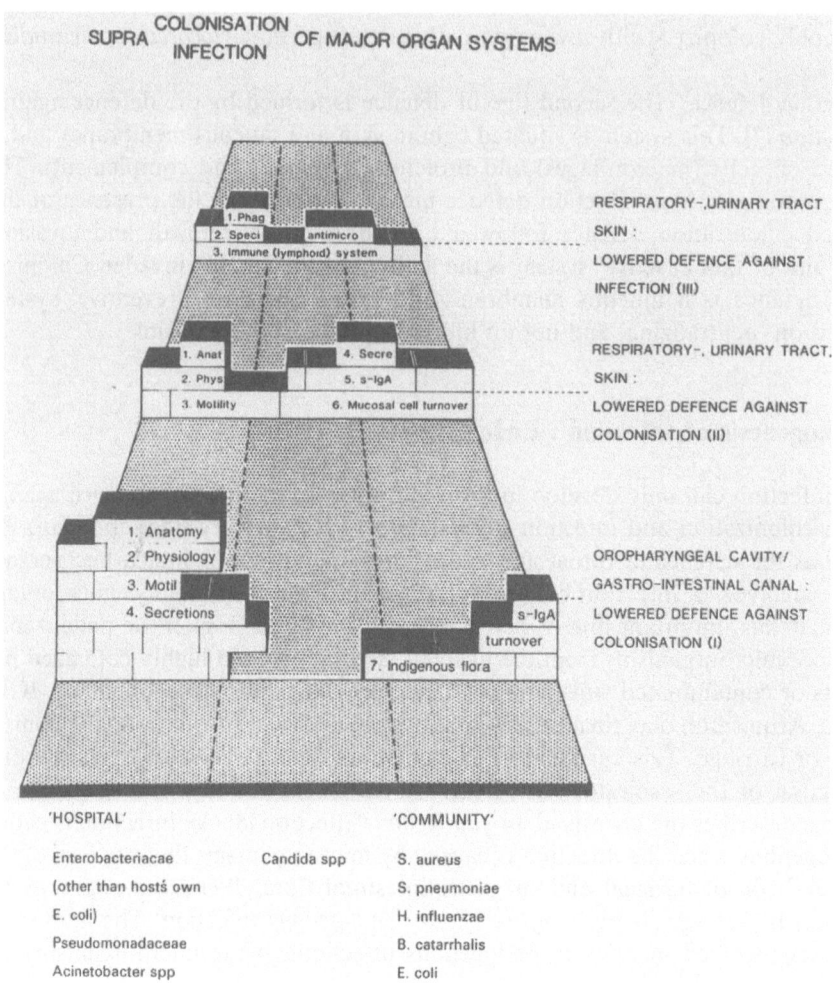

Fig. 2. Schematic representation of the impaired defence – all three lines of defence are affected – against aerobic microorganisms in a severely traumatized patient

one week of ICU stay. Secretions from lower airways, urinary tract and wounds yield microorganisms in 70% of the ICU patients needing intensive care for more than five days. Approximately half of the long-term ICU patients develop one or more infections within the first week of ICU stay. These three lines reflect impairment of colonization defence of oropharynx and gastro-intestinal tract, decreased defence of respiratory tract, urinary tract and skin and failing defence against infection. The ICU patient is a typical host in whom these two lines of defence are impaired: underlying disease is the most important factor compromising defence against both colonization and infection. The mucociliary escalator ceases to function, the urinary flow is impaired, and skin lesions are often present. The ICU patient does not swallow or chew and peristalsis is absent.

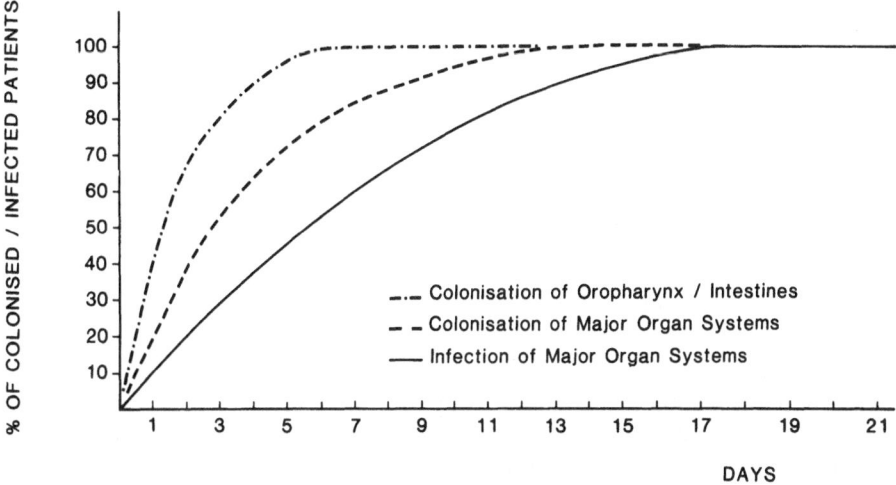

Fig. 3. Percentage of colonized and infected ICU patients versus length of stay in ICU

Medical interventions such as surgery, intubation and catheterization further decrease the defence against aerobic microorganisms. The combination of underlying disease and medical interventions results first in colonization of the throat and gastro-intestine with 'hospital' bacteria mainly from other patients and/or the environment. This carrier state may then be followed by colonization of the lower airways, urinary tract and wounds, possibly leading to infection.

Concept of Selective Flora Elimination

The aim of parenteral administration of antimicrobials is the support and enhancement of the defence against infection (last barrier in Fig. 2). To increase the defence of respiratory tract, urinary tract and skin, antimicrobials are administered endotracheally, antibiotics are instilled in the bladder and wounds are covered by creams mixed with antimicrobial agents (2nd barrier in Fig. 2). All these methods are found to be associated with a high incidence of relapse and superinfection.

The philosophy of selective flora elimination is based on the concept of the enhancement of defence of throat and gastro-intestinal tract against colonization [10]. The aim of this technique is the prevention of oropharyngeal and/or gastro-intestinal carriage formation. In a patient already colonized, selective flora elimination aims at eradication of the carrier state. Emphasis is laid on the treatment of oropharyngeal cavity and gastro-intestinal tract (first barrier in Fig. 2). Selective flora elimination is based on *long-term topical antibiotic application*, in order to prevent/eliminate carriage of 'hospital' flora (fundamental 1), enhancing colonization defence (fundamental 2) and interfering with the endogenous pathogenesis (fundamental 3). Carriage of 'community' flora is eradicated by *short-term parenteral antibiotic application*. Moreover, this parenteral antibiotic should cover 'early' colonization/infection of lower airways, urinary tract and skin by both 'community' and 'hospital' acquired microorganisms.

Long-term topical antibiotic application: Which criteria should antimicrobials fulfil to be used for selective elimination of oropharyngeal and gastro-intestinal flora? The antimicrobial spectrum should cover all 'hospital' microorganisms. The spectrum should not include the indigenous (mostly) anaerobic flora, in order to establish a flora elimination 'as selective as possible.' The antibiotics should have low MBCs for potentially pathogenic aerobes, because there are no leukocytes in the lumen of the oropharynx and gastro-intestinal tract to assist antimicrobials. They should be non-absorbable. to achieve constant high intraluminal antibiotic levels, which are not being gradually decreased by absorption; absorption of antibiotics is unnecessary and unwanted for most of the time of treatment. They should show minimal inactivation by salivary and fecal compounds. The interactions between saliva and faeces, bacteria and antibiotics determining the microbiologically active salivary and fecal concentrations are of great importance in the ultimate outcome of selective elimination [11]. Selective elimination of oropharyngeal flora occupies a central position, particularly in the intubated patient. Apart from antimicrobial factors such as spectrum and interactions, the contact time between antimicrobials and microbes is critical. Pharmaceutical technological application forms such as gel and paste may contribute to successful oropharyngeal flora elimination.

An oral non-absorbable antibiotic programme consisting of polymyxin E (colistin), tobramycin and amphotericin B (PTA regimen) is found to fulfil to a high degree the criteria required for efficient elimination of the eight 'hospital' microorganisms and of the yeast *Candida* species [12, 13]. A sticky paste of carboxymethylcellulose mixed with 2% PTA is applied to the buccal mucosa and a PTA

Table 3. Mode of administration of prophylactic regimen based on a combination of topical and systemic antimicrobials

---

1. *Topical antimicrobials   (whole ICU stay)*
   A mixture of polymyxin E, tobramycin and amphotericin B (PTA regime) is administered in:

   a) *oropharyngeal cavity:*
      - paste: carboxy methyl cellulose (ORABASE®)
      - mixed with 2% of PTA
      - a small volume (1/4 g) on a gloved finger, is applied to buccal mucosa
      - four times daily

   b) *gastrointestinal canal:*
      - suspension
      - PTA: polymyxin E   100 mg
             tobramycin   80 mg
             amphotericin B   500 mg
      - 9 ml of mixture is administered through the gastric tube.
      - four times daily.

2. *Systemic antimicrobial   (first four days)*
   cefotaxime iv 50–100 mg/kg/day

---

suspension (100 mg of polymyxin E or colistin, 80 mg of tobramycin and 500 mg of amphotericin B) is administered via a nasogastric tube, both four times a day (Table 3).

Short-Term Parenteral Antibiotic Application

The considerations which led us to choose a third generation cephalosporin, cefotaxime, are as follows:

- an adequate spectrum of activity;
- good pharmacokinetic properties;
- little or no effect on the indigenous flora; and
- no side effects such as rash or clotting disturbances.

Systemic cefotaxime is given in a dose of 50-100 mg/kg/day, started immediately on admission and continued for four days (Table 3).

Effect of Selective Flora Elimination on Colonization and Infection in ICU Patients

The results obtained with selective flora elimination as prophylaxis are promising [12, 13]. A dramatic fall of infection rate – from 81% to 16% – was observed; and pneumonia and septicemia by 'hospital' bacteria were virtually eliminated.

We have evaluated the therapy of established pneumonia by appropriate systemic antibiotics combined with the concomitant use of the selective flora elimination. In an open prospective study of twenty-five patients a cure rate of 96% was observed. These preliminary results suggest that the cure rates of established 'hospital' acquired pneumonia may be higher if elimination of the source of supply, the oropharyngeal carrier state, as well as the focus of infection is achieved [14].

At present several clinical studies in different centres are being conducted and the results can be expected in the near future. If the results of this novel approach are confirmed by these studies, it may well prove to be a major step forward in the control of infection in ICU.

Acknowledgements: We are indebted to Mrs. B. Kitchen for typing the manuscript, and to Dr. E. M. Leonard for critically reviewing the paper.

References

1. van Saene HKF, Stoutenbeek CP (1987) Selective decontamination. J Antimicrob Chemother 20:462-465
2. Goodpasture HC, Romig DA, Voth DW, Liu C, Brackett CE (1977) A prospective study of tracheobronchial flora in acutely brain-injured patients with and without antibiotic prophylaxis. J Neurosurg 47:228-235

3. Shield MJ, Hammill·HJ, Neale DA (1979) Systematic bacteriological monitoring of intensive care unit patients. The results of a twelve month study. Intensive Care Med 5:171–186
4. Mackowiak PA (1982) The normal microbial flora. N Engl J Med 307:83–93
5. Buck AC, Cooke EM (1969) The fate of ingested *Pseudomonas aeruginosa*. J Med Micro 2:521–525
6. Brun Buisson C, Meakins JL (1983) Host defence mechanisms in the acutely ill patient. In: McA Ledingham I, Hanning CD (eds) Recent advances in critical care medicine. Churchill Livingstone, Edinburgh pp 97–111
7. Miller SE, Miller CL, Trunkey DD (1982) The immune consequences of trauma. Surg Clin North Am 62:167–181
8. van Uffelen R, van Saene HKF, Fidler V, Lowenberg A (1984) Oropharyngeal flora: source of colonization of the respiratory tract in patients on artificial ventilation. Intensive Care Med 10:233–237
9. van Saene HKF, Stoutenbeek CP, Miranda DR, Zandstra DF, Langrehr D (1986) Recent advances in the control of infection in patients with thoracic injury. Injury 17:332–335
10. van Saene HKF, Stoutenbeek CP, Miranda DR, Zandstra DF (1983) A novel approach to infection control in the intensive care unit. Acta Anaesthesiol Belg 3:193–208
11. van Saene JJM, van Saene HKF, Stoutenbeek CP, Lerk CF (1985) Influence of faeces on the activity of antimicrobial agents used for decontamination of the alimentary canal. Scand J Infec Dis 17:295–300
12. Stoutenbeek CP, van Saene HKF, Miranda DR, Zandstra DF (1984) The effect of selective decontamination of the digestive tract on colonization and infection in multiple trauma patients. Intensive Care Med 10:185–192
13. van Uffelen R, Rommes JH, van Saene HKF (1987) Preventing lower airway colonization and infection in mechanically ventilated patients. Crit Care Med 15:99–102
14. Stoutenbeek CP, van Saene HKF, Miranda DR, Zandstra DF, Langrehr D: Nosocomial gram-negative pneumonia in critically ill patients. A 3-year experience with a novel therapeutic regimen. Intensive Care Med 12:419–423

Effect of Selective Decontamination on Colonization and Infection Rate in Intensive Care Patients

C. P. Stoutenbeek, H. K. F. van Saene, and D. F. Zandstra

Infection Rate

Patients admitted to the Intensive Care Unit (ICU) for the treatment of failure of vital organ systems have a severely impaired defence against infection. Infection is the major cause of multiple organ failure and late mortality in the ICU. Considering the magnitude of the problem, there are surprisingly few, detailed studies on infection in the ICU. The infection rate is determined mainly by four factors:

1. *The underlying disease:* after clean elective surgery (e.g. in cardiac surgical units) the infection rate is 13%; in general surgical ICUs it is reported to be approximately 23–28% and in traumatological ICUs it is as high as 45% [1, 2].
2. *Invasive techniques for monitoring and life-support:* the most frequent site of infection is the respiratory tract in intubated patients. After five days of mechanical ventilation the rate of pneumonia is more than 60% [3]. The other common sites of infection in intensive care patients are the urinary tract in patients with indwelling urinary catheters and bloodstream infections associated with the use of intravenous and intra-arterial catheters.
3. *Duration of stay in the ICU:* the infection rate is directly correlated with the duration of stay in the ICU, although this relationship has not been thoroughly investigated. Some studies found that more than 80% of patients staying one week or more in the ICU developed one or more infections [4, 5]. Although many infections occur very early in the course of the treatment, infection often initiates a vicious circle of (multiple) organ failure, necessitating a prolonged ICU-stay which in turn increases the risk of infection.
4. *Epidemiological factors:* the ICU is the single largest identifiable source of nosocomial infection in most hospitals. The large-scale of broad-spectrum antibiotics in the ICU is responsible for selecting multiple drug-resistant endemic bacteria in the ICU [6]. Clustering critically ill patients in such an environment and understaffing contribute to the spread of infections.

Conventional Infection Prevention

The guidelines for prevention of nosocomial infections as recommended by the Center for Disease Control (CDC), Atlanta, Georgia, USA (Category I) include:

- discipline
- handwashing and hand-disinfection
- adoption of CDC-guidelines for nursing techniques
- adoption of CDC isolation techniques
- sufficient personnel/patient relation
- disinfection procedures
- control program for antibiotic therapy and prophylaxis.

Most of these preventive measures are directed either at elimination of exogenous (environmental) sources or at prevention of *cross-infection* i.e. an infection caused by a microorganism that is transferred directly or indirectly from one person to another [7].

A control program for antibiotic therapy and prophylaxis is considered to be essential. Restriction of the use of parenteral antibiotics is accomplished by adhering to the following principles: (a) systemic antibiotic prophylaxis is *not* indicated in intensive care patients; (b) colonization is *not* treated; (c) specific systemic antibacterial therapy is given only on strict clinical and bacteriological indications [7].

Although efficient disinfection procedures have eliminated many exogenous sources of infection, the implementation of the CDC-guidelines have not resulted in a significant reduction of the infection rate in the past ten years. The generally accepted restrictive antibiotic policy has been very disappointing with respect to morbidity and mortality from infections, while the problem of emergence of multiple drug-resistant strains in the ICU remains a major concern in many hospitals.

Infection Rate with Conventional Infection Prevention Policy

A study was undertaken in a group of high-risk patients to determine (a) the effect of the length of stay in the ICU on the colonization and infection rate (b) the pathogenesis of infections (c) the effect of antibiotic treatment on the type of microorganisms causing infections.

Fifty-nine mechanically ventilated polytrauma patients, staying five days or more in the ICU were retrospectively studied [8]. In these patients a restrictive antibiotic policy was conducted and the conventional infection prevention measures were strictly adhered to. Bacteriological monitoring consisted of surveillance cultures of throat, rectum, tracheal aspirate, catheter urine (and wounds). Samples were taken on admission (baseline) and thereafter three times a week.

The effect of the length of stay in the ICU on the colonization and infection rate:
Most patients were rapidly colonized in the oropharynx or intestines by one or more hospital-acquired Gram-negative bacilli (GNB) during ICU-stay. Potentially pathogenic microorganisms (PPM) were isolated from 69% of cultures of tracheal aspirate and from 35% of urinary specimens.

The infection rate was very high (81%), predominantly respiratory and urinary tract infections, septicemia and wound infections (Table 1). Most patients had

Table 1. Infection rate in 59 mechanically ventilated polytrauma patients, staying 5 days or more in the ICU and treated with a conventional infection prevention policy

Site	Total	Gram +	Gram −	endogenous
Infected patients	48 (81%)			
Respiratory tract	35 (59%)	24	25	95%
Blood	25 (42%)	20	13	70%
Urinary tract	19 (32%)	9	13	97%
Wounds	15 (25%)	10	8	88%
Total infections	94	63	59	

more than one infection and Gram positive microorganisms were found as frequently as Gram-negative bacteria.

Pathogenesis: Infections can be either *exogenous* or *endogenous*. Exogenous infections are caused by PPM from outside the patient, whereas endogenous infections are caused by PPM from the patients own microflora, in particular from the oral or intestinal flora. In this group exogenous sources were only important as causes of septicemia (30%) whereas almost all other infections were endogenous i.e. the same PPM was first found in the oral or intestinal flora and then at the site of infection. However, many of the endogenous infections were caused by PPM that did not belong to the 'normal' resident flora, but which were hospital-acquired PPM colonizing the oropharynx or intestines. Therefore a distinction was made between primary and secondary endogenous infections: *primary endogenous* infections are defined as infections caused by PPM that belong to the 'normal' resident flora and *secondary endogenous* infections as infections caused by hospital-acquired PPM that have secondarily colonized the oropharynx or intestines. Although in the latter, the causative PPM are exogenous, but because there is a multiplication-phase in the oropharynx or intestines which is essential in the pathogenesis, these infections are called 'secondary endogenous'. Moreover, this distinction has important consequences for the prevention.

Effect of antibiotic policy: Although the antibiotic policy was meant to be restrictive, 86% of patients received antibiotic therapy for suspected or proven infections, mostly within the first week. The antibiotic therapy was associated with a high incidence of superinfections. Fourteen patients (24%) developed 18 superinfections. Seventeen different antibiotics were used. In all cases antibiotics had to be changed either because the infecting organisms were found to be resistant to the drug or because an infection with a new organism had developed. Most superinfections were caused by multiply-resistant and Gram-negative organisms which were selected in the oral or intestinal flora. All respiratory tract infections, wound infections, urinary tract infection and 3 out of 7 septicemias were secondary endogenous infections. Five patients (8%) died in the ICU with infection, despite appropriate antibiotic therapy [9].

Selective Decontamination of the Oropharynx and Intestines

A novel approach to infection prevention is based on the hypothesis that endogenous infections can be prevented by selective elimination of PPM from the oral or intestinal flora with topical non-absorbable antibiotics, whilst preserving the anaerobic flora as much possible (see contribution of van Saene in this volume). The preservation of the endogenous flora is based on the consideration that apart from the low pathogenicity of anaerobic microorganisms and enterococci, these microorganisms contribute to normal physiology and to the defence against colonization by exogenous PPM [10]. The topical non-absorbable antibiotics used are *Polymyxin E, Tobramycin and Amphotericin B (PTA regimen)*.

Clinical Studies

The clinical study consisted of three parts:

1. In the first study patients were treated with topical administration of antibiotics only in the gastrointestinal tract;
2. in the second study topical antibiotics were administered both in the gastrointestinal canal and in the oral cavity;
3. in the third study systemic antibiotic prophylaxis was given (in addition to selective flora suppression) to prevent primary endogenous infections.

Intestinal decontamination: A 9 ml mixture of polymyxin E 100 mg, tobramycin 80 mg, amphotericin B 500 mg was given through the gastric tube four times daily. In case of gastric suction, the gastric tube was clamped during one hour following administration. The results of this study showed that although the incidence of infections of the urinary tract and of wounds decreased, no reduction of oropharyngeal colonization or pulmonary infections was achieved.

Oral and intestinal decontamination: A sticky paste (Orabase) containing 2% PTA was applied to the buccal mucosa four times a day in addition to intestinal decontamination. This study showed that the oral antibiotics ointment was very effective to prevent secondary colonization of the oral cavity and this resulted in a significant reduction of secondary endogenous pulmonary infections. However, the incidence of primary endogenous infections, which were caused predominantly by *Staphylococcus aureus, Streptococcus pneumoniae* or *Haemophilus influenzae* remained as high as before [11]. Apparently the effect of flora suppression came too late to prevent these pulmonary infections by these primary endogenous PPM (community-flora).

Systemic antibiotic prophylaxis: Systemic antibiotic prophylaxis was given in addition to selective decontamination of the oral cavity and gastro-intestinal canal. Initially the systemic prophylaxis was continued until all PPM were eliminated from the oral and intestinal flora, after first year the duration of systemic prophylaxis has been reduced to 4 days. Cefotaxime was chosen as parenteral antibiotic because its spectrum include both "community" and "hospital" flora, it has little effect on the endogenous flora and and it has a broad therapeutic range with few side effects. A systemic antibiotic prophylaxis should cover both "community" and "hospital"-flora because patients who are primarily admitted to the ICU (such as multiple trauma patients) generally have a 'normal' flora on admission, but referred patients or patients who received antibiotics prior to admission may be colonized by hospital-flora.

A Two-Year Prospective Study

In the surgical ICU of the Groningen University hospital, selective flora suppression in combination with cefotaxime prophylaxis has been used since June 1982 in all patients staying longer than three days. In a prospective open trial 120 multiple trauma patients requiring prolonged mechanical ventilation and staying five days or more in the ICU were studied.

The results of this study [10, 12] showed that secondary colonization of the oropharynx by exogenous PPM could completely be prevented by the application of orabase with PTA. Elimination of PPM from the intestinal flora was effective after approximately 7 to 10 days; secondary colonization of the intestines by exogenous PPM was sharply reduced. PPM were found in only 9% of tracheal aspirate cultures and in 10% of urinary specimens.

The infection rate decreased to 18%. Most infected patients had only one infection. None of the patients developed septicemia caused by *Enterobacteriaceae* or *Pseudomonadaceae* during ICU-stay (Table 2). This antibiotic regimen is particularly effective for prevention of pneumonia: only 7 patients (6%), who were mechanically ventilated up to 69 days (mean 10 days) developed pneumonia. Only six different antibiotics were used for prophylaxis or therapy. No patient was treated with anti-pseudomonas penicillins [9]. Three patients (2.5%) died during their ICU-stay from irreversible cerebral trauma and no patient died of infection [12].

Table 2. Infection rate in 120 mechanically ventilated polytrauma patients treated with selective decontamination and cefotaxime prophylaxis

Site	Total	Gram +	Gram −
Infected patients	21 (18%)		
Respiratory tract	7 (6%)	4	2
Urinary tract	4 (5%)	3	1
Blood	9 (8%)	9	—
Wounds	5 (4%)	1	5
Total infections	25	17	8

Emergence of Resistance

The major concern when introducing this technique, was the hypothetical risk of selection of strains resistant against cefotaxime or tobramycin, which would render these valuable therapeutic agents useless. During a period of 30 months of continuous use of the same antibiotics the emergence of resistance against these antibiotics was studied.

No increase in drug-resistant PPM was found [13]. Primary or secondary colonization of the oropharynx or intestines by polymyxin E-insensitive strains (*Proteus* spp.) was found in 8% of patients. Tobramycin-resistant strains were found in 4% of patients. All strains except one were sensitive to the *combination* of tobramycin and polymyxin E. Emergence of resistance against tobramycin and polymyxin E is rare due to (a) the disinfectant-like mechanism of action of polymyxin E and (b) the lack of inducible bacterial enzymatic systems mediating resistance against these antibiotics (c) the use of high doses of non-absorbable antibiotics to assure a continuously high intraluminal antibiotic level and finally (d) the use of a combination of two antibiotics to decrease the change of resistant mutants.

Colonization with cefotaxime-resistant strains (*Pseudomonas, Enterobacter* and *Acinetobacter* spp.) occurred primarily in the intestines (10% of patients) but in 14 out of 17 patients these strains were eliminated by the topical antibiotics within 1 week. The remaining three patients (2%) developed colonization of the respiratory and urinary tracts with cefotaxime-resistant PPM. Cefotaxime-resistant *S.aureus* has not been found so far. Emergence of resistance is thought to develop at sites where high bacterial concentrations are present in combination with low antibiotic concentrations. Systemic antibiotics are secreted via saliva, bile and mucus and attain low concentrations in the oropharynx and intestines and thus create ideal circumstances for selection of resistant strains. This can be prevented by topical antibiotics which will eliminate PPM that might become resistant or are resistant to the systemic antibiotic.

The control of emergence of resistance makes the antibiotic policy in the ICU much simpler. Switching of antibiotics because of suprainfections is seldom necessary and therefore the number of different systemic antibiotics that have to be used systemically is sharply reduced. The most important consequence is the possibility to use systemic prophylaxis for an extended period of time, without risk of induction of resistance even when using a third-generation cephalosporin such as cefotaxime.

Conclusions

- Secondary endogenous infections by aerobic Gram-negative PPM and yeasts can almost completely be prevented by selective decontamination of the oropharynx or intestines with topical non-absorbable antibiotics;
- Primary endogenous infections can largely be prevented by systemic antibiotic prohylaxis;

– The selection of resistant strains and the subsequent superinfections associated with the use of systemic antibiotic prophylaxis or therapy can be prevented by selective decontamination.

References

1. Brown RB, Hosmer D, Chen HC, et al (1985) A comparison of infections in different ICUs within the same hospital. Crit Care Med 13:472–476
2. Daschner FD, Frey P, Wolff G, Baumann PC, Suter P (1982) Nosocomial infections in intensive care wards: a multicenter prospective study. Intensive Care Med 8:5–9
3. Cross AS, Roup B (1981) Role of respiratory assistance devices in endemic nosocomial pneumonia. Am J Med 70:681–685
4. Northey D, Adess ML, Hartsuck JM, Rhoades ER (1974) Microbial surveillance in a surgical intensive care unit. Surg Gynecol Obstet 139:321–325
5. Thorp JM, Richards WC, Telfer AB (1979) A survey of infection in an intensive care unit. "Forwarned is forarmed". Anaesthesia 34:643–650
6. Weinstein RA, Kabins SA (1981) Strategies for prevention and control of multiple drug-resistant nosocomial infection. Am J Med 70:449–454
7. Soddart JC (1983) Hospital-acquired infections. In: Tinker J, Rapin M (eds) Care of the critically ill patient. Springer, Berlin Heidelberg New York Tokyo, pp 873–884
8. Stoutenbeek CP, van Saene HKF, Miranda DR, Zandstra DF (1984) The effect of selective decontamination of the digestive tract on colonization and infection in multiple trauma patients. Intensive Care Med 10:8185–8193
9. Stoutenbeek CP, van Saene HKF, Miranda DR, Zandstra DF, Binnendijk B (1984) The prevention of superinfection in multiple trauma patients. J Antimicrob Chemother 14 (B):203–211
10. Waaij van der D, Berghuis-de Vries JM, Lekkerkerk-Wees van der JEC (1971) Colonization resistance of the digestive tract in conventional and antibiotic-treated mice. J Hyg Camb 69:405–411
11. Stoutenbeek CP, van Saene HKF, Miranda DR, Zandstra DF, Langrehr D (1987) The effect of oropharyngeal decontamination using topical nonabsorbable antibiotics on the incidence of nosocomial respiratory tract infections in multiple trauma patients. J Trauma 27:357–364
12. Stoutenbeek CP, van Saene HKF, Miranda DR, Zandstra DF, Binnendijk B (1985) A novel approach to antibiotic prophylaxis in multiple trauma patients. In: Infections en milieu chirurgical. Eds P. Viar. Librairie Arnette, Paris 381–391
13. Stoutenbeek CP, van Saene HKF, Zandstra DF (1987) Effect of oral nonabsorbable antibiotics on the emergence of resistance in an intensive care unit. J Antimicrob Chemother 19:513–520

Pathogenesis of Gram-Negative Bacterial Infections

J. F. P. Schellekens and J. Verhoef

Introduction

Gram-negative microorganisms such as Enterobacteriaceae and Pseudomonaceae normaly belong to the flora of the digestive tract. This close and peaceful coexistence may reflect a relatively low virulence of the bacteria, although under certain circumstances, invasion of the blood stream can occur. This may cause a life-threatening disease with circulatory shock, acute respiratory distress and multiple organ failure, often resulting in a fatal outcome.

During the last decades the incidence of gram-negative bacteremia has increased. This increase is correlated with a larger population of hospitalized patients whose defense mechanisms are impaired for various reasons [1, 2]. In fact, gram-negative microorganisms have assumed a major role in clinical infections. In view of the significant morbidity and mortality the need for prophylactic and therapeutic developments is urgent.

Therefore, the complex interactions between host and bacteria have been subjected to extensive research. In this summary, the current concepts on the acquisition of gram-negative bacteremia and the role of endotoxin, a constituent of the bacterial cell wall, in the development of septic shock will be preceded by a brief description of clinical and pathophysiological aspects of the disease. We will also focus on a new therapeutic approach, e.g. the use of antiserum against *Escherichia coli* J5 during severe gram-negative infections.

Clinical and Pathophysiological Aspects

Sudden onset of chills with spiking fever is thought to be a classical symptom of bacteremia, usually followed by an episode of vasodilatation with hypotension and oliguria. However, gram-negative bacteremia should also be considered whenever a patient suddenly becomes anxious and confused, whereas failure to develop fever is commonly observed in a debilitated patient. Other hidden signs of bacteremia can be (hyperventilation with) respiratory alkalosis, hypoglycemia, thrombopenia and leukopenia [1, 2]. When a clearcut septicemia develops, circulatory shock, respiratory distress and diffuse intravascular coagulation may supervene. Of crucial importance in septic shock is the inadequate tissue perfusion and insufficient utilization of oxygen at the cellular level [3]. Irreversible cell damage will finally supervene. Most fatalities occur within 48 hours after onset of symptoms.

Pathophysiological significance has been attached to the role of activated components of the complement system, the kallikrein-kinin system, the coagulation and the arachidonic acid cascade [4]. Interactions between activated mediators, leukocytes and platelets result in the generation of vasoactive and potentially toxic substances. Aggregation of blood cells in the capillaries and increase in capillary permeability, leading to extravasation of protein rich fluid into the extracellular space, may be important mechanisms.

Mortality rates of gram-negative bacteremia average around 30% and are mainly related to the severity of underlying disease. When septic shock develops – in 20 of 60% of cases – fatality rates increase to 50% or more [1, 2]. In general, with respect to acquisition of gram-negative bacteremia, some form of debilitation of host defense appears to precede the contribution of bacterial virulence factors. In the development of septic shock, a substantial role has emerged for endotoxin, a constituent of the gram-negative cell wall.

Acquisition of Gram-Negative Bacteremia

Gram-negative bacteremia is most frequently observed as a complication in patients hospitalized for various disorders such as hematological and solid neoplasms, diabetes mellitus, renal insufficiency, cirrhosis, extensive trauma or major surgery [1, 2]. Often these patients also receive chemotherapy, immunosuppressive or broad spectrum antibiotic therapy, and undergo invasive procedures such as intravascular catheterization and endotracheal intubation. These disorders, drugs and supportive procedures, separately or in combination, are associated with alteration of one or more host defense mechanisms. For instance, the administration of cytotoxic drugs to leukemic patients causes granulocytopenia, lesions of the mucosal lining of the digestive tract and failure to mount an antibody response, rendering this category of patients most susceptible to the development of gram-negative bacteremia [5]. The application of antibiotics can lead to disturbance of the resident anaerobic flora, promoting overgrowth of (resistant) strains of aerobic gram-negative organisms [6].

Bacteremia following urinary tract infection can be observed in otherwise non-debilitated patients. Indeed, specific bacterial virulence factors may be of paramount importance in the pathogenesis of urinary tract infections. However, invasion of the bloodstream frequently develops in association with some form of debilitation of local defense, such as after introduction of catheters or is due to disorders which cause obstruction of urine flow [7].

In many cases gram-negative bacteremia originates from an obvious infectious site, e.g. peritonitis, intra-abdominal abscess, pyelonephritis, or pneumonia. However, no primary focus can be detected, especially in presence of severely impaired host defense [1, 2]. In some of these cases, minimal lesions of colonized mucosal surfaces are thought to constitute the port of entry. Often the microorganisms cultured from the blood and the primary infection site are also present in the endogenous flora of the patient. Epidemiological studies have revealed that in a considerable portion of these cases the implicated microorganism has become part of the endogenous flora during hospitalization [8]. Such strains may be resistant to multiple antibiotics.

The most frequently isolated mircoorganisms are *E. coli* (in 30 to 40% of cases), *Klebsiella, Pseudomonas, Proteus* and *Serratia* [1, 2]. Virulence of individual strains may differ, especially in local infections, as illustrated by the specific association of upper urinary tract infections with some *E. coli* types, and infections with *Pseudomonas* species in patients with extensive burn injury or cystic fibrosis. However, the cell wall of all relevant strains of gram-negative bacteria contains factors of virulence as those that will be discussed below.

Bacterial Surface Components as Virulent Factors

The gram-negative cell wall consists of an inner cytoplasmic membrane, an intermediate peptidoglycan layer, a phospholipid-protein bilayer and an outermost lipopolysaccharide layer [9]. Lipopolysaccharide (LPS) of all relevant strains shares a remarkable similar glycolipid structure consisting of lipid A covalently bound to a core polysaccharide. Linked to the core, the polysaccharide side chain (O-antigen) exhibits type specificity. The LPS molecules are anchored by the lipid A region in the phospholipid bilayer with the polysaccharide (O-antigenic) side chains directed outwards. Some strains (e.g. many types of *E. coli* and *Klebsiella*) contain a surrounding capsular polysaccharide (K-antigen). In addition, flagellar structures for motility may be present, and pili or fimbriae for adherence to surfaces.

Important virulence factors favoring invasion are those properties of microorganisms that resist serum bactericidal activity and phagocytosis. In this respect, the presence and type of O- and K-antigens are important [10]. Rough strains, defined by their deficiency in O-antigenic side chains, are sensitive to the bactericidal activity of the complement system. Several smooth O-antigens containing strains are resistant to lysis in serum, possibly due to modifying effects of the O-antigenic side chains on complement fixation and activation. Unencapsulated (K^-) rough and smooth strains are in general readily phagocytosed by granulocytes and monocytes in the presence of complement alone. For encapsulated (K^+) strains in addition to complement, specific (anti-K) antibodies are required for phagocytosis. In the absence of specific antibodies the capsule is thought to inhibit the complement fixation at the surface by interference with activating properties of the underlying LPS components [11].

The outcome of gram-negative bacteremia is usually independent of the strain or type of causative microorganisms [1, 2]. Once survival in the bloodstream occurs, all strains and types are capable of exhibiting "endotoxic" activities.

Endotoxin

Endotoxins are LPS-protein complexes contained in the cell walls of gram-negative bacteria. Various methods have been described to extract the endotoxin from the gram-negative cell envelope, each of them yielding a material biologically active, rich in LPS, with variable amounts of protein [12]. Lipid A appears essential for most biological activities of endotoxin. However, the lipid A-associated protein and the polysaccharide side chains modify effects and may separately exhibit biological activities [13].

Of all mammalian species studied, men and rabbits are the most sensitive to the effects of endotoxin. Experiments in man are by necessity restricted to parameters (e.g. pyrogenicity) that pose minimal risk to the subject [14, 15]. Leukocytosis secondary to the release of granulocytes from the bone marrow can be observed after the intravenous administration of very low amounts of endotoxin. A slightly higher dose evokes a febrile response, concomitant with subjective symptoms such as headache and nausea. Interestingly, a relative tolerance to the febrile and subjective toxic effects develops in two discernable phases. The first tolerance phase can be observed after about 48 hours, and is specific for endotoxins as a class, without inter-endotoxin specificity. In rabbits, this first phase of pyrogenic tolerance has been attributed to the development of refractoriness of liver macrophages (Kupffer cells) to the endotoxin induced release of endogenous pyrogen. A second tolerance phase emerges after 72 hours and is largely specific for the homologous endotoxin, in accordance with the appearance of antibodies [14, 15].

Endotoxins exhibit potent adjuvant properties predominantly by induction of a selective proliferation of B-lymphocytes and their differentiation into antibody-secreting plasma cells. An endotoxin-induced increase in tumoricidal activity has been attributed to direct activation of macrophages [13]. The immunostimulatory and tumoricidal effects have led to the use of endotoxins in therapy. However, the induction of beneficial effects was severely hampered by the potent toxic activities of endotoxin.

In animal experiments, endotoxins are capable to induce hypotension with circulatory collapse, fever, dermal necrosis (localized Schwartzman reaction), diffuse intravascular coagulation and renal cortical necrosis (generalized Schwartzman reaction), thrombopenia and leukocytosis or leucopenia [13]. Several mediator systems, such as the arachidonic acid cascade (prostaglandins, leukotrienes), the complement system and the Hageman factor-dependent pathways, including the kallikrein-kinin system, are activated [4, 13].

Part of these reactions must be considered as indirect effects, triggered by direct effects of endotoxin on a limited number of cellular and humoral targets. Much attention has been devoted to the direct effects of endotoxin on cells of lymphoid origin. Research in this area was greatly facilitated by the discovery of the endotoxin resistant C3H/HeJ mouse strain. In these mice expression of the endotoxic effects of LPS (and lipid A) appears to be regulated by a simple gene [16]. In one experiment it could be observed that both sensitivity as well as resistance to LPS can be transferred by bone marrow cells [17]. Monocytes and macrophages are bone marrow-derived cells and can be directly activated by minimal amounts of endotoxins [18]. Activation can lead to increased tumoricidal activity, increased pro-coagulant activity and increased secretion of enzymes, monokines (e.g. lymphocytic activating factor), prostaglandins and interferon. Lymphocyte-activating factor stimulates the differentiation of B cells and increases the number of B cell precursors capable of responding tot T-cell help. The potent adjuvant properties of endotoxin could therefore – at least in part – be mediated by soluble factors generated by macrophages and monocytes. In addition, it has been suggested that some of the pathophysiological effects of endotoxin result from activation of these lymphoid cells [18].

A direct effect of endotoxin on the complement system has been described by several investigators and contitutes an important host defense mechanism [13]. Lipid A can bind Cl directly leading to an antibody-independent activation of the classical pathway. The polysaccharide region of LPS can activate the alternative pathway by a lipid A-independent, antibody-independent mechanism, and has a modulating effect on the expression of lipid A binding and activation of Cl. Therefore, the spectrum of complement activation of various endotoxins can differ, depending on the structure of the polysaccharide side chain. Endotoxin-induced lysis of platelets has been established to be mediated by complement activation [13]. The generation of the potent chemotactic factor C5a promotes migration and activation of leucocytes. The endotoxin molecule also can act as a negatively charged surface, facilitating activation of Hageman factor (factor XII). Through this activated factor not only the coagulation pathways, but also other pathways of inflammation can be activated [19, 20].

References

1. Kreger BE, Craven DE, Carling PC, McCabe WR (1980) Gram-negative bacteremia III. Reassessment of etiology, epidemiology and ecology in 612 patients. Am J Med 68:332–343

2. Kreger BE, Craven DE, McCabe WR (1980) Gram-negative bacteremia. IV. Re-evaluation of clinical features and treatment in 612 patients. Am J Med 68:344–355

3. Weil MH (1977) Current understanding of mechanisms and treatment of circulatory shock, caused by bacterial infection. Ann Clin Res 9:181–191

4. Kalter ES (1984) Inflammatory mediators and acute infections. Resuscitation 11:133–140

5. Armstrong D (1980) Infections in patients with neoplastic disease. In: Verhoef J, Peterson PK, Quie PG (eds) Infection in the Immunocompromised Host; Pathogenesis, Prevention and Therapy, Elsevier/North Holland, Amsterdam, pp 129–158

6. Van der Waay D (1983) Colonization resistance. In: Easmon CSF, Gaya H (eds) Second Int Symp Infections in the Immunocompromised Host, Academic Press Inc, London, pp 55–60

7. Stamm WE, Martin SM, Bennett JV (1977) Epidemiology of nosocomial infections due to gram-negative bacilli: aspects relevant to development and use of vaccins. J Infect Dis 136 (suppl):S151–S160

8. Schimpff SC, Young VM, Greene WH, Vermeulen GD, Moody MR, Wiernik PH (1972) Origin of infection in acute non-lymphocytic leukemia: significance of hospital acquisition of potential pathogens. Ann Intern Med 77:707–714

9. Costerton JW, Ingram JM, Cheng K-J (1974) Structure and function of the cell envelope of gram-negative bacteria. Bacteriol Rev 38:87–110

10. Van Dijk WC, Verbrugh HA, Peters R, Van Erne-van der Tol ME, Verhoef J (1979) *Escherichia coli* K antigen in relation to serum-induced lysis and phagocytosis. J Med Microbiol 12:123–130

11. Horwitz MA, Silverstein SC (1980) Influence of the *Escherichia coli* capsule on complement fixation and on phagocytosis and killing by human phagocytes. J Clin Invest 65:82–94

12. Galanos C, Lüderitz O, Rietschel ET, Westphal O (1977) Newer aspects of the chemistry and biology of bacterial lipopolysaccharides, with special references to their lipid A compo-

nent. In: Goodwin TW (ed) Int Rev Biochem vol 14. University Park Press, Baltimore, pp 239–386

13. Morrison DC, Ulevitch RJ (1978) The effects of bacterial endotoxins on host mediation systems. Am J Pathol 93:527–618
14. Greisman SE, Hornick RB (1973) Mechanisms of endotoxin tolerance with special reference to man. J Infect Dis 128 (suppl):S265–S276
15. Wolff SM (1973) Biological effects of bacterial endotoxins in man. J Infect Dis 128 (suppl):S259–S264
16. Watson J, Kelly K, Whitlock CH (1980) Genetic control of endotoxin sensitivity. In: Schlesinger (ed) Microbiology-1980. American Society for Microbiology, Washington DC, pp 4–10
17. Michalek SM, Moore RN, McGhee JR, Rosenstreich DL, Merkenhagen SE (1982) The primary role of lymphoreticular cells in the mediation of host responses to bacterial endotoxin. J Infect Dis 146:746–750
18. Morrison DC (1983) Bacterial endotoxins and pathogenesis. Rev Infect Dis 5 (suppl):S733–S747
19. Morrison DC, Cochrane CG (1974) Direct evidence for Hageman factor (factor XII) activation by bacterial lipopolysaccharides (endotoxins). J Exp Med 140:797–811
20. Kalter ES, Van Dijk WC, Timmermans A, Verhoef J, Bouma BN (1983) Activation of purified plasma prekallikrein triggered by cell wall fractions of *Escherichia coli* and *Staphylococcus aureus*. J Infect Dis 148:682–691

Sepsis in Children: Different Pathophysiology, Different Treatment?

P. R. Holbrook

Introduction

Children are neither small adults nor big neonates. Sepsis is a disease condition which exemplifies this adage. Nearly every aspect of the problem of sepsis demonstrates differences between children and adults. In this discussion an attempt to highlight these differences and outline their significance will be made.

Definition and Incidence

As in adults, shock in children is the condition of circulatory and metabolic dysfunction wherein the circulation fails to deliver sufficient nutrients to the tissues which require them. Most frequently, the disorder results from a failure of the circulation to deliver the nutrients to the appropriate tissues (reduced cardiac output or maldistribution of flow). Occasionally it results from a failure of the tissues to appropriately utilize the nutrients.

Because of the many of the same factors found in the adult patient population, the incidence of septic shock in children is increasing. These include more invasive procedures, more immunosuppressed patients, and longer survival of patients treated for previously lethal diseases. Furthermore, better recognition of the early findings of shock have increased the opportunities for the clinician to treat the condition. The details of each of these factors differs in children. Some increase is also due to more virulent, or less treatable organisms, a factor which has had particular relevance in the nursery.

Etiology and Primary Response

The same bacteria and fungi which cause sepsis in the the old affect the young as well. However, the young are susceptible to additional agents which do not seriously affect the adult (e.g. Group β beta-hemolytic Streptococcus and a host of viruses). The significance of group β Streptococcus as a threat highlights some of the differences between children and adults. Entry of the organism into the body, opsonization, phagocytosis, and intracellular killing are all different (at least in vitro) in the neonate [1].

The presence of microorganisms in the body triggers the host immune defenses. Developmental changes occur in both humoral and cellular immune responses over the course of childhood. The most obvious is the progressive accumulation of immunologic experience, which accounts for the susceptibility of the child to *Hemophilus influenza* infections. Humoral factors including complement and inmmunoglobulins are different at birth than later, and this determines, partially, the susceptibility of the host at certain times. The child spends part of his life in a state of relative immunodeficiency.

In addition to humoral changes both numbers and functional properties of granulocytes and lymphocytes change with age. The ability of these cells to process invasion of microorganisms of various types is different from that of adults.

Other factors related to infection which are unique to childhood include anatomic differences of both size (e.g. the middle ear as a source for sepsis), and configuration (congenital anatomic defects) and different underlying disease states (e.g. necrotizing enterocolitis, childhood acquired malignancies, etc.).

Sepsis

As the infection progresses, a point is reached when sepsis occurs. The host's response to the invading organism is complex by this time. This response is reviewed elsewhere [2, 3]. The net result is a cascade of chemical, hormonal, metabolic, and hemodynamic changes which result in the clinical picture of sepsis. While few data have accumulated regarding most of these changes in children, what is known casts light on potential differences in children.

The clinical presentation of sepsis in older children is not significantly different from that of adults. The adult oriented physician will need to recognize the early neurologic findings of septic shock in children (irritability, somnolence, restlessness or poor feeding), but otherwise, the picture is comparable.

The newborn often shows minimal clinical signs of sepsis. Mild hyper-or hypothermia, increased sleepiness, irritability, poor feeding, or, commonly, an observation by the mother that the child "just isn't acting right" may be the only harbingers. Tachypnea is usually present and the clinician is referred to standard tables of respiratory rates for comparison. With time even the very young will show cardiovascular collapse though treatment may be fruitless by then.

Studies on the cardiopulmonary response in older septic children [4] indicate similar changes to those found in adults. Comparable data in neonates is not available.

Treatment

Treatment of shock in children involves the same general principles as that of adults (resuscitation, eradication of the focus of infection and general life support). Resuscitation includes fluid administration to a degree sufficient to ensure adequate preload, and the clinician caring for the child should not be timid in providing appropriate fluids. The addition of inotropic agents, as necessary, is ideally withheld until an adequate filling volume is established. The current goal of therapy in our unit is to maximize oxygen delivery. Often, oxygen consumption may be increased by increasing delivery. Adult studies indicate that for those patients who increased consumption to a point but then leveled off despite further increases in oxygen delivery, mortality was much lower than in those in whom no plateau was reached [5].

Eradication of the focus is the *sine qua non* for recovery. Extensive studies may be necessary to identify the focus in children, but, once identified, all efforts must be made to sterilize it or further therapy will be fruitless. Foci of infection more commonly encountered in children than in adults include the meninges, the ears, and the skin.

Cardiac life support in the septic child includes fluids, and inotropes keeping in mind the differences in pharmacology in the developing child [6]. Invasive monitoring of the cardiovascular system, even in small children, has become the norm. Cardiovascular parameters which distinguish between survivors and non-survivors have been defined [7]. The use of multiple agents is not uncommon. Early application of intubation and mechanical ventilation is recommended, as is correction of hematologic and biochemical abnormalities (especially glucose).

Corticosteroid therapy, long debated, appears not to be indicated in the treatment of sepsis [8, 9], although data unique to children are not available. In earlier studies steroids appeared to reverse the hypotension more rapidly than control therapies, suggesting that a window of opportunity might be made available.

Because of the numerical and functional deficiencies of neonatal white cells, transfusions of these cells have been advocated. Benefit has been shown in adults only in the persistently neutropenic patient who has documented gram negative infection [10]. In neonates and infants the studies are controversial, and they involve small numbers of patients. It is important to remember both the risk and the cost of this form of therapy.

Exchange transfusion can increase neutrophil counts in neonates septic with group β Streptococci [11], can clear endotoxin in a group of neonates who were probably septic [12], and results in an apparent reversal of shock in anecdotal cases of neonatal sepsis. The number of "evil humors" which could be cleared with this technique is significant and a randomized controlled study is indicated.

Extracorporeal membrane oxygenation (ECMO), is anecdotally reported to aid the septic newborn [13]. Antiserum to endotoxin [14, 15] has not been attempted in children.

Conclusion

Children respond differently to different septic threats in the environment than do adults. The exploration of the mechanisms underlying the differences in the child's response to an invading organism may lead to improved understanding of sepsis in all age groups. Until this broader understanding occurs, the clinician must be mindful of the differences so that the child can be approached appropriately.

References

1. Wilson CB (1986) Immunologic basis for increased susceptibility of the neonate to infection. J Pediatrics 108:1–12
2. Sibbald WJ, Sprung CL (Eds) (1986) Perspective on Sepsis and Septic Shock: New Horizons by The Society of Critical Care Medicine, Fullterton, California. Library of Congress Catalog Number:85-63141
3. Zimmermann JJ, Dietrich KA (1987) Current perspective on Septic Shock. Pediatr Clin North Am 34:131–163
4. Pollack MM, Fields AI, Ruttimann UE (1984) Sequential cardiopulmonary variables of infants and children in septic shock, Crit Care Med 12:554–559
5. Bihari D, Smithies M, Gimson A, Tiner J (1987) The effects of vasodilation with prostacyclin on oxygen delivery and uptake in critically ill patients. N Engl J Med 317:397–403
6. Zaritsky AL, Eisenberg MG (1986) Ontogenetic considerations in the pharmacotherapy of shock. In: Critical Care State of the Art Vol 7, pp 485–527
7. Pollack MM, Fields AI, Ruttimann UE (1985) Distribution of cardiopulmonary variables in pediatric survivors and non survivors of septic shock. Crit Care Med 13:454–459
8. Bone RC, Fisher CJ, Clemmer TP, et al (1987) A Controlled clinical trial of high-dose methylprednisolone in the treatment of severe sepsis and septic shock. N Engl J Med 317:653–658
9. Veterans Administration Study Group (1987) Effect of high-dose glucocorticoid therapy on mortality in patients with clinical signs of systemic sepsis. N Engl J Med 317:659–665
10. Strauss RG (1984) The role of granulocyte transfusions. Am J Ped Hem/Onc 6:247–252
11. Hall RT, Shigeoka AO, Hill HR (1983) Serum opsonic activity and peripheral neutrophil counts before and after exchange transfusion in infants with early onset group β Streptococcal septicemia. Ped Infect Dis 2:356–358
12. Togari H, Mikawa M, Iwanaga T, et al (1983) Endotoxin clearance by exchange blood transfusion in septic shock neonates. Acta Paediatr Scand 72:87–91
13. Short BL, Pearson GD (1986) Neonatal extracorporeal membrane oxygenation: a review. J Int Care Med 1:47–54
14. Ziegler EJ, McCutchan JA, Fierer J, et al (1982) Treatment of gram-negative bacteremia and shock with human antiserum to a mutant Escherichia coli. N Engl J Med 307:1225–1230
15. Baumgartner JD, Glauser MP, McCutchan JA, et al (1985) Prevention of gram negative shock and death in surgical patients by antibody to endotoxin for glycolipid. Lancet 2:59–63

Acute Respiratory Failure

Adult Respiratory Distress Syndrome: Changing Concepts of Clinical Evolution and Recovery

A. Artigas

Introduction

The adult respiratory distress syndrome (ARDS) is an acute and severe alteration in lung structure and function characterized by hypoxemia, stiff lungs with
low functional residual capacity, and diffuse radiographic infiltrates due to increased lung capillary permeability [1, 2]. Since first described in 1967 [3], the
syndrome has been associated with high mortality, and despite clinical and laboratory investigations, survival rates remain virtually unchanged [1]. Patients with
ARDS may die from severity of lung impairment and common complications.
Whether hypoxemia is the usual cause of death in patients with ARDS is controversial. However, supportive measures such as mechanical ventilation with
positive end-expiratory pressure (PEEP) [4] or extracorporeal membrane oxygenation [5], although technically successful in increasing arterial oxygenation, have
had no obvious effect on reducing mortality. However, LFPPV-ECCO$_2$ R seems
promising in selected patients [6]. This suggests a need to focus on the prevention or treatment of other aspects of the syndrome in addition to respiratory
supportive measures, such as the analysis of the natural history and factors contributing to death.

Diagnosis of ARDS

The definition of ARDS includes only the most severe cases of permeability pulmonary edema. The diagnosis of ARDS depends on the presence of certain clinical, radiological and physiological criteria, i.e.: increased pulmonary compliance, increased V_D/V_T and recent bilateral and diffuse radiographic infiltrates in the absence of left atrial hypertension. Those patients with chronic obstructive pulmonary disease are usually excluded from the diagnosis of ARDS.
The physiologic criteria are not universally accepted and vary widely among investigators. Those authors who include stiff lungs as a diagnostic criterion of
ARDS generally use a total thoracic compliance less than 50 ml/cm H_2O [7]. The
criteria for alterations in gas exchange vary from PaO_2 less than 50 mm Hg to 75
mm Hg with a fraction of inspired oxygen (FiO_2) of 0.5 or greater [1, 2, 9]. Others use the ratio of arterial to alveolar partial pressure of oxygen (PaO_2/PAO_2)
of less than 0.2 [7] or a PaO_2/FiO_2 ratio less than 150 [10]. Criteria for pulmonary wedge pressure to exclude hydrostatic pulmonary edema vary from less than
12 cm H_2O, to less than 18 mmHg. For comparative purposes the physiologic

criteria to diagnose ARDS should be standardized. Definition of ARDS by absolute exclusion of increased hydrostatic pressure is undesirable because it does not allow for concommittant occurrence of permeability edema and high microvascular pressures [2]. Diffuse bilateral pulmonary infiltrates are sometimes not detected in X-ray control at the beside [11] and need more sophisticated techniques, such as CT scanning. The clinical signs and symptoms of onset of ARDS (respiratory distress, cyanosis, hypoxemia, and decreased lung compliance) usually precede radiographic lung infiltrates by a few or several hours, depending on the type and severity of lung injury [11]. In early and less extensive lung injury, consolidation may be regional and patchy, and is also modified by airway pressure and lung volume [12].

Recently, Sturm et al. (unpublished data) demonstrated that extravascular lung water (EVLW) was the best single parameter to define and detect ARDS. The combination of oxygenation index, lung compliance and pulmonary artery pressure could predict whether the EVLW was greater or less than 10 ml/kg in 78.3% cases with a high specificity (96.5%) in diagnosing ARDS.

Unfortunately, we do not possess the means to diagnose ARDS in its early stages. Mild hypocapnia is common in ARDS as in hypoxemic respiratory failure due to other causes. Furthermore, many patients who are at high risk of developing ARDS have severe transitory hypoxemia but never progress to the complete syndrome. Pepe et al. [9] found that 55% of patients considered at high risk for ARDS who developed "critical hypoxemia" did not progress to ARDS.

The intuitive impression of many clinicians is that most patients in risk groups such as trauma, who develop pulmonary infiltrates and require mechanical ventilation are treated successfully with a higher survival rate than reported in the majority of published studies [7, 10]. This discrepancy suggests the possibility that entry criteria for ARDS in published studies have increasingly selected an atypical population with a high incidence of severe underlying disease or multiple extrapulmonary organ system failure [13].

Two criteria, severe hypoxemia (arterial alveolar/ratio < 0.3) and a simultaneous measurement of pulmonary artery wedge pressure, may have increasingly introduced bias into published clinical studies, selecting a small subset of patients with an unusually poor prognosis. Therefore, in order to have ARDS in a publishable series, poor gas exchange refractory to PEEP and high FiO_2 must be present and a pulmonary artery catheter must be in place. Because of increasing awareness of an uncertain risk/benefit ratio of the use of pulmonary artery catheters, different groups apply PEEP to reduce FiO_2 to a non-toxic level without invasive hemodynamic monitoring. If the supportive initial therapy is effective, these patients will not be included as ARDS. To better assess the real prognosis criteria for ARDS may need to be modified. Elimination of data from pulmonary arterial catheters will raise a risk of occasional inadvertent inclusion of patients with a component of unsuspected cardiogenic edema. However, it may be necessary to accept these limitations to assess prognosis more accurately and evaluate new treatments. The selection of a high percentage of moribund patients with severe underlying organ failure or irreversible underlying diseases will virtually guarantee that drugs undergoing therapeutic trials will not improve outcome. In a recent multicentric study in Europe, patients with severe hypoxemia ($FiO_2 \geqslant 0.5$, PEEP 5 cmH_2O, $PaO_2 < 75$ mmHg) were separated into two groups in relation to response to initial treatment. The "hypoxemic group" represents patients whose hypoxemia had improved 24 hours later without invasive cardiovascular monitoring. The "severe ARDS" group represents patients with an unresolved hypoxemia 24 hours later requiring a Swan-Ganz catheter to confirm a pulmonary wedge pressure lower than 18 mmHg. The Swan-Ganz catheter should only be used in patients with ARDS when other organ system failure obscures assessment of intravascular volume and improvement in gas exchange proves difficult.

Until an accurate and clinical method is available to measure lung vascular permeability, identification of ARDS will continue to be based on clinical criteria which correspond to the moderate and severe forms of the classification of acute respiratory failure (ARF) proposed by the Massachusetts General Hospital (MGH) Specialized Center of Research in Adult ARF [14].

Etiology

ARDS occurs following a variety of overwhelming insults or risk factors. Some of the non-pulmonary conditions associated with ARDS are shock, sepsis, non-pulmonary trauma, drug overdose, pancreatitis, uremia, eclampsia, central nervous system disease, emboli, burns and massive transfusion. Those pulmonary conditions associated with ARDS include aspiration, lung contusion, infection, radiation, toxic gases, and near-drowning. Sepsis and trauma are the most common causes of ARDS but may vary from one hospital to another depending on admission policies and clinical specialty practice. In a medical ICU, bacterial, viral and aspiration pneumonia patients would predominate, whereas such patients account for only 29% of ARDS admissions in a surgical ICU [14].

Precipitating conditions and specific cause-effect relationships of ARDS often cannot be identified, and the early pathogenetic mechanisms are probably diverse [15]. The initial insult reaches the lower respiratory tract via the airway or circulation, but regardless of the early pathogenetic mechanisms, the physiologic and morphologic manifestations of ARDS become indistinguishable with time. Many processes that fit criteria for ARDS may not be associated with the classical pathologic changes. For example, high altitude pulmonary edema clears rapidly with O_2 administration or with a return to lower altitudes [16]. Intravenous narcotic-associated pulmonary edema, neurogenic pulmonary edema, and hanging-associated pulmonary edema are other atypical forms [16-19]. These atypical ARDS conditions may be neurologically and/or vascularly mediated, and may represent a different process from that associated with traumatic injury or sepsis [16].

Clinically, diffuse bilateral pneumonias and contusions can fit the criteria of ARDS, and so it is often difficult to distinguish one from the other. Intubated and mechanically ventilated patients usually become colonized with nosocomial bacteria within a few days after admission and develop a pulmonary superinfection contributing to maintain or worsen acute lung injury [8, 10, 20].

Incidence and Risk Factors

The frequency of ARDS is difficult to establish. It is estimated that approximately one ARDS occurs yearly per 17 general hospital beds or represents 7% of all combined admissions to the ICU [14]. The 1972 NHLBI Task Force on Respiratory Disease estimated that 150000 cases of ARDS (excluding pneumonia and cardiac pulmonary edema) occur annually in the United States [21]. The incidence of moderate and severe ARDS seems to have decreased over the last few years, perhaps due to initial preventive treatment of patients at-risk with modern methods of lung expansion, mechanical ventilation with PEEP, chest physiotherapy, effective and prompt treatment of shock, avoiding and excessive positive fluid balance, and early recognition and therapy of the precipitating factors of ARDS [14].

What is the risk of ARDS developing from one or more of the predisposing causes? At the MGH the at-risk group (133 patients) principally included patients suffering abdominal or extra-abdominal sepsis, chest trauma, long bone or pelvic fractures, and 36.9% subsequently developed ARF; 12 patients (9.1%) developed ARDS and all died [14]. Fowler et al. [7] in a one year study evaluated the conditions of patients presenting any of the following: sepsis, burns, long bone or pelvic fractures, DIC, cardiopulmonary bypass, acute pneumonia requiring intensive care, multiple blood transfusions, or pulmonary aspiration. From a total predisposed population of 993 patients, only 68 (7%) subsequently developed the syndrome. An additional 20 patients not meeting the pre-defined risk factor criteria also developed ARDS. They were able to identify 77% of patients developing ARDS at their institutions. The risk of ARDS varied from 1.7% after cardiopulmonary bypass to 35.6% after pulmonary aspiration. The incidence of ARF following cardiopulmonary bypass or non-thoracic trauma (5.3%) as well as hypertransfusion (4.6%) was relatively lower than with pneumonia (11.9%) and DIC (22.2%). Patients with direct pulmonary injury sich as aspiration or pneumonia tended to have higher incidence rates than patients with indirect injuries such as burns or hypertransfusion. There is a strong relationship between the number of predisposing conditions and incidence rates of the syndrome, with a cumulative risk of 5.8% for patients with a single risk in contrast to an incidence of 24.6% in patients with two or more predisposing factors [7].

The Seattle study [9] was carried out at a single hospital, Harborview Medical Center, using different entry criteria. While the Denver study used relatively broad entry criteria, the Seattle study was designed to identify high-risk population. The majority of patients were trauma victims, and only patients with endotracheal intubation were examined. In addition, stricter criteria were used to define the putative risk factors. The incidence of ARDS was 34% of 136 consecutive patients. During the same study period, 30 other patients met the criteria for ARDS, indicating a 61% sensitivity for finding ARDS when using the chosen criteria for risk. The results of these two studies are summarized in Table 1. While comparison is difficult, partly because of the differences in study design, there were remarkable similarities and complementary findings between the two studies. For example, when similar risk criteria were examined, such as those used for aspiration of gastric contents or multiple long-bone factures, the risk for

Table 1. Incidence of ARDS following clinical risks[a]

Clinical condition	Incidence of ARDS	
	Pepe et al. [9] (Seattle)	Fowler et al. [7] (Colorado)
Sepsis		
Bacteremia	–	9/239 (4%)
Sepsis syndrome	5/13 (38%)	–
Aspiration of gastric content	7/23 (30%)	16/45 (36%)
Bone fractures	1/12 (8%)	2/38 (5%)
Multiple transfusions		
10 units/24 hours	–	9/197 (5%)
10 units/6 hours	4/17 (24%)	–
Cardiopulmonary bypass	–	4/237 (2%)
Burns	–	2/87 (2%)
ICU-acquired pneumonia	–	10/84 (12%)
Disseminated intravascular coagulation	–	2/9 (22%)
Pulmonary contusion	5/29 (17%)	–
Near-drowning	2/3	–
Pancreatitis	1/1	–
Prolonged hypotension	0/1	–

[a] These data refer to patients with only a single risk event.

ARDS was fairly identical. On the other hand, when comparing bacteremia with sepsis syndrome, the relative differences in risk became very obvious, particulary when these were the only apparent risk factors involved (4% versus 38%, respectively). At the same time in both studies the incidence of ARDS rose exponentially when multiple risk factors were involved, whether or not these risk factors are related to each other (Table 2). In the initial Seattle study, ARDS developed in 18% of those with one factor, 42% of those with two, and 85% of those with three risk factors (p < 0.001), independently of the degree of oxygenation.

Although a good initial oxygenation decreases the risk of ARDS, it is no guarantee against its development particularly when multiple factors are involved [22]. The degree of hypoxemia correlates with the risk for ARDS in an almost

Table 2. Effect of multiple risk conditions on the incidence of ARDS

No risk factors	Pepe et al. [9] (Seattle) No (%)	Fowler et al. [7] (Colorado) No (%)	ISS of ARDS patients [9]
One	10/56 (18%)	54/936 (6%)	33 ± 12
Multiple	19/32 (59%)	14/57 (25%)	40 ± 13
Total	29/88 (33%)	68/993 (7%)	38 ± 13

ISS = injury severity score (Seattle study).

linear fashion (about 60% with PaO_2/FiO_2 <150, 40% with 150 to 280, and 20% with greater than 280).

In the initial Seattle study, the injury severity score (ISS) correlated very well with the development of ARDS (p<0.005) but there was no significant correlation between the ISS and the number of risk factors present in the trauma patients developing ARDS (Table 2). Recognizing that ISS, initial oxygenation and individual risk factors all correlate with the development of ARDS, the Seattle group developed an equation to predict the patient's chances of developing ARDS. They were able to demonstrate, in a select group of patients, that above a certain cut-off index score, a predictive accuracy of about 80% can be achieved; over half the patients developing ARDS can be identified above this cut-off score, while only 5% to 10% of those not developing ARDS have such high scores. Therefore, combining physiologic, anatomic and categorical risks is more helpful, though not always specific, for predicting ARDS. It is hoped that with the addition of other variables known to be important in predicting ARDS, the specificity of such techniques can be improved, and can perhaps be extended to the hospital.

In subsequent work done at Harborview, a continuing prospective study has been expanded to include those patients with head injury, liver disease, and drug overdose, whether they had received endotracheal intubation or not [22]. Although the risk of ARDS diminished slightly to an overall incidence of 24% in the 658 patients examined over the subsequent three and a half year period, this resulted in 85% successful identification of all patients who developed ARDS.

ARDS is frequently associated with septicemia. Fein et al. [23] and Kaplan et al. [24] reported an incidence of 18% and 23%, respectively, in patients with documented sepsis. This is usually preceded by hypotension, and thrombocytopenia significantly worsens the prognosis. Recently Montgomery et al. [10] reported an ARDS incidence of 37% in a large number of at-risk patients.

Prediction of ARDS by Circulatory Mediators

Much of the recent research carried out to establish the pathophysiology of ARDS has been centered around early identification of at-risk patients [22]. Most agree that therapy must begin early and particularly before multiple organ involvement occurs. Accordingly, better markers are needed. One of the approaches to accomplishing early identification has been to find a readily measurable plasma factor that could predict which patients with the appropriate risk factors would develop an ARDS. There is still a need to identify an early and easily measured plasma factor that would help to predict which patients at risk for ARDS will develop ARDS. It is intuitively obvious that the biochemical or cellular events leading to ARDS are in progress long before the full-blown clinical manifestations are appreciated.

Hypothesis for mechanisms of cell-dependent acute lung injury have been that activated platelets, neutrophils, lymphocytes and macrophages would sequester in the lung, forming micro-thrombi and then release toxic oxygen products, proteolytic enzymes, chemo-attractant substances and products of the arachidonic cascade that could injure the lung. However until now, no single type of cells able to produce acute lung injury has been identified. Leukopenia and trombocytopenia are not specific of patients at risk.

Despite intense research to find markers for ARDS in at-risk patients, very little predictive association with such mediators has been found. Clinical studies have found that measurement of complement activation in plasma does not specifically detect which patient will develop ARDS [22]. The role of arachidonic acid metabolites in acute lung injury is not clearly defined and no definitive evidence for cause and effect relationships has been found. Clinical studies demonstrate that high levels of proteases associated to low antiproteases levels do not seem to be reliable predictors of ARDS but may be considered as risk factors. Kallikrein appears to be present and active in lung lavage from patients with ARDS, and not in patients with other lung injuries [25, 26]. These investigators suggest that plasma kallikrein mediated reactions may contribute to the pathogenesis of ARDS and that the presence of the kallikrein-like activity implies activation of Hageman factor in the lungs of ARDS patients and activation of blood coagulation system. Inhibitors of blood coagulation (Antithrombin III, Protein C, alpha-2-macroglobulin) are consumed or inactivated with lower plasmatic level in at-risk and ARDS patients [27] (Fig. 1).

Recently, Hollgren et al. presented results of a study examining serum lactoferrin levels in high risk patients [28]. Although lactoferrin levels were elevated in the study group as a whole, the patients who subsequently developed ARDS had significantly higher serum levels than did non-ARDS patients.

Markers of endothelial injury factor VIII and prostacyclin are elevated in patients with acute lung injury. Patients with ARDS had a marked increase in the rapid migrating component of factor VIII while patients at risk without lung injury showed a normal pattern [29]. Plasma fibronectin is neither sensitive nor specific in predicting who will develop ARDS.

Angiotensin converting enzyme (ACE) might be an index of the extent of endothelial damage in ARDS. Fourrier et al. [30] found that ACE measurement

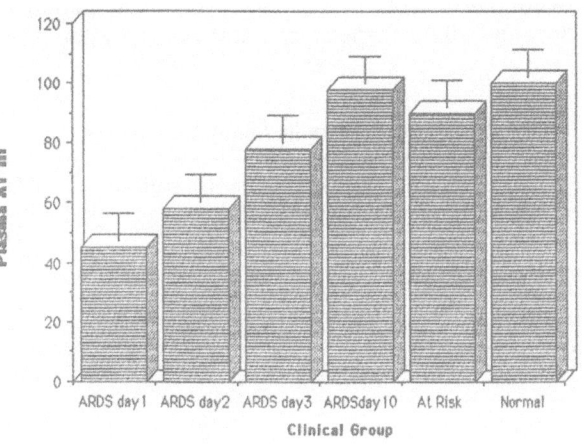

Fig. 1. Blood coagulation inhibitor antithrombin (AT) III in 20 healthy volunteers, 15 at-risk patients and 25 with ARDS at admission in ICU. Note a marked and early decrease of antithrombin III in ARDS patients. Patients atrisk showed lower levels than normal controls

was not useful in predicting ARDS high-risk patients, although levels after development of ARDS did correlate with the severity of lung injury.

In conclusion, changes in certain serum biochemical assays probably reflect the inflammatory response of the lungs in at-risk patients.

Mortality and Prognostic Factors

Despite nearly two decades of progress in supportive care for patients with ARF, recent studies and reviews continue to report a high mortality rate ranging between 41% and 74% in patients with ARDS [7–11, 23, 31] and as high as 90% in patients with both sepsis and ARDS [17]; the majority of these patients die within 14 days of onset of the syndrome [7]. This pessimism in the clinical literature could be due to entry criteria for ARDS selecting an atypical population with a high incidence of pre-existing diseases and a high mortality rate. Using broad clinical ARDS criteria Rinaldo found a mortality rate of 30% including trauma patients and all patients under 30 years of age without multiple organ system failure [13]. The mortality rate of the hypoxemia group in the European study on ARDS is 38.7%, lower than mortality of the severe ARDS group which is 69% (Table 3).

Although no substantial evidence has yet been provided, it is believed that the outcome of ARDS probably depends on the following basic factors: the intensity of the initial acute lung injury; the precipitating cause of ARDS and its response to treatment; and the occurrence of complications and further lung injury. Most deaths in the first days can be attributed to the underlying illness or injury. The majority of late deaths has been related to complications, mainly to septicemia. Fowler et al. reported a similar high mortality rate in all etiologic groups [7]. However, the initial pathogenetic mechanisms are different depending on the etiology (septicemia vs trauma) and the means of injury (airway vs circulation). The highest mortality rates were due to acute lung injury caused by diffuse infectious processes and pneumonias. ARF following chest trauma or associated with local abdominal or urinary sepsis carried an intermediate risk of death. Diffuse peritonitis and severe acute pancreatitis reaches mortality rates of 86% and 100%, respectively, and may be related to surgical problems. When in-

Table 3. Survival data from the European ARDS study

	No patients	Survivors	Non-survivors
Group A (PaO$_2$ > 75 mmHg with FiO$_2$ ⩾ 0.5 + PEEP 5 cmH$_2$O)	191	117 (61.3%)	74 (38.7%)
Group B (PaO$_2$ < 75 mmHg with FiO$_2$ ⩾ 0.5 + PEEP 5 cmH$_2$O)	400	124 (31%)	276 (69%)
Total	591	241 (40.8%)	350 (59.2%)

fectious ARDS develops in an immunocompromised host the survival is very low [32].

Irreversible respiratory failure is responsible for only 10–16% of ARDS deaths because of failure to maintain a degree of oxygenation and carbon dioxide elimination compatible with life [10, 12]. At autopsy, the lungs of these patients were severely destroyed. In contrast, Fowler et al. [7] reported that respiratory insufficiency was the major contributor in at least 75% of the deaths.

Different authors have recently studied the different factors and indicators of poor prognosis in ARDS patients [10, 12, 31]. The main factors which correlate with survival are age and the extent of multisystem failure [33, 34]. Among patients over 65 years of age, 81% died. The mortality rate is directly related to the number of complications, and increases to 86% when 3 or more complications are present. The survivors incurred an average of 1.4 complications whereas non-survivors developed an average of 2.6 complicating factors ($p < 0.005$). Shock and acute renal failure were associated to high mortality of 92% and 94%, respectively.

The most frequent complications appearing during the course of ARDS are shock and acute renal failure associated with a mortality over 90%. The majority of late deaths are related to sepsis syndrome present in 73% of ARDS patients [10, 33], where the predominant source is the lung. Several investigators indicate that sepsis syndrome, rather than respiratory failure, is the leading cause of death in patients with ARDS [8–10, 23, 24, 33].

Linear discriminant analysis has been performed for several physiologic cardiopulmonary variables during the first days of ARDS and correlation with the mortality to define prognostic factors has been analyzed. In the NHLBI ARDS studies [35] no variable or combination of variables were able to determine the survival or death for all groups. However, in the subgroup of patients with the highest mortality, effective compliance, alveolar-arterial O_2 difference (AaDO$_2$) and buffer-base deviation were the best predictors. All patients with an effective compliance below 25 ml/cm H$_2$O on the first day died [12].

Fowler et al. [31] recently found four variables significantly associated with mortality: presence of less than 10% band forms on the initial peripheral blood smear, persistent acidemia with arterial pH less than 7.40, calculated HCO$_3^-$ less than 20 mg/dl, and blood urea nitrogen greater than 65 mg/dl. After eliminating those variables that did not contribute significantly to mortality in the presence of the others, only low band forms, low pH, and low HCO$_3^-$ were significantly associated with increased mortality.

There is no difference in the initial gas exchange and hemodynamic variables between survivors and non-survivors, indicating a similar degree of pulmonary deterioration in the initial phase of ARDS [33, 37, 38] (Table 4). However, it is necessary to evaluate gas exchange parameters as prognostic factors in relation with the response to PEEP and the course of ARDS. Only the survivors presented a significant decrease in $\dot{Q}s/\dot{Q}t$ after PEEP had been applied [36], and a higher mortality rate was found by Lamy et al. [38] in patients having a "fixed shunt" with more severe and irreversible alterations in pulmonary morphology. The oscillations in arterial PO$_2$ and AaDO$_2$ indicate the evolution of the ARDS and may allow a prognosis. The persistence of values of AaDO$_2$ higher than 500

Table 4. Gasometric and hemodynamic data on admission in ARDS patients (mean ±SD)

	Survivors (n = 11)	Non-survivors (n = 24)	p-Value
FiO$_2$	0.75± 0.18	0.73± 0.18	NS
PaO$_2$ (torr)	86.4 ± 27.2	71.9 ± 32.5	NS
PaCO$_2$ (torr)	39.1 ± 12.6	37.3 ± 9.7	NS
VE (L/min)	13.8 ± 4.0	13.7 ± 3.3	NS
PEEP (cmH$_2$O)	8.1 ± 4.6	3.7 ± 3.9	<.025
Q̇sp/Q̇t (%)	27.0 ± 7.0	32.0 ± 10.0	NS
P(A-a)O$_2$ (torr)	402.7 ±120.8	414.7 ±126.5	NS
MSAP (mmHg)	85.4 ± 13.6	81.7 ± 9.4	NS
HR (beats/min)	109.0 ± 23.3	121.4 ± 17.6	NS
MPAP (mmHg)	21.3 ± 4.7	21.3 ± 3.2	NS
WP (mmHg)	9.6 ± 3.0	10.2 ± 2.9	NS
Cardiac output (L/min)	6.9 ± 2.7	5.6 ± 1.3	NS

VE = minute ventilation; MSAP = mean systemic arterial pressure; HR = heart rate; MPAP = mean pulmonary artery pressure; WP = wedge pressure; NS = non significant.

mmHg at FiO$_2$ 1, is a predictor of fatal outcome and associated to mortality in 100 per cent. Jardin et al. [39] proposed a respiratory severity index which considers the level of PEEP and FiO$_2$ and demonstrated a predictive value within the second day of treatment [34, 39]. A progressive increase of PaCO$_2$ in spite of increased ventilatory volume, an increase of V_D/V_T ratio over 70%, an increase of arterial-end-tidal CO$_2$ difference and a persistent high pulmonary vascular resistance are factors of poor prognosis, associated to morphological changes in the pulmonary circulation [36]. Determination of severity of illness or injury can be made by acute physiologic scores. Simplified acute physiologic score described by Le Gall et al. [40] can predict the prognosis in an intermediate phase of ARDS [33] (Fig. 2). This is due to major derangements of physiologic systems in non-survivors, and is clinically evidenced by a large number of complications.

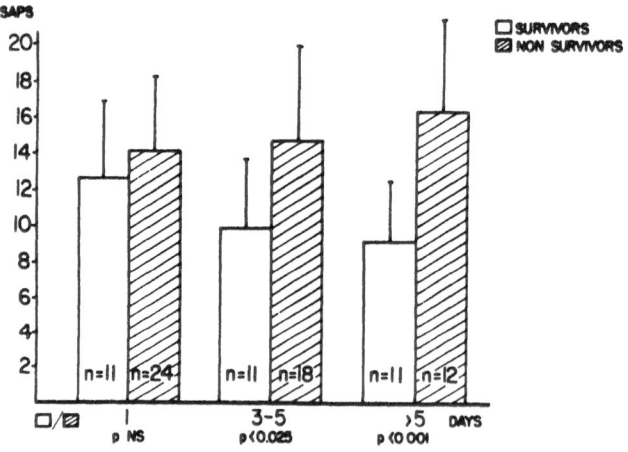

Fig. 2. Evolution of Simplified Acute Physiological Score (SAPS) in 35 ARDS patients

Biochemical and cellular mediators can predict the prognosis of ARDS. In a prospective study where different mediators were analyzed, antithrombin III, protein C, alpha-2-macroglobulin presented differences between survivors and non-survivors in an early phase of ARDS (Table 5). Progressive normalization of different biological variables leads to an improvement of ARDS [27, 41].

Long Term Recovery

Given the catastrophic degree of respiratory failure, the early presence of fibrosis in lung biopsy, the high mortality, and the high cost of trying to save these patients, what is the long term recovery rate of those who do survive?

Surprisingly, survivors of ARDS usually lose relatively little pulmonary function and are frequently able to return to their prior activities within 6 to 12 months after hospital discharge. Thus, the very poor short-term prognosis of ARDS is balanced by the potential for excellent long-term quality of life in survivors. Information on 237 ARDS survivors has been reported in 27 articles, but the discrepancy in the results is due to differences regarding severity of acute lung injury, follow-up times, premorbid pulmonary status, prior cigarette smoking, presence of nosocomial pneumonia, severity of hypoxemia and amount of oxygen received during mechanical ventilation [42–45]. Some of these factors are difficult to assess and many reports do not provide information on the different factors that can influence the results of the pulmonary function tests. Most ARDS survivors did not have prior pulmonary function tests, since they had been relatively healthy. Ideally, it would be reassuring to know that the pre-ARDS pulmonary function was normal before attributing the alterations of lung function to residue of ARDS. Table 6 indicates the number of patients and type of information provided in each report.

The most common types of physiologic defects reported in survivors of ARDS are: restrictive ventilatory defect, small airways obstruction, airway hyperreactivity, decrease gas exchange with a decrease in DLCO and hypoxemia with exer-

Table 5. Early prognostic factors (at 24 h) in ARDS

	Survivors (n = 13)	Non-survivors (n = 12)	P
Fibrinogen µg/l	5.47 ± 1.15	5.54 ± 2.40	NS
FDP µg/ml	8.2 ± 8.8	16.7 ± 23.5	NS
α_2 Macroglobulin (Ag) %	64.2 ± 17.4	52.4 ± 18.6	<0.05
α_2 Macroglobulin (Cs) %	66.2 ± 23.7	49.8 ± 24.3	<0.05
AT-III %	55.5 ± 11.9	41.2 ± 13.1	<0.02
Protein C %	47.9 ± 20.9	35.6 ± 14.9	<0.05
Factor VIII %	461.0 ± 195.0	639.0 ± 233.0	NS
Platelet Count, $10^3/mm^3$	168.0 ± 120.0	175.0 ± 96.0	NS
$P(A-a)O_2/PAO_2 + 0.014$ PEEP	0.87 ± 0.11	0.85 ± 0.12	NS
Simplified acute physiological score	14.0 ± 2.8	13.8 ± 3.3	NS

Table 6. Data available in various studies on ARDS survivors[a]

Authors/Year	Ref.	No of Patients	Age	Sex M/F	Clinical status	Chest Roentgeno-gram	Volume & Flow	Airways Resistance	Gas exchange Rest	Gas exchange Exercise	Gas exchange Shunt	D_LCO[b]
Ashbaugh et al. (1967)	[3]	9	34		*				*			
Interiano et al. (1972)	[46]	1	27	1/0		*		*			*	*
Downs and Olsen (1974)	[47]	1	16	0/1	*		*			*	*	*
Fine et al. (1974)	[48]	1	46	1/0		*	*	*		*		
Llamas (1974)	[49]	1	35	1/0	*	*	*					*
Yernault et al. (1975)	[50]	7	19	1/6	*	*	*					*
Glauser and Smith (1975)	[51]	1	42	1/0		*	*					
Lakshminarayan et al. (1976)	[52]	10	22	5/5	*	*	*	*		*	*	*
Klein et al. (1976)	[53]	10									*	
Fallat et al. (1976)	[54]	30								*	*	
Richardson et al. (1976)	[55]	2	61	2/0		*	*			*		*
Douglas and Downs (1977)	[56]	10	36	8/2	*	*	*			*	*	*
Rotman et al. (1977)	[57]	6	30	4/2	*	*	*	*		*		*
Yahaw et al. (1978)	[58]	15	26	13/2	*	*	*			*		*
Leechawengwong et al. (1979)	[59]	2	25	2/0	*	*	*					*
Bachofen and Bachofen (1979)	[60]	6	20	5/1	*	*	*	*		*		
Jenkinson and George (1980)	[61]	2	25	1/1		*	*					
Shaw et al. (1981)	[62]	2	43	2/0	*	*	*		*	*		*
Elliot et al. (1981)	[63]	13	30	6/7	*	*	*		*	*	*	*
Xaubet et al. (1981)	[64]	9			*	*	*				*	*
Bell et al. (1983)	[65]	25										*
Halevy et al. (1983)	[66]	18	39	12/6	*	*	*					*
Lakshminarayan et al. (1981)	[67]	3	28	1/2	*	*	*					*
Hudson (1984)	[68]	1	42	1/0	*	*	*					*
Artigas et al. (1984)	[42]	27	40	14/13	*	*	*		*	*		*
Buchser et al. (1985)	[69]	9		7/2		*	*	*	*	*	*	*
Elliot et al. (1985)	[70]	16	32			*	*				*	*

a Modified from Albert W. M. et al. [44]

b D_LCO = diffusing capacity for carbon monoxide.

cise or at rest. The pathology of ARDS reveals edema, congestion, alveolar exudates, hyaline membranes, cellular proliferation and fibrosis. It is not surprising that in the early phase of recovery, pulmonary function tests commonly reveal a restrictive pattern. Table 7 shows reported abnormalities of lung volumes, flow rates and DLCO at different intervals of time of recovery. Approximately one third of patients had restrictive physiology and half a decreased DLCO in the first 3 months. With time the restrictive pattern usually resolves and the DLCO rises toward normal. Restrictive ventilatory defect seems to be more related to polytrauma ARDS patients with thoracic trauma and rib fractures [71]. Decreases of expiratory flow rates may occur due to either increased airway resistance or loss of elastic recoil.

Most ARDS survivors had no airflow obstruction demonstrated by decreased forced expiratory volume in one second (FEV_1), decreased FEV_1/forced vital capacity (FVC) ratio. However, a significant number had reduced mid-expiratory flow rates (FEF_{25-75}) often accompanied by increases of RV, FRC, and RV/TLC ratio, with a marked ($>20\%$) improvement during the bronchodilator test, suggesting air trapping due to changes in the small airways. These data are best illustrated in the series of 27 severe ARDS survivors, non-smokers, without chest trauma and at 14 ± 8 months recovery period, studied by Artigas and colleagues [42] (Fig. 3).

Metacholine challenge testing and eucapnic hyperventilation revealed airways hyperreactivity in all cases with prior improvement of mid-expiratory flow rates over 20% after the inhalation of 200 μ of salbutamol. Pratt and associates noticed peribronchiolar and alveolar duct inflammation and fibrosis in patients dying from ARDS in the ECMO study, many of whom had received prolonged high levels of oxygen [72]. They suggested that this inflammatory process may be due, at least in part, to the oxygen itself. The clinical significance of the small airway obstruction and hyperreactive airways is not clear [73]. It would be logical to use bronchodilators for any clinical symptoms of obstruction.

Most patients have normal resting arterial blood gases, although some survivors have a diminished $PaCO_2$ and a few have hypoxemia ($PaO_2 < 80$ mmHg). Table 8 represents the mean values of 27 ARDS survivors, non-smokers, at rest and during exercise breathing air and pure oxygen [42]. The resting shunt fraction ($\dot{Q}s/\dot{Q}t$) was $4.5\pm2.6\%$ and alveolar-arterial oxygen gradient $AaDO_2$ was sligthly increased in 17 cases. These abnormalites in gas exchange are not due to

Table 7. Pulmonary function test results in survivors of ARDS[a]

	3 months (n = 34)	3 to 6 months (n = 23)	6 months (n = 105)
Restrictive pattern (TLC < 80%)	11 (32%)	6 (26%)	20 (19%)
Obstructive pattern (normal FEV_1 and $FEF_{25-75} < 70\%$)	4 (12%)	4 (17%)	17 (16%)
DLCO < 80%	15 (44%)	7 (57%)	22 (21%)
Normal	15 (44%)	13 (57%)	68 (65%)

[a] Data complied from the references listed in Table 6.

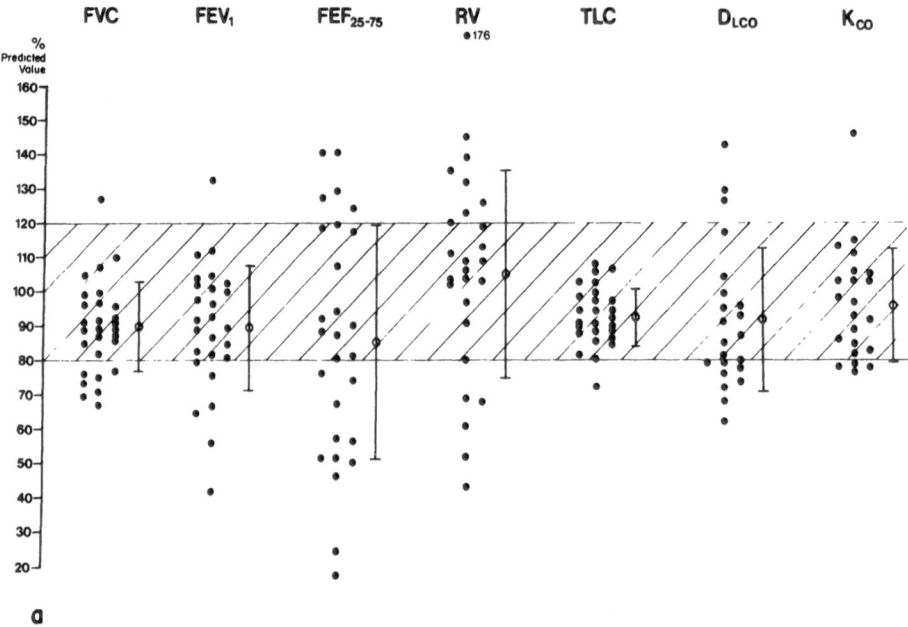

Fig. 3. Expiratory flow rates (FEV$_1$, FEF$_{25-75}$) lung volumes (FVC, RV, TLC) and lung diffusing capacity (DLco, Kco) in 27 ARDS survivors, without previous chronic lung disease or cigarette smoking, at 14±8 months after hospital discharge. Normal values were considered between 80% and 120% of their predicted values. Mean values are normal, but 11 patients showed a FEF$_{25-75}$ lower than 80% of the predicted value. Low DLco values normalized when the diffusing capacity was calculated in relationship to alveolar ventilation (DLco/V$_A$ = Kco)

emphysema because correction of the DLCO for alveolar volume results in normal values. Was this due to chronic vascular obstruction, or to the vascular remodeling that occurs during recovery from ARDS? Elliot et al. [63] demonstrated a normal response of decreasing V$_D$/V$_T$ during exercise as a function of CO$_2$ production, indicating that late chronic vascular obstruction is not an explanation for the decreased DLCO and gas exchange abnormalities. Buchser and co-workers [69] found that diffusing capacity and membrane transfer factor corrected for lung volume were normal, whereas the pulmonary capillary blood volume was significantly decreased to a mean of 49%, suggesting that most of the

Table 8. Gas exchange in 27 ARDS survivors

	Air	FiO$_2$1 (for 20 min)	Exercise (40 W for 10 min)
PaO$_2$, mmHg	84.0 ±10.0	569.0 ±31.0	82.0 ±10.0
PaO$_2$, mmHg	39.0 ± 3.0	38.0 ± 4.0	40.0 ± 2.0
pH	7.39± 0.02	7.42± 0.76	7.38± 0.01
Bicarbonate, mEq/l	23.7 ± 1.2	24.7 ± 0.7	23.2 ± 1.1
SaO$_2$, %	96.1 ± 1.0	99.9	95.7 ± 0.2

gas exchange abnormalities are not due to loss of alveolar gas exchange surface or to diffusion limitation of oxygen transfer, but to the decrease in, or abnormal arrangement of capillaries after ARDS.

Late pulmonary vascular hemodynamics at rest or during exercise in ARDS survivors have not been explored as there is little clinical indication for hemodynamic assessment after recovery. Non-invasive radionuclide techniques may help in the future to elucidate the hemodynamic evolution and the presence of fibrin deposits in the pulmonary circulation among ARDS survivors.

Acknowledgements: The author acknowledges the skillful assistance of Ms. Caroline Newey, Ms. Cuca Ayesta and Ms. Isabel Domenech in preparing the manuscript.

This work is supported by FISS grants No 83/809 and 87/909.

References

1. Petty TL, Fowler AA (1982) Another look at ARDS. Chest 82:98–104
2. Loyd JE, Newman JH, Brigham KL (1984) Permeability pulmonary edema: diagnosis and management. Arch Intern Med 144:143–147
3. Ashbough DG, Bigelow DB, Petty TL, Levine BE (1967) Acute respiratory distress in adults. Lancet 2:319–323
4. Pepe PE, Hudson LD, Carrico CJ (1984) Early application of positive end expiratory pressure in patients at risk for the adult respiratory distress syndrome. N Engl J Med 311:281–286
5. Zapol WM, Snider MT, Hill JD, et al (1979) Extracorporeal membrane oxygenation in severe acute respiratory failure. A randomized prospective study. JAMA 242:2193–2196
6. Gattinoni L, Pesenti A, Mascheroni D, et al (1986) Low-frequency positive-pressure ventilation with extracorporal CO_2 removal in severe acute respiratory failure. JAMA 256:881–886
7. Fowler AA, Hamman RF, Bood JT, et al (1983) Adult respiratory distress syndrome: risk with common predisposition. Ann Intern Med 98:593–597
8. Bell RC, Coalson JJ, Smith JD, Johanson WG (1983) Multiple organ system failure and infection in adult respiratory distress syndrome. Ann Intern Med 99:293–298
9. Pepe PE, Potkin RT, Reus DH, Hudson LD, Carrico CJ (1982) Clinical predictors of the adult respiratory distress syndrome. Am J Surg 144:124–130
10. Montgomery B, Stager MA, Carrico CJ, Hudson LD (1985) Causes of mortality in patients with the adult respiratory distress syndrome. Am Rev Respir Dis 132:485–489
11. Staub NS, Hogg JC (1981) Clinical measurement of lung water content. Chest 79:3–4
12. Maunder RJ, Shuman WP, McHugh JW, Marglin SI, Butler J (1986) Preservation of normal lung regions in the adult respiratory distress syndrome. Analysis by computed tomography. JAMA 255:2463–2465
13. Rinaldo JE (1986) The prognosis of the adult respiratory distress syndrome. Inappropiate pessimism? Chest 90:470–471
14. Pontoppidan H, Hüttemeier PC, Quinn DA (1985) Acute respiratory failure: etiology, demography and outcome. In: Zapol WM, Falke K (eds) Acute Respiratory Failure. Dekker M, New York, pp 1–21
15. Rinaldo JE, Rogers RM (1982) Adult respiratory distress syndrome: changing concepts of lung injury and repair. N Engl J Med 306:900–909
16. Hudson LD (1982) Causes of the adult respiratory distress syndrome: clinical recognition. Clin Chest Med 3:195–212

17. Colice GL, Haley JA (1984) Neurogenic pulmonary edema. Am Rev Respir Dis 130:941–948
18. Fischman CM, Goldstein MS, Gardner LB (1977) Suicidal hanging. An association with the respiratory distress syndrome. Chest 71:225
19. Jackson FN, Rowland V, Corssen G (1980) Laryngospasm-induced pulmonary edema. Chest 78:819
20. Andrews CP, Coalson JJ, Smith JD, Johanson G (1981) Diagnosis of nosocomial bacterial pneumonia in acute, diffuse lung injury. Chest 80:254–258
21. Lung Program, National Heart and Lung Institute (1972) Respiratory diseases: task force on problems, research approaches, needs, Washington, D.C. Government Printing Office, pp 171. (DHEW publication number (NIH) 73–432)
22. Maunder RJ (1985) Clinical prediction of the adult respiratory distress syndrome. Clin Chest Med 6:413–426
23. Fein AM, Lippmann M, Holtzman H, Eliraz A, Goldberg SK (1983) The risk factors, incidence, and prognosis of ARDS following septicemia. Chest 83:40–42
24. Kaplan RL, Sahn SA, Petty TL (1979) Incidence and outcome of the respiratory distress syndrome in gram-negative sepsis. Arch Intern Med 139:867–869
25. Idell S, Cohen AB (1985) Bronchoalveolar lavage in patients with the adult respiratory distress syndrome. Clin Chest Med 6:459–472
26. Schapira M, Gardaz JP, Py P, et al (1985) Prekallikrein activation in the adult respiratory distress syndrome. Bull Eur Physiopathol Respir 21:237–241
27. Fontcuberta J, Artigas A, Sala N, et al (1986) Inhibitors of blood coagulation in adult respiratory distress syndrome. Intens Care Med 12:224
28. Hollgren R, Borg T, Venge P, et al (1984) Signs of neutrophil and eosinophil activation in adult respiratory distress snydrome. Crit Care Med 12:14–18
29. Carvalho AC, Bellman SM, Saullo VJ, et al (1982) Altered factor VIII in acute respiratory failure. N Engl J Med 307:1113–1119
30. Fourrier E, Chopin C, Wallaert B, et al (1985) Compared evolution of plasma fibronectin and angiotensin-converting enzyme levels in septic ARDS. Chest 87:191–195
31. Fowler AA, Hamman RF, Zerbe GO, Benson KN, Hyers TM (1985) Adult Respiratory Distress Syndrome: prognosis after onset. Am Rev Respir Dis 132:472–478
32. Estopa R, Torres A, Kastanos N, Rives A, Agusti A, Rozman C (1984) Acute respiratory failure in severe hematologic disorders. Crit Care Med 12:26–28
33. Mancebo J, Artigas A (1987) A clinical study of the adult respiratory distress syndrome. Crit Care Med 15:243–246
34. Artigas A, Mancebo J (1987) Etiology and multiple organ system failure as prognostic factors in ARDS. In: Vincent JL (ed) Update 1987. Springer, Berlin Heidelberg New York London Paris Tokyo (Update in Intensive Care and Emergency Medicine, vol 3, pp 163–169)
35. National Heart, Lung and Blood Institute, Division of Lung Diseases (1979) Extracorporeal Support for Respiratory Insufficiency: A Collaborative Study. NIH, Bethesda, Maryland
36. De Latorre FJ, Estopá R, Artigas A (1983) Intercambio gaseoso como factor pronóstico en el síndrome de distress respiratorio de l adulto. Med Intensiva 7:1–6
37. Artigas A, Estopa R, De Latorre FJ (1981) Hemodynamic and gas exchange disorders as prognostic factors in the adult respiratory distress syndrome (Abstract). Crit Care Med 9:199
38. Lamy M, Fallat RJ, Koeniger E, et al (1976) Pathologic features and mechanisms of hypoxemia in adult respiratory distress syndrome. Am Rev Respir Dis 114:267–284
39. Jardin F, Prost JF, Bazin M, Desfond P, Ozier Y, Margairez A (1982) Modalités évolutives du syndrome de détresse respiratoire aigüe de l'adulte: Valeur pronostique d'un indice de gravité tiré de l'oxygénation artérielle. Nouv Press Med 11:29–33
40. Le Gall JR, Loirat P, Alperovitch A (1983) Simplified acute physiological score for intensive care patients, Lancet 2:741
41. Artigas A, Fontcuberta J, Castella J, Rutllant M (1985) Coagulation disorders in the adult respiratory distress syndrome. In: Vincent JL (ed) Update in Intensive Care and Emergency Medicine. Springer, Berlin Heidelberg New York Tokyo (Anesthesiology and Intensive Care Medicine, vol 178, pp 84–88)

42. Artigas A (1984) Evaluation pulmonaire des malades survivant à un syndrome de détresse respiratoire aiguë de l'adulte. In: Lemaire F (ed) Le syndrome de détresse respiratoire aiguë de l'adulte. Masson, Paris, pp 125–136

43. Ingbar DH, Matthay RA (1986) Pulmonary sequelae and lung repair in survivors of the adult respiratory distress syndrome. Crit Care Clin 2:629–665

44. Alberts WM, Priest GR, Moser KM (1983) The outlook for survivors of ARDS. Chest 84:272–274

45. Lakshminarayan S, Hudson LD (1978) Pulmonary function following the adult respiratory distress syndrome. Chest 74:489–490

46. Interiano B, Stuard ID, Hyde RW (1972) Acute respiratory distress syndrome in pancreatitis. Ann Intern Med 77:923–927

47. Downs JB, Olsen GN (1974) Pulmonary function following adult respiratory distress syndrome. Chest 65:92–93

48. Dine NL, Myerson DA, Myerson PJ, et al (1974) Near-drowing presenting as the adult respiratory distress syndrome. Chest 65:347–349

49. Llamas R (1974) Adult respiratory distress syndrome: Report of survival after two episodes. Chest 65:468–469

50. Yernault JC, Englert M, Sergysels R (1977) Follow-up of pulmonary function after "shock lung". Bull Eur Physiopathol Respir 13:241–248

51. Glauser FL, Smith WR (1975) Pulmonary interstitial fibrosis following near drowning and exposure to short term high oxygen concentration. Chest 68:373–375

52. Lakshminarayan S, Stanfor RE, Petty TL (1976) Prognosis after recovery from adult respiratory distress syndrome. Am Rev Respir Dis 113:7–16

53. Klein JJ, Van Haeringen JR, Shurter HJ (1976) Pulmonary function after recovery from the adult respiratory distress syndrome. Chest 69:350–355

54. Fallat RJ, Tucker HJ, Segovia L (1976) Lung function in long term survivors from severe respiratory distress syndrome. Am Rev Respir Dis 113:118A

55. Richardson JV, Light RW, Baskin TL, et al (1976) Late pulmonary function in survivors of adult respiratory distress syndrome. South Med J 69:735–737

56. Douglas ME, Downs JB (1977) Pulmonary function following severe acute respiratory failure and high levels of positive end expiratory pressure. Chest 71:18–23

57. Rotmann HH, Lavelle RF, Jr, Dimcheff DG (1977) Long term physiologic consequences of the adult respiratory distress syndrome. Chest 72:190–192

58. Yahav J, Lieberman P, Molho M (1978) Pulmonary function following the adult respiratory distress syndrome. Chest 74:247–250

59. Leechawenfgwong M, Berger HW, Jayamanne DS (1986) Long term serial follow-up after two episodes of heroin-induced adult respiratory distress syndrome. Mt Sinai J Med 35:119–121

60. Bachofen M, Bachofen H (1979) Der Heilungsverlauf des schweren "adult respiratory distress syndrome". Schweiz Med Wochenschr 109:1982–1989

61. Jenkinson SG, George RB (1980) Serial pulmonary function studies in survivors of near drowning. Chest 77:777–780

62. Shaw RA, Whitcomb ME, Schonfeld SA (1981) Pulmonary function after adult respiratory distress syndrome associated with Legionnaire's disease pneumonia. Arch Intern Med 141:741–742

63. Elliott CG, Morris AH, Cengiz M (1981) Pulmonary function and exercise gas exchange in survivors of adult respiratory distress syndrome. Am Rev Respir Dis 123:492–495

64. Xaubet A, Naulart Ll, Estopa R, Rodriguez Roisin R, Agusti Vidal A (1981) Evolución clínica, radiológica y funcional respiratoria del síndrome de distres respiratorio del adulto (ARDS). Med Clin (Barc) 76:291–295

65. Bell RC, Prihoda TJ, Andrews CP, et al (1983) Long term pulmonary function in survivors of adult and respiratory distress syndrome and clinical determinant of abnormalities (abstract) Chest 84:343

66. Halevy A, Sirik Z, Adam YG, et al (1984) Long-term evaluation of patients following the adult respiratory distress syndrome. Respir Care 29:132–137

67. Lakshminarayan S, Hudson LD (1981) Pulmonary function following adult respiratory distress syndrome. Semin Respir Med 11:160–164

68. Hudson LD (1983) Prognosis: Immediate and long-term sequelae of acute respiratory failure. Respir Care 2:663–671
69. Buchser E, Leuenberger P, Chiolero R, et al (1985) Reduced pulmonary capillary blood volume as a long term sequel of ARDS. Chest 87:609–611
70. Elliott CG, Rasmussen B, Crapo RD, et al (1985) Predictors of pulmonary function abnormalities after adult respiratory distress syndrome. Chest 88:638 (Abstract)
71. Hanning CD, Ledingham E, Ledingham IMcA (1980) Late respiratory sequelae of blunt chest injury. Intens Care Med 6:26 (Abstract)
72. Pratt PC, Volmer RT, Shellburne JD, et al (1979) Pulmonary morphology in a multihospital collaborative extracorporeal membrane oxygenation project. I. Light microscopy. Am J Pathol 95:191–214
73. Simpson DL, Goodman M, Spector SL (1978) Long term follow-up and bronchial reactivity testing in survivors of the adult respiratory distress syndrome. Am Rev Respir Dis 117:449–454

Role of Arachidonic Acid Metabolism in ARDS

D. R. Morel

Introduction

Arachidonic acid (AA), an unsaturated fatty acid directly from the diet or indirectly from the metabolism of linoleic acid, is released from the breakdown of cell membrane phospholipids by the action of the enzyme phospholipase A_2. Numerous stimuli, ranging from simple mechanical to specific chemical stimulation may activate what has been named the arachidonic acid cascade. Phospholipase A_2 itself can be inhibited by corticosteroids and local anesthetics which therefore are able to modulate the generation of AA.

Arachidonic acid is metabolized through two major metabolic pathways (Fig. 1). The cyclooxygenase enzyme converts free AA into a cyclized endoperoxide intermediate PGH_2 which is further metabolized to the bisenoic prostaglandins PGD_2, PGE_2 and $PGF_{2\alpha}$, to thromboxane A_2 (TxA_2), or to prostacylin (PGI_2). The generation of these active metabolites is for the most part a function of the availability of the precursor substrate rather than of the activity of a specific enzyme. However, the relative amount of each of these metabolites depends on specific enzymes, especially prostacyclin synthetase and thromboxane synthe-

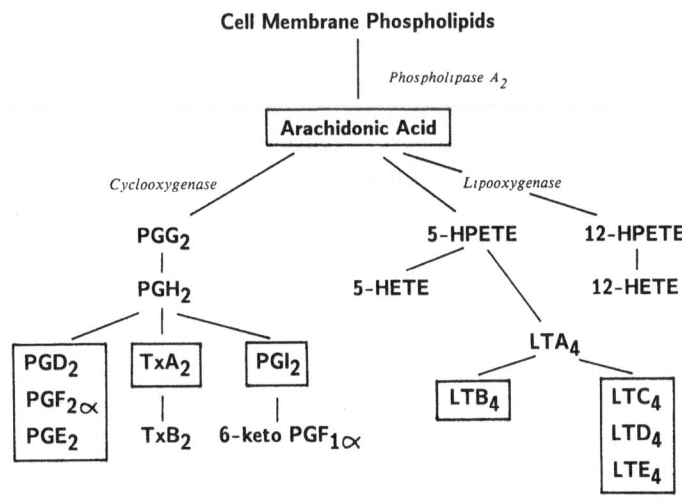

Fig. 1. Simplified metabolic pathways of arachidonic acid. Metabolites enclosed in boxes are considered to be the acitve mediators of this cascade

tase. Prostacyclin is synthetized mainly by endothelial cells, whereas thromboxane is mainly produced by platelets, peripheral blood polymorphonuclear (PMN) leukocytes and macrophages.

The alternative oxidative pathway of AA is initiated by several lipooxygenases, especially the 5-lipooxygenase, generating the chemotactic leukotriene B_4 (LTB$_4$) and the sulfidopeptide leukotrienes LTC$_4$, LTD$_4$, and LTE$_4$.

Several metabolites of both pathways of the AA cascade (which are referred to collectively as eicosanoids) are potent vasoactive and proinflammatory mediators that may reasonably be implicated in the pathogenesis of the adult respiratory distress syndrome (ARDS). However, to assess a potential role of a mediator to the pathogenesis of ARDS, several criteria should be fulfilled. First, the appearance of a significant increase in the concentration of the potential mediator should be found in local body fluids and/or in the circulating blood of patients with ARDS or animal models of the human disease. Second, the administration of the active mediator to experimental animals should reproduce consistent pathophysiologic effects similar to the ones observed during the human syndrome, and the degree of the effects should be correlated with increasing concentrations of the mediator. Third, by either inhibiting the synthesis or by antagonizing its effects at receptor sites one should be able to attenuate or even completely inhibit the pathological effect attributed to the mediator, again establishing a dose-response relationship. The aim of this chapter is to review whether these criteria have been fulfilled in the numerous experimental studies working with animal models as well as in clinical investigations in patients with ARDS and thus to evaluate the relative importance of these eicosanoids in the pathogenesis of ARDS.

Biological Effects of Arachidonic Acid Metabolites Relevant to ARDS

Thromboxane A$_2$

In vitro studies have demonstrated that TxA$_2$ causes rapid, irreversible platelet aggregation and the associated platelet release reaction [1]. It also provokes contraction of vascular and tracheal smooth muscle [2]. TxA$_2$ has a half-life of only 30–40 sec in aquous media at physiological temperature and pH [1]. It is then further metabolized to the biologically inactive and stable TxB$_2$ which can be measured by radioimmunoassay and therefore serves to document the generation of TxA$_2$.

Because of its short biological half-life, the physiological effects of TxA$_2$ have been difficult to document in vivo, but it appears from numerous studies infusing stable precursors of TxA$_2$ or specific end-organ antagonists, that TxA$_2$ is the most potent endogenous vasoconstrictor thus far known. In addition, despite its short half-life, its effects are multiplied by the fact that locally activated platelets will release additional TxA$_2$ which will in turn aggregate other uninvolved platelets, therefore leading by a positive feedback mechanism to a spatial and temporal propagation of the initial local process.

Prostaglandins

The primary protaglandins PGD_2, PGE_2 and $PGF_{2\alpha}$ have been shown to produce vaso- and bronchoconstriction in most species, with a large variation in the magnitude of the response among species [3]. In humans, the bronchoconstrictor effects of these prostaglandins has been demonstrated [4]. Since there are no specific inhibitors of these prostaglandins available, their respective role in physiological and pathological situations has been difficult to establish. Their synthesis is blocked by cyclooxygenase inhibitors (e.g. nonsteroidal antiinflammatory agents) which also block TxA_2 and PGI_2. At present, most investigators attribute a minor role to these primary prostaglandins in pathological situations when compared to TxA_2 and PGI_2.

Prostacyclin (PGI_2) has opposite effects to TxA_2. It inhibits platelet aggregation and disaggregates ADP-induced platelet clumps, both in vitro and in vivo [5]. Furthermore, PGI_2 is major pulmonary and systemic vaso- and bronchodilator and is the only metabolic product of AA that dilates the mature pulmonary vascular bed [6]. The dilator property of PGI_2 is not readily apparent under physiologic circumstances because the pulmonary bed is already in a dilated state.

PGI_2 is hydrolyzed within 3 to 8 minutes to the stable inactive metabolite 6-Keto-$PGF_{1\alpha}$, which serves as indicator of the in vivo formation of the active compound. In contrast to PGI_2, the metabolism of the primary prostaglandins to inactive metabolites is limited by the availability of an active transport mechanism enabling uptake of these prostaglandins from the pulmonary vascular bed into endothelial cells. During ARDS, a decreased metabolic function of the pulmonary endothelial cells will decrease the uptake of primary prostaglandins [7], possibly resulting in increased vaso- and bronchoconstriction. Furthermore, the decreased lung endothelial surface occurring during ARDS will decrease the amount of the continuous synthesis of prostacyclin, which normally maintains the pulmonary circulatory bed in a dilated state, therefore increasing pulmonary arterial pressure.

Prostaglandins have also been shown to be able to increase vascular permeability, although being much less active than histamine or bradykinin [8, 9]. They nevertheless appear to cause a marked potentiation of endogenous inflammatory reactions which is probably due to local vasodilation and/or contraction, resulting in an increased hydrostatic pressure gradient and local edema formation.

Leukotrienes

Unlike the prostaglandins, some of which play important roles as biological regulators, the action of lipooxygenase products appear to be exclusively of a pathological nature. The metabolites of 5-HPETE (Fig. 1) are biologically active substances that have been named leukotrienes and which appear to be potent mediators of immediate and subacute hypersensitivity reactions [10]. The leukotrienes are synthetized by a large variety of cell types, including circulating PMN leukocytes, alveolar macrophages, and lung mast cells. LTB_4 is a potent chemotactic and chemokinetic factor for human PMN leukocytes, and promotes the release of leukocytic lysosomial enzymes, whereas the sulfidopeptide leukotrienes LTC_4, LTD_4, and LTE_4 are potent vaso- and bronchoconstrictors and alter the permeability and tone of the microvasculature in skin and other tissues [11]. In addition, the leukotrienes modulate also the release of cyclooxygenase metabolites, especially TxA_2 [12, 13], as well as histamine [14], indicating that at least part of their effects may be related to the formation of other mediators in vivo.

Arachidonic Acid

In intact-chest cat and dog lungs, a rapid AA infusion produces a dose-related vaso- and bronchoconstriction, whereas a slow infusion produces a vaso- and bronchodilation [15]. Both the pressor and dilator responses to AA are blocked by the cyclooxygenase inhibitor indomethacin. These results indicate first that the pulmonary vascular effects of AA are solely mediated by cyclooxygenase metabolites, and second, that the enzymatic formation of the constrictor TxA_2 and the dilator PGI_2 is a function of PGH_2 availability. As AA substrate is increased, it exceeds the level of saturation of PGI_2 synthetase, but not that of TxA_2 synthetase, resulting in a high TxA_2/PGI_2 ratio and a constrictor response, whereas during a slow infusion, a low PGH_2 concentration results in a low TxA_2/PGI_2 ratio with a dilator response [15]. This interesting phenomenon may provide a possible explanation for the divergent responses between acute and subacute models or clinical situations inducing the activation of the AA cascade.

In chronically instrumented awake sheep, rapid intravenous infusion of purified sodium AA increases pulmonary vascular resistance in a dose-related fashion [16]. This effect is inhibited by prior cyclooxygenase blockade, indicating that the effect of AA is mediated through the formation of prostaglandin endoperoxides, including TxA_2. In addition, in this model as well as in isolated perfused canine [17] or guinea pig lungs [18], AA infusion does not increase lung vascular permeability, suggesting that in an intact pulmonary circulation the vasoactive cyclooxygenase metabolites do not increase pulmonary microvascular permeability and that exogenous AA is not converted to sufficient amounts of proinflammatory 5-lipooxygenase metabolites such as to attribute a significant role to leukotrienes in this situation. In addition, these recent studies have demonstrated that the site of the pulmonary vasoconstriction is postcapillary [17, 18] and that it depends on the generation of TxA_2 from lung parenchymal cells as well as from blood-formed elements [18].

In rabbits, a rapid intravenous injection of sodium AA has been shown to produce sudden death due to prominent coronary artery vasospasm and massive vascular thrombosis [19]. This effect is prevented by pretreatment with thromboxane synthetase inhibitors [20], further indicating that TxA_2 is the active mediator and that other bisenoic prostaglandins or lipooxygenase metabolites are not involved during acute reactions induced by exogenous AA administration.

Increased Body Fluid Levels of Arachidonic Acid Metabolites in Animal Models of ARDS and in Patients with ARDS

Animal Models

There is a large evidence that the AA cascade is activated by numerous stimuli which are present at the onset or during the course of ARDS. First, several experimental conditions that are associated with respiratory failure have been shown to influence the production of PGI_2, including alveolar hypoxia [21, 22] pulmonary vasoconstriction induced by angiotensin II [23], increased flow and sympathetic stimulation [24], or simply stretching of the pulmonary endothelium by hyperinflation and positive end expiratory pressure [25].

Second, in animal models of acute lung injury following PMN leukocyte activation by various stimuli including intravenous infusion of activated complement [26], phorbol myristate acetate [27], oleic acid [28] or endotoxins [29, 30], induction of intravascular generation of oxygen radicals [31], or following pulmonary embolism [32], there is a large increase in the concentration of the stable TxA_2 metabolite TxB_2 in plasma or pulmonary lymph associated with these different experimental situations. Furthermore, the time course between increased TxB_2 levels and pulmonary vasoconstriction and/or altered gas exchange and lung mechanics strongly suggests a cause-effect relationship, attributing the observed physiologic responses to thromboxane. Finally, in all of these experimental conditions, a selective pretreatment with either a cyclooxygenase- or thromboxane-synthetase inhibitor prevented both the rise in TxB_2 and the pulmonary vascular effect. However, thromboxane inhibition could not prevent the subsequent lung injury manifested by an increased pulmonary vascular permeability.

In contrast to the cyclooxygenase metabolites of AA, the pathogenic role of the 5-lipooxygenase-derived leukotrienes in vivo is difficult to evaluate because of the rapid "inactivation" of these substances in plasma or whole blood. Indeed their concentrations have been measured in far larger quantities in physiological salt solutions than in blood. This may be due to the fact that leukotriene binding by albumin appears to be a mechanism which may confine the leukotriene action to the site of their origin [33]. Furthermore, the lack of selective leukotriene synthetase inhibitors and specific end-organ antagonists, most of them being either unstable or nonspecific, i.e. inhibiting also other AA metabolites or having other nonspecific effects such as being free radical scavengers, makes it difficult to determine the respective role of leukotrienes in pathological situations.

Although the generation of sulfidopeptide leukotrienes, the active components of SRS-A, is usually associated with hypersensitivity reactions, there is recent evidence that leukotrienes may also be implicated in nonimmunologic reactions, such as endotoxemia [29, 34, 35], brain ischemia [36], or mechanical and thermal trauma [37]. Bremm et al. [35] first demonstrated that human PMN granulocytes incubated with endotoxins and lipid A release significant amounts of LTC_4 and LTD_4. In their classical chronically instrumented awake sheep model given intravenous E. coli endotoxin, the group of Brigham et al. measured increased lung lymph levels of the inactive lipooxygenase metabolites 5-HETE [34] as well as 12-HETE [29] during the 2–3 hours following the induction of acute endotoxemia. Recently however, the same group could not find evidence of release of sulfidopeptide leukotrienes measured by radioimmunoassay in sheep lung lymph, and pretreatment of the animals with the lipooxygenase inhibitor diethylcarbamazine did not significantly modify the response to endotoxin by and measured variable [38], indicating that lipooxygenase products of AA are probably not major active mediators of endotoxemia in vivo.

ARDS Patients

Recently, several investigators have documented elevated plasma TxB_2, or 6-keto $PGF_{1\alpha}$ concentrations in patients with ARDS or sepsis [39–44]. Reines et al. indicated that in patients dying from septic shock, the venous plasma concentration of TxB_2 [39] or 6-keto $PGF_{1\alpha}$ [40] was significantly higher than in survivors of septic shock or patients without shock. Similarly, Lamy et al. found highly abnormal TxB_2 plasma values on at least one occasion in 70% of their ARDS patients [40], with a significant correlation between the degree of ARDS and TxB_2 levels, therefore confirming the previous observation associating high TxB_2 levels and clinical severity. However, the large variance of intra- and inter-patient plasma TxB_2 or 6-keto $PGF_{1\alpha}$ concentrations and the fact that on one hand some patients without ARDS have high levels and that on the other hand about 25% of ARDS patients have no significant elevation of TxB_2 [41] makes it difficult to attribute a consistent effect of these cyclooxygenase metabolites to the pathophysiology of ARDS or septic shock. The occasional concomitant use of non-steroidal anti-inflammatory drugs given for hyperthermia during the course of these clinical studies and the possible confounding influence of other inhibitory or excitatory mechanisms of eicosanoid generation may partly explain the observed variability, but it seems more likely that in these clinical situations, in contrast to the experimental animal models of ARDS, plasma levels of 6-keto $PGF_{1\alpha}$ or TxB_2 are nonspecific and late markers of ARDS or sepsis, rather than determinant pathophysiologic mediators.

Supporting this hypothesis, two recent studies have investigated the acute hemodynamic and gasometric effects of dazoxiben, a selective thromboxane synthetase inhibitor, in patients who had developed ARDS [43, 44]. Although the drug was able to significantly reduce TxB_2 levels as well as platelet TxB_2 production, both studies indicate that no significant change in pulmonary hemodynamics, gas exchange, or extravascular lung water were observed following drug administration. These results of course do not rule out that TxA_2 may play a significant role in the initiation of the pulmonary hypertension or platelet aggregation and activation in human ARDS, but large prospective, controlled investigations using specific pretreatment agents in patients at risk of developing this syndrome are needed to determine the exact role of TxA_2 and PGI_2 in the pathogenesis of ARDS.

Because of the difficulty to characterize lipooxygenase products of AA in plasma (as already mentioned for animal investigations), it is still too early to evaluate the relative role of these potent proinflammatory metabolites in human

ARDS. There are a few reports mentioning elevated edema fluid levels of LTC_4 and LTD_4 in humans. Creticos et al. [45] first documented a dose-dependent release of sulfidopeptide leukotrienes in nasal fluids of ragweed-sensitive patients challenged with pollen grains. Stenmark et al [46] identified leukotrienes in pulmonary lavage fluids of neonates with hypoxemia and pulmonary hypertension, and finally Matthay et al [47] found elevated concentration of LTD_4 in pulmonary lavage fluids of ARDS patients, while the concentrations of LTC_4, TxB_2 and prostaglandin E_2 were not significantly different than in patients with cardiogenic pulmonary edema. These studies confirm the in vitro and animal experiments producing the release of 5-lipoxygenase metabolites during various inflammatory reactions in humans. However, further studies with large prospective specific inhibitor studies will be required to define whether the leukotrienes play a significant pathogenic role and may contribute to the permeability defect occurring in ARDS or whether these mediators are only an epiphenomenon (at least in this syndrome).

Conclusions

During the past decade, numerous experimental studies have demonstrated the activation of the AA cascade, resulting particularly in increased plasma levels of cyclooxygenase metabolites, associated with acute respiratory insufficiency induced in various animal models of ARDS. In some situations, the inhibition of selective metabolic pathways of the AA metabolism resulted in the attenuation or even complete prevention of specific physiologic effects, particularly the vasoactive effects, implying a pathophysiological role attributed to these metabolites. However, the clinical course and the mediator profile observed in patients with ARDS is quite different from the ones seen in animal models in which respiratory distress is induced within minutes or a few hours, so that the relevance of the various models may be questioned.

Some recent studies with fecal peritonits rat models have emphasized the difference in the profile of AA metabolites between the acute overwhelming compared to the more gradual development of an endotoxic or septic process. Whereas TxA_2 has been demonstrated to be the major determinant mediator of the early pulmonary hypertensive response to the bolus endotoxin infusion in various animal species, including primates, and may be implicated for its lethal outcome at least in rats [48], subacute models of fecal peritonitis are not accompanied by similar increases in thromboxane [49, 50]. Interestingly, 6-keto $PGF_{1\alpha}$, which is also increased during acute endotoxemia, shows a later (6-24 hr) peak after induction of subacute shock, which is a pattern resembling much more the human course and mediator profile [40, 51]. It is conceivable that elevated plasma TxA_2 levels occur only when the septic process is severe enough to cause death, a hypothesis supported by human investigations in which a correlation between occasional high plasma TxB_2 levels and the severity of the septic process has been described [39]. These data suggest that AA metabolites, contrary to the generally accepted view resulting particularly from the various acute endotoxin-sepsis models, may not be major determinants of septicemia and acute respiratory failure, but rather a nonspecific host's response to injury [29, 49, 50].

In conclusion, whereas there is no doubt that the AA metabolism may be stimulated during various pathological conditions found in the time course of ARDS and that both cyxclooxygenase and lipooxygenase metabolites fulfill the criteria for a mediator of an acute inflammatory process such as seen during ARDS, it is still too early to tell whether they are significantly implicated in the *pathogenesis* of ARDS in humans. To date, is seems more likely that AA metabolites (at least alone) are not primary pathogenic factors in the development of ARDS, since inhibition of the cyclooxygenase metabolism has been shown to prevent only the acute and transient pulmonary vasoconstriction in experimental animals, and to be ineffective in patients with established ARDS. Furthermore, inhibition of the lipooxygenase pathway in animal models of ARDS had no significant effect on the development of lung injury induced by endotoxin infusion. Since in humans no similar pretreatment studies have been reported so with specific antagonists will be necessary to determine the exact role of AA metabolites in the pathogenesis of ARDS.

References

1. Hamberg MJ, Svensson J, Samuelsson B (1975) Thromboxanes: a new group of biologically active compounds derived from prostaglandin endoperoxides. Proc Natl Acid Sci USA 72:2994–2998
2. Svensson J, Hamberg M, Samulsson B (1975) Prostaglandin endoperoxides. IX. Characterization of rabit aorta contracting substances (RCS) from guinea pig lung and human platelets. Acta Physiol Scand 94:222–228
3. Hyman AL, Mathé AA, Lippton HL, Kadowitz PJ (1981) Prostaglandins and the lung. Med Clin North Am 65:789–808
4. Mathé AA, Hedqvist P (1975) Effects of prostaglandins $F_{2\alpha}$ and E_2 on airway conductance in healthy sujects and asthmatic patients. Am Rev Respir Dis 111:313–320
5. Hyman, AL, Kadowitz PJ (1979) Pulmonary vasodilator activity of prostacyclin (PGI_2) in the cat. Circ Res 42:404–409
6. Kadowitz PJ, Chapnick BM, Feigen LP, Hymann AL, Nelson PK, Spannhake EW (1978) Pulmonary and systemic vasodilator effects of the newly discovered prostaglandin, PGI_2. J Appl Physiol 45:408–413
7. Gillis CN, Pitt BR, Wiedemann HP, Hammond GL (1986) Depressed prostaglandin E_1 and 5-hydroxytryptamine removal in patients with adult respiratory distress syndrome. Am Rev Respir Dis 134:739–744
8. Williams TJ, Morley J (1973) Prostaglandins as potentiator of increased vascular permeability in inflammation. Nature 246:215–217
9. Komoriya K, Ohmori H, Azuma A, Kurozumi S, Hashimoto Y (1978) Prostaglandin I_2 as a potentiator of acute inflammation in rats Prostaglandins 15:557–564
10. Samuelsson B, Hammarstrom S. Murphy RC, Borgeat P (1980) Leukotrienes and slow reacting substance of anaphylaxis (SRS-A). Allergy 35:375–381
11. Hedqvist P, Dahlen SE, Gustafsson L, Hammarstrom S, Samuelsson B (1980) Biological profile of leukotriene C_4 and D_4. Acta Physiol Scand 110:331–333
12. Noonan TC, Malik AB (1986) Pulmonary vascular response to leukotriene D_4 in unanesthetized sheep: role of thromboxane. J Appl Physiol 60:765–769
13. Piper PJ, Samhoun MN (1982) Stimulation of arachidonic acid metabolism and generation of thromboxane A_2 by leukotrienes B_4, C_4 and D_4 in guinea-pig lung in vitro. Br J Pharmac 77:267–275

14. Peters SP, Siegel MI, Kagey-Sobotka A, Lichtenstein LM (1981) Lipooxygenase products moulate histamine release in human basophils. Nature 292:455-457
15. Kadowitz PJ, McNamara DB, She HS, Spannhake EW, Hyman AL (1981) Arachidonic acid responses in the lung. Bull Europ Physiopath Resp 17:659-673
16. Ogletree ML, Brigham KL (1980) Arachidonate raises vascular resistance but not permeability in lungs of awake sheep. J Appl Physiol 48:581-586
17. Townsley MI, Korthius RJ, Taylor AE (1985) Effects of arachidonate on permeability and resistance distribution in canine lungs. J Appl Physiol 58:206-210
18. Selig WM, Noonan TC, Kern DF, Malik AB (1986) Pulmonary microvascular responses to arachidonic acid in isolated perfused guinea pig lung. J Appl Physiol 60:1972-1979
19. Silver MJ, Hoch W, Kocsis JJ, Ingerman CM, Smith JB (1974) Arachidonic acid causes sudden death in rabbits. Science 138:1085-1087
20. Puig-Perellada P, Planas JM (1977) Action of selective inhibitors of thromboxane-synthetase on experimental thrombosis induced by arachidonic acid in rabbits. Lancet 1:40
21. Said SI, Yoshida T, Kitamura S, Vreim C (1974) Pulmonary alveolar hypoxia: release of prostaglandins and other humoral mediators. Science 185:1181-1183
22. Sprague RS, Stephenson AH, Lonigro AJ (1984) Prostaglandin I_2 supports blood flow to hypoxic alveoli in anesthetized dogs. J Appl Physiol 56:1246-1251
23. Voelkel NF, Gerber JG,m McMurtry IF, Nies AS, Reeves JT (1981) Release of vasodilator prostaglandin, PGI_2, from isolated rat lung during vasoconstriction. Circ Res 48:207-213
24. Ellsworth ML, Gregory TJ, Newell JC (1983) Pulmonary prostacyclin production with increased flow and sympathetic stimulation. J Appl Physiol 55:1225-1232
25. Berend N, Christopher KL, Voelkel NF (1982) The effect of positive end-expiratory pressure on functional residual capacity: role of prostaglandin production. Am Rev Respir Dis 126:646-647
26. Perkowski SZ, Havill AM, Flynn JT, Gee MH (1983) Role of intrapulmonary release of eicosanoids and superoxide anion as mediators of pulmonary dysfunction and endothelial injury in sheep with intermittent complement activation. Circ Res. 53:574-583
27. Newman JH, Loyd JE, Ogletree ML, Meyrick O, Brigham KL (1984) Cyclooxygenase inhibition during phorbol-induced granulocyte stimulation in awake sheep. J Appl Physiol 56:999-1007
28. Olanoff LS, Reines HD, Spicer KM, Halushka PV 61984) Effects of oleic acid on pulmonary capillary leak and thromboxanes. J Surg Res 36:597-605
29. Ogletree ML, Begley CJ, King GA, Brigham KL (1986) Influence of steroidal and nonsteroidal anti-inflammatory agents on the accumulation of arachidonic acid metabolites in plasma and lung lymph after endotoxemia in awake sheep. Am Rev Respir Dis 133:55-61·
30. Snapper JR, Hutchison AA, Ogletree ML, Brigham KL (1983) Effects of cyclooxygenase inhibitors on the alterations in lung mechanics caused by endotoxemia in the unanesthetized sheep. J Clin Invest 72:63-76
31. Tate RM, Morris HG, Schroeder WR, Repine JE (1984) Oxygen metabolites stimulate thromboxane production and vasoconstriction in isolated saline-perfused lungs. J Clin Invest 74:608-613
32. Utsunomiya T, Krausz MM, Levine L, Shepro D, Hechtman HB (1982) Thromboxane mediation od cardiopulmonary effects of embolism. J Clin Invest 70:361-368
33. Voelkel NF, Stenmark KR, Reeves JT, Mathias MM, Murphy RC (1984) Actions of lipooxygenase metabolites in isolated rat lungs. J Appl Physiol 57:860-867
34. Ogletree ML, Oates JA, Brigham KL, Hubbard WC (1982) Evidence for pulmonary release of 5-hydroxyeicosatetraenoic acid (5-HETE) during endotoxemia in unanesthetized sheep. Prostaglandins 23:459-468
35. Bremm KD, König W, Spur B, Crea A, Galanos C (1984) Generation of slow-reacting substance (leukotrienes) by endotoxin and lipid A from human polymorphonuclear granulocytes. Immunology 53:299-305
36. Moskowitz MA, Kiwak KJ, Hekimian K, Levine L (1984) Synthesis of compounds with properties of leukotrienes C_4 and D_4 in gerbil brains after ischemia and reperfusion. Science 224:886-889

37. Denzlinger C, Rapp S, Hagmann W, Keppler D (1986) Leukotrienes as mediators in tissue trauma. Science 230:330–332
38. Zadoff AD, Kobayashi T, Brigham KL, Newman JH (1986) Diethylcarbamazine on pulmonary vascular response to endotoxin in awake sheep. J Appl Physiol 60:1380–1385
39. Reines HD, Halushka PV, Cook JA, Wise WC, Rambo W (1982) Plasma thromboxane concentrations are raised in patients dying with septic shock. Lancet 2:174–175
40. Halushka PV, Reines HD, Barrow SE, Blair IA, Dollery CT, Tambo W, Cook JA, Wise WC (1985) Elevated plasma 6-keto-prostaglandin $F_{1\alpha}$ in patients in septic shock. Crit Care Med 13:451–453
41. Lamy M, Deby-Dupont G, Pincemail J, et al (1985) Biochemical pathways of acute lung injury. Bull Eur Physiopathol Respir 21:221–229
42. Deby-Dupont G, Radoux L, et al (1982) Release of thromboxane B_2 during adult respiratory-distress syndrome and its inhibition non steroidal anti-inflammatory substances in man. Arch Int Pharmacodyn 259:317–319
43. Leeman M, Boeynaems JM, Degaute JP, Vincent JL, Kahn RJ (1985) Administration od dazoxiben, a selective thromboxane synthetase inhibitor, in the adult respiratory distress syndrome. Chest 87:726–730
44. Reines HD, Halushka PV, Olanoff LS, Hunt PS (1985) Dazoxiben in human sepsis and adult respiratory distress syndrome. Clin Pharmacol Ther 37:391–395
45. Creticos PS, Peters SP, Adkinson NF, et al (1984) Peptide leukotriene release after antigen challenge in patients sensitive to ragweed. N Engl J Med 310:1626–1630
46. Stenmark KR, James SL, Voelkel NF, Toews WH, Reeves JT, Murphy RC (1983) Leukotriene C_4 and D_4 in neonates with hypoxemia and pulmonary hypertension. N Engl J Med 309:77–80
47. Matthay MA, Eschenbacher WL, Goetzl EJ (1984) Elevated concentrations of leukotriene D_4 in pulmonary edema fluid of patients with the adult respiratory distress syndrome. J Clin Immunol 4:479–483
48. Cook JA, Wise WC, Halushka PV (1980) Elevated thromboxane levels in the rat during endotoxic shock. Protective effects of imidazole, 13-azaprostanoic acid, or essential fatty acid deficiency. J Clin Invest 65:227–230
49. Butler RR Jr, Wise WC, Halushka PV, Cook JA (1983) Gentamycin and indomethacin in the treatment of septic shock: effects on prostacyclin and thromboxane A_2 production. J Pharmacol Exp Therap 225:94–101
50. Fink MP, Gardiner WM, Roethel R, Fletcher JR (1985) Plasma levels of 6-keto $PGF_{1\alpha}$ but not TxB_2 increase in rats with peritonits due to cecal ligation. Circ Shock 16:297–305
51. Rie M, Peterson M, Kong D, Quinn D, Wathins D (1983) Plasma prostacyclin increases during acute human sepsis. Circ Shock 10:232–239

Leukocytes-mediated Pulmonary Injury

O. Chiara, P. Giomarelli, and B. Biagioli

Introduction

Advances in the care of patients after trauma or emergency surgical interventions have improved survival. The use of intensive care facilities such as mechanical ventilatory assistance, pharmacological hemodynamic support, parenteral nutrition, dialysis and hemofiltration, have permitted a better control of the response to this acute physiologic insult. However, in spite of these improved results the number of deaths from progressive, sequential and multiple organ failure (MOF) has increased [1-3].

In a retrospective analysis of 132 patients consecutively admitted to the intensive care unit of our institution, 38 patients (28.8%) developped MOF. In 8 patients, the initial injury was hypovolemic shock after trauma or nonseptic surgical procedures. In 30 patients the acute physiologic insult was intra-abdominal sepsis. Respiratory failure was present in all patients with MOF. ARDS requiring artificial ventilation developed in 2 patients (25%) of the hypovolemic group and in 19 patients (63%) with intraperitoneal sepsis. In no patient in the hypovolemic group but in 10 patients with sepsis, death was a direct consequence of intractable respiratory failure (Table 1). Therefore acute non-cardiogenic pulmonary edema represents a frequent problem in patients with MOF, with a mortality exceeding 50%. Previous reports [4, 5] have indicated that MOF and ARDS may be linked to a generalized auto-destructive inflammation involving a prolonged activation of polymorphonuclear granulocytes.

Table 1. Incidence and mortality of MOF and ARDS in 132 patients consecutively admitted to the intensive care unit

Total No. of patients with MOF: 38

Initial injury	Hypovolemia	Sepsis
No. of patients	8	30
Incidence of ARDS	2 (25%)	19 (63%)
Mortality	1 (12%)	22 (73%)
Mortality related to ARDS	0	10 (33%)

Role of Leukocytes in Pulmonary Injury

Evidence suggesting that neutrophils may contribute to the pathogenesis of ARDS derives from a number of observations. Microscopic studies demonstrate neutrophil accumulation together with damaged lung endothelial cells and detailed ultrastructural examinations reveal neutrophils penetrating endothelial junctions in patients with ARDS [6, 7,]. Increased number of neutrophils and their products are usually found in lung lavage fluids from patients with ARDS [8, 9]. Neutrophils possess many properties which may alter the structure and function of alveolar capillary membrane. It is well accepted that activates leukocytes release substances that increase endothelial permeability. These substances include arachidonic acid metabolites, proteases, platelet activating factors and oxygen radicals. With respect to oxygen radicals, these are metabolities of oxygen usually involved in the destruction of mocroorganisms ingested by phagocytes [10, 11].

An uncontrolled activation of phagocytes may lead to overproduction of oxidants which cause tissue injury when discharged in the extracellular environment in large quantities.

Experimentally, the first step in tissue damage is endothelial alteration with increased permeability and interstitial edema. The interaction of oxidants with biomembranes generate chemotactic agents which activate other circulating neutrophils and tissue macrophages. These mechanisms maintain and amplify inflammatory response after the initial stumulus thus leading to a self-perpetuating autodestructive process [12–16].

Recently also clinical studies in patients with ARDS have provided unequivocal evidence for the release of oxidants into the pulmonary tissues of affected individuals [17, 18]. While the role of neutrophils in the pathogenesis of lung injury is now well accepted, controversies remain about the mechanisms of leukocyte activation. Clinical or subclinical sepsis has been invoked as the underlying cause of organ failure. Therefore sepsis is not always recognized in patients with MOF and ARDS by bacteriological investigation and also by post mortem evaluation. On the other hand, procedures like extracorporeal circulation are known to produce significant complement-mediated leukocyte activation [19] causing only rarely the development of ARDS.

Experimental Models

Many authors have suggested experimental models of leukocytes-induced pulmonary injury obtained by a variety of activating agents. Live bacteria and endotoxin have been reported to produce lung injury characterized by thromboxane-induced pulmonary hypertension and neutrophil-induced increased permeability. Oxygen radicals have been hypothesized to be the mediator of endothelial damage [20]. Various experimental reports have suggested that neutrophils contribute importantly to the pathogenesis of lung injury due to pure oxygen breathing. Fox et al. [21] developed a model of an acute non-cardiogenic edematous lung damage in rats exposed to hyperoxia (more than 95% O_2) for at least three days. The same group demonstrated subsequently that alveolar macrophages exposed to hyperoxia release factors that stimulate neutrophil chemotaxis, adherence to endothelium and oxygen radicals production.

Phorbol myristate acetate (PMA) is another potent stimulant of neutrophils, experimentally used to produce lung damage. This substance induces a marked release by neutrophils of oxygen radicals and has been demonstrated to be a causative factor of edematous injury both in vivo and in isolated lungs. PMA has been useful to study pathogenetic mechanisms and to test antioxidant treatments. Obviously, PMA may not be considered a possible causative factor of clinical ARDS.

The systemic activation of the complement system has been reported to play a role in the pathogenesis of the inflammatory lung desease. Complement activation results in the biologically active fragment C_5a, which has been shown to be a potent mediator of inflammatory events involving neutrophils such as lysosomal enzymes release and oxygen radicals generation. This model of neutrophil activation may be obtained directly through the intravascular injection of the C_5a peptide or indirectly through the in vivo generation of C_5a using the intravenous injection of cobra venom factor or zymosan-activated plasma [22]. Using experimental models of complement activation, various authors reported transient decrease of leukocyte count associated with moderate hypoxemia and pres-

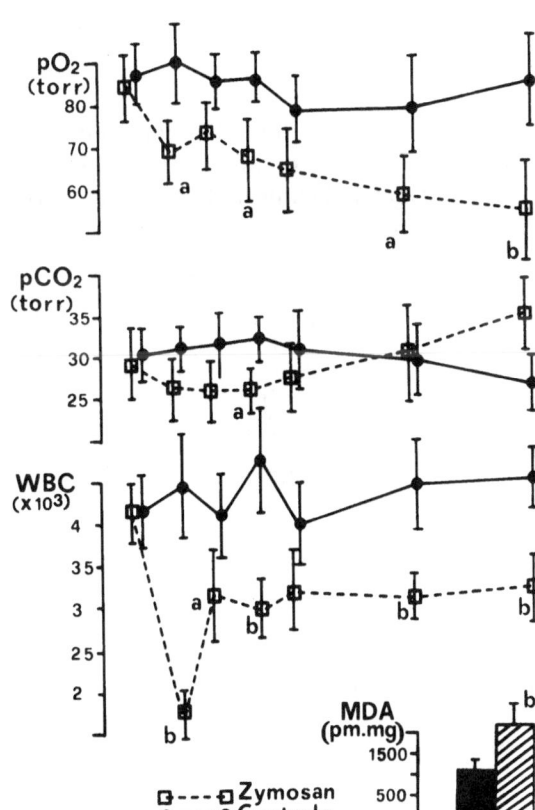

Fig. 1. PaO₂, PaCO₂, white blood cells (WBC), and malondialdehyde (MDA) levels (mean values ±SD) in 23 rabbits with intraperitoneal suspension of zymosan and paraffin compared with 7 rabbits treated with paraffin alone. Evaluations at day 0, 1, 2, 3, 4, 7 and 10

ence of leukoemboli and interstitial edema in the lung. However, these experiments usually consider only a few hours of observation which do not resemble clinical ARDS. Recently Goris et al. [23] presented an experimental model in rats of chronic organ failure using the intraperitoneal injection of a sterile suspension of zymosan and paraffin. The lung of the rats killed after 12 days showed interstitial and intravascular edema and increased number of intracapillary granulocytes and macrophages. In order to mimic clinical evolution of MOF and ARDS we applied the same preparation in rabbits, focusing our attention on physiologic, morphologic and biologic changes of lungs. In ten days, the rabbits showed an initial decrease of white blood cells, a progressive hypoxemia and a late increase in carbon dioxide (Fig. 1). The measurement of oxygen radicals activity was performed through the estimation in lung homogenates of malondialdehyde (MDA), a final degenerative product of lipid peroxidation. The levels of MDA were significantly higher in animals injected with intraperitoneal zymosan than in controls. Ultrastructural studies evidenced interstitial edema and increased cellularity of alveolar septa with accumulation into capillaries of degranulated neutrophils and macrophages. This model demonstrates that a prolonged and massive complement-mediated activation of leukocytes in the absence of sepsis is sufficient to produce lung alterations similar to that of ARDS.

Conclusions and Therapeutic Considerations

This presentation outlines that the central role of leukocytes and oxygen radicals in the pathogenesis of lung injury is now largely accepted and supported by both experimental and clinical observations. Various mechanisms of neutrophils acti-

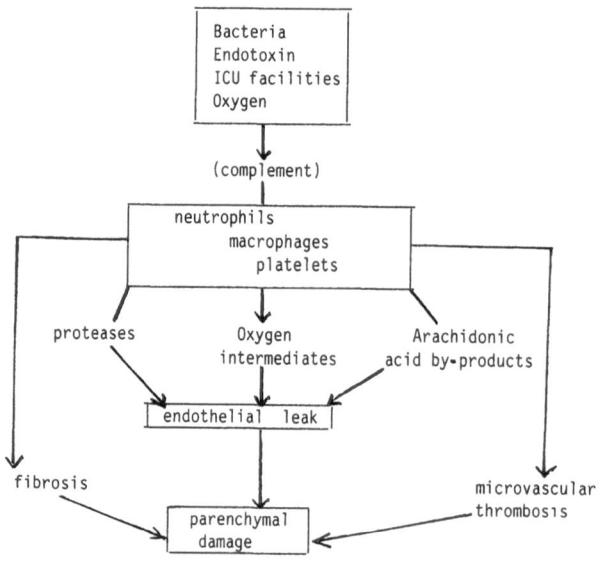

Fig. 2. Mechanisms of cellular injury

vation may be proposed. Sepsis is an important causative factor which has to be actively searched for when suspected and controlled by means of antibiotics and surgery. The presence of traumatized or necrotized tissues, the long term utilization of mechanical ventilation or hemodialysis, the prolonged use of indwelling catheters with transient episodes of endotoxemia and the prolonged use of high oxygen concentrations may play an important role in the development of uncontrolled inflammation and parenchymal damage (Fig. 2).

Pharmacological strategies to prevent ARDS and MOF are actually oriented in two directions i.e to block the stimulation or to block the effects of the mediators. Glucocorticosteroids in high doses are very effective in shutting down the inflammatory response. The problem in their use is that the entire system is inactivated both systemically and locally predisposing the host to overwhelming infections [24]. Nonsteroidal antinflammatory drugs, like indomethacin or ibuprofen have shown experimentally to ameliorate pulmonary function by inhibiting eicosanoid production. However long-term survival is minimally affected. On the contrary the prostanoid PGE_1 has been shown to enhance survival in ICU patients with ongoing ARDS in a prospective randomized double-blinded study [25]. Further observations indicated that the drug seems more effective in traumatized patients while it fails to prevent ARDS in septic patients. Presently the efficacy of PGE_1 is being evaluated in various clinical and experimental trials.

The second general approach in the prevention of ARDS is to block the effects of mediators. Because oxidants are considered as the major cytotoxic agents produced in response to inflammatory stimuli, many potential treatment protocols involve the use of specific (catalase) or aspecific (abscorbic acid, beta-carotene) antioxidants. Another theoretical possibility, which is actually a research topic, is to enhance the endogenous levels of antioxidants to prevent cytotoxicity. Results are too preliminary to evaluate the efficacy of any of these approaches in the critically ill patient.

References

1. Fry DE, Pearlstein L, Fulton RL, Polk HC (1980) Multiple System Organ failure. The role of uncontrolled infection. Arch Surg 115:136–140
2. Baue AE, Chaundry IH (1980) Prevention of multiple system failure. Surg Clin North Am 60:1167–1178
3. Carrico CJ, Meakins JL, Marhall JC, Fry DE, Maier RV (1986) Multiple organ failure Syndrome. Arch Surg 121:196–208
4. Goris RJA, Boekhorst TPA, Nuytnick JKS, Gimbrere JSF (1985) Multiple organ failure. Generalized autodestructive inflammation. Arch Surg 120:1109–1115
5. Nuytnick JKS, Goris RJA, Redl H, Schlag G, Van Munster PJJ (1986) Postraumatic complications and inflammatory mediators. Arch Surg 121:886–890
6. Bachofen M, Weibel ER (1982) Structural alterations of lung parenchima in the adult respiratory distress syndrome. Clin Chest Med 3:35–56
7. Barry BE, Crapo JD (1985) Patterns of accumulation of platelets and neutrophils in rat lungs during exposure to 100% and 85% oxygen. Am Rev Respir Dis 132:548–555
8. Lee CT, Fein AM, Lippmann M, Holtzman H, Kimbel P, Wienbaum G (1981) Elastolytic activity in pulmonary lavage fluid from patients with adult respiratory distress syndrome. N Engl J Med 304:192–196

9. Hunninghake GE, Gadek JE, Kaeanami O, Ferrand VJ, Crystal RG (1979) Inflammatory in health and disease: evaluation by bronchoalveolar lavage. Am J Pathol 97:149-206
10. Babior BM (1978) Oxygen dependent microbial killing by phagocytes. N Engl J Med 298:659-668
11. Klebanoff SJ (1980) Oxygen metabolism and the toxic properties of phagocytes. Ann Intern Med 93:480-489
12. Babior BM (1984) Oxidants from phagocytes: agents of defense and destruction. Blood 64:959-966
13. Jacob HS, Craddock PR, Hammerschmidt DE, Moldow CF (1980) Complement induced granulocyte aggregation. An unsuspected mechanism of disease. N Engl J Med 302:789-794
14. Sacks T, Moldow CF, Craddock PR, Bowers TK, Jacob HS (1978) Oxygen radicals mediate endothelial cell damage by complement stimulated granulocytes: an in vitro model of immune vascular damage. J Clin Invest 61:1161-1167
15. Harlan JM (1985) Leukocyte-endothelial interactions. Blood 65:513-525
16. Tate RM, Van Benthuysen KM, Shasby DM, McMurtry IF, Repine JE (1982) Oxygen-radical-mediated permeability edema and vasoconstriction in isolated saline perfused rabbit lungs. Am Rev Respir Dis 126:802-806
17. Cochrane CG, Spragg RG, Revak SD, Cohen AB, McGuire WW (1983) The presence of neutrophil elastase and evidence of oxidation activity in bronchoalveolar lavage fluid of patients with adult respiratory distress syndrome. Am Rev Respir Dis 127:525-527
18. Baldwin SR, Devall LJ, Simon RH, Grum CM, Ketai LH, Boxer LA (1986) Oxidant activity in expired breath of patients with adult respiratory distress syndrome. Lancet 4:11-14
19. Parker DJ, Cantrall JW, Karp RB, Stroud RM, Digerness SB (1972) Changes in serum complement and immunoglobins following cardiopulmonary variables. Surgery 71:824-830
20. Staton GW, Snider MT, Hales CA, Wathins WD (1981) Low dose endotoxin in vivo results in hydroxyl radical formation and stimulation of prostaglandin release. Am Rev Respir Dis 123:199-204
21. Fox RB, Hoidal JR, Brown DM, Repine JE (1981) Pulmonary inflammation due to oxygen toxicity: involvement of chemotactic factors and polymorphonuclear leukocytes. Am Rev Respir Dis 123:521-523
22. Webster RO, Larsen GL, Mitchell BC, Goins AJ, Henson PM (1982) Absence of inflammatory lung injury in rabbits challenged intravascularly with complement-derived chemotactic factors. Am Rev Respir Dis 125:335-340
23. Goris RJA, Boekholtz WKF, Van Bebber IPT, Nuytinck JKS, Schilling PHM (1986) Multiple organ failure and sepsis without bacteria. An experimental model. Arch Surg 121:897-901
24. Claman HN (1983) Glucocorticosteroids: anti-inflammatory mechanisms. Hosp Prac Off 18:123-124
25. Holcroft JW, Vassar MJ, Weber CJ (1986) Prostaglandin E_1 and survival in patients with the adult respiratory distress syndrome. Ann Surg 203:371-378

PGE$_1$ Administration in ARDS

A. Paes Cardoso, J. Leal, and F. Rua

Introduction: Characteristics of PGE$_1$

Eicosanoids are unsaturated hydroxylated fatty acids with 20 carbon atoms. Among these extremely potent and ubiquitous compounds are prostaglandins, thromboxanes and leukotrienes.

The series of prostaglandins E originates from the metabolism of the arachidonic acid through the cyclo-oxygenase pathway. The elements of this series (PGE$_{1-2-3}$) differ only by the number of double bounds in lateral chains [1]. These differences are of extreme importance when featuring its physiologic action. So PGE$_1$ is given preference for the treatment of respiratory failure, first because of its potent vasodilator effect on the pulmonary circulation, second because it is almost totally metabolized on a single passage through the lung, and third because of its short half-life which makes it relatively safe in continuous intravenous infusion, even in critically ill patients, as any adverse effects disappear after reduction or discontinuation of the drug [2].

On account of these specific characteristics, the intravenous administration of PGE$_1$ determines high pulmonary and low peripheral concentrations, avoiding adverse side effects, such as systemic hypotension, but still supporting, in these concentrations, the desired peripheral inflammatory response for more efficient healing and resistance to infection [3]. PGE$_1$ is inhibited by non-steroid and anti-inflammatory drugs, such as aspirin, indomethacin and ibuprofen.

Use of PGE$_1$ in ARDS

ARDS is a complex syndrome, still responsible for a very high mortality rate in the intensive care units, despite the existence of the sophisticated mechanic and pharmacologic support [4]. The prevention of multiple organ failure, more commonly associated with sepsis and trauma, is the most important issue which concentrates the attention of clinical investigators, enhancing the value of ARDS and multiple organ failure predictors, with a wiew to establish an effective preventive strategy. The development and the fineness of the process at tissue level, creates the need for sophisticated diagnostic techniques and the use of selective therapies. This justifies the interest in the study of arachidonic acid biologically active metabolites as mediators of respiratory failure, and the therapeutic value of prostaglandins in this process.

The need for criteria to define ARDS is implicit in its concept of non-cardiogenic pulmonary edema. The multiplicity of clinical and laboratorial criteria of ARDS ought to be simplified and made uniform excluding the more fallible components. We therefore suggest the following criteria:

1. Clinical situation compatible with the establishment of ARDS, or with a clear risk factor, excluding other possible causes of pulmonary dysfunction [5];
2. Severe hypoxemia, despite high FiO_2 or PaO_2/FiO_2 index equal to or less than 150, requiring mechanical ventilation;
3. Chest roentgenogram consistent with ARDS [5];
4. Absence of clinical signs of congestive heart failure and wedge pressure lower than 18 mmHg;
5. Effective compliance equal to or less than 50 ml/H_2O (usually 20 or 30).

However, very strict criteria can be fallible, and both experience and clinical common sense, seem essential in this appreciation.

It is important to schematize briefly the mechanisms of ARDS for a better understanding of the mechanisms of action of PGE_1 in this syndrome. One still lacks a precise understanding of the basic process and of the mediators involved in the inflammatory response in the lung, resulting in capillary endothelial lesion and permeability pulmonary edema, although it seems undeniable that the granulocytes play a key role in this process [7]. The complement activated by endotoxins or proteinases releases its fragments (C_3a, C_5a), which act on the activated neutrophils, which in turn aggregate and adhere to the capillary endothelium, producing large quantities of toxic oxygen radicals and proteinases [8–10], especially elastase [9].

Prostanoids released by leukocytes and alveolar macrophages, actively interfere in the process, with a potent vaso-constrictor action and platelet aggregation (thromboxane A_2). Leukotrienes strongly promote leukocyte agregation and bronchoconstriction (LC_4 and LD_4), which favour the permeability defect of the capillary endothelium [11].

Complement activation through the Hageman factor leads to profound alterations of the coagulation, especially platelet aggregation, fibrinolysis inhibition and formation of microthrombi. At the same time there is fibroblasts proliferation and development of fibrosis [10].

Recent clinical and laboratorial studies in acute respiratory failure [5], confirm the involvement of circulating prostaglandins and activated complement (C_3a, C_5a), and the very important role of granulocytes aggregation in ARDS. Interactions between these factors are very complex in ARDS. C_3a, C_5a fragments of the complement are significantly increased in the critically ill patients. Granulocyte aggregation is also significantly increased in these patients with ARDS, as compared to those without, even though in both groups there is a better aggregation response than in the control group [5]. The authors considered that the increased granulocyte aggregation in critically ill surgical patients (mediated by activated complement and/or excess of $TBxA_2$) may lead to the capillary lesion. In the future, leukotrienes may be considered as final mediators of capillary permeability and important point of this system [5].

The series of prostaglandins E, especially PGE_1 and prostacyclin (PGI_2), have a neutralizing action in this process, with inhibition of the activation of polymorphonuclear leukocytes, adherence to the vascular endothelium (PGI$_2$), inhibition of activation and platelet aggregation (PGE$_1$, PGI$_2$), and fibrinolysis (PGI$_2$), apart from the vasodilating action and "cytoprotection" (PGE$_1$, PGI$_2$) [4–16], This would result in the following effects:

– improvement in the microcirculatory blood flow, with prevention of tissue hypoxia;
– reduction in the injury of endothelium;
– hemodynamic improvement due to pulmonary vasodilation [4].

However PGE$_1$ activity is clearly dose-dependent, so that some authors doubt on its anti-inflammatory efficacy in the lungs, at the doses adopted in clinical practice (30 ng·kg^{-1}·min^{-1}). This could thus lead to an increase of the inflammatory response to inflammatory stimulants. If this assuption is valid, we can lose by anti-inflammatory inefficiency of the drug, but we gain a better response from immunodepressed patients, with a normalization of the dysfunctional neutrophils, and a clinical improvement (Holcroft's lecture, Porto 1987).

Experimental and Clinical Studies

In October 1985, a prospective randomized placebo-controlled double blind trial proved that PGE, therapy, for a maximum of 7 days, could improve 30 days survival in surgical patients with ARDS [3]. As a rule, there was an improvement in the pulmonary function, despite sometimes a transient decrease of the PaO$_2$/FiO$_2$ index, related to the reduction of the hypoxic pulmonary vasoconstriction. However, the increase of the lung blood flow caused by the pulmonary vasodilation, may contribute to the cure of the pulmonary lesions [3]. Severe hepatic and renal failure contributed to mortality. Despite the vasodilating effect of this drug, no considerable systemic hypotension, nor clear side effects such as bleeding or systemic infections increase were detected, with the doses used.

Other studies in patients with ARDS showed the hemodynamic benefits in the administration of PGE$_1$ therapy, with coronary and peripheral (to a less degree) vasodilation, leading to decreases in pulmonary arterial pressure and systemic vascular resistance, and increases in cardiac index, oxygen delivery and oxygen uptake [13, 17]. In other studies, the benefical effects of PGE$_1$ in ARDS were also related to a reduction in right ventricular afterload and an improvement in tissue oxygenation [14].

Actually, all studies nowadays concentrate on the complex problem of the improvement in tissue oxygenation with PGE$_1$, and the diagnosis and correction of covered tissue hypoxia, in an attempt to prevent ARDS and multiple organ failure.

Tissue Hypoxia

The pathway of oxygen from the airways to the mitochondria includes various stages, which may be compromized in illness, by lung and heart failure, O$_2$ transport alterations and tissue perfusion defects [15]. In ARDS, hypoxemia caused by lung failure, leads to a decrease of O_2 delivery (DO_2) which we try to solve by using mechanical ventilation, increasing cardiac output and improving O_2 transport.

However, oxygenation problems in ARDS are also at the tissue level, as a reduced oxygen extraction capacity does not compensate the decrease of O_2 delivery, forcing the O_2 uptake ($\dot{V}O_2$) to fall. This abnormal supply dependency may exist despite normal or increased overall delivery. In physiological conditions this supply dependency exists only when delivery is reduced below a critical threshold (around 8.2 ml/min/kg). [15]. In both ARDS and Sepsis, a $\dot{V}O_2$ plateau is only achieved at very high DO_2 levels (around 21 ml/min/kg), reflecting high metabolic needs [9, 12]. This decrease in O_2 extraction, may be due to blood flow abnormalities at regional or microcirculation levels, or even to the existence of peripheral microembolism. The increase of $\dot{V}O_2$ may be due to the use of oxygen in oxidizing pathways other than mitochondria, such as the production of free radicals. In fact, the presence of an abnormal supply dependency at an early ARDS stage suggests alteration in O_2 diffusion, not limited to the lung. In other words, the factors responsible for the pulmonary endothelium injury may also affect the periphery. In sepsis, a depression of the vascular reponse to catecholamines may also alter de O_2 extration capacity by heterogeneity of the capillary distribution of blood flow [15]. These alterations lead to an inadequate oxygenation of the peripheral tissues, which is sometimes difficult to recognize, and which bears a very important role in the development of multiple organ failure.

The macrocirculatory parameters do not properly reflect tissue oxygenation [9] and therefore tissue hypoxia may co-exist despite apparently adequate PaO_2, arterial pressure and cardiac output. The $P\bar{v}O_2$ value may also be misleading in presence of altered distribution of blood flow in the microcirculation. Therefore, the diagnosis of a covert tissue hypoxia is extremely important to the critically ill patient. It can be obtained by the oxygen flux test, which is based on the abnormal increase of oxygen uptake, in response to an increase in oxygen delivery by oxygen or PEEP, inotropic agents, or vasodilators such as prostaglandins [4]. The more the O_2 uptake increases, the larger will be the debt of O_2 in the tissues. Vasodilators, such as nitroprussiate may worsen the blood flow distribution so that preference is given to the use of prostaglandins, which apart from a vasodilator action, also have a neutralizing effect of the harmful mediator systems, as well as a cytoprotector effect with an improvement of tissues oxygenation [4]. The detection of hidden tissue hypoxia is of extreme importance as its results are extremely deleterious, and can be aggravated in situations where the complement system is already activated, most probably leading to irreversible multiple organ failure [9].

Our results based on a study on the administration of PGE_1 in patients with severe respiratory dysfunction under mechanical ventilation confirm so far the available data concerning the clinical investigation on the subject.

Thus, considering the average effects of PGE_1 a very clear increase of the cardiac index was found immediately after the first dose of 30 $ng \cdot kg^{-1} \cdot min^{-1}$ of PGE_1, with reduction of the right ventricular afterload due to pulmonary vasodilation and decrease of pulmonary vascular resistance. Responses in PaO_2 and $\dot{Q}s/\dot{Q}t$ to this situation were variable. Systemic vascular resistance showed a clear decrease on the first 24 hours of PGE_1 administration. Pulmonary artery pressure usually decreased, and mean arterial pressure initially decreased and later tended to be stable. There was a marked increase in O_2 delivery, which was more accentuated at the end of the first day, with parallel increase of O_2 uptake, followed by the relative stabilization of the values. O_2 extraction showed, as a rule, a slight but progressive increase. $P\bar{v}O_2$ values were not stable.

In two patients, inhibition of ADP-induced platelet aggregation was not observed during PGE_1 infusion. Fibrinolytic studies, euglobulin lysis time, and TPA are under investigation (M. Campos 1987).

These results seems encouraging and a basis for our ongoing clinical trial on the subject.

References

1. Cunha Ribeiro LM, Almeida Dias A, Goncalves FS, et al (1987) The importance of collagen and ADP in thromboxane A_2 formation. Arq Med 1:123-132
2. Long WA, Rubin LJ (1987) Prostacyclin and PGE treatment of pulmonary hypertension. Am Rev Respir Dis 136:773-776
3. Holcroft JW, Vassar MJ, Weber CJ (1985) Prostaglandin E_1 and survival in patients with ARDS. Ann Surg 371-378
4. Bihari DJ (1985) Prevention of multiple organ failure in the critically ill. Crit Care Med 13:26-39
5. Slotman GJ, Burchard KW, Yellin SA, Williams JJ (1985) Prostaglandin and complement interaction in clinical acute respiratory failure. Arch Surg 121:271-274
6. Petty TL, Fowler AA (1982) Another look at ARDS. Chest 82:98-104
7. Andreadis N, Petty TL (1985) ARDS problems and progress. Am Rev Respir Dis 132:1344-1346
8. Vassar MJ, Holcroft JW (1985) Arachidonic acid metabolites in lung injury in sepsis and trauma, pp 259-263
9. Goris RJA (1987) ARDS and multiple organ failure. Intens Care News. Excerpta Med Amsterdam pp 1-7
10. Lamy M, Deby-Dupont G, Pincemail J, et al (1985) Biochemical pathways of acute lung injury. Bull Eur Physiopath Respir 21:221-229
11. Slotman GJ (1987) The role of Prostaglandins in ARDS. In: Vincent JL (ed) Update 1987. Springer, Berlin Heildelberg New York London Paris Tokyo (Update in Intensive care and emergency Medicine, vol 3, pp 135-140)
12. Bihari D, Smithies M, Gimson A, Tinker J (1987) Effects of vasodilation with prostacyclin on oxygen delivery and uptake in critically ill patients. N Engl J Med 317:397-403
13. Shoemaker W, Appel PL (1985) Prostaglandin E_1 in ARDS. Surgery 275-281
14. Tokioka H, Kobayashi O, Ohta Y, Wakabayashi T, Kosaka F (1984) Acute effect of prostaglandin E_1 on pulmonary circulation and oxygen delivery in ARDS. Intens Care Med 11:61-64
15. Schumaker PT, Cain SM (1987) Concept of a critical oxygen delivery. Intens Care Med 13:223-229
16. Brecht T, Eryilmaz-Ayaz M (1985) Hemodynamic changes during intraarterial administration of prostaglandin E_1 in healthy subjects. Adv Prostagl Thromboxane & Leukotriene Res 13:355-357
17. Kaijser L, Eklund B, Joreteg T (1981) Hemodynamic effects of PGE_1 and PGE_2 in man. Prostaglandins in Clin Med Proceed Intern Symp Chicago Year Book Med Publish, Inc

Inhalation Injury

J. M. Beeley and R. J. Clark

Introduction

The lungs present a massive interface between the body and its external environment; in man, the area equates roughly to that of a tennis court and is some seventy times the surface area of the skin. This paper confines itself to the early effects of inhaling volatile or gaseous irritants and does not consider the long-term lung damage resulting from repeated inhalation of particulate matter such as silica.

Acute damage to the airways and lung parenchyma occurs when irritant chemicals are inhaled during industrial accidents such as the Bhopal disaster or as combustion products from fires; chemical irritants have been dispersed deliberately as lung-damaging weapons; there are now reports of pulmonary damage following solvent abuse and inhalation of drugs [1].

Reports on fire victims dominate the collected literature on inhalation injury: these include mortality statistics, clinical observations, measurements of lung function and treatment schedules; most descriptions of lung morphology relate to findings at necropsy. Attempts to identify lung injury as the principal cause of death in fire victims must exclude those whose deaths occurred within the fire due to incineration, hypoxia or chemical intoxication. Deaths generated by carbon monoxide, hydrogen cyanide, neurotoxins or alcohol serve only to remind us that immediate survivors may require urgent resuscitation and specific therapy. Little can be learned from studying the pulmonary histopathology of inhalation injury when it is sustained alongside cutaneous burns which may themselves lead to the development of multi-organ failure and lung damage. Although the pulmonary vasculature is itself a target organ, damage to the parenchyma and airspaces produces the overt clinical manifestations of inflammation or of therapeutic excess.

For these reasons, there has been little progress towards developing effective treatments for inhalation injury during an era in which burns therapy has been rapidly advanced. This is particularly regrettable as the presence of inhalation injury in burned patients is known to increase mortality [2]. Unfortunately, the literature describing inhalation of irritant gases as singleton insults is sparse, though sufficient to establish that catastrophic lung damage can result [3]. Studies of inhalation injury in the absence of burns will help in the design of appropriate treatment schedules and determine whether current burns management needs modification in those patients with coincidential irritant lung damage.

Inhalation Injury Agents

Singleton Irritants

Lung damage is sometimes provoked by the inhalation of a single irritant chemical. Reports of such cases include patients exposed to chlorine, sulphur dioxide, oxides of nitrogen and isocyanates released in an industrial setting. There are also graphic descriptions of the victims of mustard gas, phosgene and chlorine poisoning during the First World War. Use of similar agents has been reported more recently in the conflict between Iran and Iraq. It is inevitable that histological studies most commonly concern mortal cases but, in broad terms, they describe changes in the oropharynx and throughout the respiratory tract. Though the distribution of damage varies with the physical properties and concentration of the inhaled chemical, the pattern of damage is broadly similar; this is not surprising because the bronchial mucosa and alveoli tend to respond to various insults in a uniform manner [4].

Mixed Irritants

When fire-smoke is inhaled, it exposes the lung to a mixture of irritant chemical which vary according to the composition of the material and the conditions under which it burns; the dense black smoke from kerosene contains predominently carbon particles but only low concentrations of irritants and has been shown to be relatively innocuous [2]; in contrast, wood smoke is harmful chiefly because of its high aldehyde content [5] while burning synthetic materials yield a large range of highly reactive hydrocarbons which have been identified by mass spectroscopy [6]. The solubility and concentration of irritant agents determine the distribution of damage in major airways, bronchi and alveoli. Although the term "respiratory burn" appears frequently in the literature on fire victims, thermal injury rarely damages the lower respiratory tract because there is rapid cooling of the inspired gas in the upper airways [7].

Particles

Unless they are very hot, carbon particles in smoke are not themselves damaging to the lung [2] but may adsorb chemical irritants which cause injury at sites of deposition which are determined by particle size.

Intoxicant Gases

Both carbon monoxide and hydrogen cyanide are almost ubiquitous components of fire-smoke and their concentrations are interrelated [8]. These gases are the major causes of early mortality, often leading to neurological incapacitation and subsequent death by preventing escape from the fire. Work by Zikria et al. [2]

in animal models suggested that carbon monoxide itself probably does not produce histological pulmonary damage or pulmonary edema, but there is now some conflicting evidence. The importance of blood carboxyhemoglobin levels has recently been fully reviewed [9]: it appears that they do not correlate particularly well with the tissue burden of carbon monoxide but are useful predictors of the likely timescale of morbidity in survivors of fires [10], probably because they are markers of associated exposure to irritants.

Oxygen

Hyperoxia is a rare cause of primary lung damage which may occur in specialist workers such as divers. Breathing high oxygen concentrations at normobaric pressures for several hours causes abnormalities of lung function in normal subjects; additionally, severe histological damage and death have been produced by oxygen in experimental animals [11]. The hazards of pulmonary oxygen toxicity are well recognised in the intensive therapy unit.

Water

Morphological changes are found in the lungs of victims of fresh and sea-water drowning; the practical management of near-drowning is substantially different from that of other inhalation injuries and is not considered further. However, it is worthy of note that a high humidity attending the inhalation of hot gases increases morbidity [12] by augmenting their thermal capacity: this may be particularly relevant where water is used to douse a fire.

Recognition of Injury

Early awareness of possible inhalation injury in fire victims and others exposed to irritant gases is crucial if prompt measures are to be applied in management. The numerous accounts of pulmonary edema occurring many hours after inhalation of irritant chemicals are particular reasons for vigilence and caution [13]. Although some chemicals, such as phosgene, appear particularly likely to produce pulmonary edema, others such as zinc chloride are characterized more by the early development of lung fibrosis.

The literature records a high incidence of pulmonary damage amongst those who have sustained burns in confined spaces, especially those with circumoral burns. Other markers of probable inhalation injury include singed nostril hairs, edema of the uvula and inflammation of the pharynx; conjunctival irritation is a good index of exposure to irritants. Patients with stridor, hoarseness, dyspnea, viscid sputum production or retrosternal soreness are at particular risk. Lung crackles and wheezes normally antecede radiological evidence of lung damage.

The presence of carbon monoxide in most fire-smokes leads to raised carboxyhemoglobin (HbCO) levels: measurements on admission to hospital enable

HbCO concentrations at the time of exposure to be estimated from a nomogram [8]; high levels usually indicate significant associated exposure to irritant gases. Broome et al have recently drawn attention to a paradox in which a considerable tissue burden of carbon monoxide may be associated with relatively low HbCO levels [9]. This should be suspected when there is a history of disturbed consciousness, neurological impairment or abnormal behaviour.

Lastly, the measurement of blood gases and respiratory function tests identify the current pulmonary physiological disturbance. However, apparently acceptable PaO_2 levels may mask significant oxygen desaturation of hemoglobin due to the binding of carbon monoxide. Measurements of ventilation and perfusion, or tests of airways clearance, have been used in fire victims to evaluate the nature of any lung damage [14], but probably do not influence the routine early management of acutely ill patients.

Management

Elimination of Carbon Monoxide

It cannot be overstressed that the early recognition and treatment of carbon monoxide poisoning have a major effect on outcome [9]. To achieve the requisite 100% inspired oxygen concentration, it is necessary either to intubate the patient or to use a tight-fitting face mask supplied with high flow-rates of oxygen through a demand valve. Serious poisoning merits the administration of hyperbaric oxygen. In fires involving polymers, significant carbon monoxide exposure is frequently a marker of cyanide poisoning and the use of specific cyanide antidotes should be considered. Cyanide poisoning is a further justification for hyperbaric therapy [9].

Upper Airways Obstruction

Upper airway obstruction must be sought actively whenever inhalation injury is suspected. If respiratory distress is already severe, airway access may have to be secured by intubation without prior assessment; if possible, this should be achieved initially by rigid bronchoscopy under general anesthetic, which allows rapid assessment without compromising respiratory support. It is important to be aware that relief of obstruction, particularly by tracheostomy, may be followed by fulminant pulmonary edema [12]. The ability to safely remove extensive slough through the rigid bronchoscope may allow subsequent endotracheal intubation and obviate a tracheostomy, which is best avoided in patients with neck burns due to the considerable risk of introducing infection.

In patients with lesser symptoms, early fiberoptic bronchoscopy under local analgesia is indicated to assess sub-glottic edema, tracheal or bronchial injury; it may be attended by lavage of luminal debris [15]. In those who appear well and are cooperative at presentation, serial spirometry and flow-volume loops will help to identify a need for subsequent bronchoscopy.

Bronchospasm

Bronchospasm is sometimes the major effect of an inhalation incident and usually responds well to treatment with beta-2 adrenergic agonists. Since bronchospasm is difficult to distinguish from direct mucosal injury (and may well be a component of it), bronchodilators should probably be given routinely to all inhalation victims. If they are able to cooperate, such patients should have objective measurements of airflow limitation performed serially. There is a case for giving corticosteroids to anyone with a history of asthma who has been exposed to an inhalation hazard.

Oxygen Therapy

Since high inspired levels of oxygen may themselves be damaging [11], depressed arterial oxygen partial pressures should be raised to about 8kPa (60 torr) but probably not much higher. In the event of concurrent carbon monoxide or cyanide poisoning, this consideration may be overidden by the need for a period of hyperbaric therapy to reverse cellular dysfunction. In a critically ill patient, measurements of arterial and venous oxygen contents together with cardiac output provide better information about tissue oxygenation than does the arterial oxygen saturation alone.

Mechanical Ventilation

Mechanical ventilation may have to be instituted urgently in response to the rapid onset of pulmonary edema which can occur even after a latent period of several days from injury. Ventilation is indicated for progressive respiratory failure and should be instituted in anticipation of, rather than in response to, rapid deterioration. Unfortunately, information is not available in the literature to clarify which is the most appropriate technique of ventilation; for example, it has been shown that peak inspiratory pressures of 50 cm water during ventilation of normal sheep with 40% oxygen produces lung damage over a 48 hour period [16]. We speculate that the damaged lung may be especially prone to additional injury from mechanical ventilation. Even the safety of positive end expiratory pressure (PEEP), which is usually advocated to correct regional ventilation-perfusion mismatch, has been questioned.

As already mentioned, an oral or nasal endotracheal tube is preferable to a tracheostomy and provides good protection against proximal airways narrowing while allowing effective endobronchial toilet. This can be achieved by regular use of a soft endobronchial suction catheter and the frequent instillation of small volumes of sterile normal saline. Fiberoptic bronchoscopy via the endotracheal tube allows repeated examinations and directed toilet; the temptation to overuse this method should be resisted.

Humidification

Adequate humidification of inspired gases is of particular importance in the presence of abnormal ciliary clearance and inflammatory slough. It has been shown to markedly improve mortality in experimental animals subjected to smoke inhalation [12].

Fluid Balance

It is the presence of extensive cutaneous burns alongside inhalation injury which dictates the administration of intravenous fluids. The quantity of fluid required is usually calculated according to the area of the burn and the time elapsed since injury. Several similar formulas are available as guidance, varying mainly in their time-profiles for replacement and in the composition of the fluids used [17].

Diffuse lung injury is associated with increased permeability of the alveolar-capillary barrier and probably the small airways [18]. Overinfusion of fluid is likely to cause pulmonary edema, an effect of greater significance if protein also escapes and reduces the normal plasma oncotic gradient. Concern about the potential exacerbation of this protein leak by the administration of plasma led to the widespread use of crystalloids for fluid replacement during the Vietnam war. Various papers describe a very high incidence of both pulmonary and cerebral edema among casualties in that conflict who died after hospitalisation [19] and we believe strongly that the use of massive volumes of crystalloids (often 15–20 litres in a few hours) was responsible.

During the Falkland Islands conflict, casualties with burns frequently had concomitant inhalation injuries. Fluid replenishment was initiated in such patients using a colloid: crystalloid ratio of 1:1, but switched to the infusion of polygeline alone during the first 24 hours after injury. Difficult circumstances led to incomplete fluid replacement during the early post-burn period; the deficit was later calculated from the hematocrit (Hct) and made good with colloid infusion [20]. Fluid was administered until the Hct fell to 44%, which probably represented a slight undercorrection of volume deficits for physically active men whose Hct would normally be close to 40%. There were no cases of pulmonary edema or renal failure.

The administration of crystalloids to inhalation-injured animals has been shown to precipitate pulmonary edema. The outcome of ARDS has recently been shown to be adversely associated with increased body weight [21], which is probably a marker of over-loading with fluids. In burns, we favour the predominant use of colloids for volume replacement and advise extreme caution with the use of crystalloids if lung damage coexists.

Much has still to be learned about the handling of fluids leaked into the pulmonary interstitium. The role of lymphatic drainage in protecting against alveolar edema is probably crucial and there is conflicting evidence that the lymphatic flow from the lung is influenced by the pattern of respiration [22, 23]. In the presence of a compromised alveolar-capillary barrier, extra-vascular and alveolar fluid accumulation is exquisitely sensitive to alterations of the pulmonary capillary volume and hydrostatic pressure. Measurements of pulmonary capillary wedge pressure and cardiac output assist in balancing the requirement for a low pulmonary capillary pressure against that of maintaining peripheral oxygen delivery. In the absence of invasive techniques, the empirical use of a diuretic often produces a brisk response if pulmonary edema is present and is rarely harmful, despite theoretical concerns.

Infection

There is no place for the routine administration of prophylactic antibiotics. It is well recognized that the damaged respiratory epithelium and associated slough are a rich soil for the development of infection. Burned patients invariably have wound colonisation with pathogens and this provides an obvious source of organisms. Disturbing the integrity of the respiratory tract with mechanical ventilation adds to the risk of nosocomial or auto-infection. All procedures breaching the ventilation circuit should be performed with scrupulous asepsis and the avoidance of contamination of wet components with Pseudomonas should be assiduous. Antibiotics should only be given when there is clear evidence of infection, preferably supported by laboratory evidence. Appropriate specimens should be obtained prospectively and treatment should never be started without their acquisition. Treatment will often have to be instituted on a "best guess" basis and will usually include broad-spectrum cover. Antibiotics should not be continued indefinitely and the indications for changing or stopping therapy should be considered daily.

Drug therapy

Principles

It is now 20 years since Asbough, Bigelow and Petty introduced the concept of the adult respiratory distress syndrome (ARDS) to encompass the sequential lung damage which follows a variety of insults. Since then, appreciation of the roles of cells and mediators leading to final common pathways of damage and repair [24] has encouraged therapy with agents which interfere with the inflammatory cascade. The mechanisms of inhalation injury probably have much in common with those of ARDS; to date, controlled studies reporting the successful use of drugs to treat inhalation injury have been confined to animal models using corticosteroids or ibuprofen. Any other drugs which prove beneficial in ARDS will merit trial in models of inhalation injury.

Corticosteroids

A reduction of mortality in rats exposed to woodsmoke was reported by Dressler et al. [3] when large doses of methylprednisolone were administered one hour after smoke exposure. Beeley and co-workers [25] recently described a marked improvement in survival of rabbits exposed to a single fire-smoke constituent, acrolein, when single or repeated doses of methylprednisolone (40mg/kg) were given by intramuscular injection starting half an hour after injury. Both series of experiments were designed to mimic a fire victim's entrapment in smoke and subsequent escape to receive early treatment. The latter study specifically ensured that carbon monoxide could not have contributed to death: extensive histological scrutiny surprisingly revealed no difference in the extent or severity of damage between active and placebo-treated animals. Beeley et al postulated that the improved mortality was due to prophylaxis against hypoxia-induced cardiac dysrrhythmias, or by a favourable effect of corticosteroids on pulmonary vasoconstriction or bronchial obstruction. During subsequent studies, we have observed profound stridor in acrolein-exposed animals and suspect that the major benefit from corticosteroids was in ameliorating the effects of upper airways obstruction.

Prompted by the experimental evidence above, the authors recommended early corticosteroid treatment for victims of smoke inhalation during the Falklands conflict. Sixty-nine patients, many with attendent burns, were judged to have sustained respiratory damage from smoke and were treated variously with 1–2g methylprednisolone intravenously; further doses were administered in some cases [20]. There were no deaths and no cases of pulmonary edema. The patients included 14 with burns in excess of 25% body surface area and the absence of any cases of overwhelming sepsis or ARDS was reassuring. However, these observations were uncontrolled and there is now good evidence in the literature that corticosteroids confer no benefit in ARDS. Because corticosteroids suppress systemic defence against infection and diminish bacterial clearance from the lung [26], there remains much hesitency in recommending their use in fire-victims.

The role of corticosteroids thus remains unclear and further studies are necessary to establish their place: despite the lack of controlled clinical evidence to support their use in patients, we believe that further animal work is justified to explore the mechanisms by which corticosteroids influence the response to injury from singleton agents. We speculate that the early inhibition of alveolar macrophage activity might reduce the release of mediators of further damage, but that prolonged depletion of these cells predisposes to infective complications. If clinicians feel justified in using corticosteroids in the treatment of inhaltion injury, we suggest they restrict therapy to one intravenous bolus dose.

Eicosanoids

A recent paper by Shinozawa et al. [27] describes how treatment of rats with ibuprofen after smoke exposure prevented pulmonary edema. In an elegant study they exposed the animals to a synthetic smoke comprising hot carbon particles to which the fire-smoke constituent hydrochloric acid had been added. In contrast, indomethacin failed to provide similar protection against edema. The authors discuss probable mechanisms by which ibuprofen protects against lung injury via its influence on arachidonic acid metabolism. Their results, which showed a selective generation of prostacyclin without an increase in thromboxane production, suggest that prostacyclin also offers promise as treatment for inhalation injury. The differential effects of ibuprofen and indomethacin highlight the need for subtle manipulation of eicosanoid metabolism to achieve desirable results.

Conclusion

In reviewing the extensive literature on inhalation injury, we observe that the majority of reports concern fire victims; such patients, who have sustained damage to the respiratory tract from inhaling smoke, are also prone to the indirect pulmonary complications of cutaneous burns.

Upper airways damage must always be sought and dealt with before critical occlusion occurs. We have emphasized that it is crucial to identify and treat attendant intoxication with carbon monoxide and other incapacitating chemicals. Humidification is essential when the airway lining and mucociliary escalator are compromised. We recognize a requirement for research into the effects of oxygen and mechanical ventilation on the already-damaged lung so that potential enhancement of injury may be avoided. There remains a conflict of opinion on the best type of fluid to replace losses from associated cutaneous burns, especially because this may influence fluid shifts across a damaged alveolar-capillary barrier. The lung lymphatics appear crucial in protecting against alveolar flooding and ways of enhancing lymphatic clearance should be sought. Of the many drugs which influence the inflammatory cascade, few have been trialled in inhalation injury: we have discussed some evidence that corticosteroids and selective modulators of the eicosanoid pathways may be beneficial. Other agents, such as free radical scavengers and serine proteinase inhibitors, are obvious candidates for further work. We have not dealt with the medium-timescale threat of fibrosis which may prove amenable to prophylaxis, remodelling or reversal with modulators of collagen metabolism.

The prospects for effective treatment of inhalation damage are limited. The medical profession should not ignore its role in pressing for the development and use of fire-resistant materials and those with less-toxic combustion products. The introduction of personal protective equipment (as is being proposed in commercial airliners) is likely to save more lives than the pharmacological manipulation of those who have already sustained pulmonary damage.

References

1. Glassroth J, Adams GD, Schnoll S (1987) The impact of substance abuse on the respiratory system. Chest 91:596-602
2. Zikria BA, Ferrer JM, Flock HF (1972) The chemical factors contributing to pulmonary damage in 'smoke poisoning'. Surgery 71:704-709
3. Dressler DP, Skornik WA, Kupersmith S (1976) Corticosteroid treatment of experimental smoke inhalation. Ann Surg 183:46-52
4. Bowden DH (1981) Reaction of the lung to injury. In Scadding JG, Cumming G (eds) Scientific foundations of respiratory medicine, 1st edn. Heinemann, London, pp 529-545
5. Thorning DR, Howard ML, Hudson LD, Schumacher RL (1982) Pulmonary response to smoke inhalation. Morphologic changes in rabbits exposed to pine wood smoke. Hum Pathol 13:355-364
6. Wooley WD (1982) Smoke and toxic gas production from burning polymers. J Macromol Sci Chem A17:1-33
7. Moritz AR, Henriques FC, McLean R (1945) The effects of inhaled heat on the air passages and lungs: an experimental investigation. Am J Pathol 21:311-331
8. Clark CJ, Campbell D, Reid WH (1981) Blood carboxyhaemoglobin and cyanide levels in fire survivors. Lancet i:1332-1335
9. Broome JR, Skrine H, Pearson RR (1988) Carbon monoxide poisoning - forgotten not gone! Br J Hosp Med (in press)
10. Zikria BA, Budd DC, Floch F, Ferrer JM (1975) What is clinical smoke poisoning? Ann Surg 181:151-156
11. Katzenstein AA, Bloor CM, Leibow AA (1976) Diffuse alveolar damage. The role of oxygen, shock and related factors. Am J Pathol 85:210-228
12. Stone HH, Rhame DW, Corbitt JD, Given KS, Martin JD (1967) Respiratory burns. Ann Surg 165:157-168
13. Di Vincenti RC, Pruett BA, Reckler JM (1971) Inhalation injuries. J Trauma 11:109-121
14. Petroff PA, Hander EW, Clayton WH, Pruett BA (1976) Pulmonary function studies after smoke inhalation. Am J Surg 132:346-351
15. Clark CJ, Reid WH, Telfer ABM, Campbell D (1983) Respiratory injury in the burned patient. Anaesthesia 38:35-39
16. Kolobow T, Moretti MP, Fumagalli R, et al (1987) Severe impairment in lung function induced by high peak airway pressure during mechanical ventilation. Am Rev Respir Dis 135:312-315
17. Settle JAD (1982) Fluid therapy in burns. J Roy Soc Med 75 (suppl):6-11
18. Staub NC (1979) Pathways for fluid and solute fluxes in pulmonary edema. In: Fishman AP, Renkin EM (eds) Pulmonary edema. American Physiological Scociety, Maryland, pp 113-124
19. Simmons RL, Heisterkamp CA, Collins JA, Bredenburg CE, Martin AM (1969) Acute pulmonary edema in battle casualties. J Trauma 9:760-775
20. Chapman CW (1983) Burns and plastic surgery in the South Atlantic Campaign 1982. J Roy Nav Med Serv 69:71-79
21. Simmons RS, Berdine GG, Seidenfeld JJ, et al (1987) Fluid balance and the adult respiratory distress syndrome. Am Rev Respir Dis 135:924-929
22. Warren MF, Drinker CK (1942) The flow of lymph from the lungs of the dog. Am J Physiol 136:207-221
23. Jefferies AL, Hamilton P, O'Brodovich HM (1983) Effect of high frequency oscillation on lung lymph flow. J Appl Physiol: Respirat Environ Exercise Physiol 55:1373-1378
24. Haslett C, Henson PM (1988) Resolution of inflammation. In: Clark RAF, Henson PM (eds) Molecular and cell biology of wound repair. Plenum, New York, pp 185-211
25. Beeley JM, Crow J, Jones JG, Minty B, Lynch RD, Pryce DP (1986) Mortality and lung histopathology after inhalation injury. Am Rev Respir Dis 133:191-196
26. Skornik WA, Dressler DP (1974) The effects of short term steroid therapy on lung bacterial clearance and survival in rats. Ann Surg 179:415-421
27. Shinozawa Z, Hales C, Jung W, Burke J (1986) Ibuprofen prevents synthetic smoke-induced pulmonary edema. Am Rev Respir Dis 134:1145-1148

Respiratory Muscle Insufficiency in Neuromuscular Disorders

M. Estenne

Introduction

Acute ventilatory failure is a frequent occurrence in many neuromuscular disorders. It may appear at the onset of the disease, as in the acute inflammatory stage of poliomyelitis, in the Guillain-Barré syndrome, or in an episode of myasthenia gravis. Many neuromuscular disorders can also lead to chronic respratory insufficiency, which often contributes significantly to the cause of the death. Respiratory failure in these conditions is not simply due to the direct effect of weakness of the respiratory muscles leading to inability to inflate the lungs and alveolar hypoventilation. A variety of additional pathogenic mechanisms are important [1]. These include

1. alterations in the mechanical properties of the lung and chest wall,
2. inability to cough and impaired clearance of secretions,
3. dysfunction of the "respiratory centers", and
4. ventilation-perfusion inhomogeneity.

An analysis of the pathophysiology of the respiratory insufficiency in neuromuscular disorders requires therefore to give proper emphasis to each of these factors.

Lung Volumes

Numerous studies on various neuromuscular disorders have shown that vital capacity (VC) is often reduced as a consequence of respiratory muscle weakness, and that it decreases regularly with progression of the disease. The decrease in VC was initially attributed to the direct effect of weakness of inspiratory and expiratory musscles. Recent studies have demonstrated, however, that although VC is highly correlated with the strength of the respiratory muscles, the reduction in VC is greater than anticipated for the degree of muscle weakness [2, 3]. This is essentially related to alterations in the mechanical properties of the lung and chest wall.

Functional residual capacity (FRC) generally tends to be low in seated patients with chronic neuromuscular disorders, whereas residual volume is within normal limits or slightly elevated [4, 5]. Total lung capacity (TLC) is usually reduced. It is worth emphasizing that the pattern of lung volumes in these patients is influenced by the severity and the distribution of muscle weakness, and possibly also by the basic abnormality of the neuromuscular disease.

Pulmonary Mechanics

Longstanding weakness of the respiratory muscles is associated with characteristic alterations of the static pressure-volume curve of the lung:

1. lung recoil pressure at TLC is low in relation to the normal value;
2. lung recoil pressure is increased at any absolute lung volume below TLC;
3. pulmonary compliance is reduced and
4. lung recoil pressure at FRC is normal or decreased [4, 5].

The cause of the reduction in lung distensibility is uncertain but it must be emphasized that in most cases this alteration is present without any radiographic changes suggesting parenchymal disease. Three factors are theoretically capable of affecting lung compliance in otherwise normal lungs when weakness of the respiratory muscles exists: dispersed alveolar collapse, generalized increase in the surface tension of the alveolar lining layer, and stiffening of the elastic fibers within the lungs. Although the relative role played by these factors is still unknown, it is likely that chronic alveolar collapse due to inability to inflate the lungs completely accounts for part of the reduction in pulmonary compliance observed in patients with neuromuscular disorders [6].

Chest Wall Mechanics

Statics

Different methods have been used to assess chest wall compliance in patients with various neuromuscular disorders and traumatic tetraplegia. These methods have yielded virtually identical results and demonstrate that chest wall compliance is decreased to about two thirds of normal values [7, 8]. These measurements apply to the entire chest wall, but it seems reasonable to speculate that the alterations in compliance of the two chest wall compartments, i.e. the rib cage and the diaphragm-abdomen, may vary according to the type of neuromuscular disease and the distribution of the muscle weakness. For example, it has been recently shown in patients with traumatic lesion of the lower cervical cord that the rib cage is abnormally stiff whereas the distensibility of the diaphragm-abdomen compartment is increased [8]. The decrease in rib cage compliance is likely to result from paralysis of the intercostal muscles which markedly reduces rib cage expansion during inspiration [9], and hence leads to stiffening of tissues and ankylosis in the thoracovertebral and costosternal joints. On the other hand, the increase in abdominal compliance is due to paralysis of the abdominal muscles.

Further contributing factors to the decrease in chest wall compliance can be the development of scoliosis, in particular in patients in the latter stages of muscular dystrophy, and fibrotic changes or spasticity in the rib cage muscles, as occurs in patients with late tetraplegia.

Dynamics

In addition to the alterations in the static mechanical properties of the chest wall, patients with neuromuscular disorders frequently show marked distortions of the chest wall during resting breathing. In patients with traumatic tetraplegia, the upper part of the rib cage moves inward during inspiration because the fall in pleural pressure generated by the intact diaphragm is not counterbalanced by the contraction of the parasternal intercostal and scalene muscles which normally occurs during inspiration [9]. Fortunately, the paradoxical motion of the upper rib cage tends to disappear in some patients in the months after injury, presumably due to the development of rib cage stiffness [10].

In neuromuscular disorders involving the diaphragm, the chest wall is also markedly distorted during breathing. Complete paralysis of the diaphragm is indeed associated with a paradoxical inward movement of the abdomen during inspiration, which is particularly obvious in the supine posture.

In summary, the reductions in lung volumes seen in patients with chronic weakness of the respiratory muscles are attributable to a combination of muscle weakness and alterations in the mechanical properties of the lung and chest wall. They are further increased by the distortions that the chest wall undergoes during quiet breathing. The decreases in lung and chest wall compliance, together with the distortions of the chest wall, will also increase the work of breathing and place at an even greater disadvantage those patients who have less respiratory muscle power than normal persons.

Airway Mechanics – Mechanics of Cough

Although the intrinsic properties of the airways are normal in patients with neuromuscular disorders, maximum expiratory flow rates at large volumes (which are largely dependent on the force and velocity of expiratory muscle contraction) are usually decreased. However, because maximum expiratory flow can be achieved over most of the VC with rather low driving pressures, the descending limb of the maximum expiratory flow volume (MEFV) curve and the FEV_1/VC ratio (FEV_1 = forced expiratory volume in 1 sec) are usually normal or even supranormal [3, 4]. In contrast, the effectiveness of cough is much reduced because of the lack of high flow velocities which depend on the dynamic compression of central airways produced by large positive pleural pressures. As a result, there is chronic retention of secretions within the lungs and patients with neuromuscular disorders have a high prevalence of bronchopulmonary infections.

It is generally thought that in patients with lower cervical cord transection, the expiratory flows during cough are primarily dependent on the elastic recoil of the lung and chest wall because all rib cage and abdominal expiratory muscles are paralyzed [11]. We have recently demonstrated, however, that these patients are still able to empty the lungs actively by contracting the clavicular bundle of the pectoralis major muscle. This bundle remains active when the spinal lesion is located below C_5 and acts to deflate the upper part of the rib cage. Tetraplegic subjects invariably contract the clavicular portion of the pectoralis major during expiration below FRC [12], and during cough (M. Estenne and A. De Troyer, personal communication). It is possible therefore that training the pectoralis major muscle may increase the pleural pressures developed during coughing and hence improve the clearance of airway secretions in these patients.

Ventilatory Drive

Patients with neuromuscular disorders breathe faster and with a smaller tidal volume than healthy subjects [4]. The mechanism of this altered pattern of breathing is unclear. It might be related to stimulation of lung receptors due to the presence of diffuse microatelectasis. Alternatively, tachypnea could be related to afferent signals from the weakened respiratory muscles themselves. In favor of the second hypothesis is the observation that tachypnea is usually present when the respiratory muscle weakness is caused by a generalized neuromuscular disorder, but is absent in traumatic tetraplegia. Although diffuse microatelectasis is likely to develop in both conditions, afferent information from the diseased respiratory muscles cannot reach the respiratory centers when there is a transection of the spinal cord.

Specific dysfunction of the respiratory centers undoubtedly occurs in bulbar poliomyelitis. Alterations in the central control mechanisms have also been suggested in a number of neuromuscular disorders, as myotonic dystrophy, acid maltase deficiency and other nonspecific myopathy. It should be stressed, however, that it is exceedingly difficult to assess the function of the respiratory centers when there is respiratory muscle weakness.

Ventilation and Gas Exchange

The initial change in blood gases in patients with respiratory muscle weakness is a fall in PaO_2 [4]. Decreased PaO_2 coexists with an increase in the alveolar-to-arterial tension difference for oxygen, indicating a mismatch of ventilation to perfusion within the lungs, presumably due to dispersed alveolar collapse.

Initially the tachypnea causes an increase in minute ventilation and, although the dead space rises, there is also an increase in alveolar ventilation, resulting in alveolar and arterial hypocapnia. As weakness progresses, the bellows action of the chest decreases and tidal volume decreases further. As tidal volume falls, an increasing proportion of total ventilation is wasted in dead space ventilation and consequently alveolar ventilation is reduced first to normal and then to low levels. This results in hypercapnia and further arterial hypoxemia. The development of hypercapnia may be a late event, or may appear relatively early in the course of the disease. For reasons which are not fully understood, the development of weakness of the diaphragm appears to be important contributing factor to chronic CO_2 retention in neuromuscular disorders [13].

References

1. De Troyer A, Pride NB (1985) The respiratory system in neuromuscular disorders. In: Roussos C, Macklem PT (eds) The thorax part B. Marcel Dekker Inc, New York, pp 1089–1121
2. Braun NMT, Rochester DF (1979) Muscular weakness and respiratory failure. Am Rev Respir Dis 119(2):123–125
3. De Troyer A, Borenstein S, Cordier R (1980) Analysis of lung volume restriction in patients with respiratory muscle weakness. Thorax 35:603–610
4. Gibson GJ, Pride NB, Newsom Davis J, Loh LC (1977) Pulmonary mechanics in patients with respiratory muscle weakness. Am Rev Respir Dis 115:389–395
5. De Troyer A, Heilporn A (1980) Respiratory mechanics in quadriplegia. The respiratory function of the intercostal muscles. Am Rev Respir Dis 122:591–600
6. De Troyer A, Deisser P (1981) The effects of intermittent positive pressure breathing on patients with respiratory muscle weakness. Am Rev Respir Dis 124:132–137
7. Estenne M, Delhez L, Heilporn A, Yerneult JC, De Troyer A (1983) Chest wall stiffness in patients with chronic respiratory muscle weakness. Am Rev Respir Dis 128:1002–1007
8. Estenne M, De Troyer A (1986) Effect of tetraplegia on chest wall statics. Am Rev Respir Dis 134:121–124
9. Estenne M, De Troyer A (1985) Relationship between respiratory muscle EMG and rib cage motion in tetraplegia. Am Rev Respir Dis 132:53–59
10. Morgan MDL, Gourlay AR, Silver JR, William SJ, Denison DM (1985) Contribution of the rib cage to breathing in tetraplegia. Thorax 40:613–617
11. Siebens AA, Kirby NA, Poulos DA (1964) Cough following transection of spinal cord at C6. Arch Phys Med Rehab 45:1–8
12. De Troyer A, Estenne M, Heilporn A (1986) Mechanism of active expiration in tetraplegia. N Engl J Med 314:740–744
13. Newsom Davis J, Goldman M, Loh L, Casson M (1976) Diaphragm function and alveolar hypoventilation. Q J Med 45:87–100

Severe Asthmatic Crisis

Ventilation-Perfusion Relationships in Acute Asthma

R. Rodriguez-Roisin and J. Roca

Historical Background

Until recently, little work has been done to investigate ventilation-perfusion ($\dot{V}A/\dot{Q}$) relationships in human asthma. This is important because, in the absence of alveolar hypoventilation, arterial PO_2 (PaO_2) is generally considered to directly reflect the degree of $\dot{V}A/\dot{Q}$ inequality in this condition. In fact, although $\dot{V}A/\dot{Q}$ mismatching plays a key role in asthma, little information exists concerning the characteristics of the distribution of $\dot{V}A/\dot{Q}$ ratios in patients with asthma. One main reason is the difficulty in assessing $\dot{V}A/\dot{Q}$ abnormalities. PaO_2 alone is difficult to use as a reliable indicator of the amount of $\dot{V}A/\dot{Q}$ mismatch because of variability and uncertainty in cardiac output and minute ventilation in human asthma [1]. Indeed, patients with asthma are commonly treated with bronchodilators (usually methylxanthines and adrenergic agents) which may increase cardiac output which in turn increases PaO_2 for a given amount of $\dot{V}A/\dot{Q}$ mismatching. Thus, clinicians could be misled by the assumption that PaO_2 in this situation reflects only $\dot{V}A/\dot{Q}$ abnormalities. Consequently, the finding of nearly normal values for PaO_2 may preclude the conclusion that the patients' lungs are almost devoid of gas exchange inequality, even in presence of nearly normal airflow rates. In any case, PaO_2 *per se* cannot give information about the pattern of $\dot{V}A/\dot{Q}$ distributions.

Until recently, two main approaches have been used to study the abnormalities of pulmonary gas exchange during human asthma. First, numerous studies using the Riley-Cournand analyses [2] confirmed that arterial hypoxemia was mainly induced by both $\dot{V}A/\dot{Q}$ abnormalities and true right-to-left shunt [3, 4]. Second, topographic approaches of pulmonary ventilation and perfusion with radioactive tracers during asthma have also shown maldistribution of each of these [5, 6]. However, the latter two techniques are limited in their ability to assess accurately the amount of $\dot{V}A/\dot{Q}$ mismatching. While the Riley-Cournand approach has the advantage of simplicity because of its three compartment lung model, it does not provide a detailed full picture of $\dot{V}A/\dot{Q}$ distribution within the lung. Alternatively, topographic approaches are limited by the spatial resolution of external counting techniques that average the radioactivity through a given lung field. Besides, the range of $\dot{V}A/\dot{Q}$ mismatch measured by these two methods is much less than that actually present within the normal lung and generally tends to underestimate functional $\dot{V}A/\dot{Q}$ inequality.

Extent and Pattern of $\dot{V}A/\dot{Q}$ Inequality in Patients with Mild to Moderate Asthma

In 1978, Wagner et al. [1] first documented distributions of $\dot{V}A/\dot{Q}$ ratios in patients with bronchial asthma using a multiple inert gas elimination technique [7]. This technique estimates distributions of ventilation and perfusion and has the potential to define and assess more accurately the gas exchange characteristics of the lung than either of the previous approaches. Specifically, the inert gas method estimates the degree of $\dot{V}A/\dot{Q}$ mismatching and provides a frequency distribution of lung units to allow the shape of this distribution to be determined. Furthermore, it is the only approach which gives a detailed picture and complete information of all the pulmonary and extrapulmonary factors which may influence pulmonary gas exchange.

In this study [1], $\dot{V}A/\dot{Q}$ inequality was measured in six asymptomatic patients with bronchial asthma and in a seventh patient during an acute exacerbation of asthma. Thus, while six patients had some residual mild airway obstruction as measured during forced spirometry (forced expiratory volume in one second (FEV_1) range, 66–96% predicted), one was experiencing a very severe airflow obstruction with a FEV_1 of 0.5 L (11% predicted). PaO_2 was generally 80 mm Hg or more with a normal $PaCO_2$. The most striking findings were related to measurements of distribution of $\dot{V}A/\dot{Q}$ ratios, revealing substantial $\dot{V}A/\dot{Q}$ mismatching and, moreover, bimodal patterns of distributions of $\dot{V}A/\dot{Q}$ ratios in all except one patient. In this patient, $\dot{V}A/\dot{Q}$ distribution was narrow and unimodal, similar to that seen in young healthy nonsmoking subjects, except for the presence of a small (less than 5%) shunt. The results showed than the two modes of gas-exchanging units in the lung consisted of one population centered around a normal $\dot{V}A/\dot{Q}$ ratio of 1.0, and a second one centered around low $\dot{V}A/\dot{Q}$ lung units betwen 0.01 and 0.1, containing approximately 20% of the cardiac output; true shunting, i.e. $\dot{V}A/\dot{Q}$ ratios of zero, was not observed. In each of these six patients, bimodality was shown on all repetitive measurements. Areas of high $\dot{V}A/\dot{Q}$ units were not seen in any patient. Interestingly, the extent and pattern of $\dot{V}A/\dot{Q}$ inequality in these quite asymptomatic asthmatic patients did not bear a close relationship to the severity of airflow obstruction. One interesting observation was that breathing 100% O_2 did not change pattern or extent of $\dot{V}A/\dot{Q}$ inequality nor convert any low $\dot{V}A/\dot{Q}$ ratio areas into unventilated lung (shunt) in four of the patients, suggesting no release of hypoxic pulmonary vasoconstriction. Finally, a further transient impairment of $\dot{V}A/\dot{Q}$ mismatch occurred following inhalation of isoproterenol consistent with a fall in PaO_2, which occurred simultaneously with an increase in cardiac output.

Four years later, Young et al. [8] analyzed the pattern and time course of $\dot{V}A/\dot{Q}$ distributions in six individuals with exercise induced asthma. Bimodal perfusion distributions during exercise challenge, that caused a greater than 20% decrease in FEV_1 or in peak expiratory flow rate (PEFR) together with mild to moderate hypoxemia (PaO_2 range, 59–90 mm Hg), were shown in only two of six patients. Again there was no relationship between the decrease in FEV_1 or PEFR and the amount of $\dot{V}A/\dot{Q}$ inequality. These data were reproduced experimentally in dogs using different bronchoconstrictive agents [9]. Furthermore, it was possible to develop a repetitive animal model of bronchoconstrictions using aerosolized methacholine, that was characterized by highly reproducible severe changes in $\dot{V}A/\dot{Q}$ distributions similar to those observed in human asthma [10]. Similar results were also observed in asthmatic children either with exercise-induced asthma [11] or after histamine challenge [12]. However, a striking finding of gas exchange in childhood asthma was the presence of a bimodal ventilation distribution including one mode centered within normal $\dot{V}A/\dot{Q}$ areas (but with increased blood flow to regions with $\dot{V}A/\dot{Q}$ units between 0.1 and 1) and the other within regions of high $\dot{V}A/\dot{Q}$ ratios (greater than 10). The magnitude of the latter mode correlated well to the degree of airway obstruction and PaO_2. Shunt was insignificant and low $\dot{V}A/\dot{Q}$ (lower than 0.1) mode was not seen. Corte and Young [13] measured distributions of $\dot{V}A/\dot{Q}$ ratios in 10 asthmatic patients with moderately severe disease (FEV, range, 22–58% predicted; PaO_2 range, 65–87 mm Hg). Interestingly, six patients with minimal $\dot{V}A/\dot{Q}$ maldistribution (but with airflow obstruction close to that in the four remainders with marked $\dot{V}A/\dot{Q}$ mismatching) displayed a substantial worsening of $\dot{V}A/\dot{Q}$ relationships while breathing 100% O_2; shunt remained very small. In contrast to the work of Wagner and coworkers [1], these data suggest that most patients with moderately severe asthma released hypoxic pulmonary vasoconstriction. Recently, Wagner et al. [14] investigated the prevalence and variability of $\dot{V}A/\dot{Q}$ mismatching in 26 stable, symptomatic patients with chronic asthma, weekly over a period of nine weeks using a noninvasive approach of the multiple inert gas elimination technique [15]. Basically, $\dot{V}A/\dot{Q}$ inequality was present in the vast majority of them and were due mainly to development of areas of low $\dot{V}A/\dot{Q}$ mode.

Pathogenesis of $\dot{V}A/\dot{Q}$ Inequality

Wagner et al. [1] have suggested that the consistently predominant bimodal blood flow distribution with small or nonexistent shunt seen in human asthma may reflect collateral ventilation. Bronchial asthma is a disease where mucus plugging and/or wall edema combined with active bronchoconstriction leading to obstruction of distal small airways. However, the alveolar units distal to the obstructed airway are slightly ventilated through collateral pathways (Lambert channels; Köhn poros; other communications). Thus, a widespred diffuse lesion with peripheral, small airways obstruction, but with collateral ventilation from relatively less affected lung units precludes shunting, could account for bimodality in perfusion distribution. This may also explain the failure of units with low $\dot{V}A/\dot{Q}$ areas to develop shunt during 100% O_2 breathing. Alveolar units susceptible to collapse under these conditions may have their inspired volume increased through collateral ventilation, so that they remain open. Because of worsening in $\dot{V}A/\dot{Q}$ distributions while airflow rates were returning to normal, it was also suggested that gas abnormalities in bronchial asthma were related more to mucus plugging and/or wall edema in small, peripheral airways than to reversible bronchoconstriction. The hypothesis of collateral ventilation would be further supported by macroscopic abnormalities evident at postmortem examination in animal models [9, 10]. On the one hand, in the only one dog with substantial shunt, a mucous plug was occluding a lobar bronchus [9] (only the occlusion of a lobar or larger bronchus in the dog lung increases shunt [16]). On the other hand, all dogs with airway secretions at necropsy had more blood flow to low $\dot{V}A/\dot{Q}$ areas than the others [10]. This was again consistent with the hypothesis that the perfusion of low $\dot{V}A/\dot{Q}$ units is due to completely obstructed alveolar units ventilated through collateral pathways. A striking finding in childhood asthma was the presence of a high $\dot{V}A/\dot{Q}$ mode [11], considered as an additional abnormal mode due to exercise challenge rather than caused by a normal $\dot{V}A/\dot{Q}$ mode moved to a high $\dot{V}A/\dot{Q}$ area by increased ventilation. This high $\dot{V}A/\dot{Q}$ mode might reflect regions of pulmonary hyperinflation with increased alveolar pressure, which in turn would give rise to areas of zone 1 (alveolar pressure exceeding pulmonary capillary pressure) with reduction in capillary blood flow. This is of importance because high $\dot{V}A/\dot{Q}$ mode has only been reported in few clinical conditions, such as pulmonary emphysema [17] and mechanical ventilation using a positive end expiratory pressure [18]. Finally, an interesting observation was that PaO_2 ranged from normal to mild-moderate values in the presence of substantial $\dot{V}A/\dot{Q}$ mismatching in the vast majority of patients, indicating that hypoxemia also depends on other variables, such as cardiac output, minute ventilation and O_2 consumption. An increase in the former two parameters and/or a fall in the latter increases mixed venous PO_2 which in turn increases PaO_2. The use of the multiple inert gas elimination technique has therefore facilitated our understanding of the complex interaction between these extrapulmonary factors in the presence of moderately severe $\dot{V}A/\dot{Q}$ inequality.

$\dot{V}A/\dot{Q}$ Mismatching in Acute Severe Asthma

Recently, our group has repeatedly measured $\dot{V}A/\dot{Q}$ ratios distributions in patients with acute severe asthma [19, 20]. Acute severe asthma followed the definition given by TJH Clark ten years ago, that is *an acute episode of asthma of increased severity failing to respond to more than average treatment,* which is synonymous of the more classical term *status asthmaticus* [21]. Part of these investigations have been possible by the use of the peripheral venous sampling which allows serial assessment of $\dot{V}A/\dot{Q}$ distributions [15]. This approach allows frequent repetitive measurements without sampling arterial blood. Using the peripheral venous method, the best parameter of $\dot{V}A/\dot{Q}$ inequality is expressed through the second moment of the pulmonary blood flow (log SDQ) and ventilation (log SDV). This variable, taken on a natural log scale (log SD), represents an index of $\dot{V}A/\dot{Q}$ mismatching and should be therefore regarded only as a descriptor of abnormality in pulmonary blood flow (Q) or ventilation (V) [14]. More simply, the normal limits of log SD for Q or V range from 0.3 through 0.6. A value of 1.0 represents moderate amounts of $\dot{V}A/\dot{Q}$ inequality, which in the theoretical analysis made by West [22], corresponds to a PaO_2 of less than 60 mm Hg and $PaCO_2$ around 45 mm Hg. For severe $\dot{V}A/\dot{Q}$ mismatch, i.e. log SDQ euqals to 1.5, PaO_2 would be 40 mm Hg and $PaCO_2$ 57 mm Hg, respectively. Interestingly, the vast majority of data collected over the last ten years using the inert gas elimination technique indicates that the index or amount of dispersion for blood flow (log SDQ) appears more abnormal than for ventilation (log SDV) [15]. This is consistent with the pathophysiology of abnormalities found in human asthma where airway obstruction may cause areas of low $\dot{V}A/\dot{Q}$ units, so called "low $\dot{V}A/\dot{Q}$ mode", that are perfused but poorly ventilated. As a result, this must worsen blood flow dispersion more than that of ventilation.

Figure 1 illustrates the extent, pattern and time course of $\dot{V}A/\dot{Q}$ distributions in a representative individual with *status asthmaticus*. She was a young female, aged 28 years, first admitted severe asthma attack. She had mild asymptomatic asthma over the last three years and was not under regular treatment. Her chest X-ray was normal and she had no fever nor other associated diseases. On admission, she had resting breathlessness, intense cough, tachypnea, tachycardia, pulsus paradoxus, accessory muscle use, and also diffuse wheezing on auscultation. PEFR was 120 L/min and FEV, 1.18 L (34% predicted). While breathing room air, PaO_2 was 38 mm Hg, $PaCO_2$ 43 mm Hg, pH 7.39, and alveolar-arterial difference for O_2 ($AaDO_2$) 58 mm Hg. She required hospitalization for more than 48 hours and was treated with intravenous theophylline and steroids, inhaled salbutamol, fluids and continuous oxygen therapy. During the follow-up study, the clinical course and the duration of hospitalization were evaluated by attending physicians not directly involved in the study. Measurements were made in the sitting position, breathing room air, at the same time during the day, and 3 hours after giving any oral bronchodilating drug. On entry, 12 hours after her admission (A) (left) the patient showed considerable amount of $\dot{V}A/\dot{Q}$ inequality, with a clearly bimodal pattern in blood flow distribution and a broadly unimodal ventilation distribution. As a result, both the index of dispersion of blood flow (log SDQ, 1.48) and of ventilation (log SDV, 0.98) were substantially increased. On the other hand, the percentage of perfusion to low $\dot{V}A/\dot{Q}$ areas was 35% while shunt was absent. There were no areas of high $\dot{V}A/\dot{Q}$ ratios (between 10

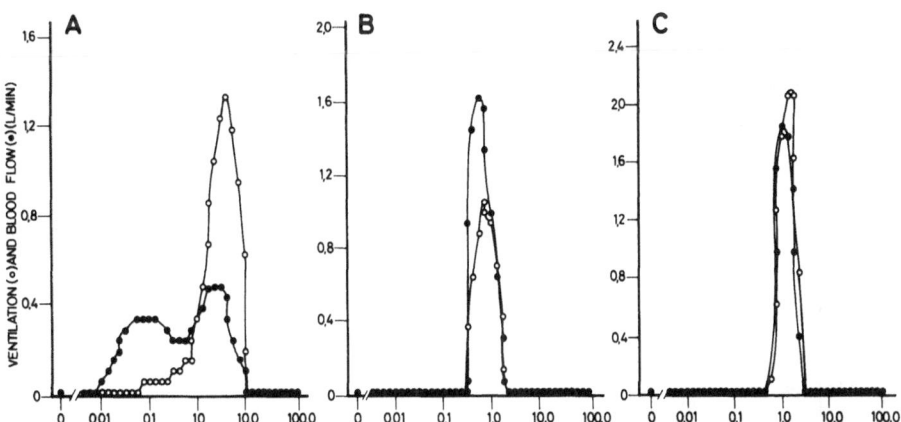

Fig. 1. Serial measurements of $\dot{V}A/\dot{Q}$ distribution in a representative patient with acute severe asthma. **A:** Within 24 hours of admission: **B:** Last of hospitalization; **C:** One month after discharge from hospital (for explanation, see text)

and 100), and inert dead space was low (23% of ventilation). During the seven days of hospitalization, she improved clinically and spirometrically. Thus, at the fifth day PEFR doubled (245 L/min); in addition, $\dot{V}A/\dot{Q}$ inequality (not shown in Fig. 1) improved: log SDQ was 0.99, log SDV was 0.87, and low $\dot{V}A/\dot{Q}$ mode averaged 13% of cardiac output. However, perfusion distribution was still bimodal. At the seventh day, the patient was discharged from hospital in good clinical condition (B) (middle). She was still treated with oral steroids and inhaled bronchodilators. At this time, $\dot{V}A/\dot{Q}$ mismatching was practically normal with a slightly increased log SDQ (0.67) and a normal log SDV (0.49). Both blood flow and ventilation distributions were narrowly unimodal. There was no shunt or low $\dot{V}A/\dot{Q}$ mode, and inert dead space was 33%. Finally, four weeks after discharge (C) (right) the patient was completely asymptomatic (PEFR, 560 L/min). Gas exchange also was normal, as shown in the figure, with narrowly unimodal blood flow and ventilation distributions (log SDQ, 0.29 and log SDV, 0.27). During the first hours of the acute episode, the patient was given 100% O_2 for 30 minutes. As a consequence, the bimodal blood flow distribution pattern almost doubled in shape. Both log SDQ and low $\dot{V}A/\dot{Q}$ mode increased (from 1.48 to 1.99, and from 35% to 41%, respectively) while log SDV remained unchanged (from 0.98 to 0.93); shunt fraction was not seen. In other words, there was a dramatic worsening in $\dot{V}A/\dot{Q}$ mismatching. Of further note was the lack of any correlation between central (FEV, and PEFR) or peripheral (MMFR) airflow rates and conventional (PaO$_2$) or inert (log SDQ) gas exchange data throughout the study.

Figure 2 includes $\dot{V}A/\dot{Q}$ ratio distributions in a 47 year old patient with very severe status asthmaticus within the first four hours of treatment with mechanical ventilation. This patient, asthmatic since he was teenager, was regularly treated with inhaled salbutamol and beclomethasone and oral theophylline. The patient was sedated and paralyzed (left), with a normal minute ventilation, but an increased cardiac output. PaO$_2$ was within normal limits (PaCO$_2$, 38 mm Hg; pH, 7.43). There was a substantial $\dot{V}A/\dot{Q}$ inequality such that both blood flow

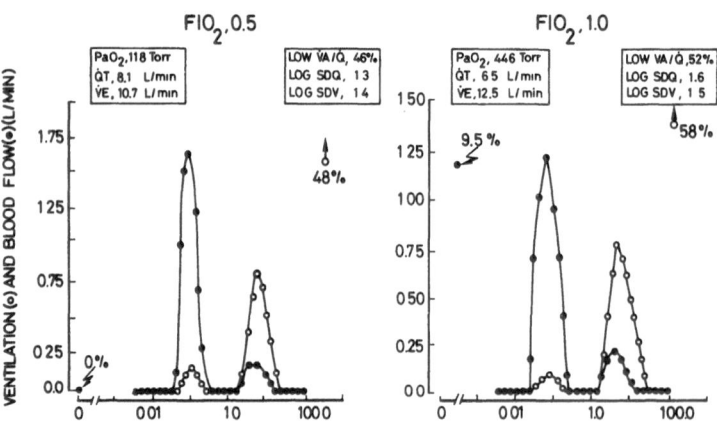

Fig. 2. $\dot{V}A/\dot{Q}$ distributions at maintenance FiO$_2$ (left) and during 100% O$_2$ (right) in a patient with acute severe asthma treated by mechanical ventilation (for explanation, see text)

and ventilation distributions displayed a clearly bimodal pattern. Indices of dispersion were severely increased (log SDQ, 1.3 and log SDV, 1.4, respectively). While shunt was absent, almost half the cardiac output was distributed to low $\dot{V}A/\dot{Q}$ units (46%). Interestingly, there was a mild high $\dot{V}A/\dot{Q}$ mode (9%) and inert dead space was increased (48%). While breathing 100% O_2 during 30 minutes (right), there were several interesting changes. On the one hand, cardiac output moderately decreased and minute ventilation slightly rose; although PaO_2 also increased (up to 446 mm Hg), it lower than expected. On the other hand, $\dot{V}A/\dot{Q}$ dramatically worsened. Shunt emerged, averaging 9.5% of cardiac output and both log SDQ and low $\dot{V}A/\dot{Q}$ mode increased, log SDV and high $\dot{V}A/\dot{Q}$ mode remaining essentially unchanged; inert dead space increased as well. As a result, the bimodal pattern of both distributions became more apparent than during maintenance FiO_2.

Pathogenesis and Clinical Implications of $\dot{V}A/\dot{Q}$ Inequality in Acute Severe Asthma

These results deserve several comments. First, patients with acute severe asthma have the most abnormal gas exchange characteristics of the $\dot{V}A/\dot{Q}$ spectrum in bronchial asthma, namely a substantial amount of $\dot{V}A/\dot{Q}$ mismatching where shunt is negligible. Bimodality in blood flow distribution, with no or little shunt, was a cardinal feature during the acute asthma attack, irrespective of treatment. This agrees with earlier investigations in both human beings [1] and animals [9] and gives further support to the key role played by collateral ventilation. Second, the dissociation between spirometry and gas exchange date (PaO_2 and $\dot{V}A/\dot{Q}$ inequality) reinforces the view that airflow rates mainly reflect obstruction of large airways, while $\dot{V}A/\dot{Q}$ inequality is more related to the abnormalities in peripheral, small airways where mucus plugging and/or bronchial wall edema are more relevant. Third, the areas of high $\dot{V}A/\dot{Q}$ mode are negligible in patients with *status asthmaticus*. As pointed out previously, this suggests that high $\dot{V}A/\dot{Q}$ areas observed in patients with chronic airflow obstruction, such as chronic obstructive pulmonary disease (COPD), rather than a functional finding related to air trapping and regional hyperinflation, may mainly reflect pulmonary emphysema, where the high $\dot{V}A/\dot{Q}$ mode follow from capillary bed destruction. Fourth, the administration of 100% O_2 in associated with a marked worsening in $\dot{V}A/\dot{Q}$ inequality suggesting release of hypoxic pulmonary vasoconstriction. In other words, in acute severe asthma there is a considerable hypoxic pulmonary vascular response as opposed to some asymptomatic asthmatics. More importantly, in the patient with the most life-threatening condition of *status asthmaticus,* who needed mechanical ventilation, there was a ten-fold increase in shunt during 100% O_2 breathing. To our knowledge, this is the only clinical condition in pulmonary medicine where such shunt increase is seen [23]. This would be in agreement with the analysis made by Dantzker and coworkers [24] showing the development of shunt due to eventual reabsorption atelectasis. This would also suggest that collateral ventilation becomes inefficient during 100% O_2 breathing in this kind of patients to prevent the alveolar collapse with critical inspiratory

$\dot{V}A/\dot{Q}$ ratios [24]. However, during low FiO_2 breathing collateral ventilation would remain as the most powerful mechanism to protect the lungs from development of shunt. In any case, an observation of considerable clinical interest is that substantial $\dot{V}A/\dot{Q}$ mismatch may exist in patients with acute severe asthma with relatively little change in PaO_2.

References

1. Wagner PD, Dantzker DR, Iacovoni VE, Tomlin WC, West JB (1978) Distributions of ventilation-perfusion ratios in asthma. Am Rev Respir Dis 118:511-24
2. Riley RL, Cournand A (1949) 'Ideal' alveolar air and the analysis of ventilation-perfusion relationships in the lungs. J Appl Physiol 1:825-47
3. McFadden EF, Lyons HA (1968) Arterial-blood gas tension in asthma. N Engl J Med 278:1027-33
4. Knudson RJ, Constantine HP (1967) An effect of isoproterenol on ventilation-perfusion in asthmatic versus normal subjects. J Appl Physiol 22:402-6.
5. Heckscher T, Bass H, Oriol A, Rose B, Anthonisen NR, Bates DV (1968) Regional lung function in patients with bronchial asthma. J Clin Invest 47:1063-70
6. Orphanidou D, Hughes JMB, Myers MJ, AL-Suhali A-R, Henderson B (1986) Tomography of regional ventilation and perfusion using Krypton 81m in normal subjects and asthmatic patients. Thorax 41:542-51
7. Wagner PD, Saltzman HA, West JB (1974) Measurement of continuous distributions of ventilation-perfusion ratios: theory. J Appl Physiol 36:588-99
8. Young IH, Corte P, Schoeffel RE (1982) Pattern and time course of ventilation-perfusion inequality in exercise-induced asthma. Am Rev Respir Dis 125:304-11
9. Rubinfeld AR, Wagner PD, West JB (1978) Gas exchange during experimental canine asthma. Am Rev Respir Dis 118:525-36
10. Rodriguez-Roisin R, Bencowitz HZ, Ziegler MG, Wagner PD (1984) Gas exchange responses to bronchodilators following methacholine challenge in dogs. Am Rev Respir Dis 130:617-26
11. Freyschuss U, Hedlin G, Hedenstierna G (1984) Ventilation-perfusion relationships during exercise-induced asthma in children. Am Rev Respir Dis 130:888-94
12. Hedlin G, Freyschuss U, Hedenstierna G (1985) Histamine-induced asthma in children: effects on the ventilation-perfusion relationship. Clin Physiol 5:19-34
13. Corte P, Young IH (1985) Ventilation-perfusion relationships in symptomatic asthma. Response to oxygen and clemastine. Chest 88:167-75
14. Wagner PD, Hedenstierna G, Bylin G (1987) Ventilation-perfusion inequality in chronic asthma. Am Rev Respir Dis 136:605-12
15. Wagner PD, Smith CM, Davies NJH, McEvoy RD, Gale GE (1985) Estimation of ventilation-perfusion inequality by inert gas elimination without arterial sampling. J Appl Physiol 59:376-83
16. Metcalf JF, Wagner PD, West JB (1978) Effect of local bronchial obstruction on gas exchange in the dog. Am Rev Respir Dis 117:85-95
17. Wagner PD, Dantzker DR, Dueck R, Clausen JL, West JP (1979) Ventilation-perfusion inequality in chronic obstructive pulmonary disease. J Clin Invest 59:203-16
18. Dueck R, Wagner PD, West JB (1977) Effects of positive end-expiratory pressure on gas exchange in dogs with normal and edematous lungs. Anesthesiology 47:359-66
19. Ballester E, Reyes A, Rodriguez-Roisin R, et al (1986) Ventilation-perfusion relationships in acute severe asthma. Effects of intravenous and aerosolized salbutamol. Am Rev Respir Dis 133:A178
20. Roca J, Ramis Ll, Rodriguez-Roisin R, Ballester E, Montserrat JM, Wagner PD (1988) Serial relationships between $\dot{V}A/\dot{Q}$ inequality and spirometry in acute severe asthma requiring hospitalization. Am Rev Respir Dis (in press)

21. Clark TJH (1977) Acute severe asthma. In: Clark TJH, Godfrey S (eds) Asthma. Chapman and Hall Ltd, London, pp 303-23
22. West JB (1969) Ventilation-perfusion inequality and overall gas exchange in computer models of the lung. Respir Physiol 7:88-110
23. Lemaire F, Matamis D, Lampron N, Teisseire B, Harf A (1985) Intrapulmonary shunt is not increased by 100% oxygen ventilation in acute respiratory failure. Bull Eur Physiopathol Respir 21:251-56
24. Dantzker DR, Wagner PD, West JP (1975) Instability of lung units with low $\dot{V}A/\dot{Q}$ ratios during O_2 breathing. J Appl Physiol 38:886-95

Clinical Assessment of Severe Asthma

J. C. Yernault and C. Lenclud

Introduction

Most commonly bronchial asthma presents clinically as attacks of breathlessness and/or chest tightness (that the physician calls dyspnea) accompanied by cough and wheezing. The pathophysiological characteristic of the asthma attack is a reduction of the intrathoracic airway lumen resulting from a contraction of the airway smooth muscle, an edematous and inflammatory thickening of the mucosa and submucosa together with accumulation of viscous secretions within the lumen. In order to maintain ventilation the respiratory muscles have to work harder and develop large negative intrapleural pressure swings during inspiration (and sometimes positive pressure during expiration).

The anatomical lesions being inequally distributed, ventilation becomes inhomogeneous and ventilation-perfusion inequalities explain the arterial hypoxemia. Both hypoxemia (via a stimulation of the carotid chemoreceptors) and reflex mediated via the vagus nerve (for instance stimulation of the irritant receptors) increase the overall ventilation so that hypocapnia occurs. However, with further $\dot{V}A/\dot{Q}$ mismatching and prolongation of intense respiratory muscle work, pump failure may develop so that $PaCO_2$ becomes again normal and eventually increases. This is the case in about 10% of the patients presenting to an emergency room with an asthma attack [1]. Hypoxemia and large intrathoracic pressure swings result in cardiovascular adjustments with tachycardia and sometimes pulsus paradoxus [2]. In view of the above events the severity of an asthma attack can be judged from several aspects which are more or less related.

The Measurement of Dyspnea

Earlier attempts to quantify the severity of dyspnea in asthma were in fact evaluating the functional abililty of the patient [3]. However, dyspnea is a sensation that can be quantified by psychophysical methods [4], such as the Borg scale [5]. Dyspnea generally occurs when the respiratory effort approaches the maximal possible effort, the important parameters to consider being the peak pressure (compared to the maximal pressure that the inspiratory muscles can generate) as well as the duration and speed of contraction. However, for a given level of airway obstruction the intensity of dyspnea may vary considerably between individuals, which can be explained by variations in the level and pattern of breathing, by differences in respiratory muscles operating characteristics, by differences in perceptual sensitivity as well as by psychological and emotional factors. The visual analogic and the Borg scales are therefore most useful to evaluate the changes occurring in a given patient than to compare different patients.

The following points must be kept in mind when using dyspnea as an index of asthma severity:

- The ability to discriminate changes in airway resistance (Raw) is a constant fraction of the initial value: this implies that a subject with chronically increased Raw becomes less perceptive to small variations in Raw than a subject with a normal Raw during the intercrisis period. In addition there is also a temporal habituation effect so that a severe chronic airway obstruction may not be detected by the patient [5, 6].
- About 1/3 of the asthmatics are "poor perceivers", but they can be trained to improve their perceptiveness by simultaneously rating their dyspnea and measuring their peak expiratory flow [7].
- The patient is more able to evaluate changes in peak expiratory flow (PEF) induced by an inhaled bronchodilator than the physician [8].
- The dyspnea of the asthmatic predominates during inspiration [9] in contrast to a still common belief.

From all the above considerations it follows that it is important to rate the intensity of dyspnea and to evaluate its response to treatment, but than it cannot be relied only on it to judge the severity of airway obstruction.

The Quantification of Wheezing

Wheezes are high-pitched continuous sounds with frequencies above 200 Hz and duration of at least 250 msec. They are produced by oscillations of airway walls set-up by turbulence of air moving through a narrowed lumen. The pitch of the wheeze is determined by the mass and elasticity of the oscillating wall and not by the length and caliber of the airway [10]. They are better transmitted through airways than through lung parenchyma and chest wall and consequently are better heard over the trachea than over the chest wall [11].

Wheezing is not always noted during exacerbations of asthma, although in most cases it is heard over the entire chest wall in both phases of the respiratory cycle. During milder exacerbations wheezes can be heard only over the trachea during expiration. In the severe asthmatic with hyperinflation the disappearance of wheezing may indicate a very low flow rate (and not an improvement!); at that time listening at the patient's open mouth may still detect audible wheezes. In the patient without a noisy breathing during tidal volume respiration, wheezing can be detected during a forced expiratory maneuver, the duration of which can be measured. At the time wheezing is disappearing specific airway conductance (sGaw) is normalized, but significant airway obstruction is present as reflected by a decreased FEV_1 [12].

The problems in evaluating the severity of wheezing come from a large intra- and interobserver variability in assessment [13]. However this can now be over-mounted by computer-analysis of sound recordings made with an electronic ste-thoscope [14, 15] which has shown that wheeze duration as a proportion of the respiratory cycle and the peak sound frequency parallels the degree of broncho-constriction. With a microphone fixed over the suprasternal notch [16] and fur-ther refinement in computer analysis we are now able to monitor the presence or absence of wheezing for more than 18 hours in a given subject and to obtain on line measurement of the percent of time occupied by wheezing as well as of the frequency of the wheezes. The application of that procedure in the clinical situ-ation is currently being evaluated.

The Value of Inspection and Palpation

Large intrathoracic negative swings may be suspected from supraclavicular and intercostal retraction during inspiration. The increased inspiratory work of breathing can be detected by palpating a more than usual vigorous contraction of the scalenes (the "respiratory pulse") and by visualizing the use of the sterno-mastoid muscles; at that time sGaw is lower than 0.05 cm $H_2O^{-1} \cdot s^{-1}$. However, all the patients with severe airway obstruction do not necessarily use their acces-sory muscles [12]. Patients electing to remain seated in their bed also have a severe airway obstruction [17].

Expiratory effort may be judged in a lying subject from the palpation of an active contraction of the abdominal muscles. During the most severe attacks dys-synchronous breathing and eventually paradoxical abdominal motion can occur, which indicate diaphragm dysfunction and imminent pump failure.

The respiratory rate (fR) is a very simple but useful measurement to be per-formed, since fR increases with the increasing severity of an asthmatic attack, a fR above 30/min being associated with a poor prognosis [18]. However, monitor-ing fR during the night does not recognize patients with a morning dip [19].

The Measurement of Airway Obstruction

It is clear from the above considerations that a through clinical examination and precise evaluation of symptoms do not always suffice to correctly evaluate the severity of airway obstruction, which must therefore be directly measured. Even the less well-equipped physician can measure the time of a forced expiration and must routinely use a mini-peak flow meter. However, repeated forced expiratory manoeuvers are not always well tolerated by an acutely dyspneic patient and can by themselves aggravate airway obstruction. It might therefore be better to rely on non invasive measurements of airway resistance obtained during normal tidal breathing eventually at the bedside; despite its theoretical limitations an inter-ruption method can be useful to monitor the response to treatment.

Symptoms and Signs of Altered Gas Exchange

Arterial hypoxemia is the rule during an asthma attack but is partially compensated by hyperventilation so that it is usually not deep enough to induce a clinically detectable (central cyanosis) fall in hemoglobin saturation. Moreover the respiratory alcalosis shifting the oxyhemoglobin dissociation curve towards the left acts to preserve a better saturation. Consequently cyanosis during an asthma attack is a rare event that always indicate profound hypoxemia [20] and monitoring by pulse oximetry can be useful only in these severe cases.

Hypocapnia and alkalosis may be severe enough to induce symptoms such as dizziness and hand paresthesias. In those patients who do not wheeze these symptoms can be very misleading so that the diagnosis of asthma can be overlooked if bronchial hyperreactivity is not demonstrated by adequate bronchoprovocation tests. In the most severe cases hypercapnia may induce diaphoresis and various degrees of alteration of consciousness which always indicate a very serious situation.

The Cardiovascular Signs

Tachycardia is the most common cardiac abnormality observed during an asthma attack; it closely parallels the degree of hypoxemia [20]. An error to avoid is to consider tachycardia as secondary to abusive inhalation of beta-agonists such an interpretation would refrain from further beta-mimetics administration, which remain the first choice therapy [21].

Electrocardiographic changes add little [22], except when arrhythmias are present, which are usually induced by severe hypoxemia and/or metabolic (lactic) acidosis [23]. In the most severe cases of airflow limitation and hyperinflation, pulsus paradoxus may develop. It is better detected by auscultation than by simple palpation of the radial artery: an inspiratory drop of the systemic systolic blood pressure higher than 15 mm Hg must be considered as an additional sign of very severe airway obstruction [12, 18].

To conclude we have now the instruments to properly evaluate the severity of an asthma attack; none of them is perfect so that it is preferable to rely on several indexes:

- The patient can rate the severity of his breathlessness and its evolution under treatment.
- We have the means to quantify and follow up wheezing.
- A close observation of the patient can detect the signs of an increased respiratory work and the precursors of a pump failure.
- The degree of airway obstruction can and should be measured in each case.
- The abnormalities in arterial blood gases are poorly reflected, clinically, tachycardia being the best simple indicator.
- Development of pulsus paradoxus always indicates a severe airflow limitation.

Despite recent progress in understanding the pathophysiology of asthma and its clinical manifestations, it remains difficult to predict which patient has to be hospitalized for an asthma attack [24, 25].

References

1. Mc Fadden ER Jr, Lyons HA (1968) Arterial blood gas tension in asthma. N Engl J Med 278:1027–1032
2. Knowles GK, Clark TJH (1973) Pulsus paradoxus as a valuable sign indicating severity of asthma. Lancet 2:1356–1359
3. Center DM, Make BJ (1981) Management of severe asthma. In: Brody JS, Snider GL (eds) Current topics in the management of respiratory diseases. Churchill Livingstone, New York pp 15–34
4. Altose MD (1987) Psychophysies – An approach to the study of respiratory sensation and the assessment of dyspnea. Am Rev Respir Dis 135:1227–1228
5. Burdon JGW, Juniper EF, Killian KJ, Hargreave FE, Campbell EJM (1982) The perception of breathlessnes in asthma. Am Rev Respir Dis 126:825–828
6. Orehek J, Beaupré A, Badier M, Nicoli MM, Delpierre S (1982) Perception of airway tone by asthmatic patients. Bull Eur Physiopathol Respir 18:601–607
7. Higgs CMB, Richardson RB, Lea DA, Lewis GTR, Laszlo G (1986) Influence of knowledge of peak flow on self assessment of asthma: studies with a coded peak flow meter. Thorax 41:671–675
8. Shim CS, Williams MH (1980) Evaluation of the severity of asthma: patients versus physcicians. Am J Med 68:11–14
9. Morris MJ (1981) Asthma-expiratory dyspnoea? Br Med J 283:838–839
10. Hollingsworth HM (1987) Wheezing and stridor. Clin Chest Med 8:231–240
11. Loudon R, Murphy RLH Jr (1984) Lung sounds. Am Rev Respir Dis 130:663–673
12. Mc Fadden ER, Kiser R, de Groot WJ (1973) Acute bronchial asthma: relations between clinical and physiological manifestations. N Engl J Med 288:221–225
13. Pasterkamp H, Wiebicke N, Fenton R (1987) Subjective assessment versus computer analysis of wheezing in asthma. Chest 91:376–381
14. Baughman RP, Loudon RG (1984) Quantitation of wheezing in acute asthma. Chest 86:718–722
15. Baughman RP, Loudon RG (1985) Lung sounds analysis for continuous evaluation of airflow obstruction in asthma. Chest 88:364–368
16. Charbonneau G, Racineux JL, Sudraud M, Tuchais E (1983) An accurate recording system and its use in breath sound spectral analysis. J Appl Physiol 55:1120–1127
17. Brenner BE, Abraham E, Simon RR (1983) Position and diaphoresis in acute asthma. Am J Med 74:1005–1009
18. Fischl MA, Pitchenik A, Gardner LB (1981) An index predicting relapse and need for hospitalization in patients with acute bronchial asthma. N Engl J Med 305:783–789
19. Morgan AD, Rhind GB, Connaughton JJ, Catterall JR, Shapiro CM, Douglas NJ (1987) Breathing patterns during sleep in patients with nocturnal asthma. Thorax 42:600–603
20. Rebuck AS, Read J (1971) Assessment and management of severe asthma. Am J Med 51:788
21. Rossing TH, Fanta CH, Mc Fadden ER Jr, and the Medical House Staff, Brigham and Women's Hospital (1983) Effect of outpatient treatment of asthma with beta agonists on the response to sympathico-mimetics in an emergency room. Am J Med 75:781–784
22. Mc Fadden ER Jr (1986) Clinical physiologic correlates in asthma. J Allergy Clin Immunol 77:1–5
23. Appel D, Rubenstein R, Schrager K, Williams MH Jr (1983) Lactic acidosis in severe asthma. Am J Med 75:58C
24. Rose C, Murphy JG, Schwartz JS (1984) Performance of an index predicting the response of patients with acute bronchial asthma to intensive emergency department treatment. N Engl J Med 310:573
25. Centor RM, Yarbrough P, Wood JP (1984) Inability to predict relapse in acute asthma. N Engl J Med 310:577

Can Fatal Asthma Be Prevented?

P. Barriot, B. Riou, and P. Duroux

Introduction

Asthma in France is a common disease which affects approximately 3 to 4 percent of the population and carries considerable morbidity. But, only in the past 50 years has fatal asthma been recognized. It represents a rare complication of asthma, but it assumes considerable importance because of the high prevalence of asthma. The socio-economic impact of death caused by asthma is important, because the mortality rate from asthma is high and has increased over the past 25 years in many developed countries despite new treatment regimes, and because many of these deaths occur in young and otherwise healthy people. Moreover, most deaths from asthma appear to be largely preventable. The aim of this chapter is to summarize current findings concerning fatal asthma, and our own recent experience in its prevention.

Epidemiology

The mortality rate from asthma differs from one country to another (Fig. 1). Differences in prevalence of asthma were thought to explain differences in the

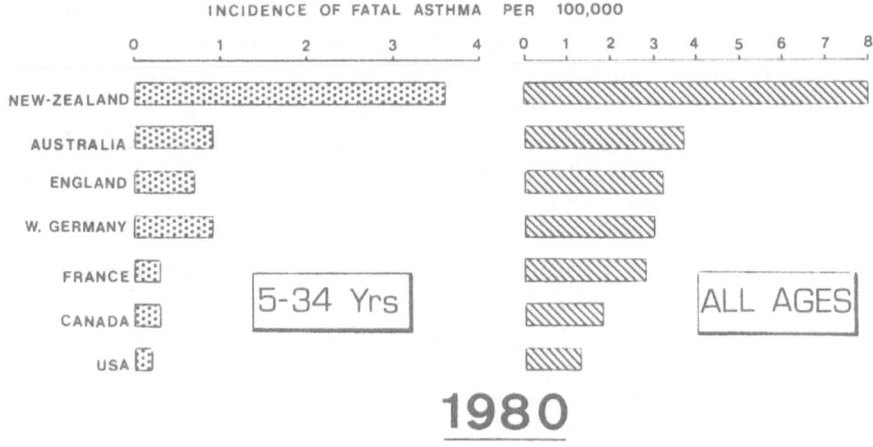

Fig. 1. Deaths from asthma in various countries, in five- to 34-year old patients and in patients of all ages during the year 1980. (From Riou et al., L'asthme mortel, Rev Mal Resp; in press)

mortality rate [1]. The highest mortality rates occur in New-Zealand, whereas the lowest rates have been reported in the USA. In Europe, mortality rates appear to be similar in England and Wales, West Germany, and France, i.e. 3 to 4 deaths per 100 000 habitants. Since the 1960s, many studies have addressed the problem of the increasing mortality rate from asthma [2], and now there is some agreement that this trend is real and cannot be explained by differences in disease classification, or inaccurate death certificates. Moreover, a recent study [3] has shown a further increase in mortality during 1974–84 in England and Wales. The reason why fatalities from asthma have increased remains unknown but the possibility that its prevalence and severity have changed cannot be excluded.

There are few studies which document fatal asthma in a large asthmatic population. An early study by MacCracken [4] reported a mortality rate of 500/ 100 000 whereas Alderson and Loy [5] have recently reported a mortality rate of 250/100 000; Blair [6] reported a mortality rate of 50/100 000 in asthmatic children.

Fatal asthma may occur in the hospital, as a complication of status asthmaticus. The mortality rate of status asthmaticus ranges from 39% [7] to 0% [8]. A 10 to 15% mortality rate in patients with status asthmaticus requiring mechanical ventilation is not unusual. A final point concerns the outcome of patients who suffered from status asthmaticus and were discharged alive from the hospital. Bousser et al. [9] have reported a mortality of 41% in these patients, 8 years after hospital discharge.

Risk Factors for Fatal Asthma

Many studies [2] have attempted to identify factors which characterize asthmatic patients who are at high risk of death but most of them did not include control groups. Nevertheless two recent studies [10, 11] that included control groups have confirmed earlier findings. A long history of asthma, a previous life-threatening attack, recent emergency hospital admission, poor medical management, poor compliance with treatment, lack of adequate objective evaluation of the severity of airway limitation, poor perception of airway limitation, and delay in hospital admission, are thought to be risk factors [2, 10, 11]. Nevertheless, fatal asthma may occur suddenly in patients not having any recognized risk factors. In our study [12], only 10% of patients with fatal asthma required mechanical ventilation previously, and in 43% no contributing factor was found.

Since the 1960s, the increase in deaths from asthma has been attributed to an increase in the use of pressurized aerosols containing sympathomimetic agents [2]. However, major errors in methodology were discovered in these earlier studies, and the relationship between fatalities from asthma aerosols containing sympathomimetic agents has been questioned by recent and well-conducted studies. Esdaile et al. [13] have reviewed this problem and concluded that the causal link between fatal asthma pressurized aerosols containing sympathomimetic was not supported by any scientific evidence. The consequences of earlier alarmist reports are still present, and many explain why many patients and physicians are still reluctant to use pressurized sympathomimetic aerosols extensively.

A poor perception of the severity of airflow limitation by the asthmatic patients has been emphasized in cases of fatal asthma. Rubinfeld and Pain [14] have shown that 15% of asthmatic patients were unable to detect a 50% limitation of airflow. Nevertheless, most of the studies which concluded in poor self-assessment of the severity of the attack also underline the long delay in hospital admission, which is not under the asthmatic patient's control. There is evidence that asthmatic patients are capable of assessing their condition:

1. in the retrospective portion of our study [12], we observed that 9% of asthmatic patients who called our prehospital emergency care unit died;
2. in the prospective part of our study, 85% of asthmatic patients who called had a peak expiratory flow value less than 150 ml/min demonstrating that they were actually critically ill.

Psychological factors appear to be important also since they affect medical management, compliance, and behavior during a severe attack of asthma.

Characteristics of the Fatal Attack of Asthma

Many fatal attacks of asthma have a sudden unexpected onset. Deaths have been reported to occur within 30 min in 25% [2] to 65% [12] of patients. This suggests that fatal asthma is not necessarily related to a prolonged attack and that fatal asthma is often due to sudden severe attacks "out of a clear blue sky" as stated by Stableforth [15]. The rapid onset of a fatal asthma attack might explain the "inaccurate" assessment of disease severity by the asthmatic patient. Moreover, Arnold et al. [16] suggested that adequate prevention of fatal asthma depends on the rapidity of onset. If fatal attacks progress slowly, it is safe to concentrate on improved management of the patient at home, whereas, if fatal attacks develop more rapidly, improvement in pre-hospital measures is more appropriate.

Prevention of Fatal Asthma

Retrospective studies [2] have suggested that up to 80% of deaths from asthma could be prevented, since in most cases potentially avoidable factors could be identified. However, only two studies [14, 16] have actually sought ways to decrease the mortality rate from asthma. Prevention of fatal asthma might be achieved at different but not exclusive levels (Table 1).

Failure to diagnose asthma precludes effective treatments. Physicians must be aware that chronic bronchitis or COPD, and asthma are not mutually exclusive. Underdiagnosis of asthma in children should be underlined: diagnosis of asthma was offered in only 12% of children who suffered at least one episode of wheezing since starting school, and in only 35% of children experiencing more than 12 episodes a year [17]. Failure to diagnose asthma deprives the patient of specific treatment and leaves him in real danger in case of any severe sudden attack.

Table 1. Recommendations to prevent fatal asthma

- Improvement in recognition of asthma, especially in children
- Education of physicians
- Recognition of patients at high risk for fatal asthma
- Education of asthmatic patients
  - knowledge of asthma and its treatment
  - self-management skills
  - how and when to call for emergency help
- Improvement in therapy
  - preventive therapy
  - symptomatic treatment
  - self-control using peak-flow meter
- Improvement in prehospital management of emergency calls
  - self-referral admission services [19]
  - systematic prehospital emergency care plans [12]
- Adequate hospital care of status asthmaticus [8]
- Reappraisal of patients who experienced near-fatal asthma [19]

The education of asthmatic patients is of major importance. Physicians must explain the purpose of each treatment (relief or prevention of symptoms) and the need to continue treatment even when the patient feels well. Teaching patients how to use inhalers is of paramount importance, but it has been shown that many patients are unable to use conventional pressurized aerosols efficiently even after careful training. In these patients, new devices, such as aerochambers, facilitate aerosol administration. Physicians must teach the asthmatic patient self-management skills: administering a short individually-adapted course of corticosteroid when he recognized sufficient deterioration, recognition of symptoms requiring emergency medical assistance, self-management of a severe attack until the physician's arrival, including self-injection of a subcutaneous sympathomimetic agent (Bricanyl) in those patients suffering from rapid severe attacks. Definition of conditions requiring a call for emergency assistance are very important. The efficacy of both treatments, for prevention and for relief of an attack, and especially self-administered treatment during a severe attack, must be evaluated by objective measurement of airflow limitation using a home peak-flow meter.

Training of all physicians likely to encounter asthmatic patients is obviously necessary. A recent European audit of asthma therapy has shown large differences in physicians' view on how to treat asthma, the main contrast involves physicians in Britain and Scandinavia who prefer β-agonists in inhalation and corticosteroids, and, on the other hand, those in France, Portugal, and some other countries who favor administration of theophylline and desensitization [18]. It must be pointed out that undertreatment (i.e. insufficient use of inhaled β-agonists and corticosteroids) was recognized as a main risk factor for fatal asthma [2]. Corticosteroids should always be envisaged to treat patients who experience a life-threatening asthma attack. General practioners must verify the efficacy of emergency treatment of an asthma attack in the patient's home using a peak-flow meter.

The only two studies [12, 19] which actually decreased the mortality rate from asthma sought to improve the prehospital management of emergency call. As a matter of fact, delay at any stage of care is an important factor involved in deaths from asthma [2, 12]. Crompton et al. [19] have developed a self-admission service for asthmatic patients and reported a lower mortality rate from asthma (0,3%) than that observed in patients who used other asthma services (0.6%). But, this scheme is probably useful only in cooperative patients, and Anderson et al. [20] failed to demonstrate any improvement in the mortality rate when applying such a system of self-refferal to a population of asthmatic children. We have initiated a prospective study [12] in an effort to decrease the incidence of fatal asthma, with improvement in the prehospital management of emergency calls from asthmatic patients. This study was based on the following assumption: asthmatic patients who call an emergency care unit actually are having a severe attack that might be fatal. Thus, standardized behavior was decided, whatever the apparent severity of the attack: team of firemen (mean delay of arrival 5 min) and an ambulance with a physician (mean delay 10 min) were immediately dispatched to the asthmatic patient and he was taken to the hospital. In this manner, we obtained a 6-fold reduction in the mortality rate from asthma (Fig. 2), and during a 6-month period, 17 patients who experienced cardiorespiratory arrests were successfully resuscitated and were discharged from the hospital alive.

Conclusion

Fatal asthma clearly remains as a major health problem affecting young people and accounting for more than 1500 dealths per year in France. Moreover, mortality rates from asthma appear to have increases, despite new treatment regimes whereas mortality rates from other respiratory diseases have decreased at the

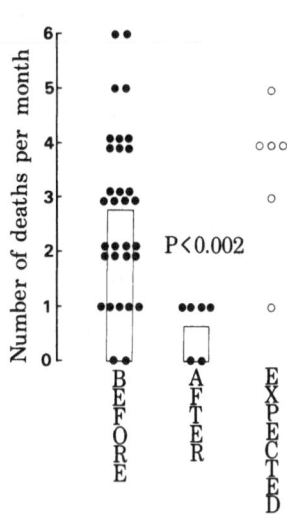

Fig. 2. Comparison of the mortality rate from asthma before (mean 2.75 deaths/month) and after (mean 0.66 deaths/ month) our recommendations in the prehospital management of emergency calls from asthmatic patients. Dotted rectangle and open circles represent the expected mortality rate if patients who experienced near-fatal asthma had not been resuscitated (mean 3.5 deaths/month). Each circle represents one month, and the rectangles the average. (From [12])

same time. Improved recognition of asthma, education of asthmatic patients and all medical personnel likely to encounter asthmatic patients, improvement in therapy, and development of patient self-referral admission services are probably necessary. But development of prehospital emergency plans are of paramount importance and can actually prevent some deaths. Emergency calls from asthmatic patients must be considered as severe attacks that may be fatal because of the lack of an accurate method to evaluate the severity of an attack that progresses rapidly, with the risk of sudden death.

References

1. Woolcock AJ (1986) Worldwide differences in asthma prevalence and mortality. Chest 90:40S–45S
2. Benatar SR (1986) Fatal asthma. N Engl J Med 314:423–429
3. Burney PG (1986) Asthma mortality in England and Wales: evidence for a further increase 1974–84. Lancet 2:323–326
4. MacCracken D (1950) Prognosis in bronchial asthma. Br Med J 1:409–412
5. Alderson M, Loy RM (1977) Mortality from respiratory disease at follow-up of patients with asthma. Br J Dis Chest 71:198–202
6. Blair H (1977) Natural history of childhood asthma: a 20-year follow-up. Arch Dis Child 52:613–619
7. Scoggin CH, Shan SA, Petty TL (1977) Status asthmaticus. A nine year experience. JAMA 238:1158–1162
8. Darioli R, Perret C (1984) Mechanically controlled hypoventilation in status asthmaticus. Am Rev Respir Dis 129:385–387
9. Bousser J, Reubet-Degat O, Jeannin L (1986) Evolution à distance des états de mal asthmatique. Réanim Soins Intens Med Urg 2:278 (Abstract)
10. Rea HH, Scragg R, Jackson R, Beaglehole R, Fenwick J, Sutherland DC (1986) A case-control study of deaths from asthma. Thorax 41:833–839
11. Strunk RC, Mrazek DA, Wolfson Furhman GS, Labrecque JF (1985) Physiologic and psychological characteristics associated with deaths due to asthma in childhood: a case-controlled study. JAMA 254:1193–1198
12. Barriot P, Riou B (1987) Fatal asthma. Chest 92:460–466
13. Esdaile JM, Feinstein AR, Horwitz RI (1987) A reappraisal of the United Kingdom epidemic of fatal asthma. Arch Intern Med 147:543–549
14. Rubinfeld AR, Pain MC (1976) Perception of asthma. Lancet 1:882–884
15. Stableforth D (1983) Death from asthma. Thorax 38:801–805
16. Arnold AG, Lane DJ, Zapata E (1982) The speed of onset and severity of acute severe asthma. Br J Dis Chest 76:157–163
17. Speight ANP, Lee DA, Hey EN (1983) Underdiagnosis and undertreatment of asthma in childhood. Br Med J 286:1253–1256
18. Vermeire PA, Wittesaele WM, Janssens E, De Backer WA (1986) European audit of asthma therapy. Chest 90:58S–61S
19. Crompton GK, Grant IWB, Bloomfield P (1979) Edinburgh emergency asthma admission service: report on 10 years' experience. Br Med J 2:1199–1201
20. Anderson HR, Bailey P, West S (1980) Trends in the hospital care of acute childhood asthma 1970–8. Br Med J 281:1191–1194

Status Asthmaticus: An Approach to Therapy

P. Goldberg and C. Roussos

Introduction

Status asthmaticus is defined as severe bronchial obstruction refractory to the "usual treatment". This description is by definition somewhat arbitrary in that it lacks any objective criteria and that "usual treatment" may differ from center to center. Therefore, it would be more appropriate to discuss the severe asthmatic in whom spirometry demonstrates marked obstruction with an FEV_1 of less than 1 liter and often of less than 700 cc.

In 1975, in the United States, an estimated 183 000 persons were admitted to hospitals for treatment of asthma; it was also estimated that asthma was the cause of death in 2000 patients [1]. In their study, Scoggin et al. [2] described 811 admissions for status asthmaticus between 1967 and 1975 to one tertiary care hospital in Denver. Of these, 21 (2.6%) required mechanical ventilation and 8 (1.0% of admissions; 38% of these mechanically ventilated) died.

Treatment

Supportive Care

Treatment is aimed both at supporting the patient and at reversing the obstruction. Because ventilation/perfusion is a constant feature with resultant hypoxemia, supplemental oxygen should be administered. The method of its delivery – masks vs prongs – should be determined by the comfort of the patient. Because diminished CO_2 responsiveness is not a feature of this disease, the amount of oxygen administered is not problematic. However, because both distilled water and cold humidification may each provoke bronchospasm the oxygen administered should be humidified with warm normal saline.

The appropriate fluid management of these patients is problematic. Many of these patients manifest evidence of dehydration with an increased propensity for mucus inspissation and bronchial lumen obstruction. At the same time, however, they may be at an increased risk for the development of pulmonary edema as described by Stalcup et al. [3]. Therefore, fluid management should be adjusted to achieve a normal serum osmolarity on the one hand and a urine output of approximately 0.5–1 ml/kg/hour.

Pharmacotherapy

Theophylline: Theophylline has long held a significant role in the therapy of severe asthma. First Mitenko and Ogilvie [4] and the Racineux et al. [5] demonstrated the long-dose relationship between serum theophylline levels and bronchodilatation. Although theophylline inhibits phosphodiesterase thereby elevating cAMP levels, there are several lines of evidence suggesting that this is not the mechanism of its bronchodilating effect [6]. Whatever the biochemical pathway its final action must be through the lowering of intracellular smooth muscle calcium levels.

Rossing et al. [7] were the first to question its efficacy in the treatment of asthma. Since that initial study there has been a mounting body of evidence [8, 9] suggesting that theophylline adds little to the bronchodilating response of appropriately used β_2-agonists while significantly adding to their toxicity.

The true role of theophylline may lie in its more recently described properties. Aubier et al. [10] demonstrated that at therapeutic levels (10–20 μg/ml) theophylline enhances diaphragmatic contractility and retards the onset of diaphragmatic fatigue. Matthay et al. [11] showed that the drug augments right ventricular ejection fraction both by a direct inotropic effect and by decreasing pulmonary vascular resistance. This latter property may assume critical importance given the increased load against which the right ventricle must pump – an increased load determined by high lung volumes, hypoxemia, and acidosis.

For patients not having taken a theophylline compound within the preceding twenty-four hours, a loading dose of 5.6 mg/kg is administered over 20–30 minutes; for those on theophylline, one-half of that loading dose is administered. The maintenance dose ranges from 0.2–0.9 mg/kg/hour depending on a host of variables which can influence theophylline metabolism. However, because of such variables and because of a very narrow therapeutic to toxic ratio, the only prudent fashion with which to safely monitor theophylline is to frequently assay serum theophylline levels.

β_2-Agonists: β_2-agonists, both resorcinols (metaproterenol, terbutaline, fenoterol) and salinigens (salbutamol) provide greater β_2 selectivity and less cardiac stimulation than their catecholamine precursors (epinephrine, isoproterenol) and are the drugs of first choice. However two major controverses still surround their use.

The first concerns the route of administration. To date, various studies comparing parenteral and aerosol administration have demonstrated conflicting results [12–15], and as yet, no consensus has been achieved on this issue. However, most studies do support the finding that whatever the relative efficacy, parenterally administered β_2-agonists result in a higher incidence of side-effects, notably tachycardia and tremor.

As unsettled is the optimal dose of the aerosol and the frequency of its administration. Walters et al. [16] examined this issue and found that while the dose response of salbutamol was linear between 1.5 mg and 7.5 mg, side effects became troublesome at a dose greater than 3.0 mg and thus recommended the latter dose. However, other authors [13] have used far greater amounts of salbutamol (10 mg) with relative inpunity.

The second issue addresses the dosing frequency. Although the duration of action of these agents is approximately 6 hours, Weber et al. [17] demonstrated that repetitive doses at 20 minute intervals produced continued bronchodilatation. It would appear from these results that aerosol dosage and frequency should be titrated to side effects and that rather large doses administered at least every 20 minutes may be administered achieving a cumulative bronchodilating effect with minimal toxicity.

Corticosteroids: While the exact dosage of glucocorticoids may be controversial, their role in the treatment of severe asthma was firmly established by Fanta et al. [18]. There are, nevertheless, multiple studies supporting or rejecting the use of high dose steroids [19–21]. In Haskell's study [19], both the high (125 mg q6h) and moderate (40 mg q6h) dose of methylprednisolone were superior to the low (15 mg q6h) in achieving bronchodilatation while the high dose achieved its effect more rapidly than the moderate dose. Because few adverse effects save for hyperglycemia, and the rare episode of psychosis accrue to the use of a short course of high-dose steroids, such a dose is advisable. Finally, to spare the sodium-water retentive and kaliuretic properties of hypocortisone, methylprednisolone is preferable.

Anticholinergics: Anticholinergics have a long history in the treatment of asthma and they were in fact, the drugs of choice prior to the clinical application of catecholamines. Because of variable local and systemic side effects, atropine has not gained wide clinical acceptance. However, ipratropium bromide, a quaternary amine with minimal systemic absorption has been widely used with little or no toxicity including the lack of any adverse effects on the viscoelastic properties of mucus [22]. Some studies have favorably compared ipratropium to β_2-agonists [23], while others [24] have clearly demonstrated the superiority of the latter. However in his recent work, Bryant [25] demonstrated that when used concurrently with ipratropium, a β_2-agonist achieved greater bronchodilatation than when used alone.

Mechanical Ventilation

Continuous Positive Airway Pressure (CPAP): In their elegant study, Martin et al. [26] demonstrated the beneficial effects of CPAP in a group of histamine induced asthmatics. They showed that the work of breathing per liter of ventilation decreases secondary to a decrease in lung resistance – at the mechanism of which they could only speculate – and by unloading the inspiratory muscles.

Asthmatics in severe exacerbation probably develop significant levels of intrinsic PEEP [27] which acting as a threshold resistor, increase the work of breathing [28]. The addition of CPAP may, therefore, decrease the work of breathing in the severe asthmatic by unloading the inspiratory muscles, decreasing lung resistance, and providing positive pressure to overcome the threshold resistor of intrinsic PEEP.

Intubation – Mechanical Ventilation: A review of the literature reveals that in asthmatics undergoing intubation and mechanical ventilation there is an increased incident of complications including barotrauma as compared to patients undergoing mechnical ventilation for other causes [2] and barotrauma in intubated asthmatic patients has been associated with an increased mortality [2], estimated at approximately 30% [29].

The factors most often incriminated as being responsible for this increased risk of barotrauma are excessive peak airway pressures and distal air-trapping. In their report, Darioli and Perret [30] addressed the former. In ventilating their asthmatic patients these authors chose to disregard the $PaCO_2$ as long as it was less then 90 mmHg while established a maximal airway pressure of 50 cm H_2O at which level the volume-cycled ventilator would switch to its expiratory phase; minute ventilation was adjusted accordingly. They reported no deaths and three episodes of barotrauma, none of which was a pneumothorax (subcutaneous emphysema 2; pneumomediastinum 1).

In a similar study, Menitove and Goldring [29] selected a maximal airway pressure of 50 cm H_2O, ignoring $PaCO_2$. They chose, however, to maintain an arterial pH of approximately 7.3 with exogenous administration of bicarbonate. They reported no deaths or barotrauma in their three cases.

This concept of cathecholamine airway responsiveness and an arterial pH of 7.3 is a theme found repetitively through the asthma literature. It is however a concept that has been extrapolated from the cardiovascular literature (α_1 and β_1 adrenergic receptors) [31] and has not been substantiated as regards β_2 receptors.

Conclusions

Most deaths from asthma are due to suboptimal therapy and not to overtreatment [32]. We have presented an approach to therapy which when appended to a hightened awareness of an attack's severity should prevent that occurrence. The β_2 selective agonists are the drugs of choice and should be used in sufficient amount and frequency, both titrated to the patient's side-effects. Large doses of glucocorticoids are advisable and should be employed early because of their delayed beneficial effects (approximately 12 hours). Ipratropium bromide may also be added.

Although there is a solid theoretical basis for its use and some prelimary clinical data CPAP must still be regarded as investigational until further data can be collected. When intubation and mechanical ventilation must be instituted, all attempts should be made to avoide excessive airway pressure in an attempt to decrease the incidence of barotrauma.

References

1. Hopewell PC, Miller TR (1984) Pathophysiology and management of severe asthma. Clin Chest Med 5:623-634
2. Scoggin CH, Sahn S, Petty TL (1977) Status asthmaticus: A nine-year experience. JAMA 238:1158-1162
3. Stalcup SA, Mellins RB (1977) Mechanical forces producing pulmonary edema in acute asthma. N Engl J Med 297:592-596
4. Mitenko PA, Ogilvie RJ (1973); Rational intravenous doses of theophylline. N Engl J Med 289:600-603
5. Racineaux JL, Troussier J, Turcant A, et al (1981) Comparison of bronchodilation effects of salbutamol and theophylline. Bull Eur Physiopathol Respir 17:799-806
6. Jenne JW (1984) Theophylline use in asthma: Some current issues. Clin Chest Med 5:645-658
7. Rossing TH, Fanta CH, Goldstein DH, et al (1980) Emergency therapy of asthma: Comparison of the acute effects of parenteral and inhaled sympathomimetics and infused aminophylline. Am Rev Respir Dis 122:365-371
8. Fanta CH, Rossing TH, McFadden ER (1982) Emergency room treatment of asthma. Relationships among therapeutic combinations, severity of obstruction and time course of response. Am J Med 72:416-422
9. Siegel D, Sheppard D, Gelb A, Weinberg PF (1986) Aminophylline increases the toxicity but not the efficacy of an inhaled beta-adrenergic agonist in the treatment of acute exacerbations of asthma. Am Rev Respir Dis 132:283-286
10. Aubier M, Detroyer A, Sampson M, et al (1981) Aminophylline improves diaphragm contractility. N Engl J Med 305:249-252
11. Matthay RA, Berger H, Davis R, et al (1979) Prolonged improvement in cardiac performance by oral long-acting theophylline in chronic obstructive pulmonary disease (Abstract). Circulation 59:11
12. Williams S, Seaton A (1977) Intravenous or inhaled salbutamol in severe acute asthma. Thorax 32:555-558
13. Lawford P, Jones BJM, Milledge JS (1978) Comparison of intravenous and nebulized salbutamol in initial treatment of severe asthma. Br Med J 1:84
14. Pierce RJ, Payne CR, Williams SJ, Denison DM, Clark TJH (1986) Comparison of intravenous and inhaled terbutaline in the treatment of asthma. Chest 79:506-511
15. Williams SJ, Winner SJ, Clark TJH (1981) Comparison of inhaled and intravenous terbutaline in acute severe asthma. Thorax 36:629-631
16. Walters EH, Cockroft A; Giffiths J, Rocchiccioli K, Davies BH (1981) Optimal dose of salbutamol respiratory solution: Comparison of three doses with plasma levels. Thorax 36:625-628
17. Weber RW, Petty WE, Nelson HS (1979) Aerosolized terbutaline in asthmatics: Comparison of dosage strength, schedule, and method of administration. J Allergy Clin Immunol 63:116-121
18. Fanta CH, Rossing TH, McFadden ER (1983) Glucocorticoids in acute asthma. A critical controlled trial. Am J Med 74:845-851
19. Haskell RJ, Wong BM, Hansen JE (1983) A double-blind, randomized clinical trial of methylprednisolone in status asthmaticus. Arch Intern Med 143:1324-1327
20. Tanaka RM, Santiago SM, Kuhn GJ, Williams RE, Klaustermeyer WB (1982) Intravenous methyprednisolone in adults in status asthmaticus. Comparison of two dosages. Chest 82:438-440
21. Raimondi AC, Figueroa-Casas JC, Roncoroni AJ (1986) Comparison between high and moderate doses of hydrocortisone in the treatment of status asthmaticus. Chest 89:832-835
22. Gross NJ, Skorodin MJ (1984) Anticholinergic, antimuscarinic bronchodilators. Am Rev Respir Dis 129:856-870
23. Ward MJ, Fentem PH, Roderick Smith WH, Davies D (1981) Ipratropium bromide in acute asthma. Br Med J 282:598-600

24. Karpel JP, Appel D, Breidbart D, Fusco MJ (1986) A comparison of atropine sulfate and metaproterenol sulfate in the emergency treatment of asthma. Am Rev Respir Dis 133:727–729
25. Bryant DH (1985) Nebulized ipratropium bromide in the treatment of acute asthma. Chest 88:24–29
26. Martin JG, Shore S, Engel LA (1982) Effect of continous positive airway pressure on respiratory mechanics and pattern of breathing in induced asthma. Am Rev Respir Dis 126:812–817
27. Fleury B, Murcino D, Talamo C, Aubier M, Pariente R, Milic-Emili J (1985) Work of breathing in patients with chronic obstructive pulmonary disease in acute respiratory failure. Am Rev Respir Dis 131:822–827
28. Rossi A, Gottfried SB, Zocchi L, et al (1985) Measurement of static compliance of the total respiratory system in patients with acute respiratory failure during mechanical ventilation. Am Rev Respir Dis 131:672–677
29. Menitove SM, Goldring RM (1983) Combined ventilator and bicarbonate strategy in the management of status asthmaticus Am J Med 74:898–901
30. Darioli R, Perret C (1984) Mechanical controlled hypoventilation in status asthmaticus. Am Rev Respir Dis 129:384–387.
31. Blumenthal JS, Blumenthal MN, Brown EB, Campbell GS, Prasad A (1961) Effect of changes in arterial pH on the action of adrenalin in acute adrenalin-fast asthmatics. Dis Chest 39:516–522
32. Benatar S (1986) Fatal Asthma. N Engl J Med 314:423–429

Right Ventricular Failure
– Pulmonary Hypertension

The Obscure Right Ventricle – A Historical Review

J. F. Dhainaut, E. Ghannad, and J. Dall'ava-Santucci

"La force du mythe est d'opposer aux légitimes inquiétudes de l'homme une illusion cohérente afin de rendre le monde compréhensible" (Ph. Gorny [1])

Introduction

The historical development of knownledge regarding the right ventricle is tightly linked to that of the cardiovascular system which is the cornerstone of under-standing of human physiology. The history of this phase of intellectual advance is long and full of intense human interest. It is also stimulating in a practical way to consider how our knowledge of the operation of the heart and blood vessels were obtained.

The Right Ventricle in the Galenical Theory

Stone and Bronze Age cultures recognized warm blood as being an essential life factor in humans. Not only injury and warfare contribute to vague notions about the primacy of blood and heart, but also the deeply emotional factors associated with widespread human sacrifice (Aztec civilization) must have profoundly in-fluenced thought on the functions of the heart and great vessels carrying blood from it [1]. The emotional change in heart action was probably the background for the ancient idea that the heart is the location of thought. The Editorial writer of Genesis referred to *"The thoughts of my heart."* Even, Aristotle, the great Greek philosophizing founder of modern science, made this same mistake.

"Les sanglots longs des violons de l'automne blessent mon coeur d'une langueur monotone ..." (Verlaine)

The old Chinese, Hindu and Egyptian physicians were reported to note the rela-tion of the heart to the pulse and to use the radial pulse to evaluate heart ac-tion.

Along the Nile Riverside ...

The old Egyptian ideas regarding heart and blood vessels were the most sophis-ticated and were included in one of the great teaching text: *"The beginning of the secrets of the physician: knowledge about the movements of the heart"* in the Ebers

Papyrus. There is nothing to suggest that the old Egyptians had any notion of heart action in relation to blood movement. There is, however, the explicit statement that the breath which enters the nose goes into the heart from the lung. This markedly affected the later development of Greek culture.

At the Greek Health Temple School ...

Hippocrates (460–375 B.C.) described the anatomy of the heart precisely with some errors in discussing the physiologic consequences of his observations: "The vessel, coming from the right ventricle (pulmonary artery), goes into the lungs to distribute nutritive spirits necessary for its nutrition ... and this right ventricle is closing to let air from the lungs come into. The left ventricle only contains air from the atria. This idea is partially based on the observation that the left ventricle when opened after death is empty and thus was thought to contain air. This left ventricle closes more tightly, because the human intelligence is born of this left part of the heart, and controls the rest of the soul ..." In addition, he developed the concept that health depends upon a balance of four humours in which blood play a major role [2].

Aristotle (384–322 B.C.), the great pupil of Plato and the tutor of Alexander the Great, made the first animals classification. He recognized the relation of form and function, thus beginning comparative anatomy, physiology and embryology. He noted the developing chick and observed that the first thing to show life is the beating heart, influencing William Harvey many centuries later.

These studies and those undertaken by Erasistratus in Alexandria have given background for the classical scheme developed by Galen.

The Dogma ...

Galen (131–201 A.C.), a brillant Greek physician from Pergamon, showed that arteries contain blood, but was so impressed by the general theory which he has in mind, that he did not understand the significance of his observation [2].

His scheme of cardiovascular function proceeds from the following: the "nutritive spirits," made by the liver from food absorbed by the intestines, are distributed by veins. Some of these nutritive spirits, via the right ventricle, pass through pores in the interventricular septum and are combined in the left ventricle with air coming from the lungs, to form "vital spirits," necessary for life and distributed in all parts of the body by arteries. This scheme became unquestionable dogma for 1500 years.

The Meditative Calm of the Middle Ages ...

During the Middle Ages, the Italian and French Schools of Anatomy gradually accumulated knowledge of the cardiovascular system as based on occasional dissection of human cadavers.

The Arab physician, Ibn-al-Nafis (d. 1289), described the pulmonary circulation anatomically, and indicated its function in cooling the blood, putting air into it, and removing "fuliginous vapors."

The Renaissance ...

Ambroise Paré (1510–1590), the great French surgeon must have realized some of fallacies of Galenical cardiovascular theory, and reintroduced ligatures for controlling blood loss from ruptured vessels.

Leonardo da Vinci (1452–1519) showed the pores of the inteventricular septum, but not as though they go directly through from the right to the left ventricle. "It is strange that the remarkable drawings and notations of Leonardo da Vinci on the heart and vessels seem to have had so little influence in their time ... Leonardo himself was so bound by tradition that he could not see the truth under his own eyes, skilled hydraulic engineer though he was [2].

In his great description of the structure of the human body in 1543, Andreas Vesalius (1514–1564), then Realdus Colombo (1516–1559) did question the dogma about tiny pores in the septum. This was beginning to be a crucial for the validity of scholastic cardiovascular theory. Actually Galen may have seen the Thebesian vessels, named for Adam Christian Thebesius (1686–1732), which drain venous sinuses from the coronary vessels. The error in the interpretation of these endocardial openings was paramount in scholastic dogma, and, fully exposed, led to its repudiation.

The Right Ventricle in the "De motu cordis et sanguinis"

"Il y a des hommes qu'il n'est pas permis d'ignorer" (Jean Rostand)

William Harvey (1578–1657) received the inspiration from anatomical demonstrations of Girolamo Fabrizzi (1537–1619). Twelve years later, he published his famous *"De motu cordis et sanguinis"* [1]. It is a remarkable manuscript of only 70 pages which, not only demonstrated the principle of modern cardiovascular physiology, but also introduced the method of quantitative reasoning to effectively prove the existence of the circulation. Despite of his occasional fumbling logic and his failure to deal effectively with the pulmonary circulation, Harvey was a pioneer and had no example to follow [2].

Toward the Scientific Knowledge ...

The Harvey's followers have progressively completed the knowledge of cardiovascular physiology. Using first described microscopes, Marcello Malpighi (1628–1694) observed the capillaries, postulated by Harvey. Raymond Vieussens (1641–1715) described the course of the coronary vessels. This is basic to an appreciation of coronary factors in cardiac dysfunction. He also discussed the back-pressure symptoms in miltral stenosis and described the first the clinical and antomic signs of right ventricular failure in *"Le Traité nouveau de la structure et des causes du mouvement naturel du coeur"* [1].

Antoine Lavoisier (1734–1794) showed the real relation between respiration, the oxygen transport of the blood and bodily heat formation.

The mechanism of pumping action was progressively evidenced by Niels Stensen (1668–1706), Jean Poiseuille (1799–1869), Franklin Mall (1862–1917) McLeod (1876–1935) ...and admirably summarized by Leonard Hill in *"The mechanism of the circulation of the blood"* (1900). Last, Werner Forssmann (b. 1904) opened the way for the accurate diagnosis of cardiac anomalies in catheterizing his own heart.

The Right Ventricle at the Twentieth Century

At the beginning of the twentieth century, there would have been very little to report about the right ventricular function. In contrast to the left ventricle, the right ventricle has been allocated to relative obscurity. This comparative neglect was apparently due to two major factors.

First, after birth, the systolic pressure required by the right ventricle to sustain systemic blood flow markedly falls. Commensurate with this reduced pressure work, the right ventricular myocardium is remodeled from a thick-walled pump to a thin-walled, low pressure displacement pump on the adult. Even when cardiac output is increased during vigourous physical exercise, the normal adult right ventricle has to generate a systolic pressure of only 30–35 mm Hg [3]. The functional significance of the right ventricle appears to be minimal.

In addition, the fact that the left ventricle has a fairly simple geometric shape and can be easily analyzed has been of major importance. In contrast the right ventricle often defies simple geometric analysis. Finally, most attention should be focused on the left ventricle, the "business" part of the heart [4].

The "Dispensable" Right Ventricle!

The right ventricle was then considered to be little more than a conduit for blood flow between the peripheral venous circulation and the pulmonary arterial tree, the "weak sister" of the left heart [5].

The theory that right ventricular pump function is not necessary to sustain a normally functioning heart is predicated by the first experimental studies performed by thoroughly cauterizing or burning the right ventricular free wall [6]. The authors observed that both the right atrial and pulmonary arterial pressures did not change, probably due to the preservation of structural coupling of the two ventricles. By virtue of this anatomic continuity, tension developed during contraction of the intact left ventricle is transmitted to the damaged right ventricle. Complete bypass of the right ventricle has been successfully exploited clinically.

However, extensive right ventricular infarction is usually followed by a severe right ventricular failure, including a low cardiac output, a pronounced rise in systemic venous presure, and peripheral edema. This is probably due to the infarcted right ventricle is less rigid and therefore less efficiently coupled to the contracting left ventricle, and often associated with additional damage of the left ventricle.

The Right Ventricle Revisited

In the hemodynamic model of exclusion of the right ventricle developed by Furey et al. [6] acute elimination of right ventricular function usually leads to a marked fall in cardiac output. When the fluid volume was increased sufficiently, cardiac output was restored to the control level, but central venous pressure markedly increase. This maneuver most dramatically illustrated the normal role of the right ventricle in maintaining a low systemic venous pressure.

Furthermore, if the resistance to right ventricular ejection was increased, then the heart did not respond well to this additional resistance, life cannot be supported for any length of time, a situation that is quite similar to the outcome observed after extensive left ventricular damage [5].

In 1979, Laver et al. [7] epitomized the clinical problem of acute right ventricular overload in a remarkable lecture. Indeed, some patients with acute pulmonary hypertension, such as pulmonary embolism, adult respiratory distress syndrome, acute thermal injury, asthma attack, acute exacerbations of chronic obstructive pulmonary disease ... develop a marked increase in right ventricular afterload. This results in increased right ventricular volumes, wall stress and myocardial oxygen consumption. If severe enough, these changes will lead to an eventual decline in cardiac output and may, therefore limit survival in acute diseases. Further, therapy commonly used in the care of the critically ill, such as ventilation with positive end-expiratory pressure, will further increase right ventricular afterload and may, despite improved gas exchange, further reduce cardiac output and tissue oxygen delivery. In addition, right ventricular dilation can, via a leftward septal shift, alter left ventricular diastolic mechanics.

In the late 1980's, we began our clinical research because we are just able to perform invasive and non-invasive evaluations of the right heart.

After a long phase of obscurity, attention to the right heart seems critically important in the successful management of various cardiac and pulmonary diseases. Most exciting aspects of the right ventricular function, however, remain to be solved.

References

1. Gorny P (1985) Histoire illustrée de la cardiologie de la préhistoire à nos jours. R. Dacosta Ed, Paris
2. Leak CD (1962) The historical development cardiovascular physiology. In: Handbook of Physiology. American Physiology Society. Washington DC. Section 2: Circulation. Vol. 1, p 11–22

3. Weber KT, Janicki JS, Shroff SG et al (1983). The right ventricle: Physiologic and pathophysiologic considerations. Crit Care Med 11:323–328
4. Frelink J (1982) Right ventricular function in adult cardiovascular disease. Prog Cardiovasc Dis 25:225–267
5. Fisk RL (1987) The right heart. Cardiovascular Clinics. (AN Brest Ed) FA Davis Co, Philadelphia
6. Furey SA, Zieske HA, Levy MN (1984) The essential function of the right ventricle. Am Heart J 107:404–410
7. Laver MB, Strauss HW, Pohost GM (1979) Right and left ventricular geometry: adjustments during acute respiratory failure. Crit Care Med 7:509–519

The Hemodynamic Effects of Artificial Ventilation*

M. R. Pinsky

Introduction

Oxygen transport to the tissues is a function both of arterial oxygen content and of cardiac output. Artificial ventilation can affect both these determinants of oxygen transport. Although it is clear that artificial ventilation may alter gas exchange by changing FiO_2, minute ventilation and Q_S/Q_T, its effects on both cardiac output and blood flow distribution are less appreciated. The heart, existing within the thorax, is a pressure chamber within a pressure chamber. Thus, changes in intrathoracic pressure (ITP) will affect the pressure gradient for blood returning to the chest (venous return) [1] and leaving the chest (left ventricular (LV) output) [2].

Similarly, as lung volumes change, pulmonary vascular resistance [3] and capacitance [4] vary, and at high lung volumes, mechanical heart-lung interactions may occur [5]. All of these changes can affect cardiac performance. Since ITP rises during positive-pressure inspiration and falls during spontaneous inspiration, the effects of positive-pressure ventilation on cardiovascular performance may not be the same as those of spontaneous ventilation, despite the fact that lung volumes may increase to a similar extent with both modes of breathing.

Neurohumoral Effects of Positive-Pressure Ventilation

Both neuroreflex mechanisms and humoral cardiac depressant substances have been shown to influence the cardiovascular response to positive-pressure ventilation [6-9]. Lung hyperinflation induces a reflex vasodilation, bradycardia, and a negative inotropic response [10]. This vasodepressor response is directly proportional to tidal volume [11, 12]. The receptors for this response, whose fibers travel in the vagus nerve, tonically inhibit the vasomotor center [13, 14]. Lung inflation also may produce humoral substances that may depress myocardial performance [15], alter the distribution of peripheral blood flow [16], and stimulate fluid retention [17]. Positive-pressure ventilation with positive end-expiratory pressure (PEEP) results in redistribution of renal blood flow with fluid retention primarily due to the fall in cardiac output. If cardiac output is main-

---

* Supported in part by a Veterans Administration Research Award.

tained constant, there is no redistribution of renal blood flow or fluid retention [18]. This effect appears to be directly related to stretch receptors in the right atrium, which stimulate secretion of ADH if atrial volume decreases [19]. PEEP also decreases splanchnic blood flow in proportion to cardiac output and alters the liver's extraction ability independent of blood flow [20].

The Oxygen Cost of Breathing

The work of breathing under normal resting conditions is minimal, accounting for approximately 5% of the total oxygen consumption. With increasing elastic loads (pulmonary edema or fibrosis) of resistive loads (bronchospasm or airway collapse), however, the respiratory muscles may use more than 50% of the total oxygen delivery [21]. This increased metabolic demand may overtax a failing cardiovascular system even if the oxygen-carrying capacity and blood volume are sufficient for resting conditions. As the work of breathing increases, blood flow to the respiratory muscles also will increase, which may compromise flow to other organs, limiting exercise capacity and remote organ function [22]. If ventilation-perfusion imbalance exists, the decreasing mixed-venous oxygen content associated with this increased oxygen consumption can cause arterial oxygen content and oxygen delivery to fall, as deoxygenated blood flows through intrapulmonary shunts. Artificial ventilation, by eliminating the work cost of breathing, will decrease oxygen consumption and may increase mixed-venous oxygen content. It is therefore possible that artificial ventilation may increase arterial oxygen content without primarily affecting either gas exchange or cardiac output.

Right Ventricular Performance

Preload

Right ventricular (RV) stroke volume is directly related to RV distending pressure when afterload is not elevated [23]. RV distending pressure is the intracavitary pressure minus extracavitary (pericardial) pressure. Extracavitary pressure rarely equals atmospheric pressure, and fluctuates widely during respiration. Thus, the accurate estimation of RV distending pressure during ventilation requires the measurement of extracavitary pressure. In practice, the pleural pressure can be used to approximate pericardial pressure. Since the pericardium does not function as a limiting membrane under most conditions, and especially during positive-pressure breathing, this approximation seems to be valid.

Recently, it has ben demonstrated in both animals [24] and humans [25] that RV distending pressure may not determine RV end-diastolic volume when RV function is normal because the RV at end-diastole is below its unstressed volume. Under these conditions, the pressure gradient between right atrium and pericardium will not change despite changes in RV preload. When pulmonary hypertension develops or in heart failure states, however, the RV functions above its unstressed volume, and RV distending pressure is proportional to RV end-diastolic volume [26, 27].

Pleural Pressure

Pleural pressure is difficult to measure, primarily because gaining access to the pleural space is difficult and methods of estimating pleural pressure are inaccurate. Although pleural pressure has been measured with chest tubes, fluid-filled catheters and collapsible soft plastic catheters, it is most accurately quantitated with air-filled, thin-walled balloon catheters, of which various types are available [28]. Esophageal pressure can be measured as an estimate of pleural pressure [29]. Although esophageal pressure follows negative swings in pleural pressure in upright humans, it may underestimate positive swings in pleural pressure, because of the stenting effect of the mediastinum or the esophagus on intraluminal esophageal pressure [30].

Intrathoracic Pressure

Intrathoracic pressure (ITP) is not uniform throughout the thoracic cavity [5]. As lung volume increases, juxtacardiac pleural pressure increases to a greater extent than lateral chest wall pleural pressure. Thus, juxtacardiac pleural pressures give the most accurate estimate of the pressure surrounding the heart when lung volumes increase. To simplify the discussion, however, we will use ITP as a common pressure throughout the pleural and pericardial space. By definition, then, RV distending pressure can be approximated as right atrial pressure (Pra) minus ITP, or transmural Pra. The driving pressure for venous return from the body to the heart, however, is determined by the pressure gradient between the systemic venous reservoirs and the right atrium, both measured relative to atmospheric pressure [1]. Since the right atrium is an intrathoracic structure, changes in ITP will directly affect Pra. Spontaneous inspiration, for example, by decreasing ITP, makes Pra more negative, thus increasing the pressure gradient between the systemic veins and the right atrium accelerating venous blood flow [31]. Under most conditions, spontaneous inspiration is associated with an increase in systemic venous return. This increase in venous return manifests itself as an inspiratory increase in both transmural Pra and RV end-diastolic volume (preload), augmenting RV stroke volume. In contrast, increasing ITP positive-pressure inspiration artificially increases Pra decreasing the pressure gradient for venous return and decelerating venous blood flow [32]. This decrease in venous return manifests itself as an inspiratory decrease in both transmural Pra and RV end diastolic volume, which in turn decreases RV stroke volume and, ultimately, cardiac output. The reciprocal change in Pra and transmural Pra (RV filling pressure) during both spontaneous (intermittent negative-pressure breathing) and intermittent positive-pressure breathing (IPPB) is shown in Figure 1. These phasic fluctuations in Pra during ventilation should not be confused with the steady-

Spontanous Breath   Positive Pressure
                           Breath

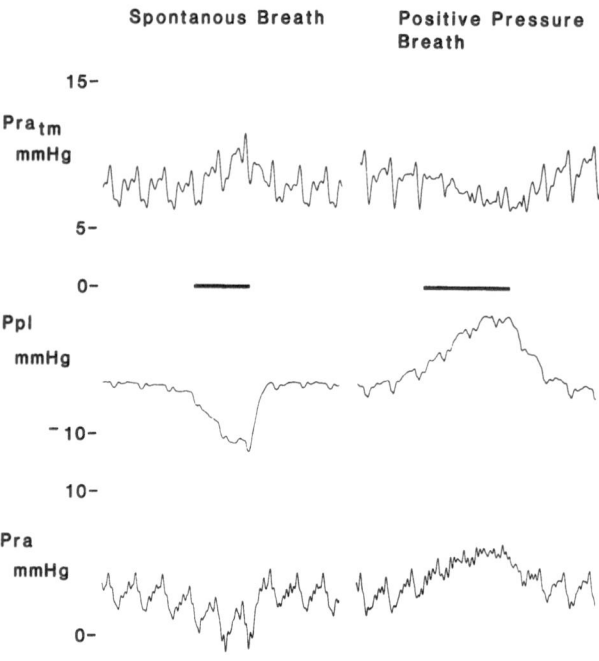

Fig. 1. Trend recordings of right atrial pressure (Pra), juxtacardiac pleural pressure (Ppl), and Pra measured relative to Ppl, called transmural Pra during a spontaneous breath *(left)* and a similar tidal volume positive pressure breath *(right)* in an intact close-chested canine model. The solid horizontal bars denote inspiration. Note the Ppl changes in an opposite fashion between spontaneous and positive pressure breaths, and that within each breath Pra and transmural Pra change in opposite directions. See text for further discussion

state effect of intravascular volume loading on Pra and transmural Pra. With volume loading, both mean Pra and transmural Pra increase, although their phasic reciprocal relation persists.

Venous Return and Intrathoracic Pressure

It follows that since the pressure gradient for venous blood flow can be defined as Pra minus the hydrostatic pressure in the small venules [1], the driving pressure for venous return can decrease from an increase in Pra, a decrease in peripheral venous pressure, or both. Accordingly, the decrease in the pressure gradient for venous return during positive-pressure breathing is exacerbated by any condition that decreases venous pressure in the periphery, such as hypovolemia or decreased vasomotor tone. Similarly, the positive-pressure ventilation-induced decrease in venous return can be minimized either by decreasing mean ITP (decreased inspiratory time or increasing inspiratory flow rate for a fixed tidal volume) to decrease man Pra [33], or by infusing volume or using vasotonic agents to increase systemic venous pressure [34]. If pulmonary parenchymal compliance is low, then a fixed increase in airway pressure does not increase ITP as much as when lung compliance is normal, because lung volume does not increase as much. Change in lung volume, not in airway pressure, determines change in ITP [35]. Thus, in patients with stiff lungs, whose lung volume changes little, artificial ventilation may have less effect on venous return and overall cardiovascular homeostasis than would be expected from the observed changes in airway pressure.

Right Ventricular Afterload

RV afterload can be defined as RV systolic wall stress, which is a function of both end-diastolic volume and systolic RV pressure [36, 37]. The RV and the pulmonary circulation are surrounded by ITP. Thus, the pressure generated by the RV during systole is more accurately defined as pulmonary artery pressure (Ppa) relative to ITP (transmural Ppa). Since both the RV and pulmonary artery sense ITP as their surrounding pressure, changes in ITP, per se, will not alter the pressure gradient for RV ejection. For example, if lung volume does not change, then increases in ITP, as occur with a Valsalva maneuver, will not alter the pressure gradient between the RV and the pulmonary artery. Only if transmural Ppa increases relative to systolic RV pressure, will RV ejection be impeded. Under these conditions, RV end-systolic volume will increase and stroke volume will initially decrease. For cardiac output to remain unchanged, RV filling pressures must also increase in order to increase RV end-diastolic volume by the Frank-Starling mechanism. Clinically, in pulmonary hypertensive states, this increase in RV end-diastolic volume occurs by intravascular fluid retention, intravascular volume loading, or both. It follows that acute elevations of transmural Ppa may profoundly compromise cardiac output by impeding RV ejection, causing the presure gradient for venous return to decrease. Transmural Ppa may increase either from a passive back-up of pressure from the LV or from increased pulmonary vascular resistance (PVR). Pulmonary hypertension resulting from LV pump failure may precipitate secondary pulmonary edema and respiratory failure and thus necessitate artificial ventilation, but it is not usually in itself a consequence of artificial ventilation.

If transmural Ppa increases during artificial ventilation, it is usually caused by increased PVR. As lung volume increases above functional residual capacity (FRC), PVR increases as alveolar vessels are compressed [4]. Overdistension of the lungs, as occurs with large tidal volume ventilation or the application of excessively high PEEP will increase PVR. Normal resting tidal volume is about 5–10 ml/kg [38] which increases PVR at end-inspiration in a normal lung by no more than 12% [39]. Accordingly, RV systolic performance changes minimally during normal ventilation [40, 41]. Therefore, changes in lung volume occurring during normal tidal volume ventilation at FRC in patients without pulmonary hypertension do not affect RV performance through increases in PVR. Artificial ventilation may actually decrease PVR. In acute respiratory failure, resting lung volumes are often below FRC and alveolar hypoxia may be present [42]. When lung volume falls below FRC, PVR also rises from compression of extra alveolar vessels. In addition, hypoxia can increase PVR by inducing vasoconstriction [43]. If artificial ventilation increases the concentration of oxygen in the alveoli or returns lung volume to its normal end-expiratory level, then PVR may decrease. Canada et al. [44] have recently demonstrated that in a dog model with normal lungs, increasing end-expiratory volumes by the use of 10 cm H_2O PEEP increases PVR, whereas similar increases in lung volume after the induction of acute respiratory failure by oleic acid decrease PVR.

Conclusions

Positive-pressure ventilation increases Pra, either by passive transmission of ITP to intrathoracic vascular structures or by RV dilation secondary to increases in PVR. Increasing Pra decreases the pressure gradient for venous return [1, 23] and decelerates venous blood flow; thus, cardiac output is often lower during IPPB than during spontaneous breathing [45]. The most common and important hemodynamic effect of artificial ventilation is to decrease cardiac output by decreasing the pressure gradient for venous return. This deleterious side effect of positive-pressure ventilation can be reduced by minimizing the increase in mean ITP or by volume resuscitation.

Left Ventricular Performance

The determinants of LV performance can be categorized as factors related to preload (end-diastolic volume), contractility, to afterload (systolic wall stress), or to heart rate (HR) [46]. By the Frank-Starling mechanism, LV stroke volume depends primarily on LV end-diastolic volume. Under normal conditions, small changes in HR or LV afterload, as may occur during positive-pressure ventilation, do not significantly change stroke volume [47].

Left Ventricular Preload

Artificial ventilation can significantly alter LV end-diastolic volume in several ways. First, if systemic venous return decreases because Pra increases, pulmonary venous blood flow and LV end-diastolic volume will eventually decrease as well. Second, changes in LV diastolic compliance will change LV end-diastolic volume for a given distending pressure. If lung hyperinflation during artificial ventilation increases the RV systolic pressure, the RV will dilate. LV diastolic volume may be compromised by RV dilation either by leftward shifting of the common intraventricular septum [48], by decreasing LV diastolic compliance (ventricular interdependence), or by limiting absolute biventricular end-diastolic volume owing to the semi rigid pericardium [49, 50]. Ventricular interdependence decreases LV diastolic compliance, thus LV distending pressure (left atrial pressure relative to pericardial pressure) for the same end-diastolic volume will increase. Marini et al. [51] measured both left atrial pressure (Pla) and pericardial pressure in dogs and found that increasing positive airway pressure decreased LV distending pressure but did not decrease diastolic compliance. When LV distending pressure was returned to control levels, LV performance returned to normal. Similarly, Rankin and colleagues [52] studied the deformational characteristics of the LV in dogs with normal lungs using ultrasonic crystals to measure the anterior-to-posterior axis and the septal-to-free-wall minor axis. They found that positive-pressure ventilation decreases LV chamber size independent of changes in RV chamber size. Therefore, ventricular interdependence is probably not a significant factor in depressing steady-state LV performance during positive-pressure ventilation unless marked cardiomegaly or large increases in transmural Ppa occur.

As lung volume increases, the expanding lungs compress the heart in the cardiac fossa [53]. Wallis et al. [5] have demonstrated that this mechanical heart-lung interaction decreases LV end-diastolic volume by increasing juxtacardiac pleural pressure and that this mechanical heart-lung interaction becomes more important as lung volume or heart size increases beyond normal limits.

Although septal shift, pericardial limitation of biventricular volume, and mechanical heart-lung interactions are different mechanisms, clinically they all maintain adequate end-diastolic LV pressure (measured relative to atmosphere) but reduce LV end-diastolic volume. Thus, all three mechanisms decrease the "effective" LV diastolic compliance, and all three respond appropriately to intravascular volume challenge. Therefore, positive-pressure ventilation may decrease LV preload either by decreasing systemic venous return or by decreasing effective LV diastolic compliance.

LV Afterload

Since the LV ejects its stroke into an aorta that has free extrathoracic drainage, changes in ITP may affect the ejecting LV independent of aortic pressure (Pa) measured relative to atmosphere. Buda et al. [2] have shown that Pa relative to ITP (transmural Pa) more accurately represents LV systolic pressure load than does LV pressure alone. For a given aortic pressure, positive swings in ITP will decrease the transmural LV pressure and decrease LV afterload, whereas negative swings in ITP will increase LV afterload (Fig. 2). Spontaneous inspiratory efforts in the setting of upper airway obstruction [54], bronchospasm [55], or decreased lung compliance [56] may significantly decrease ITP and thereby increase LV afterload by increasing the transmural LV pressure. In such patients, positive-pressure ventilation may improve LV performance by abolishing the negative swings in ITP seen during spontaneous inspiration as well as by adding positive ITP during the positive-pressure breaths. Calvin and associates [57] studied patients with severe LV dysfunction who were dependent on changes in LV afterload for changes in LV performance and relatively less responsive to changes in preload. They found that increasing ITP by adding PEEP did not depress LV function and in some patients improved LV performance. Mathru and associates [58] demonstrated that in patients with elevated LV filling pressures (> 15 torr) and presumably decreased myocardial performance, increasing ITP by applying 10 cm H_2O PEEP improve cardiac output, whereas in patients with low LV filling pressure (< 15 torr), the same amount of PEEP decreased

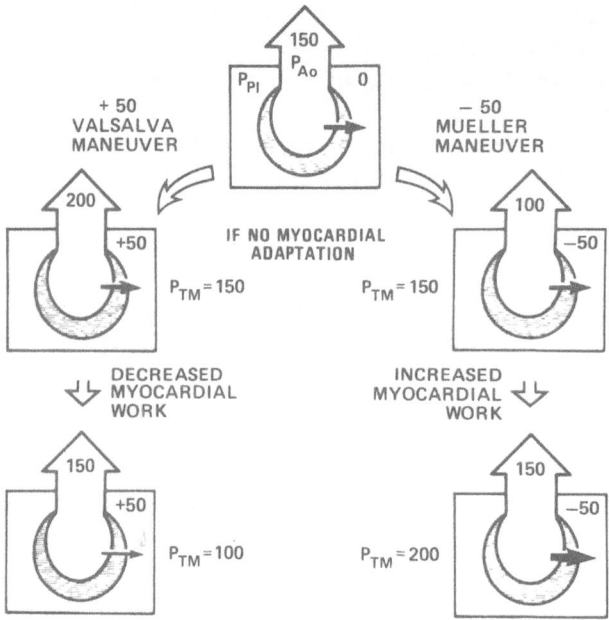

Fig. 2. This schematic diagram depicts the effects of changes in pleural pressure (Ppl) on the amount of work the heart must perform to maintain a constant aortic pressure (AoP).

The top figure represents a left ventricle surrounded by a thorax ejection blood into an extra-thoracic aorta with Ppl = 0 mm Hg, a left ventricular pressure (LVP) of 150 mm Hg will generate an AoP of 150 mm Hg. The pressure across the wall of the left ventricle (LVP-Ppl) will be 150 mm Hg.

If a 50 mm Hg Valsalva maneuver is performed with no myocardial adaptation, then LVP-Ppl and myocardial work will be constant and AoP will reflect the change in Ppl in 50 mm Hg.

To maintain a 150 mm Hg AoP, the myocardium does not have to generate as great a trans-mural pressure and LVP-Ppl will dicrease to 100 mm Hg.

For a –50 mm Hg Mueller maneuver, the opposite is true, such that to maintain an AoP of 150 mm Hg, LVP-Ppl must be increased to 200 mm Hg and the myocardium must perform more work

cardiac output. Artificial ventilation may improve LV performance for a given LV preload by either eliminating the negative swings in ITP seen during spontaneous ventilation or by increasing ITP. Both changes will decrease LV afterload.

Summary

Thus, increases in ITP will alter LV performance by decreasing both LV preload and LV afterload. To the extent that cardiac performance depends on venous return and LV end-diastolic volumes, positive-pressure ventilation will decrease blood flow. This scenario represents most clinical situations in which cardiac and respiratory functions are normal. If LV end-diastolic volume can be maintained, increases in ITP would not be expected to depress LV performance and may improve LV performance when contractility is depressed by decreasing LV afterload. This scenario represents acute heart failure and especially cardiogenic shock.

Cardiac Performance During the Ventilatory Cycle

During the ventilatory cycle, the cardiovascular system is never in a circulatory steady state, with LV and RV output equal and constant from one beat to the next. Thus, hemodynamic measurements averaged throughout the respiratory cycle or measured only at end-expiration may not represent the hemodynamic interactions present during specific phases of the respiratory cycle. Analysis of the moment-to-moment changes in intrathoracic vascular pressures and blood flow increases an understanding of the overall hemodynamic effects of artificial ventilation.

Spontaneous Ventilation

Spontaneous inspiration decreases Pra (Fig. 3) by decreasing ITP. This decrease in Pra increases the pressure gradient for venous return, which in turn increases RV filling pressure (transmural Pra), resulting in an increase in RV stroke volume and transmural Ppa on the following systole. Intrathoracic blood volume increases, and within two to three cardiac cycles, as the increased blood flow reaches the LV, transmural Pla and LV stroke volume increase as well. This phasic lag in the outputs of the two ventricles in response to respiration-induced changes in venous return to the RV is variable and dependent on the respiratory rate, tidal volume, and intravascular volume status [59]. Spontaneous inspiration, however, may concomitantly increase transmural Pla without representing the increased systemic venous return reaching the left side of the heart. Transmural Pla may increase during spontaneous inspiration by any of four mechanisms: direct transmission of the pressure pulse from the pulmonary artery (no change in preload) [34]; acceleration of pulmonary venous blood flow during inspiration, as blood is squeezed out of the alveolar vessels (increase in preload) [32]; interdependent decrease in LV diastolic compliance from the suddenly dilated RV (decrease in preload) [50, 60]; or decrease in LV ejection when negative ITP increases the LV systolic pressure load (increase in afterload) [2]. Ventilation-associated changes in aortic pressure and flow are usually less than those in the pulmonary circulation, because systemic venous return is greatly affected by small changes in Pra and the pulmonary vascular capacitance can absorb a large variation in venous blood flow [4], whereas during quiet breathing, similar changes in transmural Pa do not affect LV systolic performance [2, 37]. However, to the extent that spontaneous respiratory efforts change ITP and lung volume, affecting venous return and LV diastolic compliance, LV output also may be affected. Changes in ITP may alter the background pressure for LV ejection without altering actual output. Under these conditions, Pa decreases but aortic pulse pressure, transmural Pa, and LV stroke volume remain constant [61, 62].

196   M. R. Pinsky

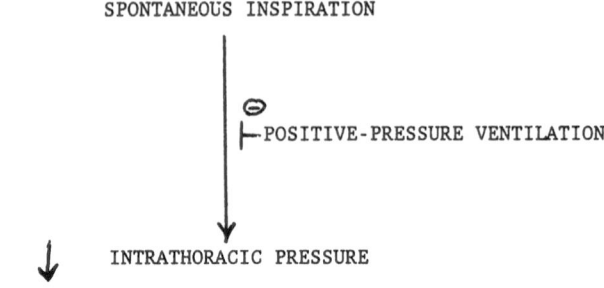

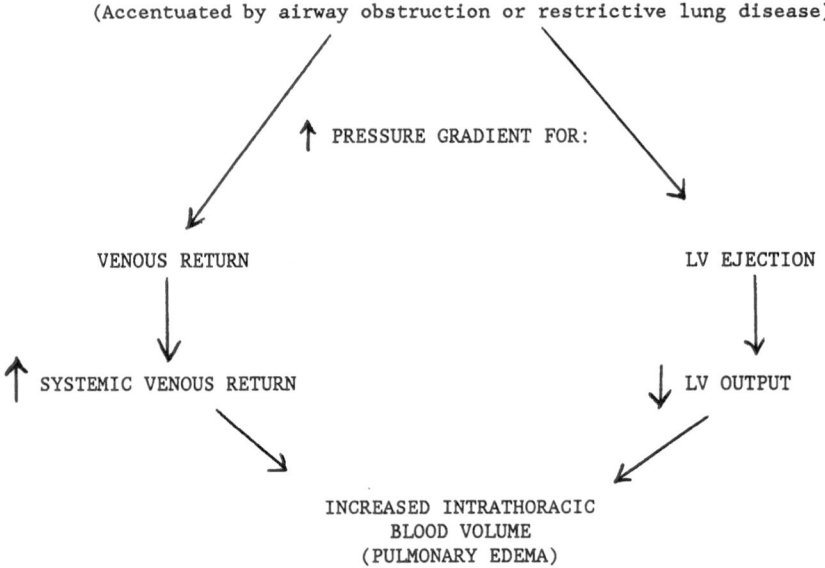

Fig. 3. Schematic representation of the forces that may promote pulmonary edema formation during spontaneous ventilation

This form of pulsus paradoxus should be contrasted with the non-respiratory pulsus seen in pericardial tamponade. In pericardial tamponade, the diastolic Pa is constant, but the aortic pulse pressure decreases with inspiration in proportion to the LV stroke volume. In the setting of decreased lung compliance or increased resistance to inspiration, spontaneous inspiratory efforts may result in large negative swings in ITP that will both increase venous return and reduce LV output. This scenario will result in an increased intrathoracic blood volume, which may promote pulmonary edema production and thus further decrease lung compliance (Fig. 3). Such a negative feed-back process has been postulated to be a cause of pulmonary edema in asthma [55] and upper airway obstruction [54]. It may also be important in the progression of pulmonary edema associated with acute myocardial infarction. Accordingly, artificial ventilation in such patients, by abolishing the negative swings in ITP, will decrease intrathoracic blood volume and can decrease LV afterload. Such a therapeutic interaction may allow for a more rapid resolution of the pulmonary edema process than otherwise would have occurred.

Positive-Pressure Ventilation

Positive-pressure inspiration increases airway pressure and distends the lungs, causing ITP to increase. The increasing ITP increases Pra, which in turn decreases venous return, RV filling pressure, and RV stroke volume. Since the pulmonary circulation is intrathoracic and has a relatively high capacitance relative to the right of the heart, transmural Pla (LV filling pressure) and LV stroke volume will not vary as much as transmural Pra and RV stroke volume during ventilation, despite similar changes in venous return and pulmonary arterial blood flow [41]. The decrease in LV stroke volume seen with positive-pressure ventilation is usually delayed by two to three beats from that of the RV and represents the decrease in systemic venous return finally reaching the left side of the heart. Such decreases in LV stroke volume will be accentuated when there is functional hypovolemia, decreased vasomotor tone, large tidal volume breathing or prolonged inspiratory time [59]. The former two factors decrease the upstream pressure for venous return and the latter two increase the back pressure to venous return [16, 34, 51, 53]. Inspiratory increases in LV stroke volume (reverse pulsus paradoxus) may also occur during positive-pressure ventilation in heart failure. Reverse pulsus paradoxus is manifested by an increase in aortic pulse pressure over end-expiratory levels [63]. Such matching of inspiration to aortic pulse pressure changes usually does not indicate relative hypovolemia, but rather decreased LV contractility and/or volume overload. Although pulsus paradoxus suggests cardiac or pulmonary pathology, it is clear from this discussion that it is not enough to ascertain that the aortic pulse pressure and systolic Pa vary with artificial ventilation, the timing of such changes and their direction relative to the cycle also are important.

Positive End-Expiratory Pressure

End-expiratory airway pressure relative to atmospheric pressure may be zero or positive, independent of the mode that generates tidal breaths. Positive expiratory (and inspiratory) airway pressure is referred to as continuous positive airway pressure (CPAP) when applied during spontaneous ventilation, and as PEEP when applied during pressure breathing. Both CPAP and PEEP are used in respiratory failure to improve gas exchange. Acute respiratory failure is often associated with a decrease in FRC [29] owing partly to lung collapse [43]. With increases in end-expiratory airway pressure, collapsed or closed lung areas may expand, allowing FRC to increase. To the extent that closed areas of lung are opened by CPAP or PEEP, PVR will tend to decrease. If collapsed alveoli reexpand, hypoxic pulmonary vasoconstriction may be reversed, further lowering PVR. If pulmonary parenchymal compliance is nonuniform owing to nonhomogenous lung disease, however, then end-expiratory airway pressure may overexpand compliant areas, leaving diseased regions collapsed. This would increase resistance to blood flow in the "healthy" lung, thereby shunting pulmonary blood flow to collapsed lung areas. Thus, the effects of CPAP or PEEP on PVR and gas exchange are variable and dependent on the degree to which each local lung volume is normalized and hypoxia relieved. As PVR decreases, RV volume and filling pressure will decrease, improving both venous return and LV filling without increasing intrathoracic blood volume. If positive airway pressure returns the lungs to a more compliant state, reducing the elastic load on the respiratory muscles, the work cost of breathing will be reduced. Venus et al. [64] were able to use CPAP without mechanical ventilation to successfully treat previously healthy young adults with the adult respiratory distress syndrome (ARDS), without causing CO_2 retention. CPAP and PEEP have similar hemodynamic effects for the same mean ITP [65, 66], but because CPAP is associated with spontaneous ventilation for a given level of end-expiratory airway pressure, mean ITP will be higher with PEEP.

Clinical Applications

When cardiac function is normal, venous return is the primary determinant of cardiac output. Increases in Pra induced by positive-pressure ventilation will decrease cardiac output by increasing the back pressure to venous blood flow. This decrease in venous return will be especially pronounced in hypovolemic states (hermorrhage or dehydration) and when vasomotor tone is decreased (sepsis, spinal shock, or autonomic blockage). In these clinical settings, increases in ITP by any means, whether induced by positive-pressure breathing, by CPAP, or by hyperinflation in patients with airflow obstruction, will be associated with a decrease in cardiac output. This decrease in venous return induced by positive-pressure breathing may be responsible for the often observed cardiovascular collapse seen in some patients immediately after endotracheal intubation and "bagging" for acute respiratory failure. Since the reduction in blood pressure and cardiac output is due to decreased venous blood flow, appropriate treatment should restore the normal pressure gradient for venous return. This can be accomplished by administering fluids, elevating the legs, applying a pressure suit (MAST), and minimizing the increase in ITP by decreasing inspiratory time, decreasing tidal volume, or using the minimal amount of PEEP necessary to keep the lung open. Intermittent mandatory ventilation by interspersing spontaneous breaths with mechanically delivered ones may minimize the increase in ITP.

When pulmonary artery pressure rises acutely, RV systolic performance can be compromized. Hyperinflation, excessive use of PEEP, pulmonary thromboembolism, and hypoxic pulmonary vasoconstriction can induce acute cor pulmonale. As Pra increases, venous blood flow decreases. The dilated RV impinges on the LV decreasing LV diastolic compliance and filling, which further decreases cardiac output. Minimizing hyperinflation by bronchodilator therapy, minimum inspiratory-to-expiratory time ratio, and minimum necessary levels of PEEP will decrease PVR. Opening closed lung areas and supplemental oxygen may reverse hypoxic vasoconstriction. However, increasing RV filling pressure by volume infusion will result in improved cardiac output in all but the most advanced forms of cor pulmonale [40, 67], and may allow time for other selective forms of therapy to become effective.

When the LV fails, intrathoracic blood volume increases, and spontaneous inspiration only increases it further. If pulmonary venous pressure is elevated either from volume overload or from severe LV failure, pulmonary edema may develop, decreasing pulmonary compliance and alveolar gas exchange, and increasing the work of breathing. If attempts to reverse these processes with perpheral vasodilators, inotropic agents, or diuretics, for example, are not successful, or when severe hypoxemia associated with pulmonary edema necessitates endotracheal intubation, positive-pressure breathing (including CPAP) may improve cardiac performance by increasing ITP and will decrease intrathoracic blood volume by decreasing venous return. Either an improvement or no change in cardiac output associated with a decreasing LV filling pressure should then occur. To the extent that extra work of breathing had impeded oxygen delivery to the rest of the body and that the positive-pressure ventilation improves alveolar gas exchange without impeding cardiac output, oxygen delivery to the tissues also will improve.

References

1. Guyton AC, Lindsey AW, Abernathy B, et al (1957) Venous return at various right atrial pressures and the normal venous return curve. Am J Physiol 189:690–715
2. Buda AJ, Pinsky MR, Ingels NB, et al (1979) Effect of intrathoracic pressure on left ventricular performance. N Engl J Med 301:453–459
3. Whittenberger JL, McGregor M, Berglund E, et al (1960) Influence of state of inflation of the lung on pulmonary vascular resistance. J Appl Physiol 15:878–882
4. Permutt S, Howell JBL, Proctor DF, et al (1961) Effect of lung inflation on static pressure-volume characteristics of pulmonary vessels. J Appl Physiol 16:64–70
5. Wallis TW, Robotham JL, Compean R, et al (1983) Mechanical heart-lung interaction with positive end-expiratory pressure. J Appl Physiol: Respirat Environ Exercise Physiol 54:1039–1047
6. Conway CM (1975) Haemodynamic effects of pulmonary ventilation. Br J Anaesth 47: 761–766
7. Grenvik A (1966) Respiratory, circulatory, and metabolic effects of respirator treatment. Acta Anaesth Scand Suppl 19
8. Shepherd JT (1981) The lungs as receptor sites for cardiovascular regulation. Circulation 63:1010
9. Widdicombe JG (1964) Respiratory reflexes. In: Fenn WD, Rabin H (eds) Handbood of Physiology, Sec. 3, Washington, D.C., American Physiological Society, pp 585–630
10. Cassidy SS, Eschembacher WL, Johnson RJ Jr (1979) Reflex cardiovascular depression during unilateral lung hyperinflation in the dog. J Clin Invest 64:620–629
11. Schrender JJ, Jansen JRC, Versprille A (1984) Contribution of lung stretch depressor reflex to nonlinear fall in cardiac output during PEEP. J Appl Physiol 56:1578–1582
12. Vatner SF, Rutherford JD (1978) Control of the myocardial contractile state by carotid chemo- and baroreceptors and pulmonary inflation reflexes in conscious dogs. J Clin Invest 63:1593–1601
13. Glick G, Wechsler AS, Epstein SE (1969) Reflex cardiovascular depression produced by stimulation of pulmonary stretch receptors in the dog. J Clin Invest 48:467–472
14. Painal AS (1973) Vagal sensory receptors and their reflex effects. Physiol Rev 53:59–88

15. Patten Mt, Liebman PR, Hechtman HG (1977) Humorally mediated decreases in cardiac output associated with positive end-expiratory pressure. Microvasc Res 13:137–144

16. Lenfant C, Howell BJ (1960) Cardiovascular adjustments in dogs during continuous pressure breathing. J Appl Physiol 15:425–428

17. Zehr JE, Hasbarger JA, Risz KD (1976) Reflex suppression of renin secretion during distention of cardiopulmonary receptors in dogs. Circ Res 38:232–239

18. Priebe HJ, Heimann JC, Hedley-Whyte J (1981) Mechanisms of renal dysfunction during positive end-expiratory pressure ventilation. J Appl Physiol 50:643–649

19. Brennan CA Jr, Malvin RL, Joachmin KE, et al (1971) Influence of right and left atrial receptors on plasma concentrations of ADH and revin. Am J Physiol 221:273–278

20. Matuschak GM, Pinsky MR, Rogers RM (1987) Effects of positive end-expiratory pressure on hepatic blood flow and performance. J Appl Physiol 62(4):1377–1383

21. Roussos C, Macklem PT (1982) The respiratory muscles. N Engl J Med 307:786–797

22. Viires N, Sillye G, Aubier M, et al (1983) Regional blood flow distribution in dog during induced hypotension and low cardiac output. J Clin Invest 72:935–947

23. Pinsky MR (1984) Instantaneous venous return curves in an intact canine preparation. J Appl Physiol: Respirat Environ Exercise Physiol 56:756–771

24. Smiseth OA, Refsum H, Tyberg JV (1984) Pericardial pressure assessed by right atrial pressure: A basis for calculation of left ventricular transmural pressure. Am Heart J 108:603–605

25. Tyberg JV, Taichman GC, Smith ER, et al (1986) The relationship between pericardial pressure and right atrial pressure: an intraoperative study. Circulation 73(3):428–432

26. Fewell JE, Abendschein DR, Carlson CJ, et al (1980) Continuous positive-pressure ventilation decreases right and left ventricular end-diastolic volumes in the dog. Circ Res 46:125–132

27. Henning RJ (1986) Effects of positive end-expiratory pressure on the right ventricle. J Appl Physiol 61(3):819–826

28. McMahon SM, Permutt S, Proctor DF (1969) A model to evaluate pleural, surface pressure measuring devices. J Appl Physiol 27:886–871

29. Milic-Emili J, Mean J, Turner JM, et al (1964) Improved technique for estimating pleural pressure from esophageal balloons. J Appl Physiol 19:207–211

30. Prewitt RM, Wood LDH (1979) Effect of positive end-expiratory pressure on ventricular function in dog. Am J Physiol 236:H534–544

31. Brecher GA, Hubay CA (1955) Pulmonary blood flow and venous return during spontaneous respiration. Circ Res 3:210–214

32. Morgan BC, Abel FL, Mullins GL (1966) Flow-patterns in cavae, pulmonary artery, pulmonary vein, and aorta in intact dogs. Am J Physiol 210:903–909

33. Braunwald E, Binion JT, Morgan WL, et al (1957) Alterations in central blood volume and cardiac output induced by positive pressure breathing and counteracted by metraminol (Aramine). Circ Res 5:670–675

34. Maloney JE, Bergel DH, Blazier JB, et al (1968) Transmission of pulsatile blood pressure and flow through the isolated lung. Circ Res 23:11–24

35. Ellman H, Denbin H (1982) Lack of a diverse hemodynamic effect of PEEP in patients with acute respiratory failure. Crit Care Med 10:711–716

36. Matthay RA, Berger HJ (1983) Non-invasive assessment of right and left ventricular function in acute and chronic respiratory failure. Crit Care Med 11:329–338

37. Suga H, Sagawa K (1974) Instantaneous pressure-volume relationships and their ration in the excised, supported canine left ventricle. Circ Res 35:117–126

38. Tobin MJ, Chadha TS, Jenouri G, et al (1983) Breathing patterns I. Normal subjects. Chest 84:202–205

39. Shuler RH, Ensor C, Gunning RE, et al (1942) The differential effects of respiration on the left and right ventricles. Am J Physiol 137:620–627

40. Piene H, Sund T (1982) Does normal pulmonary impedance constitute the optimal load for the right ventricle? Am J Physiol (Heart Circ Physiol II) 242:H154–160

41. Pinsky MR (1984) Determinants of pulmonary arterial blood flow variation during respiration. J Appl Physiol: Respirat Environ Exercise Physiol 56:1237–1243

42. Pontoppidan H, Green B, Lowenstein E (1972) Acute respiratory failure in the adult. N Engl J Med 87(Pat I):690–698

43. Ahmed T, Oliver W Jr (1983) Does slow-reacting substance of anaphylaxis mediate hypoxic pulmonary vasoconstriction? Am Rev Respir Dis 127:566-571
44. Canada E, Benumof JL, Tousdale FR (1982) Pulmonary vascular resistance correlated in intact normal and abnormal canine lungs. Crit Care Med 10:719-723
45. Cournaud A, Motley HL, Werko L, et al (1948) Physiologic studies of the effect of intermittent positive pressure breathing on cardiac output in man. Am J Physiol 152:162-174
46. Sarnoff SJ (1955) Myocardial contractility as described by the ventricular function curves: observations on Starling's Law of the Heart. Physiol Rev 35:107-122
47. Patterson SW, Piper H, Starling EH (1914) The regulation of the heart beat. J Physiol 48:465-513
48. Brinker JA, Weiss I, Lappe DL, et al (1980) Leftward septal displacement during right ventricular loading in man. Circulation 61:626-633
49. Brookhart JM, Boyd TE (1947) Local differences in intrathoracic pressure and their relationship to cardiac filling pressure in the dog. Am J Physiol 148:434-444
50. Janicki JS, Weber KT (1980) The pericardium and ventricular interaction distensibility, and function. Am J Physiol 238(Heart Circ Physiol) 7:H494-503
51. Marini JJ, Culver BN, Butler J (1981) Mechanical effect of lung distension with positive pressure in cardiac function. Am Rev Respir Dis 124:382-386
52. Rankin JS, Olsen CO, Arentzen CE, et al (1982) The effects of airway pressure on cardiac function in intact dogs and man. Circulation 66:108-120
53. Butler J (1983) The heart is in good hands. Circulation 67:1163-1168
54. Lee KWT, Downess JJ (1983) Pulmonary edema secondary to laryngospasm in children. Anesthesiology 59:347-349
55. Stalcup SA, Mellins RB (1977) Mechanical forces producing pulmonary edema in acute asthma. N Engl J Med 297:592-596
56. Milic-Emili J, Ruff F (1977) Effects of pulmonary congestion and edema on the small airways. Bull Physiol Pathol Respir 7:1181-1196
57. Calvin JE, Driedger AA, Sibbald WJ (1981) Positive end-expiratory pressure (PEEP) does not depress left ventricular function in patients with pulmonary edema. Am Rev Respir Dis 124:121-128
58. Mathru M, Rao TLK, El-Etr AA, et al (1982) Hemodynamic response to changes in ventilatory patterns in patients with normal and poor left ventricular reserve. Crit Care Med 10:423-426
59. Scharf SM, Brown R, Saunders N, et al (1980) Hemodynamic effects of positive pressure inflation. J Appl Physiol: Respirat Environ Exercise Physiol 49:124-131
60. Taylor RR, Corell JW, Sonnenblick EH, et al (1967) Dependence of ventricular distensibility on filling of the opposite ventricle. Am J Physiol 213:711-718
61. Robotham JL, Rabson J, Permutt S (1979) Left ventricular hemodynamics during respiration. J Appl Physiol: Respirat Environ Exercise Physiol 47:1295-1303
62. Wise RA, Robotham JL, Summer WR (1976) Effects of spontaneous ventilation on the circulation. Lung 159:175-192
63. Massumi RA, Mason DT, Vera Z, et al (1973) Reversed pulsus paradoxus. N Engl J Med 289:1272-1275
64. Venus B, Jacobs HK, Lim L (1979) Treatment of the adult respiratory dis-syndrome with continuous positive airway pressure. Chest 76:257-261
65. Dorinsky PM, Whitcomb ME (1983) The effect of PEEP on cardiac output. Chest 84:210-216
66. Vuori A, Jalonen J, Laaksonen V (1979) Continuous positive airway pressure during mechanical ventilation and spontaneous ventilation. Effects on central hemodynamics and oxygen transport. Acta Anaesth Scand 23:459-462
67. Sibbald WD, Driedger AA, Myers ML, et al (1983) Biventricular function in the adult respiratory distress syndrome. Hemodynamic and radionuclide assessment with special emphasis on right ventricular function. Chest 84:126-134

Respiration Within the Cardiac Cycle

J. Peters

Introduction

The interactions between the respiratory and cardiovascular systems are complex. Clinical terms as "cor pulmonale" or "cardiopulmonary unit" attest to the intimate anatomic and physiologic relationship between heart and lung. In the intact circulation changes in intrathoracic pressure and/or lung volume will simultaneously induce alterations in venous return, abdominal pressure, cardiac volumes, lung vascular restistance, lung vascular capacity, cardiac output and contractility, aortic pressure, and surface pressures surrounding the various intrathoracic vascular and cardiac structures [1]. While the analysis of steady state effects of pertubations in intrathoracic pressure such as positive or negative pressure breathing on global cardiovascular parameters in health and disease states is very important clinically, it can contribute little to our understanding of the specific mechanisms involved in cardiopulmonary interactions from a physiologic point of view. In the past ten years therefore, emphasis was laid on investigation of the effects of shorter pertubations in pleural pressure, e.g. a single spontaneous inspiratory effort with and without changes in lung volume or a single positive pressure ventilation [2-11]. This approach led to the emergence of basic concepts of cardiorespiratory interactions [see 1 for review].

However, a problem still persists even with this type of analysis: the pertubation of intrathoracic pressure extends over several cardiac cycles, i.e. it may influence cardiac filling and emptying as well as contractility at the same time, rending the experimental identification of any specific mechanism difficult.

After giving a brief summary of potential mechanisms of interaction between the ventilatory and circulatory system, this chapter will carry the analysis one step further and focus on the effects of respiration within a single cardiac cycle. By applying step changes in intrathoracic pressure confined to either diastole or systole effects on cardiac filling can be separated from those on cardiac emptying. Finally an outlook on potential future applications of these concepts will be provided with reference to clinical cardiovascular support.

Cardiopulmonary Interactions:
Anatomical and Physiological Considerations

Effects of Intrathoracic Pressure

It the heart were in a closed box with all vessels entering and leaving the cardiac chambers ligated, any increase or decrease in the surrounding pressure in the box would be reflected to the same extent in intracardiac chamber pressures when recorded with a transducer outside the box referenced to atmospheric pressure. Similarly, if the entire cardiovascular system existed in a closed box a negative or positive surrounding pressure would induce no pressure gradients along the circulation within this system. However, our cardiovascular system is compartmentalized into an intrathoracic and extrathoracic part with different pressures surrounding the vascular structures in each compartment. Furthermore, both the intrathoracic venous as well as the arterial system are connected with the extrathoracic system, so that any change in intrathoracic pressure not accompanied by an equivalent change in extrathoracic surrounding pressure must displace volume from one compartment into the other. Traditionally, the influence of changes in intrathoracic pressure on cardiac output is considered by flow analysis in terms of changes in venous return. An increase in intrathoracic pressure, e.g. by opening the chest, decreases systemic venous return [12]. While it is generally accepted that a fall in intrathoracic pressure will promote venous return toward the heart [8, 13, 14], there is no a priori reason to believe that the analogous mechanism is not operative on the arterial side of the circulation, i.e. that negative pressure impedes the egress of blood out of the thorax (vide infra).

In the intact circulation intrathoracic blood flow is directed by cardiac valves. Any elastic fluid filled tubing system with one directional valves at its ends will generate flow, when being compressed by an increase in surrounding pressure, the magnitude of flow being dependent on the amplitude and frequency of compression, capacity and flow resistance of the tubing, and viscosity of the fluid contained in the tubing. Thus we can expect unidirectional flow to occur with phasic increased intrathoracic pressures even in the absence of cardiac activity, i.e. during circulatory arrest and cardiopulmonary resuscitation, as long as the valves remain competent. An impressive example of this mechanism has been demonstrated with spontaneous coughing during ventricular fibrillation in man [15, 16].

Finally, it is not often considered that at least with great changes in intrathoracic pressure, physical compression of intrapulmonary gas may be a significant factor. During cough and chest compression with cardiopulmonary resuscitation intrathoracic pressures up to 100 mm Hg are generated [17–19] while air flow out of the lung is restricted or abolished. Assuming a functional residual capacity of 2000 ml in man, a 100 mm Hg increase in intrathoracic pressure and no gas escape from the lung, calculation from Boyle's law ($P_1V_1 = P_2V_2$) indicates a 233 ml or 11.7% decrease in lung volume. This may cause blood flow from the heart toward the alveolar pulmonary vascular compartment during chest compression.

It is possible that this mechanism plays an important yet unappreciated role in the generation of blood flow during cardiopulmonary resuscitation [20].

Ventricular Interdependence

The anatomical arrangement of the intrathoracic vascular structures in man is complicated by the fact that right and left heart are not only arranged in series, but, by virtue of the interventricular and interatrial septa as well as by the pericardium, also in parallel. Thus there are means by which filling and performance of each cardiac chamber can potentially alter the physiologic characteristics of the other three chambers. Using septum-to-free wall right ventricular (RV) and left ventricular (LV) ultrasound dimension transducer, it has been demonstrated in open chest dogs that RV distention markedly influenced the LV pressure-dimension relationship with the pericardium closed, but little with the pericardium removed [21]. Similar results were obtained in conscious dogs measuring myocardial segment length [22] and in isolated canine hearts [23]. Finally, Santamore et al. showed that inspiration results in an increase in RV volume associated with a decrease in the apparent LV compliance when LV transmural filling pressure was calculated from esophageal pressure measurements [11]. Using mathematical analysis Slinker et al. have estimated that the in parallel interaction, i.e. ventricular interdependence, is one half as important as the series interaction between the ventricles [24]. However, the calculation of cardiac volumes for analysis of ventricular interdependence from ultrasonic dimensions, implanted intramyocardial radiopaque markers, echocardiography, radionuclide ventriculography, or angiocardiography makes certain assumptions about 3-dimensional ventricular shape to reach conclusions about volume. These assumptions may not be valid, particularly under conditions of increasing lung volume. The problem is further confounded by the uncertainty what the correct ventricular surface pressures are that can be applied for the calculation of ventricular transmural pressure volume relationships during respiratory maneuvers.

Measurement of Cardiac Surface Pressures and Compression of the Heart by the Lungs

Any surface pressure in vivo is difficult to measure accurately [25] because extrapericardial mediastinal or pleural pressure measurements are poorly defined and may not reflect true intrapericardial left ventricular surface pressure. Under conditions of acutely increasing intrapericardial volume, i.e. cardiac size, extrapericardial pressure measurements may underestimate intrapericardial surface pressure [26–28]. Indeed unequal regional intrapericardial pressures on the surface of the RV and LV have been reported (Fig. 1) when different loads are placed on the right and left ventricles, respectively [29]. The problem is even more confounded by the fact that during LV systole approximately one third of the LV surface is surrounded by RV systolic pressure while the other two thirds of the LV are subjected to the regional intrapericardial pressure. It is difficult, if not impossible, therefore to calculate a reliable LV transmural pressure volume relationship using any form of surface pressure measurements.

Lung expansion with IPPV and PEEP has been demonstrated to physically compress the heart at end-expiration and end-inspiration even when the pleural space is open to atmosphere [30]. Thus spontaneous or mechanical lung inflation may exert a surface stress on the heart not appreciated by esophageal or pleural pressure measurements potentially impeding cardiac filling [31] and/or deforming cardiac shape [32–34] independent of any effects of intrathoracic pressure on venous return.

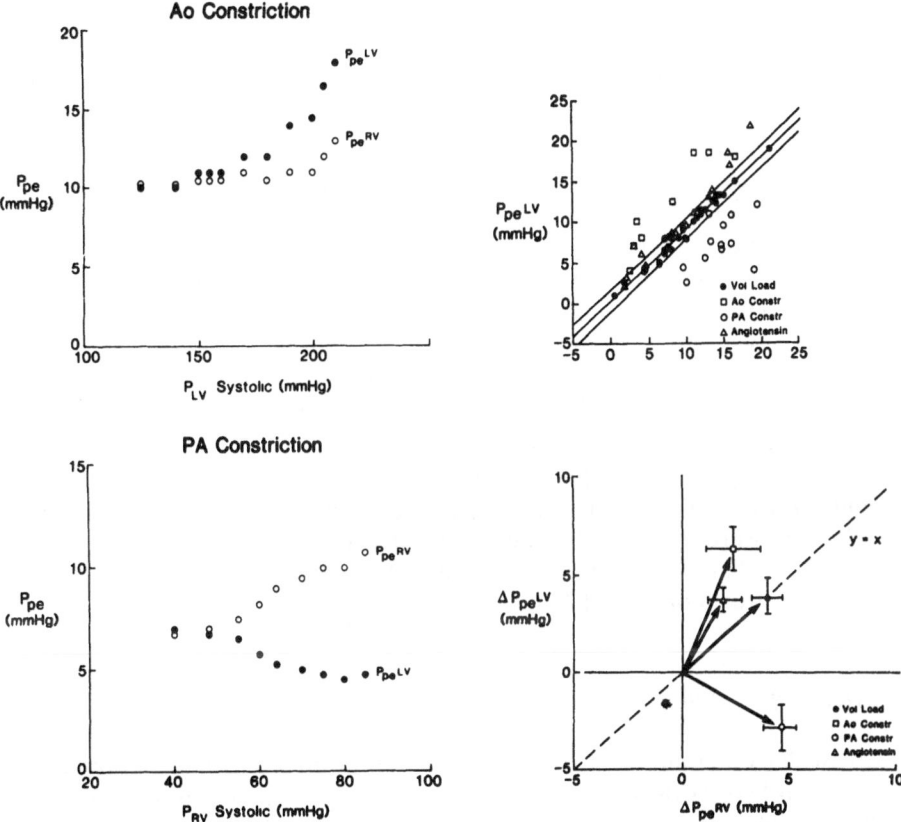

Fig. 1. Changes in regional intrapericardial pressures measured with liquid filled balloons over the left ($\Delta P_{pe}LV$) and right ($\Delta P_{pe}RV$) ventricular free wall in closed chest dogs during volume loading (Vol load), aortic constriction (Ao Constr), pulmonary artery constriction (PA Constr), and angiotensin infusion. *Panel A:* Individual data with regression line and 95% confidence limits. *Panel B:* Mean data from the preceding control values and the corresponding vectors. With volume loading surface pressures increase similarly over both ventricles. However, during aortic constriction LV surface pressure increases more than RV surface pressure, whereas PA constriction rises RV surface pressure, but actually decreases LV surface pressure. Angiotensin infusions result in a similar increase in both surface pressures. Thus an increase in ventricular size increases the surrounding pressure acting on its free wall. (From [29] with permission of the author and American Heart Association)

Effects of Lung Inflation on the Pulmonary Vasculature

Lung inflation by itself can exert effects on the circulation independent of changes in pleural pressure. Depending on the state of lung expansion the pulmonary vascular bed can act as both a variable capacitor and resistor. The alveolar capillary network is surrounded by alveolar pressure and compressed by mechanical lung inflation. Intraparenchymal extraalveolar vessels in contrast increase in size as the lung is stretched. Lung inflation therefore can expel blood from alveolar capillaries but store blood in extraalveolar vessels [35]. Depending on the prevailing zone condition of the lung, lung inflation can therefore either decrease or increase pulmonary venous blood flow [35], which in turn may influence flow into the left atrium and ventricle. Changes in pulmonary venous return to the LV may be one of several mechanisms associated with the transient change in arterial pressure observed with mechanical or spontaneous inspiration. In general, lung inflation will tend to increase pulmonary venous return with hypervolemia, but tends to decrease pulmonary venous return with hypovolemia.

The state of lung inflation can also alter pulmonary vascular resistance. Based on data obtained from isolated lungs perfused with constant blood flow, it appears that flow resistance is at a minimum at and around functional residual capacity, and increases both with atelectasis and overinflation [36, 37]. An increase in pulmonary vascular resistance would require the right ventricle to generate more work for a given cardiac output, i.e. load the right ventricle. This may be the reason why Scharf et al. [38] found an increase in a RV dimension with PEEP in the open chest dog, but a decrease when intrathoracic pressure rose with the chest closed. Pulmonary vascular resistance is also influenced markedly by the filling state of the pulmonary vasculature and the hydrostatic pressures. Under zone III conditions ($P_{PA} > P_{LA} > P_{ALV}$) left atrial pressure is the downstream pressure for the pulmonary vascular bed, whereas under zone II conditions ($P_{PA} > P_{ALV} > P_{LA}$) alveolar and not left atrial pressure constitutes the effective downstream pressure [39, 40].

Effects of Abdominal Pressure

A vascular waterfall may exist at the junction of the extrathoracic venous compartments [41]. As the diaphragm descends with spontaneous or mechanical ventilation with and without PEEP a phasic or steady state increase in intraabdominal pressure can be anticipated. This by itself may either pool blood in the intraabdominal and leg vascular compartments [42, 43] or, alternatively, redistribute blood into the intrathoracic vascular compartment [14, 44, 45] depending on the filling state of the vasculature and degree of intraabdominal pressure.

Summary

Thus multiple mechanical mechanisms operate simultaneously during spontaneous and mechanical ventilation. Their physiologic significance and interplay is only partially understood at present. There is no doubt that reflex effects from cardiopulmonary and baroreceptors will further modify the body's response to changes in intrathoracic pressure, cardiac and lung volumes, and arterial pressure [46–48]. However, as considered below different mechanisms can be isolated experimentally by applying transient pertubations in pleural pressure within a single cardiac cycle.

Respiration Within the Cardiac Cycle

In recent experiments in dogs, transient negative pertubations in intrathoracic pressure were evoked by stimulation of both phrenic nerves synchronized to the R-wave of the ECG. To evaluate effects of changes in lung volume the airway was either obstructed or unobstructed during phrenic nerve stimulation (PNS). By using appropriate electronic delays and stimulation durations it was possible to time the negative intrathoracic pressure (NITP) resulting from phrenic nerve stimulation to occur during either a single diastole or systole. If phrenic stimulation is performed after a brief period of apnea to achieve a steady hemodynamic state, effects of negative intrathoracic pressure on systolic left ventricular (LV) emptying can be analyzed to constant preload. Similarly, effects on LV filling

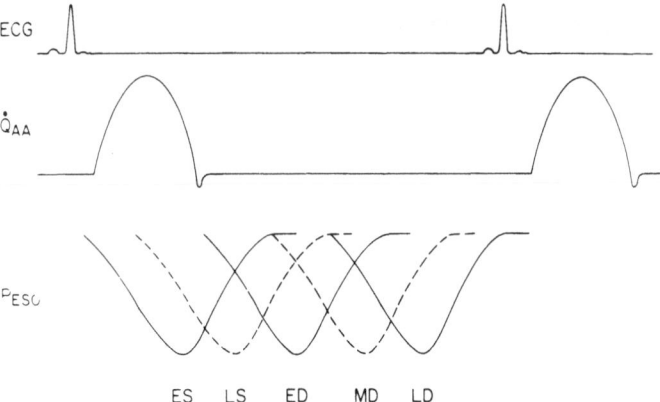

Fig. 2. Timing of the fall in esophageal pressure related to the electrocardiogram (ECG) and ascending aortic flow (Q$_{AA}$) during ECG-triggered phrenic nerve stimulations (PNS). After an apneic period to achieve a stable hemodynamic state, a single phrenic nerve stimulation was performed in early (ES) and late systole (LS) as well as in early (ED), mid (MD), and late diastole (LD) resulting in a decrease in esophageal pressure (P$_{ESO}$). With diastolic PNS esophageal pressure returned to baseline within the same diastole. Decreases in intrathoracic pressure confined to systole allowed evaluation of effects on left ventricular emptying, while decreases in diastole permitted evaluation of effects on diastolic LV filling and the ensuing LV stroke volume

can be assessed during diastole. Finally, by applying phrenic nerve stimulation in diastole, i.e. after aortic valve closure, it is also possible to study the effects of negative intrathoracic pressure on peripheral arterial flow independent of any direct cardiac effects. This experimental set-up also breaks the natural in series arrangement of the circulation by not allowing RV output to influence LV output. The time relation of the fall in intrathoracic pressure to the ECG and ascending aortic flow is shown in Figure 2.

Effects of Negative Intrathoracic Pressure on Left Ventricular Inflow

To avoid assumptions about LV geometry, LV filling was assessed continuously using a circumferential electromagnetic flow probe sewn just above the mitral valve annulus during cardiopulmonary bypass. This technique does not interfere with normal mitral valve function [49]. After the dog was weaned from bypass and the chest closed airtight diastolic phrenic nerve stimulations were performed while LV inflow and outflow were recorded on line. A typical tracing is shown in Figure 3. NITP resulted in a marked fall in mitral flow and diminished LV filling (integrated mitral flow) by an everage of 40%. Since this fall was also seen with

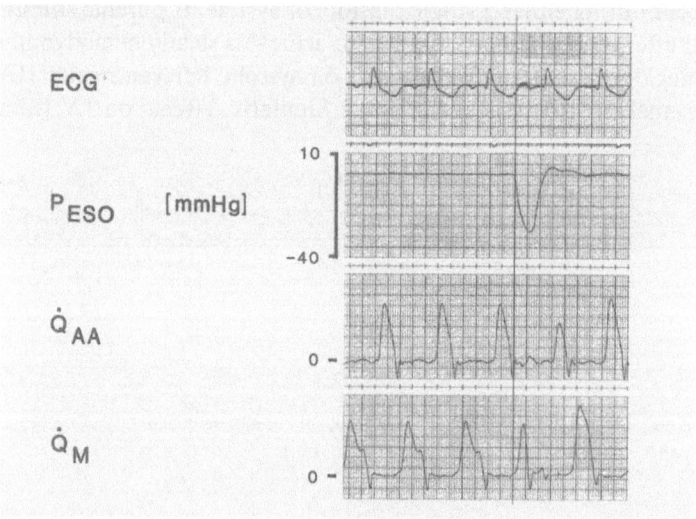

Fig. 3. Diastolic PNS with the airway obstructed and the pericardium reapproximated in a closed chest dog (recording speed: 50 mm/s). ECG-triggered PNS confined to diastole results in an immediate fall in esophageal pressure (P_{ESO}). Mitral flow (Q_M) decreases followed by a decrease in the ensuing ascending aortic flow (Q_{AA}) and LV stroke volume. Similar findings were seen with the airway unobstructed during PNS. Thus, a diastolic fall in intrathoracic pressure decreases LV inflow and thus LV preload. Since end-diastolic LV and left atrial pressures (not shown) after PNS but before the next ejection increased both relative to atmosphere and P_{ESO} a primary decrease in pulmonary venous return is ruled out. Right atrial pressure increased both relative to atmosphere and P_{ESO}, the increase being greater than the rise in left sided pressures. These findings are consistent with negative intrathoracic pressure distending the right heart and actually limiting LV filling by ventricular interdependence

the airway completely obstructed during the decrease in intrathoracic pressure an increase in lung volume cannot be responsible. Similarly, widely opening the abdomen to minimize any increase in intraabdominal pressure during phrenic stimulation and diaphragmatic descend did not abolish the fall in mitral flow. Removal of the pericardium however greatly reduced the decrease in LV filling (Fig. 4). These findings demonstrate that the pericardium mediates the fall in LV filling with decreased intrathoracic pressure, presumptively by limiting LV expansion as right heart volume increases during negative intrathoracic pressure, i.e. by ventricular interdependence. This is further supported by an increase in LV end-diastolic filling pressures relative to both esophageal and atmospheric pressures after diastolic PNS but before the ensuing ejection. Since LV volume has decreased during NITP, this finding indicates a decrease in the apparent diastolic LV compliance, again compatible with ventricular interdependence.

When NITP was applied only in either early or late diastole a differential effect on mitral flow was observed (Fig. 5). With early diastolic NITP early diastolic peak mitral flow decreased but was followed by a rebound increase in flow in late diastole as phrenic stimulation ceased and intrathoracic pressure returned towards baseline. With late diastolic NITP in contrast, only late diastolic flow diminished. This suggested that differential effects of NITP on LV filling can occur depending on the specific time NITP is applied in diastole. In another series of experiments therefore, the effects of NITP confined to either early, mid, and late diastole on the succeeding LV stroke volume were evaluated. The results are shown in Figure 6. In general, the fall in LV stroke volume was more pronounced the later in diastole the fall in intrathoracic pressure was timed to occur. This probably reflects the fact that the increase in right heart volume with early diastolic PNS is compensated partially by a relative decrease in late diastole secondary to a smaller filling gradient or by reaching a steeper portion on its pressure volume relationship. LV filling would therefore be impeded only moderately. A late diastolic bolus of increased inflow however would be superimposed on a right heart already filled and therefore increase right heart volume and decrease LV filling to a much greater extent. This finding may have clinical implications with regard to mechanical ventilation in a hypovolemic patient (vide infra).

Effects of Negative Intrathoracic Pressure on Left Ventricular Outflow

With constant end-diastolic LV pressure and volume and thus preload, negative intrathoracic pressure confined to systole resulted in a decrease in LV stroke volume. Peak systolic transmural pressure, estimated as LV minus esophageal pressure, increased. Despite less blood leaving the left ventricle during LV ejection, intrathoracic descending aortic diameters measured directly by piezoelectric crystals sewn onto the aortic adventitia simultaneously increased (Fig. 7), indicating an increased aortic (and LV) systolic transmural pressure with negative intrathoracic pressure. Since contractility changes are unlikely to occur within 150 ms, these findings are consistent with negative intrathoracic pressure impos-

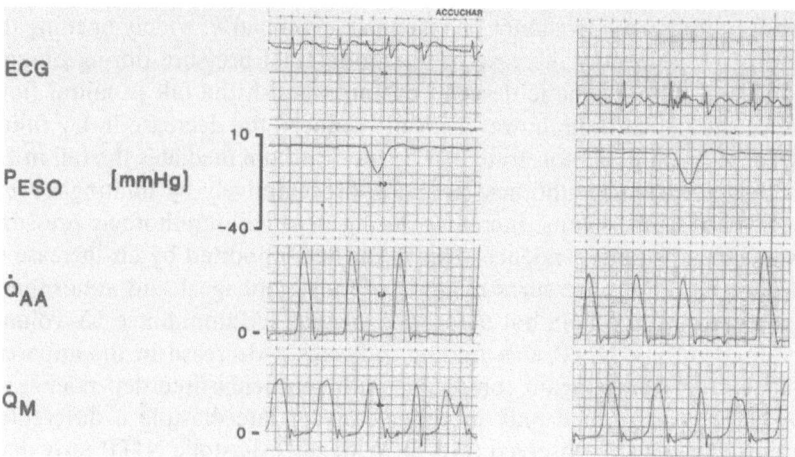

Fig. 4. Diastolic *(left panel)* and systolic *(right panel)* PNS with the airway obstructed and the pericardium removed in a closed chest dog (recording speed: 50 mm/s). In contrast to the situation with the pericardium on, the diastolic decrease in P_{ESO} no longer results in an appreciable fall in mitral flow. Again, these data are consistent with ventricular interdependence mediated by the presence of the pericardium limiting LV filling when intrathoracic pressure is decreased in diastole. With systolic phrenic stimulation, removal of the pericardium has no effect on the fall in ascending aortic flow (Q_{AA}). In both panels the effects of premature LV contractions on mitral flow are also seen

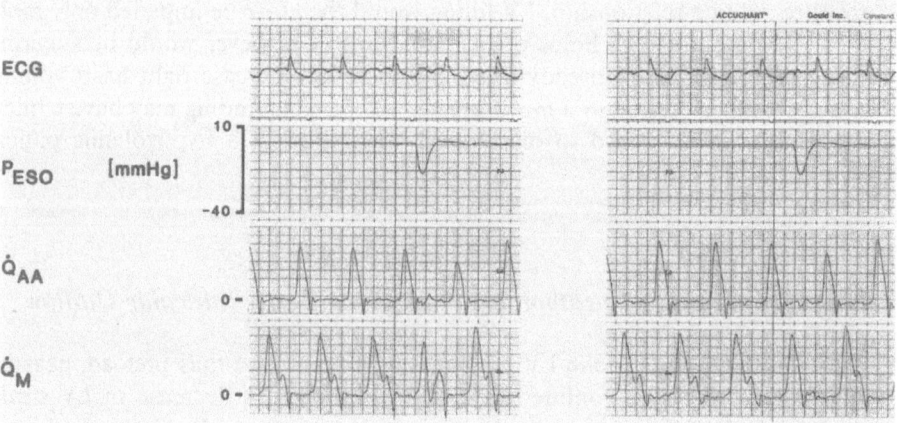

Fig. 5. PNS performed in either early *(left panel)* or late *(right panel)* diastole with the airway obstructed and the pericardium reapproximated (recording speed: 50 mm/s). With the decrease in esophageal pressure (P_{ESO}) occuring during early diastole peak mitral flow (Q_M) is reduced, followed by a non-compensatory flow increase in late diastole. With the decrease in P_{ESO} timed to late diastole, early diastolic mitral flow is unchanged, but falls during late diastole. Thus negative intrathoracic pressure can diminish LV inflow during both early and late diastole

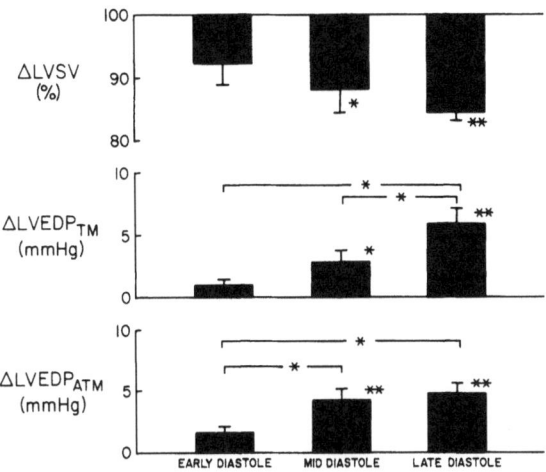

Fig. 6. Effects of early, mid, and late diastolic PNS with the airway obstructed on LV end-diastolic pressure relative to esophageal (ΔLVEDP$_{TM}$) and atmospheric pressure (ΔLVEDP$_{ATM}$) after PNS and on the ensuing LV stroke volume (ΔLVSV). Data are compared to the immediately preceding control cardiac cycle. LV stroke volume decreases with mid and even more with late diastolic PNS, while LV end-diastolic pressures rise relative to both esophageal and atmospheric pressures. The fall in stroke volume and increase in filling pressures is more pronounced the later in diastole the fall in intrathoracic pressure occurs. This may relate to a bolus increase in systemic venous return having a greater effect in increasing right heart volume and impeding LV filling in late diastole

ing an increased effective afterload on the LV. It should be emphasized that the mechanism for this increase in effective afterload is not reflected by an increased pressure gradient between LV and ascending aorta during systole but rather by an increase in the force the heart has to generate to eject a given quantity of blood out of the intrathoracic into the extrathortacic arterial compartment with negative intrathoracic pressure. From a mechanical point of view, there is no difference in the afterload imposed on the LV to pump blood out of the thorax whether the extrathoracic arterial pressure rises with a constant surrounding pressure or the pressure surrounding the LV falls with the extrathoracic pressure constant (Fig. 8). Alternatively, negative intrathoracic pressure can be thought of as increasing mean systolic LV wall stress for a given end-diastolic volume, resulting in a greater end-systolic volume.

It is likely therefore that high negative intrathoracic pressures can afterload the LV under clinical conditions such as asthma, upper airway obstruction, sleep apnea [50, 51], spontaneous breathing in the presence of a low lung compliance, and contribute to the development of pulmonary edema and cardiac failure, especially in patients with limited cardiac reserve. A major strategy therefore must be to eliminate excessive swings in negative intrathoracic pressure in these patients by appropriate respiratory therapy. Scharf et al. have demonstrated that an inspiratory effort with the glottis closed can provoke akinesia and decrease LV ejection fraction in patients with coronary artery disease, but not in healthy volunteers [52].

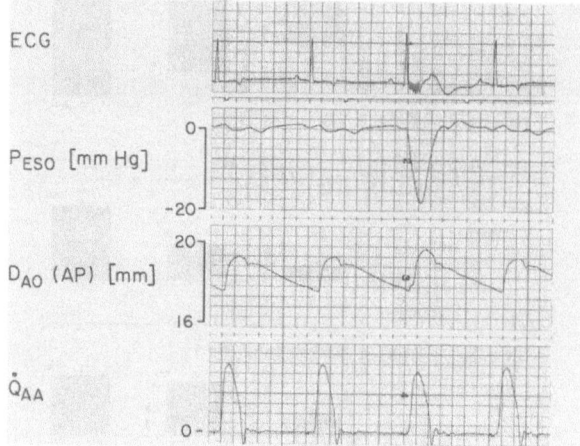

Fig. 7. Effects of phrenic nerve stimulation confined to systole (airway obstructed, paper speed: 50 mm/s). The systolic decrease in esophageal pressure (P_{ESO}) is associated with a decrease in ascending aortic blood flow (Q_{AA}) and LV stroke volume (integrated aortic flow). Since LV preload has not changed during the preceding apnea end-systolic LV volume must have increased. Anterior-posterior intrathoracic aortic dimension [$D_{AO}(AP)$] increased compared to the preceding beat indicating an incrase in aortic transmural pressure associated with negative intrathoracic pressure. Since reflex changes in LV contractility are unlikely to occur within 150 ms during an ongoing LV contraction, the only single mechanism that can explain both the decrease in stroke volume and an increase in aortic size is a rise in effective LV afterload imposed by negative intrathoracic pressure

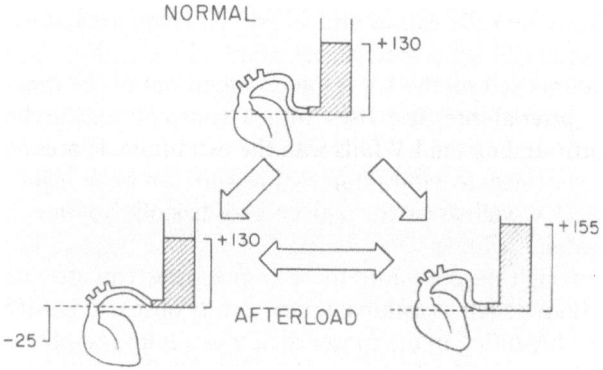

Fig. 8 Schematic demonstrating the analogy between a rise in extrathoracic arterial pressure and a fall in the pressure surrounding the left ventricle. The systolic load on the LV is indicated by the height of the ventrical fluid column above the heart level which was arbitrarily chosen to be zero. Mechanically there is no difference whether the load on the heart is increased by elevating extrathoracic arterial pressure, or lowering the pressure surrounding the heart. In both cases the net pressure to pump a given amount of blood out of the thorax is increased consistent with a rise in effective LV afterload

Positive intrathoracic pressure in contrast can be assumed to unload the LV during systole and improve systolic performance especially in patients with LV failure. In clinical practice however this effect is usually blurred by the decrease in preload with increased intrathoracic pressure. Nevertheless some clinical reports have suggested improved cardiac performance with application of PEEP in selected groups of patients [53, 54].

Effects of Negative Intrathoracic Pressure on Arterial Blood Flow and Aortic Dimensions

The finding of increased aortic diameters with systolic negative intrathoracic pressure despite a smaller LV stroke volume suggested that negative intrathoracic pressure can diminish arterial blood flow out of the thorax independent on any direct effects on LV performance. In another series of experiments therefore, the effects of negative intrathoracic pressure on the vasculature were assessed in diastole after aortic valve closure, while intrathoracic aortic diameters, descending aortic flow and extrathoracic carotid blood flow were recorded.

Consistent with impeding egress of blood flow out of the chest, NITP generally resulted in an increase in aortic dimensions and a fell in blood flow out of the thorax (Fig. 9) compared to control. In several experiments aortic and carotid blood flow was actually reversed, i.e. negative intrathoracic pressure caused aortic blood to flow from the intrathoracic arterial compartment. Thus both an impeded antegrade flow and retrograde flow can summate to distend the intrathoracic aorta. These findings were abolished when the decrease in intrathoracic pressure with phrenic stimulation was eliminated by opening the chest, but not by opening the abdomen to minimize any increase in intraabdominal pressure with diaphragmatic descend. It appears therefore that the aorta and, presumably, most of the intrathoracic arterial compartment can be viewed as an elastic container driven by changes in intrathoracic pressure. Extending this finding into the clinical area, one is tempted to speculate that it may be possible in the future to create an extravascular extracorporeal "aortic balloon pump" where aortic volume is varied by positive intrathoracic pressure within the cardiac cycle to unload a failing and/or ischemic LV.

Relation of Results with Phrenic Nerve Stimulation to Normal Respiration

Thus transient negative intrathoracic pressure appears to have a dual effect on LV performance. During diastole LV inflow is diminished by ventricular interdependence reducing LV preload, i.e. right heart distention limits LV filling. During systole LV emptying is impeded, presumptively by increasing effective LV afterload, rising end-systolic volume. Both mechanisms are independent and should contribute to the fall in LV stroke volume with spontaneous and obstructed respiration. It is clear that studies evaluating LV volumes with respiration extending over several cardiac cycles are likely to yield conflicting results.

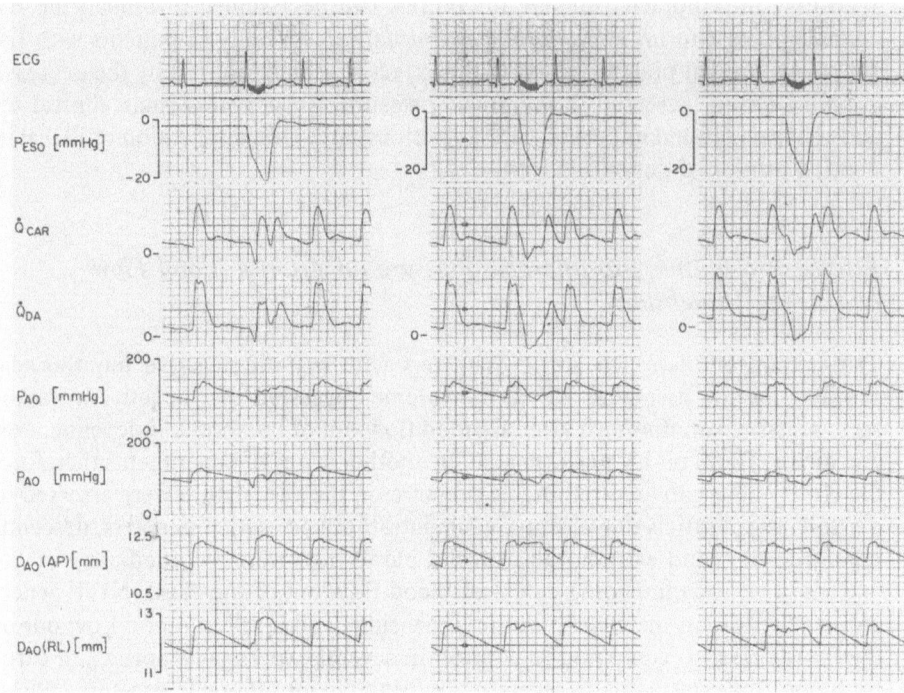

Fig. 9. Original recording (airway obstructed, paper speed: 50 mm/s). A complete cardiac cycle is scanned with phrenic nerve stimulation beginning in systole *(left panel)*, early *(middle panel)*, and late diastole *(right panel)*, while esophageal pressure (P_{ESO}), extrathoracic carotid blood flow (Q_{CAR}), intrathoracic descending aortic blood flow (Q_{DA}), aortic pressure (P_{AO}) as well as anterior-posterior [$D_{AO}(AP)$] and right-to-left [$D_{AO}(RL)$] intrathoracic are recorded. Negative intrathoracic pressure causes a retrograde Q_{CAR} and Q_{DA}, i.e. blood flows from the extrathoracic into the intrathoracic arterial compartment. This results in distention of the intrathoracic aorta. As phrenic stimulation ceases and P_{ESO} returns towards baseline, aortic diameters rapidly decrease and the blood stored in the intrathoracic arterial compartment with negative intratroracic pressure is discharged resulting in a bolus antegrade flow. With late diastolic phrenic stimulation *(right panel)* this antegrade bolus summates with the ensuing LV ejection. Thus the aorta can be considered an elastic reservoir driven by changes in pleural pressure

Finally the studies have demonstrated a third independent mechanism, i.e. negative intrathoracic pressure impeding blood flow from the intrathoracic into the extrathoracic arterial compartment and distending the intrathoracic aorta. All three mechanisms will summate to decrease peripheral arterial flow and pressure with spontaneous and obstructed respiration, i.e. pulsus paradoxus. It remains to be demonstrated that equivalent, but opposite findings are present with increased intrathoracic pressure.

Clinical Implications for Respiration Within the Cardiac Cycle

The results presented suggest that it may be possible to exploit the differential effects of changes in intrathoracic pressure within the cardiac cycle for therapeutic clinical strategies. With high frequency jet ventilation an increase in intrathoracic pressure can be generated and synchronized to the ECG with an appropriate electronic circuitry while maintaining gas exchange. If the data using a single transient fall in pleural pressure can be extrapolated to the situation where increases in intrathoracic pressure are applied to each cardiac cycle, we would expect the least impairment of cardiac filling to occur with early diastolic mechanical inspiration and the greatest improvement in LV emptying with systolic mechanical inspiration. Minimal inference with diastolic filling would be important during hypovolemia, while improved systolic emptying is an important goal during cardiac failure where the LV operates on a flat portion of the Starling curve anyway. In a steady state situation however, both factors are obviously interrelated and increases in lung volume may change diastolic LV filling [35]. Preload may also be altered by other mechanisms. Thus an alternate timing of the mechanical inspiration may prove to be optimal.

Pinsky's group in Pittsburgh has presented data along these lines of thinking. Using ECG-triggered high frequency jet ventilation in dogs end-diastolic mechanical ventilation was associated with the least deterioration in cardiac output compared to apnea. However, when a state of "LV failure" was induced by propranolol and volume administration, systolic jet ventilation was associated with the greatest hemodynamic stability [55]. Similarly, the least circulatory depression was seen with late diastolic jet ventilation during hemorrhagic shock, but, for unknown reasons, not during hypotension induced by ganglionic block with hexamethonium [56]. Extending these laboratory studies into the operating room, Pinsky et al. [57] demonstrated an increase in cardiac output with systolic jet ventilation in patients with severe cardiomyopathy awaiting cardiac transplantation, compared with jet ventilation of a similar frequency not triggered by the ECG so that inspiration occurred randomly within the cardiac cycle.

While these important data cannot pinpoint the responsible mechanisms because no ventricular volumes or ventricular function curves could be measured, they do indicate a potential for improving the failing circulation non-invasively by specific means of mechanical respiratory support. Respiration within the cardiac cycle therefore, apart from giving insights into the physiology of cardiopulmonary interactions, may enrich the anesthesiologist's or critical care physician's therapeutic armentarium within the next decade to provide not only adequate pulmonary gas exchange but also to assist the circulation by mechanical ventilation tailored to a patient's particular needs.

Acknowledgments: The author wishes to acknowledge the cooperation of his coinvestigators Drs. Baumgartner, Fraser, Robotham, and Stuart, who participated in the experimental work described in this chapter. My thanks also go to Antje Nebert for preparation of the illustrations.

References

1. Wise RA, Robotham JL, Summer WR (1981) Effects of spontaneous ventilation on the circulation. Lung 159:175–186
2. Robotham JL, Lixfeld W, Holland L, MacGregor D, Bryan AC, Rabson J (1978) Effects of respiration on cardiac performance. J Appl Physiol 44:703–709
3. Robotham JL, Rabson J, Permutt S, Bromberger-Barnea B (1979) Left ventricular hemodynamics during respiration. J Appl Physiol 47:1295–1303
4. Robotham JL, Bell RC, Badke FR, Kindred MK (1985) Left ventricular geometry during positive end-expiratory pressure. Crit Care Med 13:617–624
5. Scharf SM, Brown R, Saunders N, Green LH, Ingram RH (1979) Changes in canine left ventricular size and configuration with positive end-expiratory pressure. Circ Res 44:672–678
6. Scharf SM, Bianco JA, Tow DE, Brown R (1981) The effects of large negative intrathoracic pressure on left ventricular function in patients with coronary artery disease. Circulation 63:871–875
7. Buda AJ, Pinsky MR, Ingels NB, Daughters GT, Stinson EB, Alderman EL (1979) Effects of intrathoracic pressure on left ventricular performance. New Engl J Med 301:453–459
8. Brinker JA, Weiss JL, Lappe DL, et al (1980) Leftward septal displacement during right ventricular loading in man. Circulation 61:626–633
9. Olson CO, Tyson GS, Maier GW, Sratt JA, Davis JD, Rankin JS (1983) Dynamic ventricular interaction in the conscious dog. Circ Res 52:85–104
10. Olson CO, Tyson GS, Maier GW, Dawis JW, Rankin JS (1985) Diminished stroke volume during inspiration: A reverse thoracic pump. Circulation 72:668–679
11. Santamore WP, Heckman JL, Bove AA (1984) Right and left ventricular pressure-volume reponse to respiratory maneuvers. J Appl Physiol 57:1520–1527
12. Fermoso JD, Richardson TQ, Guyton AC (1964) Mechanism of decrease in cardiac output caused by opening the chest. Am J Physiol 207:1112–1116
13. Brecher GA, Mixter G (1953) Effect of respiratory movements on superior cava flow under normal and abnormal conditions. Am J Physiol 172:457–461
14. Mixter G (1953) Respiratory augmentation of inferior caval flow demonstrated by a low-resistance phasic flowmeter. Am J Physiol 172:446–456
15. Criley JM, Blaufuss AH, Kissel GL (1987) Cough-induced cardiac compression. JAMA 11:1246–1250
16. Niemann JT, Rosborough J, Hausknecht M, Brown D, Criley JM (1980) Cough-CPR. Documentation of systemic perfusion in man and in an experimental model: a "window" to the mechanism of blood flow in external CPR. Crit Care Med 8:141–146
17. Leith D, Butler JP, Sneddon SL, Brain JD (1986) Mechanics of breathing. Handbook of Physiology, Section 3, Volume 3, Part 1, American Physiologic Society, Baltimore, pp 315–336
18. Maier GW, Tyson GS, Olson CO, et al (1984) The physiology of external cardiac massage: high-impulse cardiopulmonary resuscitation. Circulation 70:86–101
19. Halperin HR, Tsitlik JE, Guerci AD, et al (1986) Determinants of blood flow to vital organs during cardiopulmonary resuscitation in dogs. Circulation 73:539–550
20. Beattie C (pers. comm.), 1987
21. Glantz SA, Misbach GA, Moores WY, et al (1978) The pericardium substantially affects the left ventricular diastolic pressure-volume relationship in the dog. Circ Res 42:433–441
22. Shirato K, Shabetai R, Bhargava V, Franklin D, Ross J (1978) Alteration of the left ventricular diastolic pressure-segment length relation produced by the pericardium. Circulation 57:1191–1197
23. Janicki JS, Weber KT (1980) The pericardium and ventricular interaction, distensibility, and function. Am J Physiol 238:H494–H503
24. Slinker BK, Glantz SA (1986) End-systolic and end-diastolic ventricular interaction. Am J Physiol 251:H1062–H1075
25. McMahon SM, Permutt S, Proctor DF (1969) A model to evaluate pleural surface pressure measuring devices. J Appl Physiol 27:886–891

26. Refsum H, Jünemann M, Lipton MJ, Skiøldebrand C, Carlsson E, Tyberg JV (1981) Ventricular diastolic pressure-volume relations and the pericardium. Circulation 64:997–1004
27. Smiseth OA, Frais MA, Kingma I, Smith E, Tyberg JV (1985) Assessment of pericardial constraint in dogs. Circulation 71:158–164
28. Jünemann M, Smiseth OA, Refsum H, et al (1987) Quantification of effect of pericardium on LV diastolic PV relation in dogs. Am J Physiol 252:H963–968
29. Smiseth OA, Scott-Douglas NW, Thompson CR, Smith ER, Tyberg JV (1987) Nonuniformity of pericardial surface pressure in dogs. Circulation 75:1229–1236
30. Wallis TW, Robotham JL, Kindred MK (1983) Mechanical heart-lung interaction with positive end-expiratory pressure. J Appl Physiol 54:1039–1047
31. Lloyd TC (1982) Respiratory system compliance as seen from the cardiac fossa. J Appl Physiol 53:57–62
32. Cassidy SS, Mitchell JH, Johnson RL (1982) Dimensional analysis of right and left ventricles during positive-pressure ventilation in dogs. Am J Physiol 242:H549–556
33. Cassidy SS, Ramanathan M (1984) Dimensional analysis of the left ventricle during PEEP: relative septal and lateral wall displacements. Am J Physiol 246:H792–805
34. Cassidy SS, Wead WB, Seibert GB, Ramanathan M (1987) Changes in left ventricular geometry during spontaneous breathing. J Appl Physiol 63:803–811
35. Brower R, Wise RA, Hassapoyannes C, Bromberger-Barnea B, Permutt S (1985) Effect of lung inflation on lung blood volume and pulmonary venous flow. J Appl Physiol 58:954–963
36. Whittenberger JL, McGregor M, Berglund E, Borst HG (1960) Influence of state of inflation of the lung on pulmonary vascular resistance. J Appl Physiol 15:878–882
37. Graham R, Skoog C, Oppenheimer L, Rabson J, Goldberg HS (1982) Critical closure in the canine pulmonary vasculature. Circ Res 50:566–572
38. Scharf SM, Brown R (1982) Influence of the right ventricle on left ventricular function with PEEP. J Appl Physiol 52:254–259
39. Permutt S, Bromberger-Barnea B, Bane HN (1962) Alveolar pressure, pulmonary venous pressure, and the vascular waterfall. Med Thorac 19:239–260
40. Lodato RF, Michael JR, Murray PA (1985) Multipoint pulmonary vascular pressure-cardiac output plots in conscious dogs. Am J Physiol 249:H351–357
41. Duomarco JL, Rimini R (1954) Energy and hydraulic gradients along systemic veins. Am J Physiol 178:215–220
42. Guyton AC, Adkins LH (1954) Quantitative aspects of the collapse factor in relation to venous return. Am J Physiol 177:523–527
43. Willeput R, Rondeux C, De Troyer A (1984) Breathing affects venous return from legs in humans. J Appl Physiol 57:971–976
44. Moreno AH, Burchell AR, van der Woude R, Burke JH (1967) Respiratory regulation of splanchnic and systemic venous return. Am J Physiol 213:455–465
45. Lloyd TC (1983) Effect of inspiration on inferior vena caval blood flow in dogs. J Appl Physiol 55:1701–1708
46. Fitzgerald RS, Robotham JL, Anand A (1981) Baroreceptor output during normal and obstructed breathing and Mueller maneuvers. Am J Physiol 240:H721–729
47. Malliani A, Peterson DF, Bishop VS, Brown AM (1972) Spinal sympathetic cardiocardiac reflexes. Circ Res 30:158–166
48. Ashton JH, Cassidy SS (1985) Reflex cardiovascular depression of cardiovascular function during lung inflation. J Appl Physiol 58:137–145
49. Laniado S, Yellin EL, Miller H, Frater RWM (1973) Temporal relation of the first heart sound to closure of the mitral valve. Circulation 47:1006–1014
50. Stalcup SA, Mellins RB (1977) Mechanical forces producing pulmonary edema in acute asthma. N Engl J Med 297:592–596
51. Parsons GB, Green JF (1978) Mechanisms of pulsus paradoxus in upper airway obstruction. J Appl Physiol 45:598–603
52. Scharf SM, Woods BO, Brown R, Parisi A, Miller MM, Tow DE (1987) Effects of the Müller maneuver on global and regional left ventricular function in angina pectoris with and without previous myocardial infarction. Am J Cardiol 59: 1305–1309

53. Grace MP, Greenbaum DM (1982) Cardiac performance in response to PEEP in patients with cardiac dysfunction. Crit Care Med 10:358–360
54. Mathru M, Rao TLK, El-Etr AA, Pifam R (1982) Hemodynamic response to changes in ventilatory patterns in patients with normal and poor left ventricular reserve. Crit Care Med 10:423–426
55. Pinsky MR, Matuschak GM, Bernardi L, Klain M (1986) Hemodynamic effects of cardiac cycle-specific increases in intrathoracic pressure. J Appl Physiol 60:604–612
56. Matuschak GM, Pinsky MR, Klain M (1986) Hemodynamic effects of synchroneous high-frequency jet ventilation during acute hypovolemia. J Appl Physiol 61:44–53
57. Pinsky MR, Marquez J, Martin D, Klain M (1987) Ventricular assist by cardiac cycle-specific increases in intrathoracic pressure. Chest 91:709–715

Right Ventricular Performance During Mechanical Ventilation in ARDS

F. Brunet and J. F. Dhainaut

Introduction

In 1977, Zapol and Snider [1] reported pulmonary artery hypertension in ARDS, even after correction of systemic hypoxemia. Sibbald et al. [2], as well as our group [3], demonstrated that this pulmonary artery hypertension was associated with an increased right ventricular (RV) end-diastolic volume and a decreased ejection fraction (EF). The stroke volume is preserved by the Frank-Starling mechanism as preload increases.

However, PEEP ventilation will further increase RV afterload by increasing alveolar volume and pressure, and may, despite improved gas exchange, further reduce cardiac output and tissue oxygen delivery [4]. The RV response to PEEP is often unpredictable because this response depends on many factors such as lung and thoracic compliance, previous ventricular loading conditions and myocardial function. Consequently, if PEEP therapy produces severe reductions in cardiac output despite reasonable volume expansion, the reasons may be the following:

1. decreased RV preload requiring additional volume expansion [5, 6] or low doses of dopamine [7], or the combination of the two,
2. or increased RV afterload. In this situation, volume expansion may be deleterious by inducing RV overdilation, fall in RVEF and overall cardiac performance [2].

Unfortunately, major technical problems impede assessment of the mechanisms of PEEP-induced cardiac dysfunction by conventional hemodynamic montoring. Indeed, determination of the correct reference pressure for calculating transmural pressure is very difficult because extracardiac pressure is not uniform and changes nonuniformly [6, 8–9]. Because of this problem, the measurements of RVEF and volumes only provide an adequate assessment of RV response to PEEP.

This review will discuss the scientific information pertinent to clinical approaches towards the RV performance changes secondary to PEEP therapy in patients with ARDS.

Assessment of the Effects of PEEP on RV Performance

To precisely analyze these RV performance changes, two majors technological problems must be overcome:
1. determination of the correct reference pressure for calculating transmural pressure, and
2. accurate determination of ventricular volume.

At present, no clinical study completely resolves these problems, leading to a strong note of caution in accepting definitive conclusions.

Assessment of RV Transmural Pressures

To estimate RV preload during PEEP, RV end-diastolic or mean right atrial pressures must be referenced to this extracardiac pressure. Changes in afterload are usually assumed to be proportional to pressure within the RV, which may be estimated from pulmonary artery pressure, referenced to extracardiac pressure. Similarly, to estimate changes in myocardial function assessed as end-systolic pressure-volume ratio [10, 11], end-systolic pressure must be referenced to extracardiac pressure. However, determination of extracardiac pressure for calculating transmural pressure is very difficult because this pressure is not uniform and changes nonuniformly. This nonuniformity has been well documented in several experimental studies [8, 9], strongly suggested in a recent clinical study from our ICU [6], showing poor correlation between changes in lateral pericardial and esophageal pressure in two patients with acute lung injury.

Assessment of RV Volumes

Assessment of RV volumes is also very difficult. The three currently available methods are echocardiography, radionuclide angiography and thermodilution technique. With the use of two-dimensional echocardiography, end-diastolic and end-systolic area can be measured from endocardial outlines on apical and subcostal four-chambers views. However, the RV endocardium can be traced in only 50% of patients with coronary artery disease [12]. This percentage probably decreases in critically ill patients, especially during mechanical ventilation. The choice of non-geometric methods for measuring RV volume seems the most appropriate, given its variable shape. Radionuclide angiography techniques, both first-pass and equilibrium gated blood pool, seem less subject to errors in measurement. With first-pass radionuclide angiography, data analysis is based on a few cardiac cycles. The major limiting factor of this technique is the low count rates of the raw data. The equilibrium gated technique provides informations during a longer period of time. However, the left anterior oblique position only separates activity within the two ventricles and then right atrium contributes substantially to RV counts in this position [13]. Last, the thermodilution technique seems particularly appealing for serial monitoring of RV performance [14]. Technical problems related to catheter-mounted fast-response thermistor [15, 16] seem to be solved [17].

These factors should be considered when analyzing the effects of PEEP on RV performance by currently available techniques in the ICU.

Effects of PEEP Ventilation on RV Performance in ARDS

With increasing PEEP, heart rate in general fails to rise despite a decreased RV output. The reason remains unclear [6, 18–20], but may contribute to the overall side effects of PEEP on RV performance. Thus, the entire fall in RV output is a consequence of a reduction in RV stroke volume.

Decreased RV Preload

There are a number of mechanisms whereby RV stroke volume may decrease with PEEP. Most investigators agree, however, that RV preload decreases with PEEP and decreased venous return to the right heart secondary to the increase in intrapleural pressure plays the major role [6, 18–21].

Increased RV Afterload

However, resistance to RV ejection (i.e., pulmonary vascular resistance) slightly increases with levels of PEEP higher than 10 cm H_2O [6, 18–21]. The systematic overestimation of transmural pressure discussed above should be considered when assessing results of pulmonary vascular resistance. Thus, this small increase in RV afterload is probably insignificant in such patients. However, in 6 out of 90 patients with ARDS investigated in our ICU, PEEP led to a significant increase in RV afterload (i.e., marked increase in end-diastolic volume and fall in ejection fraction). This unusual response to PEEP was associated with very low total thoracic compliance and severe acute pulmonary hypertension. The explanation for these findings is not clear. Such a response may be due to the existence of non-uniform lung disease, so that in the normally compliant areas high PEEP induces a marked increase in alveolar volume, producing a collapse of pulmonary capillaries and aggravating RV overload [22]. Further studies are required to confirm this hypothesis.

Ventricular Interference

In addition, left ventricular (LV) end-diastolic transmural pressure falls more than RV end-diastolic transmural pressure, resulting in a decrease in left to right end-diastolic pressure gradient [6, 18]. A similar fall in end-diastolic ventricular [23] and atrial [24, 25] pressure gradients have been reported in animal studies. This fact suggest that PEEP may shift the interventricular septum leftward. However, the observed decrease of RV preload parallels that of the LV, and the lack of correlation between RV and LV end-diastolic volume ratio, as developed by Viquerat et al. [20], and addition of PEEP seems to indicate that ventricular interference plays a minor role in patients with ARDS, and that reduced RV preload secondary to decreased venous return [6, 20] is the most important mechanism for decreased RV output.

The above conclusions, based on radionuclide techniques, are in contrast to those of Jardin et al. [18], utilizing two-dimensional echocardiography. These authors reported leftward displacement of the interventricular septum with PEEP. They concluded that the effects of PEEP on LV preload are primarily mediated by restriction of LV filling due to septal bulging. However, the radius of septal curvature increased significantly at both end-systole and end-diastole, only at the highest PEEP (≥ 25 cm H_2O). These high levels of PEEP probably lead to marked increase in lung volume, afterloading the RV to such a degree as to produce septal flattening and enhanced ventricular interference. It is interesting to note that such an effect on RV afterload appears at lower levels of PEEP in patients without marked lung injury, as after elective coronary bypass surgery (PEEP ≥ 15 cm H_2O) [26], or, even more so, in normal subjects (PEEP ≥ 10 cm H_2O) [27]. Fortunately, these detrimental PEEP levels are usually above those required to significantly improve arterial oxygen content of patients with ARDS [28].

Decreased RV Contractility

Some animal studies [29, 30] suggest that depressed myocardial contractility may follow PEEP therapy. However, the absence of change of end-systolic pressure-volume ratio or even leftward shift (at levels of PEEP ≥ 10 cm H_2O) of this ratio indicates that RV contractility does not decrease during PEEP [6].

Therefore, in the absence of marked changes in RV end-systolic transmural pressure, the marked fall in RV end-diastolic volume with increasing PEEP, and the complete return to pre-PEEP value after volume expansion [6] strongly support the thesis that the most common hemodynamic response to reasonable levels of PEEP in patients with ARDS, is a moderate decrease in RV preload without evidence of neither ventricular interference nor myocardial dysfunction.

Guidelines for Monitoring PEEP Therapy in ARDS

During the incremental increases of PEEP, essential monitoring includes vital signs, especially blood pressure and urinary output, continuous ECG, serial arterial blood gas measurements, and appropriate nurse and respiratory therapist availability. Appropriate monitoring of the respiratory equipement, inspiratory gas concentration, and system flow is essential, since technical malfunction is not uncommon [28].

Right Heart Catheterization Monitoring

Hemodynamic investigation by pulmonary artery catheter is advantageous in monitoring PEEP therapy, but is by no means a necessity except when more than 15 cm H_2O PEEP is required, or there is evidence of RV overload by noninvasive technique [12, 18]. Of course, when there is uncertainty regarding the diagnosis of cardiogenic vs non-cardiogenic pulmonary edema, pulmonary artery catheterization is valuable.

The clinically useful information available from this invasive hemodynamic monitoring includes:

1. measurement of cardiac output, arterial and venous oxygen content, and arterial lactate to adequately assess peripheral perfusion and oxygen requirement;
2. calculation of intrapulmonary shunt to aid the evaluation of the pulmonary effects of PEEP; and
3. RV end-diastolic volumes, or right atrial and pulmonary wedge pressures to guide the administration of intravascular volume expansion or inotropic support.

Accuracy of RV Preload

Controversy exists concerning the method for serially evaluating hemodynamic status in ARDS with PEEP. First, a major problem is determining ventricular preload (filling) from intracardiac pressures not referenced to intrathoracic or extracardiac pressure with PEEP. The data described above clearly establish that accurate assessment of ventricular preload with PEEP requires measurement of ventricular volumes, or, failing that, calculation of transmural ventricular filling pressures. When measurement of ventricular volumes is not technically feasible, accurate measurement of pleural and even esophageal pressure for calculating transmural pressure is, unfortunately, not readily available in the clinical setting. Davison et al. [31] demonstrated that momentarily interrupting PEEP therapy to perform hemodynamic measurements produces unreliable data in patients receiving PEEP ventilation for ARDS. In our clinical practice, when measurements of ventricular volumes are not technically feasible, hemodynamic measurements are performed at end-expiration under PEEP ventilation without major error in estimating ventricular filling pressure when using "reasonable" levels of PEEP, as previously recommended by Downs and Douglas [32].

Accuracy of Pulmonary Wedge Pressure

Another problem is the accuracy of pulmonary wedge pressure as a reflect of left ventricular filling pressure at ligh levels of PEEP. The associated increase in lung volume could lead to a dissociation between pulmonary wedge pressure and left atrial pressure (zone II lung), in which pulmonary wedge pressure is higher than atrial pressure. By contrast, LV end-diastolic pressure bears a close and linear relation to right atrial pressure with a slope almost equal to one [18]. In our experience, it is possible to adequately measure pulmonary wedge pressure, whatever the level of PEEP, using fluoroscopy to place the pulmonary artery catheter at the posterior part of the lung (zone III lung).

In summary, only ventricular volumes adequately assess ventricular preload. In the absence of such a measurement, right atrial and pulmonary wedge pressures measured at end-expiration (under PEEP ventilation) are a easy estimation of ventricular preload, as we assume the absence of alteration of ventricular compliance.

Airway Pressure-Related Cyclic Changes in Hemodynamics

The last problem in assessing hemodynamic status of such patients during PEEP ventilation, concerns airway pressure-related cyclic changes in both cardiac output and RVEF. Jansen et al. [33] estimated the error in the cardiac output measured by thermodilution in pigs while varying injectate time over different phases of the respiratory cycle during PEEP ventilation. The average of each series of 50 measurements done at regular intervals over the respiratory cycle showed an excellent correlation with the measurements of cardiac output by the direct Fick method. However, with PEEP, the maximum difference between the values of cardiac output randomly measured by the thermodilution method was 70% and the authors could find no truly satisfactory time within the respiratory cycle for injectate administration with PEEP. This was confirmed by Snyder and Powner [34], who recommended that the mean of measurements taken at regularly spaced intervals through the respiratory cycle be used by estimates of cardiac output by thermodilution.

In a preliminary report, Assmann and Falke [35] found that determinations of RVEF during mechanical ventilation did not represent the mean value across the ventilatory cycle and were of poor reproducibility, especially at low respiratory frequency (8 cycles/min). At low frequencies, the mean amplitude of modulation extended 49% of a partient's mean value during the ventilatory cycle (16 cycles/min: 25%, and 24 cycles/min: 10%). Conversely, both with an automatically phase-selected injection technique and during apnea, the reproducibility improved, reducing the coefficient of variation to 7%. Our clinical experience is that, if a phase selected injection is not possible, one has to rely on a series of injections which are randomly distributed during the ventilation cycle. Evaluation of RVEF can be as reliably accomplished as measuring cardiac output.

Cardiovascular Support

Correlation of hypovolemia or cardiac failure should ideally be achieved prior to initiation of PEEP therapy. Usually, an increase in blood volume [5, 6] or venous tone [7] may compensate for PEEP-induced fall in cardiac output, as long as low levels of PEEP are required to reduce hypoxemia. PEEP therapy may occasionally produce severe reductions in cardiac output despite reasonable intravascular volume expansion or low doses of dopamine. An inotropic agent such as dobutamine is then required to increase overall cardiac performance by improving RV performance, septal contraction, and hence decreasing ventricular interference [36].

Conclusion

The most common RV response to reasonable levels of PEEP in patients with ARDS is a moderate decrease in RV preload with evidence of neither marked ventricular interference nor myocardial dysfunction, and appropriate increase in intravascular fluid volume usually restores RV preload and output. While the small increase in RV afterload with PEEP is probably functionally insignificant in patients with ARDS, in those with high levels of PEEP or most with severe acute pulmonary hypertension, this element may become much more important.

References

1. Zapol WM, Snider MT (1977) Pulmonary hypertension in severe acute respiratory failure. N Engl J Med 296:476–480
2. Sibbald WJ, Driedger AA (1983) Right ventricular function in acute disease states: Pathophysiologic considerations. Crit Care Med 11:339–345
3. Brunet F, Dhainaut JF, Devaux JY, Huyghebaert MF, Villemant D, Monsallier JF (1988) Behaviour of the RV performance in patients with acute respiratory failure. Intensive Care Med (in press)
4. Lutch JS, Murray JF (1972) Continuous positive-pressure ventilation on systemic oxygen transport and tissue oxygenation. Ann Intern Med 76:193–202
5. Qvist JH, Pontoppidan H, Wilson RS, Laver MB (1975) Hemodynamic response to mechanical ventilation with PEEP: the effect of hypervolemia. Anesthesiology 42:45–55
6. Dhainaut JF, Devaux JY, Monsallier JF, Brunet F, Villemant D, Hugghebaert MF (1986) Mechanisms of decreased left ventricular preload during continuous positive pressure ventilation in ARDS. Chest 90:74–80
7. Hemmer M, Suter PM (1979) Treatment of cardiac and renal effects of PEEP with dopamine in patients with acute respiratory failure. Anesthesiology 50:392–399
8. Fewell JE, Abendschein DR, Carlson J, Rapaport E, Murray JF (1981) Continuous positive-pressure ventilation does not alter ventricular pressure volume relationship. Am J Physiol 240:H821–H826
9. Marini JJ, Culver BH, Butler J (1981) Mechanical effect of lung distension with positive pressure on cardiac function. Am Rev Respir Dis 124:382–386
10. Suga H, Sagawa K (1974) Instantaneous pressure-volume relationships and their ratio in the excited, supported canine left ventricle. Circ Res 35:117–126
11. Maughan WL, Shoudas AA, Sagawa K, Weisfeldt ML (1979) Instantaneous pressure-volume relationship of the canine right ventricle. Circ Res 44:309–315
12. Kaul S, Tei C, Hopkins JM, Shah PM (1984) Assessment of right ventricular function using two-dimensional echocardiography. Am Heart J 107:526–531
13. Berger HJ, Matthay RA (1981) Noninvasive radiographic assessment of cardiovascular function in acute and chronic respiratory failure. Am J Cardiol 47:950–962
14. Kay HR, Afshari M, Barash P, et al (1983) Measurement of ejection fraction by thermal dilution technique. J Surg Res 34:337–346

15. Maruschak G, Schauble JF (1985) Limitations of thermodilution ejection fraction: degradation of frequency response by catheter mounting of fast-response thermistors. Crit Care Med 13:679–682
16. Dhainaut JF, Brunet F, Monsallier JF, et al (1987) Bedside evaluation of right ventricular performance using a rapid computerized thermodilution method. Crit Care Med 15:148–152
17. Dhainaut JF, Brunet F, Villemant D (1987) Evaluation of right ventricular function by thermodilution techniques. In: Vincent JL, Suter PM (eds) Cardiopulmonary interactions in acute respiratory failure. Springer, Berlin Heidelberg New York London Paris Tokyo (Update in Intensive Care and Emergency Medicine, vol 2, pp 95–106)
18. Jardin F, Farcot JC, Boisante L, Curien N, Margairaz A, Bourdarias JP (1981) Influence of positive end-expiratory pressure on left ventricular performance. N Engl J Med 304:387–392
19. Prewitt RM, Oppenheimer L, Sutherland JB, Wood LDH (1981) Effect of positive end-expiratory pressure on left ventricular mechanics in patients with hypoxic respiratory failure. Anesthesiology 55:409–415
20. Viquerat CE, Righetti A, Suter PM (1983) Biventricular volumes and function in patients with adult respiratory distress syndrome ventilated with PEEP. Chest 83:509–514
21. Calvin JE, Driedger AA, Sibbald WJ (1981) Positive end-expiratory pressure (PEEP) does not depress left ventricular function in patients with pulmonary edema. Am Rev Respir Dis 124:121–128
22. Dhainaut JF, Schlemmer B, Monsallier JF, Fourestié V, Carli A (1984) Behaviour of the right ventricle following PEEP in patients with mild and severe ARDS. Am Rev Respir Dis 129:A99
23. Cassidy SS, Mitchell JH, Johnson RL Jr (1982) Dimensional analysis of right and left ventricles during positive-pressure ventilation in dogs. Am J Physiol 24:H549–H556
24. Cassidy SS, Roberson JH Jr, Pierce AK, Johnson RL Jr (1978) Cardiovascular effects of positive end-expiratory pressure in dogs. J Appl Physiol 44:743–750
25. Scharf SM, Caldini P, Ingram RL Jr (1977) Cardiovascular effects of increasing airway pressure in the dog. Am J Physiol 232:H35–H43
26. Biondi JW, Matthey RA (1986) The effect of positive end-expiratory pressure (PEEP) on right ventricular function. Am Rev Respir Dis 133:A303
27. Cassidy SS, Eschenbacher WL, Roberson CH Jr, Nixon JV, Blomqvist G, Johnson RL Jr (1979) Cardiovascular effects of positive-pressure ventilation in normal subjects. J Appl Physiol 47:453–461
28. Shapiro BA, Roy DC, Harrison RA (1984) Positive end-expiratory pressure therapy in adults with special reference to acute lung injury: a review of the literature and suggested clinical correlations. Crit Care Med 12:127–141
29. Manny J, Patten MT, Liebman PR, Hechtman HB (1978) The association of lung distention, PEEP and biventricular failure. Ann Surg 187:151–159
30. Liebman PR, Patten MT, Manny J, Shepro D, Hechtman HB (1978) The mechanism of depressed cardiac output on positive end-expiratory pressure (PEEP). Surgery 83:594–598
31. Davison R, Parker M, Harrison RA (1978) Validity of determinations of pulmonary wedge pressures during mechanical ventilation. Chest 73:352–356
32. Downs JB, Douglas ME (1980) Assessment of cardiac filling pressure during continuous positive pressure ventilation. Crit Care Med 8:285–289
33. Jansen JRC, Schreuder JJ, Bogaard JM, van Rooyen W, Versprille A (1981) Thermodilution technique for measurement of cardiac output during artificial ventilation. J Appl Physiol 50:584–591
34. Snyder JV, Powner DJ (1982) Effects of mechanical ventilation on the measurement of cardiac output by thermodilution. Crit Care Med 10:677–682
35. Assmann R, Falke KJ (1987) Cyclic modulation of thermal right ventricular ejection fraction during controlled mechanical ventilation. Intensive Care Med 13:217–218
36. Jardin F, Ozier Y, Farcot JC, Bazin M, Bourdarias JP, Margairaz A (1984) Acute right ventricular failure: treatment with dobutamine. Presse Méd 13:2563–2566

Pulmonary Gas Exchange in Pulmonary Vascular Obstruction

D. R. Dantzker

Introduction

Abnormal arterial blood gases are an invariable consequence of both acute and chronic pulmonary vascular obstruction regardless of the etiology. In diffuse lung diseases in which the pulmonary vessels are involved as part of an underlying parenchymal process it is very difficult to separate out the contribution to abnormal pulmonary gas exchange made by the vascular involvement. These would include the pulmonary occlusion seen in the adult respiratory distress syndrome (ARDS), the pulmonary hypertension which results from chronic hypoxic vasoconstriction typified by patients with chronic obstructive pulmonary disease and the vascular obliteration secondary to diffuse interstitial fibrosis. For this reason we will confine ourselves in this discussion to entities, both acute and chronic, in which involvement of the vessels predominate and thus in which the contribution of vascular obstruction is clear.

Acute Pulmonary Vascular Occlusion

Acute pulmonary vascular obstruction is almost always due to embolization of material into the pulmonary vascular bed. Depending on the composition of the embolized material the clinical findings may be dominated by diffuse alveolar injury and the presence of non-cardiogenic pulmonary edema as is seen following fat and amniotic fluid embolization or may be due to the vascular obstruction itself as with tumor, air and thromboemboli. It is this latter group we will discuss, utilizing thromboemboli as the model, since it has been the best and most completely characterized.

Acute pulmonary thromboembolism probably always results in abnormal pulmonary gas exchange. Hypoxemia is characteristic (Fig. 1). Only 13%, in one collected series of patients with angiographically proven pulmonary embolism, had an arterial oxygen tension (PaO_2) of greater than 80 torr and only 6% greater than 90 torr [1]. While most of the patients had a moderate degree of hypoxemia, 32% had a PaO_2 of less than 60 torr. Even in those patients with a normal PaO_2 there is usually a widening of the alveolar to arterial gradient for oxygen (A-a DO_2). In those patients in whom there is no prior history of cardiopulmonary disease there is a good correlation between the severity of the hypoxemia and the extent to which the pulmonary vascular bed is occluded. This relationship is not apparent, however, in patients with pre-existing disease [2]. Hypocarbia,

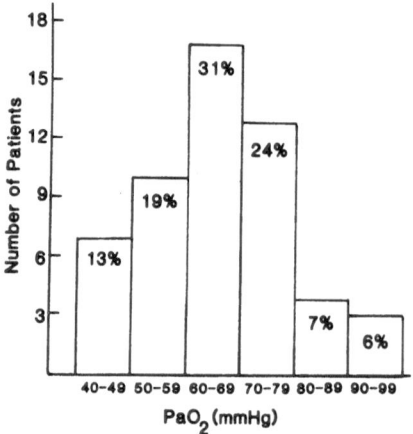

Fig. 1. The arterial PO_2 from 54 patients without previous cardiopulmonary disease and angiographically proven acute pulmonary embolism. (From [1])

even in patients with significant underlying lung disease, is a very common finding although it is not as universal a phenomenon as hypoxemia.

The results of studies which have attempted to elucidate the physiological mechanisms of this abnormal gas exchange, both in patients and animal models, have been far from consistent. In part, this is due to differences in the response of different species with regards to thrombosis and thrombolysis, as well as differences in the vasoactive mediators which may be released following embolization. In addition, the majority of animals were studied while sedated and/or mechanically ventilated which undoubtedly interfered with a normal ventilatory response. Finally the differences in the quantity and composition of the embolized material, varying from small glass beads to large homogenous thromboemboli guaranteed a inconsistent response.

Even in human studies, the results from series to series are not directly comparable due to differences in the degree of vascular occlusion, the time since the acute event, and the presence or absence of complicating cardiopulmonary disease. In addition, until the recent development of the multiple inert gas elimination technique [3], the routine variables which were used to characterize pulmonary gas exchange were inadequate to differentiate between various physiological mechanisms with sufficient sensitivity. In particular, it was impossible to clearly discriminate between pulmonary and non-pulmonary causes of hypoxemia. Using this technique, however, the physiological mechanisms have now been elucidated and demonstrated to include, to one degree or another in different clinical settings, shunt, ventilation-perfusion (VA/Q) inequality, diffusion impairment and mixed venous desaturation. Unfortunately, the pathological bases of these physiological abnormalities are still not entirely clear. Let us look at each of these mechanisms in turn.

Pulmonary Factors

Right to left shunting through the lung has been demonstrated in animal studies subsequent to both homologous thromboemboli and glass beads [4, 5] (Fig. 2a). Distributions of ventilation and blood flow qualitatively similar to those found in the experimental animals were measured in two patients with massive pulmonary emboli and marked cardiopulmonary insufficiency [6] (Fig. 2b). In two series of patients recently reported, shunt made up a variable portion of the abnormal VA/Q distributions [7, 8] (see below). The mechanism of the shunt has not been clearly established although three good possibilities have been suggested.

Post-embolic atelectasis, hypothesized to result from alterations in surface active properties of the lung due to the reduction in alveolar blood flow, are a common finding in patients with embolic disease. Reperfusion of these unventi-

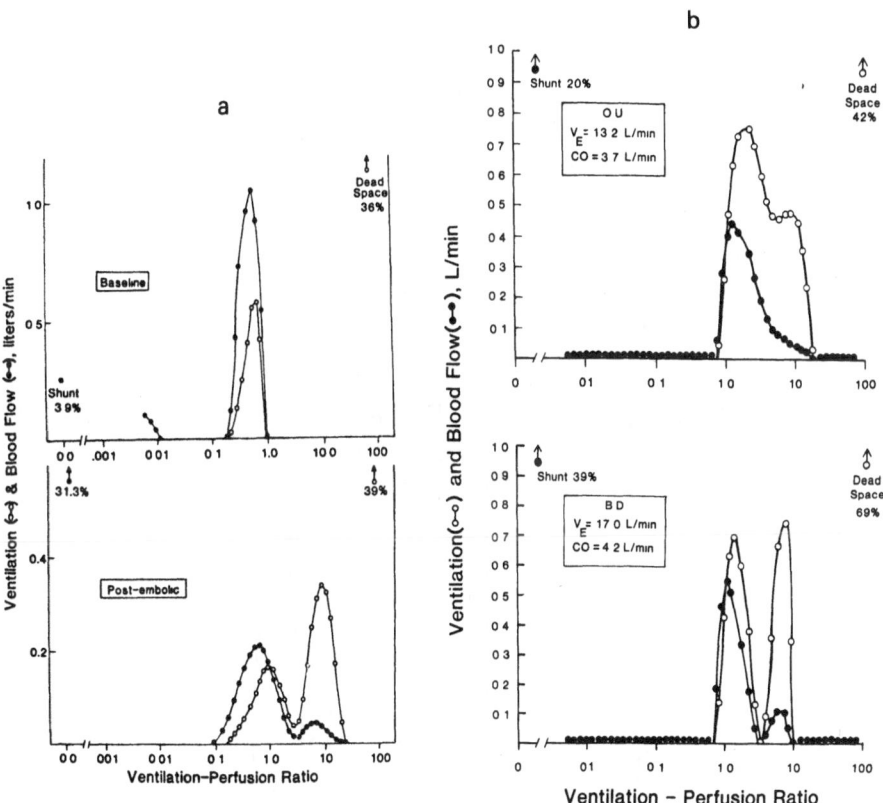

Fig. 2. a The distribution of ventilation-perfusion ratios in a dog at baseline and following glass bead embolization. The post-embolic distribution shows a dramatic increase in shunt and the appearance of lung units with high ventilation-perfusion ratios but no significant change in dead space. (From [1] with permission). **b** The distribution of ventilation-perfusion ratios in two patients with acute, massive pulmonary embolism. Similar to the findings in Figure 2a the major abnormalities are the large shunt and the presence of lung units with high ventilation-perfusion ratios. VE is the minute ventilation and CO the cardiac output. (From [6] with permission)

lated lung units due to clot dissolution or breakup would result in shunting. The observation that post-embolic hypoxemia can often be ameliorated by short periods of positive pressure breathing lends support to this as a mechanism.

The development of pulmonary edema would also lead to shunting. The edema may develop in this setting as a result of increased hydrostatic pressure in the unobstructed pulmonary vessels either due to an imbalance in the Starling forces (the increase in vascular hydrostatic pressure itself) or to physical damage to the vascular endothelium from high shearing forces resulting in an increase in vascular permeability. In one study using glass beads, the amount of shunt produced was closely correlated with the increase in pulmonary artery pressure [9]. A second possible mechanism involves the release of mediators from the clot leading to an increase in vascular permeability in the embolized regions. Animals pretreated with heparin prior to embolization with thromboemboli failed to develop edema while those not pretreated, did [10]. Which mechanism is involved may be determined by the size of the vessel occluded. Small glass beads were shown to cause edema by altering downstream permeability in the embolized vessels while larger ones increased pressure in the unobstructed vessels leading to hydrostatic edema [11].

A final mechanism demonstrated to cause shunting in this setting is the development of an intracardiac shunt. Approximately 15% of people are thought to have a potentially patent foramen ovale. Thus it is not surprising, that in the setting of acute cor pulmonale, shunting through this intracardiac connection may occur.

Mismatch of ventilation and blood flow is a potent and common cause of abnormal pulmonary gas exchange. In two recent studies of patients with acute, moderately severe (mean vascular occlusion approximately 50%) pulmonary em-

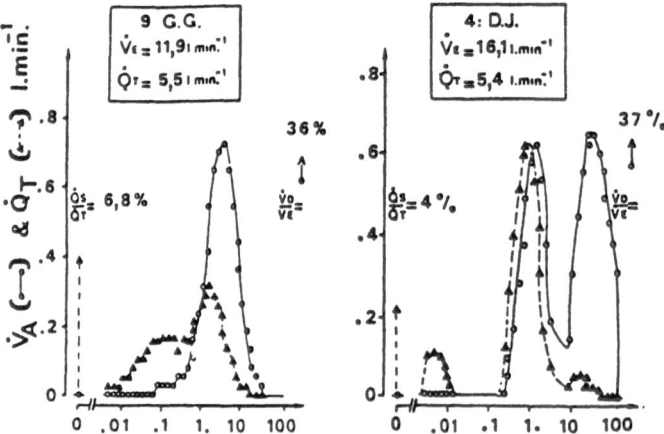

Fig. 3. The distribution of ventilation-perfusion ratios in two patients with acute pulmonary embolism. Two different patterns can be seen. Patient GG has as large amount of blood flow to lungs units with very low ventilation-perfusion ratios while the major abnormality in patient DJ is the presence of high ventilation-perfusion units. Both patients have a small amount of shunt but no increase in dead space. VA is alveolar ventilation, E is minute ventilation and Qt is cardiac output. (From [7] with permission)

boli, VA/Q inequality was shown to play an important role in the hypoxemia which developed [7, 8]. The patterns of VA/Q inequality varied from patient to patient (Fig. 3). Some had unimodel distributions which were only slightly wider than that seen in normals. Others had, as the predominant abnormality, the presence of lung units with either high or low VA/Q ratios. In some cases, modes of both high and low VA/Q ratios were present. In general, shunt played a less significant role as a cause of abnormal gas exchange, although in some patients it received as much as 15% of the cardiac output. In many of the patients with significant shunts, there was roentgenographic evidence of parenchymal lung abnormalities such as areas of atelectasis that may have accounted for the physiological findings. The dead space varied from a low of 26.5% to a high of 63.4%.

This heterogeneity of patterns of VA/Q inequality following acute pulmonary embolism is not surprising, as it was predicted from previous studies done in dogs [12]. In those animals, embolization with autologous thrombi to similar de-

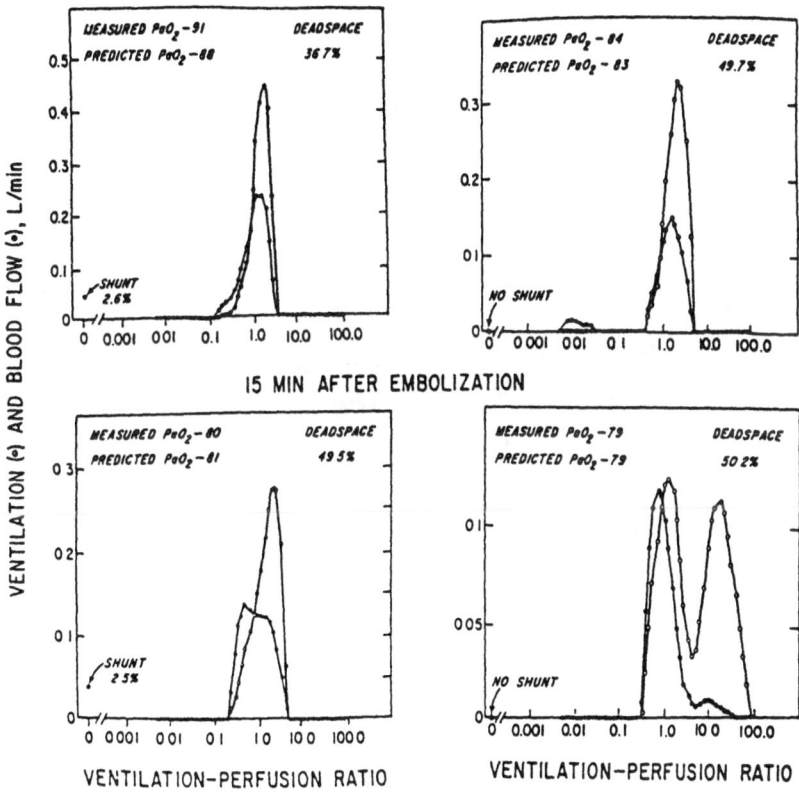

Fig. 4. The distribution of ventilation-perfusion ratios in two dogs before and after pulmonary embolization with autologous blood clot. Despite equal increases in pulmonary artery blood pressure, suggesting equal degrees of embolization, two different patterns of ventilation-perfusion inequality developed similar to that shown in Figure 3. The animal shown on the left side of the figure developed predominantly long units with low ventilation-perfusion ratios while the dog on the right developed predominantly high ventilation-perfusion units. (From [11] with permission)

grees of vascular occlusion, as judged by acute increase in pulmonary vascular resistance, led to a variety of patterns of VA/Q inequality similar to those described above (Fig. 4). Most animals developed a broadening of their distributions with modes of both low and high VA/Q ratios present. Some, however, developed modes of only low VA/Q units while others demonstrated only high VA/Q units. Shunt units were not found post embolism and significant increases in totally unventilated lung units (i.e. dead space) were not seen suggesting that total vascular occlusion is unusual.

Using a relatively simple two-compartment model, this diversity of ventilation and perfusion redistribution can be easily accounted for (Fig. 5). Partial occlusion of a large number of pulmonary vessels with diversion of only a por-

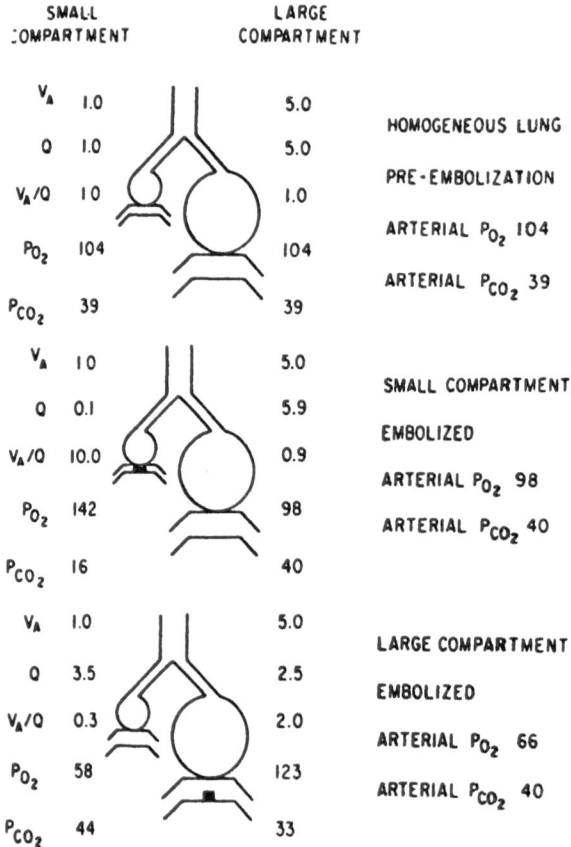

Fig. 5. Ventilation and perfusion are matched in the two-compartment lung model demonstrated in the top panel. In the middle panel, small compartment blood flow has been reduced by 90% and diverted to the large compartment, resulting in the development of a high VA/Q unit but a minimal decrease in the VA/Q of the larger compartment (1.0 to 0.9). Thus, no significant hypoxemia would develop (104 to 94 mm Hg). In the bottom panel, larger compartment blood flow has been reduced by 50% and diverted to the small compartment. This leads to 58% of the blood flow distributed to a lung unit with a VA/Q of 0.3, and significant hypoxemia develops (104 to 66 mm Hg). Mixed venous gas tensions remained constant and physiologic. (From [11] with permission)

tion of their blood flow to remaining unembolized vessels would result in over-perfusion of some lung regions creating lung units with low VA/Q ratios and thus hypoxemia. Reversing the hypoxemia created by this mechanism would require dramatic increases in minute ventilation in order to return the VA/Q ratio of the unembolized region to 1.0 unless some mechanism existed to divert the entire sum of the additional gas flow to these units. Since this marked hyperventilation would result in significant hypocapnia full compensation would undoubtedly be blunted. In this proposed scenario, neither high VA/Q ratios or an increase in dead space would develop because the occlusion of vessels was incomplete and thus only a portion of the blood flow was diverted. One may contrast this with a situation in which the thromboemboli occlude, almost totally, the vascular supply to a smaller region of the lung. The embolized region would now represent a mode of high VA/Q units but since a relatively small total amount of blood flow was diverted to the large amount of remaining unembolized lung, low VA/Q units would not develop and thus neither would hypoxemia. Combinations of these events will lead to the more commonly seen presence of both high and low VA/Q units.

In addition to this rather simplistic explanation for the observed variety of patterns, it is probable that mechanisms in addition to just mechanical redistribution of pulmonary blood flow is at work. There are well described changes in pulmonary mechanics following acute experimental pulmonary embolism resulting in a fall in lung compliance and increase in lung resistance which will alter both ventilation and perfursion distribution. In addition there are reflexes, hypoxic vasoconstriction and hypocapnic bronchoconstriction, which can minimize VA/Q inequality. These may help to explain the rapid normalization of the VA/Q distribution seen in some animal studies and the relatively normal distributions found in some patients. It should be noted, however, that in a recent report no changes in VA/Q distributions were measured in patients with acute thromboembolic disease who were given hyperoxic mixtures to breath questioning the role of hypoxic vasoconstriction in this setting [13].

Since complete equilibration between alveolar gas and end-capillary blood requires sufficient contact time, the reduced transit time which should result from a major reduction in vascular cross-sectional area might lead to impaired gas diffusion as an additional mechanism of abnormal pulmonary gas exchange. However, most studies have found that the abnormal distribution of VA/Q fully explains the abnormal blood gases which are found after acute pulmonary embolism without having to invoke diffusion impairment as an additional contributor. Nevertheless, it was recently reported that impaired diffusion could be responsible for up to 13% of the measured A-a DO_2 [7]. In situations in which cardiac output is increased, either by increased demands or pharmacologically, this mechanism could therefore play a significant role.

Non-Pulmonary Factors

For any lung unit, the alveolar and thus end-capillary PO_2 will be effected by the mixed venous blood although the magnitude of the influence will depend on it's

VA/Q [14]. The greatest effect will clearly be on shunt units and those with low VA/Q ratios. It will be much less important as the VA/Q increases above 1.0. The final consequence of this on the PaO_2 will depend on the overall VA/Q distribution. In patients with significant VA/Q inequality or shunting a low mixed venous PO_2 ($P\bar{v}O_2$) can markedly accentuate the degree of hypoxemia. In most clinical situations a low $P\bar{v}O_2$ results from a cardiac output which is inadequate for tissue O_2 demands causing increased peripheral O_2 extraction or from anemia. With normal lungs, the effect of any reduction of $P\bar{v}O_2$ on PaO_2 can be attenuated by an increase in minute ventilation which increases the VA/Q ratio of each lung unit. This protects us, for example, from developing hypoxemia during exercise. However, when VA/Q inequality is present, hyperventilation is less effective since it has only a minor effect on lung units with low VA/Q ratios and none on the shunt. For this reason, despite the hyperventilation commonly seen following acute pulmonary embolism a low $P\bar{v}O_2$ can still amplify the degree of hypoxemia that results. The importance of this non-pulmonary mechanism was well demonstrated in one recent study in which only one of ten patients studied after an acute pulmonary embolism would have been hypoxemic if their $P\bar{v}O_2$ had been normal [7]. Thus the hypoxemia which is seen following pulmonary embolism probably overestimates the degree of VA/Q inequality and shunt which is present. In addition, changes in the PaO_2 seen during the post embolism phase are as likely to signal alterations in cardiac output as a change in ventilation and blood flow distribution.

Hypocapnia

The cause of the increased minute ventilation and thus hypocapnia which is so often seen following acute pulmonary embolism is unknown. The increased ventilation is beneficial to arterial oxygenation in two ways. It returns, to some degree, the VA/Q ratio of the overperfused lung units towards normal correcting this mechanism of hypoxemia. It also blunts the effect of a low $P\bar{v}O_2$ on arterial oxygenation. However, it is unlikely that hypoxemia is the stimulus for the increased ventilation since it is seen even when the degree of hypoxemia is well below that thought necessary to elicit a response from the carotid bodies. Non-chemical stimuli such as stretch and baroreceptors are likely to be playing an important but as yet unspecified role.

Chronic Pulmonary Vascular Occlusion

Chronic pulmonary vascular occlusion without significant pulmonary parenchymal disease is due either to primary vascular disease as in primary pulmonary hypertension or pulmonary vasculitis or results from recurrent or unresolved single embolic events. The embolic material may be thrombi or may consist of foreign material such as parasites or particles injected during illicit drug use or red cells as in sickle cell anemia. While the best studied patients and thus the ones we will discuss in detail below are those with primary pulmonary hypertension and thromboembolic disease, it is likely that the physiological mechanisms of the abnormal gas exchange is common to all. In general, these patients have mild to moderate hypoxemia which worsens during exercise as well as a chronic respiratory alkalosis. The pathophysiological bases for these changes is similar qualitatively if not quantitatively to those operative in acute pulmonary vascular occlusion.

Pulmonary Factors

Despite the extensive pulmonary vascular occlusion in these patients, sufficient to increase pulmonary vascular resistance in some ten to twenty times normal with mean pulmonary artery pressures often greater than 60 mm Hg, there is only mild to moderate VA/Q inequality and small amounts of intra-pulmonary shunt [15] (Fig. 6). The total blood flow to these abnormal units is always less than 20% of the total cardiac output. Unlike patients with acute vascular obstruction there is usually no clearly defined high VA/Q mode and no increase in dead space. The etiology of the shunt and low VA/Q units is unclear but probably due, at least in part, to the overperfusion of the lung units subtended by the remaining open vessels. In addition there is likely to be abnormalities of ventilation distribution due to areas of edema from the increase in the microvascular pressures in the least involved lung or as a result of small airway occlusion secondary to bronchial compression by adjacent dilated small pulmonary arteries.

A pharmacologically induced reduction in pulmonary vascular tone is often accompanied by an increase in the degree of VA/Q inequality, in particular an increase in the blood flow to low VA/Q units or shunt [16]. This suggests that, at

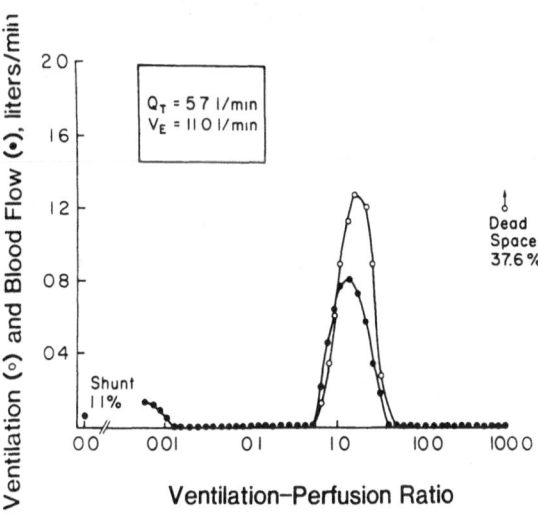

Fig. 6. The distribution of ventilation and blood flow in a 35 year old patient with chronic, recurrent pulmonary emboli and severe pulmonary hypertension. Despite the presence of extensive angiographically documented pulmonary embolism, the VA/Q distribution is essentially normal. (From [14] with permission)

least part of the vascular tone, contributes to a minimizing of the abnormal blood flow distribution. This additional tone is probably not functioning through the usual mechanism of hypoxic vasoconstriction since oxygen responsive tone is rarely seen. When severe hypoxemia is seen in these patients it is invariably associated with intra-cardiac shunting through a patient foramen ovale. There is no evidence for incomplete alveolar-endcapillary equilibration playing a significant role in the observed hypoxemia. As in patients with acute pulmonary vascular occlusion, the etiology of the respiratory alkalosis is unknown but unlikely to be secondary to carotid body output by itself.

Non-Pulmonary Factors

Patients with chronic pulmonary vascular occlusion often have a low $P\bar{v}O_2$ predominantly due to an impaired cardiac output. As in patients with acute pulmonary vascular occlusion, this amplifies the effects of the mild to moderate degrees of VA/Q inequality and shunt leading, at times, to marked hypoxemia. Conversely, improvements in cardiac output can increase the arterial PO_2. This explains the frequent observation that, despite the increased VA/Q inequality induced by pumonary vasodilators, the PaO_2 is often unaffected. Increases in cardiac output and thus $P\bar{v}O_2$ are able to compensate for the worsening match of blood flow and ventilation. Mixed venous hypoxemia is predominantly responsible for the increased oxygen desaturation characteristic of these patients during even low levels of exercise [17]. A reduction in $P\bar{v}O_2$ is a normal response to increasing tissue oxygen demands during exercise and is accentuated in patients with impaired cardiac function who are unable to augment cardiac output effectively. Interestingly, there is no worsening of the VA/Q matching during exercise and no evidence of impaired diffusion, at least at the low levels at which it has been evaluated.

Patients with chronic pulmonary vascular obliteration have an exaggerated ventilatory response to exercise with an increase in the slope of the relationship of CO_2 production and minute ventilation [18]. By increasing the overall VA/Q ratio, this "excessive ventilation" serves to lessen the impact of the falling $P\bar{v}O_2$ on the PaO_2. The stimulus for the exaggerated response, however, probably relates to the low starting $PaCO_2$. It has been demonstrated that subjects will maintain during exercise, the same $PaCO_2$ that they started with [19]. The lower the baseline $PaCO_2$, the greater the incremental increase in ventilation necessary to maintain it under conditions of increased CO_2 production. Since patients with chronic pulmonary vascular occlusion have a chronic respiratory alkalosis, it is not surprising that their exercise ventilatory response is increased.

Conclusion

The abnormal pulmonary gas exchange seen in both acute and chronic pulmonary vascular occlusion is multifactoral and similar. It is due to the presence of variable amounts of VA/Q inequality and shunt amplified by a low $P\bar{v}O_2$. In

both situations there is hyperventilation, not likely due to increased chemoreceptor drive which leads to a respiratory alkalosis. The hyperventilation serves to
mitigate some of the mixed venous induced hypoxemia especially during situations of increased oxygen utilization when the ability to increase oxygen delivery
is impaired by the increased right ventricular afterload. The impact of various
physiological stresses on the arterial blood gases depends on the relative degree
to which they influence both the distribution of blood flow and ventilation and
the mixed venous O_2 saturation.

References

1. Dantzker DR, Bower JS (1982) Alterations in gas exchange following pulmonary thromboembolism. Chest 81:495–501
2. McIntyre KM, Sasahara AA (1973) Determinants of the cardiovascular response pulmonary embolism. In: Moser K, Stein M (eds) Pulmonary Thromboembolism. Chicago, Year
   Book Medical Publishers
3. Wagner PD, Saltzman HA, West JB (1974) Measurement of continuous distributions of
   ventilation-perfusion ratios: Theory. J Appl Physiol 36:588–599
4. Caldini P (1965) Pulmonary hemodynamics and arterial oxygen saturation in pulmonary
   embolism. J Appl Physiol 20:184–190
5. Johnson A, Malik AB (1981) Effects of different-size microemboli on lung fluid and protein
   exchange. J Appl Physiol 51:461–464
6. D'Alonzo GE, Bower JS, DeHart P, Dantzker DR (1983) The mechanisms of abnormal gas
   exchange in acute massive pulmonary embolism. Am Rev Respir Dis 128:170–172
7. Manier G, Castaing Y, Guenard H (1985) Determinants of hypoxemia during the acute
   phase of pulmonary embolism in humans. Am Rev Respir Dis 132:332–338
8. Huet Y, Lemaire F, Brun-Buisson C, et al (1985) Hypoxemia in acute pulmonary embolism.
   Chest: 88:829–836
9. Young I, Mazzone RW, Wagner PD (1980) Identification of functional lung unit in the dog
   by graded vascular embolization. J Appl Physiol 49:132–141
10. Malik AB, Van der Zee H (1978) Mechanism of pulmonary edema induced by microembol-
    ization in dogs. Circ Res 42:72–79
11. Dantzker DR, Wagner PD, Tornabene VW, Alazraki NP, West JB (1978) Gas exchange
    after pulmonary thromboembolization in dogs. Circ Res 42:92–103
12. Manier G, Castaing Y, Guenard H (1986) Cardiac output adjustment to hypoxemia during
    pulmonary embolism. Am Rev Respir Dis 133:A223
13. West JB (1977) Ventilation-perfusion relationships. Am Rev Respir Dis 116:919–943
14. Dantzker DR, Bower JS (1979) Mechanisms of gas exchange abnormally in patients with
    chronic obliterative pulmonary vascular disease. J Clin Invest 64:1050–1055
15. Dantzker DR, Bower JS (1981) Pulmonary vascular tone improves VA/Q matching in obli-
    terative pulmonary hypertension. J Appl Physiol: Respirat Environ Exercise Physiol
    51:607–613
16. Dantzker DR, D'Alonzo GE, Bower JS, Popet K, Crevey BJ (1984) Pulmonary gas ex-
    change during exercise in patients with chronic obliterative pulmonary hypertension. Am
    Rev Respir Dis 130:412–416
17. D'Alonzo GE, Gianotti LA, Pohil RL, et al (1987) Comparison of progressive exercise per-
    formance of normal subjects and patients with primary pulmonary hypertension. Chest
    92:57–62
18. Oren A, Wasserman K, Davis JA, Whipp BJ (1981) Effect of CO_2 set point on ventilatory
    response to exercise. J Appl Physiol 51:185–189

Strategy in Massive Pulmonary Embolism

C. Perret

Introduction

Pulmonary thrombo-embolism is one of the most common acute pulmonary diseases observed in hospitalized patients. Its true prevalence is unknown. It is still an underdiagnosed medical condition especially in patients with pneumonia or congestive heart failure [1]. This non-recognition of pulmonary embolism has severe consequences since the mortality rate under such conditions is 30%, that is, three times higher than in treated patients. Pulmonary embolism is also an overdiagnosed disease: too often the diagnosis is based on a suggestive clinical picture or on non-specific examination findings, leading finally to undue anticoagulant therapy.

Diagnosis of Massive Pulmonary Embolism

Massive pulmonary embolism is defined either as an anatomic obstruction of pulmonary artery greater than 50% on arteriography or, as we consider in this report, a clinical condition characterized by severe physiological impairment requiring cardio-respiratory support. In this respect, it should be noted that a single, fatal pulmonary embolism is probably a much rarer phenomenon than it is believed: the apparently primary accident is often preceded by clinical signs that are overlooked or misunderstood, corresponding to earlier embolic episodes.

There is no symptom or sign characteristic of pulmonary embolism. The clinical impression is not reliable, but it is a necessary step to select patients who have to be submitted to complementary tests. ECG is of little value because of its poor specificity and sensitivity. In massive pulmonary embolism, the signs of right ventricular strain can be very transient. Arterial blood gas analysis, contrary to widespread opinion, is not useful for diagnosis. There is no significant difference between PaO_2 or $PaCO_2$ values measured in patients with suspected pulmonary embolism whether pulmonary angiography is positive or negative [2].

Chest X-ray is the most useful routine diagnostic procedure. If correctly interpreted, it can be suggestive in two thirds of the cases of massive pulmonary embolism. The four principal signs are: regional oligemia, enlarged pulmonary arteries, cardiomegaly and elevation of hemi-diaphragm. It is considered that there is some abnormality in 90% of patients. This also means that a normal chest film does not exclude pulmonary embolism.

The perfusion lung scan is a simple and safe procedure. It is of great interest to exclude the diagnosis of pulmonary embolism. A normal perfusion lung scan has the same value as a normal arteriogram. On the other hand, a positive scan is a non-specific finding. The specificity can be improved by retaining only the large segmental or labor defects, without corresponding radiological lesions. Moreover, the scan interpretation is largely subjective and disagreement among scintigraphists is common. The net result is disappointing due to the number of false positive and false negative results [3].

Combined ventilation/perfusion scan is regarded as a good method for increasing specificity. It is based on the principle that an area of decreased perfusion due to hypoxemic vasoconstriction is underventilated ($\dot{V}/\dot{Q}$ match), whereas the ventilation is assumed to be maintained when the perfusion defect results from vascular obstruction ($\dot{V}/\dot{Q}$ mismatch). But here too, the number of false positive and false negative results remain too high for it to replace angiography. In addition, it is a costly technique, heavy and difficult to apply under emergence conditions. The echocardiogram is a sensitive test but it also is unspecific. It reflects the repercussions of acute pulmonary arterial hypertension on the right heart performance.

Pulmonary angiogram is the only specific diagnostic test for pulmonary embolism and it serves as the standard of comparison for the other procedures. Nevertheless, angiography still has a bad reputation and clinicians fail to use it sufficiently. It results in therapeutic decisions more dangerous than the examination itself.

For selected patients an alternative to conventional angiography is available. This is pulmonary intravenous digital substraction angiography (IV-DSA). It is too soon yet to judge the importance of this method in the diagnosis of pulmonary embolism. Its major advantages appear to be a satisfactory visualization of the pulmonary artery tree, up to second order branches with a right atrial injection and the ability to perform the investigation with a Swan-Ganz catheter [4]. The technique has some drawbacks: it needs the patient's cooperation; it is less sensitive; it represents an expensive equipment and requires an adequate training.

Diagnostic Strategy

Taking into account all means at our disposal, we can define a strategy leading to a diagnosis of certainty with a minimum of procedures [5]. In a hospital with all procedures available, the diagnostic approach is first determined by the clinical picture (Fig. 1).

In a patient without shock, a perfusion lung scan is performed. A negative scan rules out the diagnosis of acute pulmonary embolism. If the scan shows multiple wedge-shaped segmental and/or labor defects in a patient without underlying cardio-respiratory disease or bronchospasm, we consider the diagnosis of acute pulmonary embolism as highly probable; this is also true when a radiographic infiltrate is present somewhere, provided its size is smaller than the corresponding perfusion defect. No further investigation is done and the patient is treated with heparin. When anticoagulation is contraindicated or when the scan suggests massive pulmonary embolism requiring fibrinolysis, pulmonary angiography is

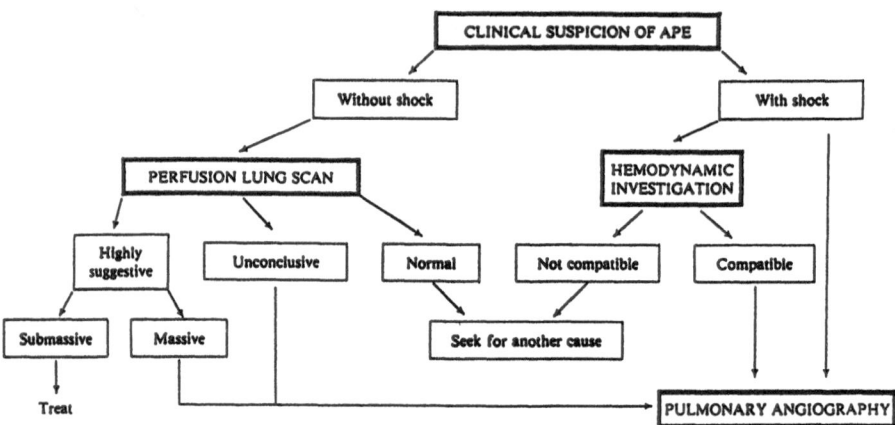

Fig. 1. Diagnostic strategy of massive pulmonary embolism

requested considering the fact that a therapeutic risk implies a clear-cut diagnosis. We usually do not perform additive ventilation lung scan, because it is an expensive procedure with a relatively small benefit, considering the low proportion of patients in whom it makes the difference. In case of intermediate or low probability scan, or in presence of known cardiopulmonary disease, we still proceed to pulmonary angiogram.

For the *patient in shock*, pulmonary angiography is mandatory since the treatment of choice is thormbolysis or even embolectomy. In order to avoid the risk of pulmonary angiography in a critically ill patient without convincing signs of pulmonary embolism, we usually perform first a bedside hemodynamic investigation, that is also useful to adjust the cardio-respiratory support therapy. If the hemodynamic picture is compatible, angiography is carried out, if necessary under partial extracorporeal circulation, in order to decrease the risks inherent in the examination.

This diagnostic strategy implies having equipment and competent staff available night and day, every day of the week. When such conditions are not present, then the diagnostic pathway is more tricky. Without angiography to objectivate pulmonary vascular obstruction, one can attempt to demonstrate thrombosis of the ilio-femoral axis by means of phlebography, Doppler or impedance plethysmography. A positive perfusion lung scan with a high degree of probability together with the demonstration of ilio-femoral obstruction by either invasive or non-invasive methods may constitute a sufficient argument to diagnose pulmonary embolism and to begin treatment. Further studies are needed to determine the sensitivity of this approach.

Therapeutic Approach

Three aspects can be considered concerning the treatment of massive pulmonary embolism.

1. Symptomatic treatment aimed at restoring adequate cardiovascular conditions;
2. Anticoagulant treatment aimed at preventing recurrences;
3. Fibrinolytic treatment and surgery aiming at rapid desobstruction of the pulmonary vascular bed.

Symptomatic Treatment

It is well known that about 2/3 of patients who die of pulmonary embolism do so within the first two hours. This means that in the hemodynamically compromised patients, symptomatic treatment must be initiated immediately on the unique basis of clinical suspicion. The aim is to restore adequate cardio-circulatory conditions in order to proceed to diagnostic procedures. Oxygen delivery is usually severely impaired due to the combination of decreased tissue perfusion and reduction in O_2 content. Hypoxemia is primarily due to ventilation/perfusion disturbances. In presence of shock, the decreased venous PO_2 amplifies the effect of venous admixture due to maldistribution. Rarely, in patients with acute heart failure and high right atrial filling pressure, intracardiac right to left shunt may develop through a patent foramen ovale. The reduction in O_2 content is associated with an acute decline in stroke index and a concomitant increase in right ventricular end-systolic and end-diastolic volumes. Several mechanisms are involved: an acute increase in right ventricular afterload as a consequence of augmented impedance, a decrease in pulmonary venous return and altered compliance of the left ventricle secondary to ventricular interference and finally right ventricular ischemia.

Under these conditions, dobutamine appears to be very effective to induce a substantial and dose dependent rise in cardiac index [6]. Dobutamine should be preferred to isoproterenol which exacerbates right ventricular ischemia by decreasing perfusion pressure and augmenting myocardial oxygen requirements. Volume expansion has also been proposed to improve cardiac output in presence of increased right ventricular afterload. However, due to the risks of further enhancing right ventricular dilatation and ventricular interference, it is recommended to initiate volume expansion slowly under hemodynamic control. When shock persists more than one hour in spite of maximal medical therapy, it is urgent to consider other treatments to obtain rapid relief of obstruction.

Prevention of Recurrences

Heparin therapy is essentially a prophylactic treatment indicated in patients with stable cardio-circulatory conditions. In patients with circulatory failure with a suggestive history and clinical picture, 15000 I.U. should be given immediately before anything else is done. Heparin treatment has no acute effect on the size of emboli and the consequences of vascular obstruction. It has two main properties: it prevents further growth of thrombi and prevents recurrence of embolism. Thus it provides the adequate conditions which allow the natural fibrinolytic system to dissolve the clot. But anticoagulation with heparin does not eliminate the source of subsequent embolisations, it does not alleviate the hemodynamic disturbances and does not prevent permanent impairment to the pulmonary vascular bed.

Thrombolysis

The ideal treatment for massive pulmonary embolism should aim at rapid dissolution of the clot, in order to recover adequate hemodynamic conditions and to restore the integrity of the vascular bed. It has been proved that thrombolytics are able to remove vascular obstruction rapidly [7, 8]. However, their use entail risks which restrict their indications.

According to a Consensus Development Panel held at the NIH [9], the following conditions must be fulfilled for considering thrombolytic therapy:

- the diagnostic is established;
- the severity of the clinical problem exceeds the risk of bleeding associated with a major contraindication;
- proper care is taken in the handling of the patient and in avoiding all but absolutely essential invasive procedures;
- there is a clear understanding of the details of therapy, including monitoring, management of bleeding complications, and the control of subsequent anticoagulation.

In some centers, thrombolysis is thought too dangerous and too costly to be considered. In others, it is applied to patients with a stable circulatory condition whenever vascular obstruction in judged serious by angiography and if there are no major countraindications. In our institution, given the recognized risks with thrombolysis, we reserved this treatment first for patients with acute, massive life-threatening pulmonary embolism who had survived the initial episode and were stabilized with supportive measures but whose immediate course was precarious. At present, the experience acquired has lead us to extend the indications for thrombolysis also to patients whose circulatory state is stable or stabilized but who have a very large obstruction (over 50%) and a positive phlebography.

The indications for thrombolysis are likely to increase in the years to come, with the development of new agents more selective than streptokinase or urokinase. In this respect, plasminogen tissue activator (rt-PA) appears to be particularly interesting [10, 11], since it has only a slight affinity for the circulating plasminogen, but on the other hand, has a very strong affinity for the plasminogen of the thrombus.

Most patients with massive pulmonary embolism will survive with maximal medical treatment. Nevertheless, some fail to respond to inotropic and respiratory support and continue to deteriorate. In these rare cases (2 to 6%) with persistent hypotensions, oliguria and low cardiac output, pulmonary embolectomy represents the last resort treatment, which must be performed within the hour of unsuccessful treatment. Pulmonary embolectomy is also indicated:

- in patients with refractory unstable cardio-circulatory conditions and absolute contraindication to thrombolysis or anticoagulation;
- in patients with cardio-respiratory arrest when external cardiac massage does not swiftly bring about acceptable hemodynamic conditions.

The reported mortality rate varies greatly from a series to the other [12]. Many factors may explain these differences and not only the skill of the surgical team.

Another interesting approach to pulmonary artery desobstruction has been proposed by Greenfield and Zocco in 1979 [13], who employed a steerable catheter device to extract clots without general anesthesia, thoracotomy or cardiopulmonary bypass. Experience is still needed to determine the actual value of this method in massive embolism.

Therapeutic Strategy

Our present strategy for treatment of massive pulmonary embolism depends primarily on the hemodynamic conditions (Fig. 2). In patients with cardio-respiratory arrest, surgery with Trendelenburg operation is the last resort treatment. In those with severe shock refractory to optimal medical treatment, pulmonary embolectomy must be performed when equipment and surgical team are immediately available. Thrombolysis represents a method of choice for patients with massive pulmonary embolism who respond to inotropic and respiratory support and have no bleeding hazards. Thrombolysis might be extended to patients with a large obstruction of the pulmonary vascular tree and proven residual thrombi in the deep veins. In all other cases, stable hemodynamic conditions enable one to wait for spontaneous fibrinolysis and heparin treatment is used to prevent a possible recurrence. In the few cases where heparin is contraindicated or ineffective, the insertion of a caval device must be considered [14].

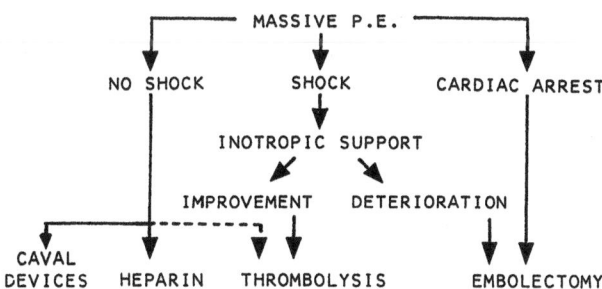

Fig. 2. Therapeutic strategy of massive pulmonary embolism

References

1. Goldhaber SZ, Henekens CH, Evans DA, Newton EC, Godleski JJ (1982) Factors associated with correct antemortem diagnosis of major pulmonary embolism. Am J Med 73:822–826
2. Menzoian JO, Williams LF (1979) Is pulmonary angiography essential for the diagnosis of acute pulmonary embolism? Am J Surg 137:543–548
3. Marsh JD, Glynn M, Torman HA (1983) Pulmonary angiography. Application in a new spectrum of patients. Am J Med 75:763–770
4. Pond GD (1985) Pulmonary digital subtraction angiography. Radiol Clin North Am 23:243–260
5. Vincent A, Poli S, Perret Cl (1984) Diagnostic approach to pulmonary embolism: our strategy. Intensive Care Med 10:85–89
6. Jardin F, Genevray B, Brun-Ney D, Margairaz A (1985) Dobutamine: A hemodynamic evaluation in pulmonary embolism shock. Crit Care Med 13:1009–1012
7. Miller GAH, Sutton GC, Kerr IH, Gibson RV, Honey M (1971) Comparison of streptokinase and heparin in treatment of isolated acute massive pulmonary embolism. Br Med J 2:681–684
8. Sharma GVRK, Burleson VA, Sasahara AA (1980) Effect of thrombolytic therapy on pulmonary-capillary blood volume in patients with pulmonary embolism. N Engl J Med 303:842–845
9. NIH consensus conference (1980) Thrombolytic therapy in thrombosis. Br Med J 280:1585–1587
10. Verstraete M, Collen D (1986) Thrombolytic therapy in the eighties. Blood 67:1529–1541
11. Sharma GV (1987) Historical overview of antithrombotic and thrombolytic therapy. Am J Med 83:2–5
12. Del Campo C (1985) Pulmonary embolectomy: a review. Can J Surg 28:111–113
13. Greenfield LJ, Zoco JJ (1979) Intraluminal management of acute massive pulmonary thromboembolism. J Thorac Cardiovasc Surg 77:402–410
14. Mansour M, Chang AE, Sindelar WF (1985) Interruption of the inferior vena cava for the prevention of recurrent pulmonary embolism. Am Surg 51:375–380

Cardiovascular Response to Acute Pulmonary Embolism

A. Artigas, R. Martinez, and A. Roglan

Introduction

Pulmonary embolism (PE) is a frequent cause of in-hospital death. Therapeutic and prophylactic measures are obviously needed but must be preceded by an accurate diagnosis and also by the evaluation of the factors that may influence its prognosis [1].

There are enough data in the literature to consider that the cardiovascular response to PE is chiefly dependent upon the degree and localization of the obstruction, the degree of hypoxia and the presence or absence of preexisting cardiopulmonary disease. Reflex pulmonary vasconstriction, right ventricular dilatation and displacement of the interventricular septum may also modulate the hemodynamic profile of PE. Furthermore two unavoidable technical facts, such as the time elapsed between the acute episode and its hemodynamic study and the limitation of angiography in diagnosing embolism in arteries of less than 2 mm in diameter, may make it difficult to obtain valuable hemodynamic and angiographic data to establish adequate diagnosis and prognosis [2]. Nevertheless, and in absence of previous cardiopulmonary disease, the degree of right ventricular strain appears to be related to the degree of obstruction as visualized in the pulmonary angiogram [3].

Preexisting Cardiopulmonary Disease

Previous cardiopulmonary disease is an important factor in determining the hemodynamic response to PE, and may therefore influence the interpretation of prognostic indices. Because the preembolic condition of the heart and lungs play such an important role in the postembolic hemodynamic status, it is worthwhile considering those patients with and without prior heart and lung disease separately. To evaluate the hemodynamic response to PE we analyzed the hemodynamic data of 57 acute PE diagnosed by pulmonary angiography: 30 patients with previous chronic lung disease and 27 with previous normal cardiopulmonary system [4]. The vascular involvement appeared to be less in CPD patients than in previously health patients, but the degree of pulmonary artery hypertension (PAH) was definitely higher, indicating the preexisting greater pressure generating capability of the right ventricle because of its adaptation to sustained pressure work (Table 1). The level of PAH was disproportionate to the degree of embolic obstruction. Small embolization may therefore be accompanied by a

Table 1. Comparative hemodynamic response to pulmonary embolism in patients with normal cardiopulmonary system and with underlying pulmonary disease

	Normal cardiopulmonary system	Underlying pulmonary disease	p
	(n = 27)	(n = 30)	
Angiographic obstruction, %	46 ± 19	34 ± 17	< 0.05
Heart rate, beat/min	103 ± 20	99 ± 23	
Right atrial pressure, mmHg	9 ± 5	7 ± 6	
Right ventricular systolic pressure, mmHg	44 ± 14	66 ± 24	< 0.01
Pulmonary artery systolic pressure, mmHg	43 ± 15	61 ± 24	< 0.01
Pulmonary artery diastolic pressure, mmHg	13 ± 6	25 ± 14	< 0.001
Cardiac index, l/min/m²	2.39 ± 1.33	2.36 ± 1.00	
Stroke volume index, ml/beat/m²	26 ± 13	24 ± 14	
Pulmonary vascular resistance index, dynes·sec·cm^{-5}·M^{-2}	1 109 ± 715	1 828 ± 970	< 0.05

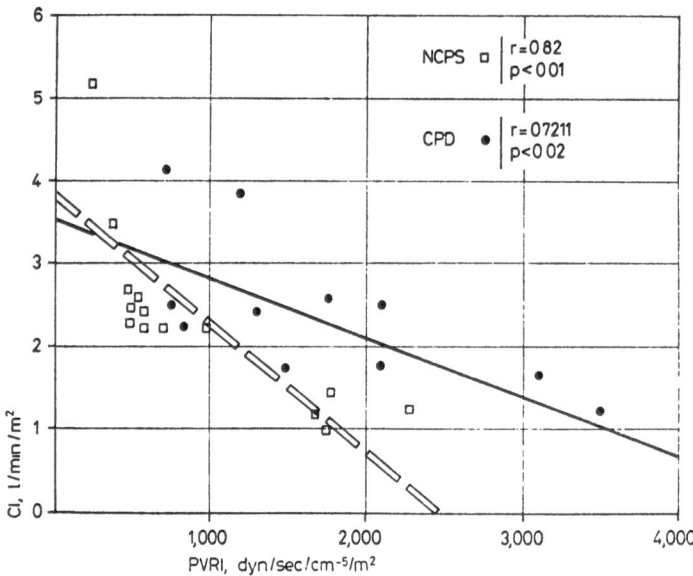

Fig. 1. Pulmonary vascular resistance index (PVRI) is plotted in the horizontal axis against cardiac index (CI). A good correlation was found between both parameters in patients with NCPS as well in patients with previous CPD

severe increase of mean pulmonary artery pressure (PAP). No correlation was found between the decrease in flow and the degree of pulmonary vascular obstruction or the level of PAH. The elevation of right atrial pressure was not a reliable index of severity of PE. The clinical translation of this is obviously the lack of accuracy in the determination of central venous pressure or simply of jugular venous pulse observation to assess the severity of the vascular obstruction. Although CPD patients would response by a higher right ventricular performance given a PE at a certain level of vascular resistance, and even after having sustained a less severe vascular obstruction, the cardiac index would also start falling, probably constituting the first sign of right ventricular failure (Fig. 1).

Hemodynamic Response in Patients with Previously Normal Cardiopulmonary System

The hemodynamic response in previously healthy patients is characterized by precapillary pulmonary hypertension, increased right atrial pressure and low cardiac index. The most frequent derangement after PE is PAH which was present in our series in 85% of patients with NCPS, whilst pulmonary capillary wedge pressure was usually normal. There is a gradient between capillary and arterial diastolic pressures which is often considered to be a diagnostic feature. PAH correlates well with the pulmonary perfusion defect and angiographic obstructions over 30–40% have been associated with PAH (Fig. 2). It is of particular interest to note that no patient in our study developed PAP in excess of

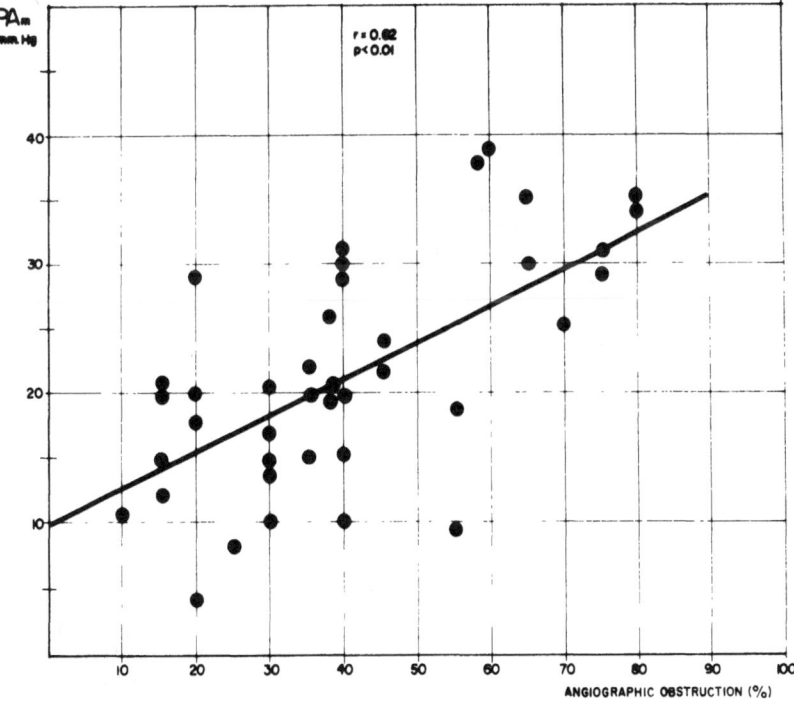

Fig. 2. The percentage of angiographic obstruction is plotted in the horizontal axis against pulmonary artery mean pressure (PAP) for 27 previously healthy patients

40 mm Hg despite sometimes massive embolic obstruction. This pressure represents the maximal capability to generate pressure from a previous normal right ventricle. Higher values may be recorded in patients with prior right ventricular hypertrophy due to chronic cor pulmonale or to left ventricular failure.

In previously healthy patients the right ventricle appears unable to generate enough pressure to overcome the increased resistance to ejection and to maintain a normal pulmonary blood flow and left ventricular filling. Cardiac output falls and right ventricular failure is manifested by a rise in end-diastolic pressure. When PAP exceeded 30 mm Hg, the right atrial pressure was consistently elevated (which could be diagnosed by a prominent neck vein distension), associated to a right shift of venous return with an increase in the mean systemic filling pressure.

Pumonary vascular resistances (PVR) are inversely related to cardiac index (Fig. 1). Variations of cardiac output must be taken into account to interpret variations of PAP and PVR. A sudden increase of PAP may be due to an increase in cardiac output rather than to extension of vascular occlusion. On the contrary, a reduction in PAP is very likely a consequence of decreased cardiac output. Linear pressure flow relationships have been consistently determined and the extrapolated pressure intercept has been argued to represent the mean closing pressure of pulmonary vasculature and thus reflect the operative downstream pressure. The slope of the linear segment of the pressure-flow line, represents the incremental PVR. Prewitt et al. [5] in an experimental model of PE, demonstrated a marked upward shift in the extrapolated pressure intercept, suggesting that the predominant mechanism explaining the increase in PAP is an

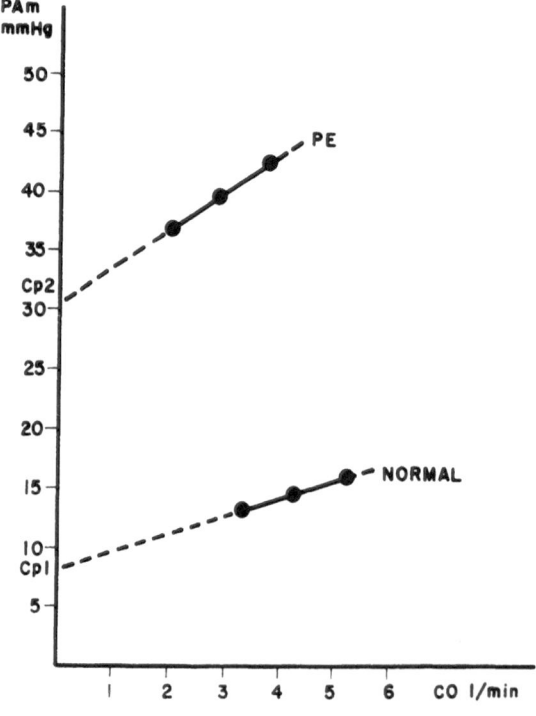

Fig. 3. Cardiac output (CO) is plotted in the horizontal axis against pulmonary artery mean pressure (PAP). Embolization produced a marked upward shift in the pressure-flow line, with a less obvious increase in the slope of the line

increase in the mean pulmonary vascular closing pressure rather than a change in PVR (Fig. 3).

When PVR is markedly increased, dilatation of the right ventricle can be assessed by echocardiography or radionuclide techniques. Volume expansion in this case may cause further deterioration in both ventricles because of an increased wall stress and oxygen consumption. Failure was explained by right ventricular ischemia because of systemic hypotension combined with right ventricular hypertension. When blood pressure is increased and right ventricular coronary blood flow is maintained constant, beneficial hemodynamic effects appeared, presumably by relieving right ventricular ischemia and increasing the capability to generate pressure [6]. Jardin et al. [7] demonstrated an initial right ventricular dilatation associated with a reduction in left ventricular volumes. With clinical improvement there is an inverse change of ventricular volumes in right and left ventricles. This change in left ventricular compliance seems to be explained by diastolic bulging of the interventricular septum.

We believe, therefore, that conclusions about the hemodynamic response of acute PE must be based on a consideration of both the inmediate preembolic cardiopulmonary status and the extent of embolic involvement. In absence of preexisting cardiopulmonary disease, the degree of cardiovascular impairment should be proportional to the degree of pulmonary vascular obstruction. When cardiovascular impairment is severe and embolic involvement is small, preexisting cardiopulmonary disease should be considered the major responsible factor. Pulmonary arteries and right heart are enlarged and right ventricular ejection fraction is reduced. Left ventricular systolic function appears unchanged, but diastolic function might be reduced by bulging. While under certain conditions volume expansion is an appropriate therapy to increase cardiac output, in acute PAH, with excessive right ventricular afterload, volume expansion may worsen both ventricular functions. When shock complicates an acute PE, initial therapy should be directed towards restoration of adequate arterial blood pressure and cardiac output, thus improving right ventricular coronary blood flow.

Acknowledgement: This work is supported by the research grant FISS 85/1301.

References

1. Dalen JE, Alpert JS (1985) Natural history of pulmonary embolism. In: Sasahara AA, Sonnenblick EH, Lesch M (eds) Pulmonary emboli. Grune Stratton, New York, pp 77–88
2. Sharma GV, Mc Intyre KM, Sharma S, Sasahara AA (1984) Clinical and hemodynamic correlates in pulmonary embolism. Clin Chest Med 5:421–437
3. Mc Intyre KM, Sasahara AA (1971) Hemodynamic alterations related to extent of lung scan perfusion defect in pulmonary embolism. J Nucl Med 12:166–170
4. Artigas A, Crexells C, Net A, Oriol A, Rutllant M (1980) Hemodynamic response to pulmonary embolism in patients with previous chronic pulmonary disease. In: Widimsky J (ed) Pulmonary embolism. Karger, Basel, pp 49–54
5. Ducas I, Girling L, Shick U, Prewitt RM (1986) Pulmonary vascular effects of hydralazine in a canine preparation of pulmonary thromboembolism. Circulation 73:1050–1057
6. Laver MB, Strauss HW, Pohost GM (1979) Right and left ventricular geometry: adjustements during acute respiratory failure. Crit Care Med 7:509–519
7. Ozier Y, Dubourg O, Farcot JC, Bazin M, Jardin F, Margairaz A (1983) Circulatory failure in acute pulmonary embolism. Intensive Care Med 10:91–97

Pathophysiology and Treatment of Pulmonary Hypertension

J. Ducas and R. M. Prewitt

Introduction

Pulmonary hypertension may be present in a variety of clinical conditions. For example, certain patients with the Adult Respiratory Distress Syndrome (ARDS) may develop severe pulmonary hypertension as a consequence of the underlying lung disease. The increase in right ventricular (RV) afterload may decrease cardiac output (CO) and tissue O_2 delivery and may impair survival [1, 2]. In another example, short-term mortality is reported to increase when hypotension complicates pulmonary emboli. For example, mortality in patients, where the diagnosis has been confirmed angiographically is reported to be 6%, increasing to greater than 30% if hypotension develops [3].

A recent canine study by Molloy et al. was designed to investigate treatment of shock in a canine model of acute embolic pulmonary hypertension [4]. Small autologous blood clots were injected intravenously over approximately 25 minutes, and mean blood pressure (BP) had fallen to 70 mm Hg (shock), dogs were treated according to prior randomization. One group served as controls and received no treatment. Another group was treated with volume expansion. A third group was randomized to treatment with isoproterenol and dogs in a fourth group were treated with norepinephrine. While isoproterenol and volume were ineffective, norepinephrine reversed the shock state and markedly improved hemodynamic status.

Table 1 illustrates hemodynamic effects of pulmonary emboli and norepinephrine. Note the marked deterioration in RV function with embolization. Norepinephrine increased blood pressure (BP) and cardiac output (CO) increased from an unmeasurable value to 2.3 $1 \cdot min^{-1}$. Hemodynamic status remained sta-

Table 1. Hemodynamic effects of norephinephrine treatment (Mean $\pm$ S.D.)

	Baseline	Treatment	15 min	60 min	30 min post norepinephrine
CO (L·min^{-1})	3.5±1.5	–	2.3±0.7	2.3±0.3	1.2±0.3
BP (mmHg)	140±22	71±2	112±25	106±16	74±28
RVEDP (mmHg)	0.7±0.8	10±1	5±5	5±3	4±2
PAP (mmHg)	13±3	62±11	55±7	50±6	43±5
PVR (mmHg·L^{-1}·min)	2.5±0.7	–	28±8	31±18	44±19

ble during one hour of continuous infusion and deteriorated after the drug was discontinued. Note the fall in BP and CO and the increase in pulmonary vascular resistance that occurred when norepinephrine was discontinued. Other studies of acute embolic pulmonary hypertension have reported hemodynamic improvement with norepinephrine [5, 6].

While in the study cited above [4], isoproterenol was ineffective in treatment of frank shock, this agent may be useful in treatment of RV dysfunction when RV afterload is less and when BP prior to treatment is not as low. To test this hypothesis, a recent study compared acute cardiopulmonary effects of norepinephrine and isoproterenol in a relatively stable model of canine pulmonary embolism, characterized by a moderate decrease in CO and BP [7]. While both drugs increased stroke volume, only isoproterenol increased CO. Corresponding to the increase in flow, RV filling pressure and pulmonary vascular resistance decreased with isoproterenol. Note that in this study, both CO and pulmonary vascular resistance remained constant with norepinephrine. The difference in hemodynamic effects of isoproterenol and norepinephrine between this study and the study by Molloy at al. cited above are probably due to differences in hemodynamic status prior to treatment.

Dantzker and Bower reported a beneficial hemodynamic response when isoproterenol was given to patients with chronic pulmonary hypertension secondary to pulmonary embolism [8]. Jardin et al. [9] recently reported results of a clinical study where dobutamine was given to patients with pulmonary embolism and systemic hypotension. Short-term infusion of dobutamine increased cardiac index in six of the ten patients, mean change from 1.7 to 2.3 $1 \cdot min^{-1}$. Mean BP prior to treatment was 81 mm Hg and was unchanged 30 minutes after onset of therapy. Mean PAP decreased slightly and there was a 25% decrease in pulmonary vascular resistance. Zapol et al. [1] reported beneficial hemodynamic effects of isoproterenol in patients with ARDS and pulmonary hypertension. In another study, Snider et al. investigated effects of isoproterenol in patients with ARDS and mild pulmonary hypertension. Isoproterenol increased CO and caused a small decrease in pulmonary vascular resistance [10].

Accordingly, when a moderate decrease in CO and/or BP complicates an increase in RV afterload, isoproterenol or dobutamine may be excellent drugs to decrease pulmonary vascular resistance, increase CO, and improve RV function.

Vasodilators may be employed to improve pulmonary hemodynamics and RV performance in pulmonary hypertension. For example, hydralazine has been reported to decrease pulmonary vascular resistance and to improve ventricular performance in patients with primary pulmonary hypertension and in patients with pulmonary hypertension secondary to chronic lung disease. Rubin et al. [11] studied the effects of oral hydralazine in chronic pulmonary hypertension and RV failure. Despite unchanged pulmonary artery pressure and decreased RV end-diastolic pressure, CO and stroke volume markedly increased with hydralazine. The authors attributed the improvement in RV function to a decrease in pulmonary vascular resistance. Similarly, other clinical studies of pulmonary hypertension report improved cardiopulmonary function with hydralazine.

A recent study compared acute cardiopulmonary effects of nitroprusside and hydralazine in a canine model of pulmonary hypertension and decreased CO

[12]. Autologous clot injection increased RV afterload and decreased CO. While both drugs decreased ventricular filling pressure and systemic vascular resistance, only hydralazine increased CO, from 1.3 to 2.7 $1 \cdot min^{-1}$. The failure for CO to increase with nitroprusside is explained by the lack of change in RV afterload; pulmonary artery pressure (PAP) and pulmonary vascular resistance (PVR) did not decrease with nitroprusside.

While several studies indicate that hydralazine may be useful in treatment of a decreased CO complicating increased RV afterload, excessive decreases in BP with subsequent deleterious consequences have been reported [13]. Accordingly, while hydralazine may be useful to decrease RV afterload and increase CO when a low output state complicates an acute increase in RV afterload, extreme care should be taken to ensure that excessive falls in BP and RV perfusion do not occur. Conceivably inotropic agents with pressor effects, such as norepinephrine, which may not increase pulmonary vascular tone, could be used in conjunction with a vasodilator if the latter is indicated. For example, one clinical study of patients with pulmonary hypertension and circulatory failure complicating mitral valve replacement reported marked improvement in hemodynamic parameters with norepinephrine and PGE_1 [14]. PGE_1 decreased pulmonary vascular resistance but caused an excessive fall in systemic BP; therefore norepinephrine was used to maintain BP and RV perfusion pressure.

Pressure-Flow Relationships of the Pulmonary Vascular Bed

In acute respiratory failure (ARDS/pulmonary embolism) RV afterload increases because of alteration in the pulmonary vascular bed; however, despite the potential importance, the pathophysiology of acute pulmonary hypertension has only recently been investigated.

Conventionally, pulmonary vascular resistance (PVR) calculated as (PAP-LV filling pressure)/CO, is assumed to reflect the flow resistive properties of the pulmonary vasculature. Changes in PVR are felt to reflect changes in effective vascular caliber. This calculation employs only a single pressure-flow (P-Q) coordinate to describe the vascular resistance and assumes that the effective pulmonary vascular outflow pressure in Zone III of West is the left ventricular (LV) filling pressure [15].

Several recent studies have used multicoordinate pulmonary vascular P-Q plots to investigate physiology and pathophysiology of the pulmonary circulation [16-18]. Over physiological flow rates this relationship has consistently been reported as linear. When plotted with pressure as the dependent variable, the slope of the P-Q relationship has the units of resistance, and to differentiate it from traditional PVR the term incremental resistance has been used. The extrapolated pressure intercept (P_i) of the P-Q relationship may define the effective outflow pressure operative at physiologic rates of flow. Several studies have confirmed that under certain conditions, P_i may exceed LV filling pressure in Zone III [16, 18] and alveolar pressure in Zone III [19].

Accordingly, in pulmonary hypertension, the elevation in PAP may be related to an increase in P_i, an increase in incremental resistance or a combination of these two factors. Similarly, vasoactive compounds may produce alterations in pulmonary hemodynamics, by altering these factors either separately or in combination.

A recent canine study investigated pulmonary vascular effects of pulmonary emboli and hydralazine [18]. To define the vascular P-Q relationship, multiple PAP-CO points were obtained by opening systemic A-V fistulas fitted with variable resistors. Before and after emboli and after hydralazine, the P-Q relationships were well described by linear regression analysis. While there was a marked increase in calculated PVR with emboli, the predominant effect of emboli was to increase the effective outflow pressure, i.e. the zero flow intercept, from 8.8 to 28.6 mm Hg. As in previous studies, hydralazine markedly increased CO, decreased calculated PVR and did not affect PAP. While incremental vascular resistance decreased with hydralazine, the predominant explanation for the improvement in pulmonary hemodynamics was a decrease in P_i (see Table 2). To test the hypothesis that the extrapolated pressure intercept reflects the effective outflow pressure, in four dogs, left atrial pressure was progressively raised by inflating a left atrial balloon at constant CO. Before embolization, increases in left atrial (LA) pressure over a given range (approximately 8 to 18 mm Hg) caused similar changes in PAP, indicating LA pressure approximated the effective outflow pressure. In contrast, after embolization, changes in LA pressure over the same range had absent to trivial effects on PAP. Accordingly, as shown by the change in extrapolated zero flow intercept, embolization resulted in a marked increase in the effective outflow pressure and created an effective vascular waterfall.

The increase in slope of the P-Q relationship with emboli, signals a corresponding change in the pressure cost for flow and is explained by a decrease in parallel vascular units and likely by a generalized increase in effective vascular tone. However, as cited above, the predominant effect of emboli was to increase the extrapolated pressure intercept. The increase in pressure intercept may be explained by a vascular waterfall model of hemodynamics in vessels with tone [20]. In such a model, an increase in vascular tone acts like an increase in surrounding pressure at a collapsible site. When pressure at this locus exceeds intravascular pressure, vascular collapse occur and a vascular waterfall is created. The surrounding pressure becomes the effective outflow pressure. When considering the numerous vessels in the lung, the overall P-Q slope represents a summation of these parallel units and the extrapolated pressure intercept the mean effective outflow pressure. As cited above, following pulmonary emboli, changes in LA pressure, the apparent downstream pressure, had little or no effect on PAP conforming with the model of a vascular waterfall. Since there was continous flow, and thus effective vascular continuity, the dissociation between LA pressure and PAP is probably not due to actual vascular collapse. Instead, results from recent work are consistent with the hypothesis that the vascular waterfall in embolic pulmonary hypertension is, at least in part, explained by a high velocity of blood flow at a critical locus, upstream from the capillary bed [21]. In six anesthetized dogs, following moderate embolic pulmonary hypertension, the effects of altered LA pressure on PAP were determined at low flow and high flow. In moderate hypertension, unlike severe pulmonary hypertension, a measurable fraction of an increase in LA pressure is recorded upstream (PAP). In both flow

Table 2. Effects of embolus and hydralazine on the slope and intercept of the pulmonary P-Q curve

	Control 1				Control 2				Hydralazine			
	r	Slope	Intercept	LVEDP	r	Slope	Intercept	LVEDP	r	Slope	Intercept	LVEDP
1	0.95	2.4	6.5	3.0	0.99	4.9^a	33.2^a	1.5	0.99	4.0	29.9^b	0.5
2	0.92	2.0	8.1	8.0	0.99	4.6^b	22.1^a	7.0	0.99	3.6^a	13.7^a	8.0
3	0.77'	1.8	8.5	6.0	0.99	4.6^b	27.3^a	4.5	0.97	2.5^b	21.5^a	8.0
4	0.82'	0.8	10.7	7.5	0.92	2.4^a	25.2^a	6.0	0.84	3.2	11.3^a	5.4
5	0.98	1.9	9.8	7.0	0.98	2.9^b	29.0^a	9.0	0.91	1.9^c	26.0^b	8.5
6	0.86'	1.9	10.7	9.0	0.94	2.6	30.2^a	8.0	0.96	1.3^c	27.3^a	12.0
7	0.95	1.3	11.0	10.0	0.99	3.5^b	30.2^a	10.0	0.95	2.6^b	23.7^a	12.0
8	0.98	2.4	5.2	7.0	0.98	2.8	31.2^a	9.0	0.99	3.5	22.5^a	4.0
Mean ±SD		1.8±0.5	8.8±2.1	7.2±2.1		3.5±1.0	28.6±3.6	6.9±4.0		2.8±0.9	22.0±6.4	7.4±4.0

All r values $P<0.01$ except ' $P<0.05$.
[a] $p<0.001$ compared to previous condition by analysis of covariance.
[b] $p<0.01$ compared to previous condition by analysis of covariance.
[c] $p<0.05$ compared to previous condition by analysis of covariance.

conditions in this study multiple PAP-LA pressure points were determined as LA pressure was varied between 4 to 18 mm Hg. In all six dogs, the slope of the PAP-LA pressure relationship was less at high flow (mean CO 5.1 $1 \cdot min^{-1}$) than at low flow (mean CO 2.0 $1 \cdot min^{-1}$). The mean slope was 0.3 at high flow and 0.5 at low flow. The venous vasculature should have been better distended in the higher flow condition. Therefored, in the high flow condition, less of the increase in LA pressure should have been dissipated in recruitment or distension of the venous bed, and the increase in PAP greater. It was postulated that the depression in transmission of LA pressure to PAP at higher flow may be due to an increasingly turbulent flow regime at a critical locus.

Another recent canine study investigated effects of pulmonary emboli and norepinephrine on P–Q characteristics [22]. Emboli increased mean incremental resistance from 1.9 to 5.5 mm $Hg \cdot 1^{-1} \cdot min$ and caused a marked upward shift in

Table 3. Results of linear regression analysis: norepinephrine group

	No.	Slope ($mmHg \cdot 1 \cdot min^{-1}$)	Intercept (mmHg)	r	p<
Before Norepinephrine	1	3.4	26	0.942	0.01
	2	4.2	36	0.981	0.001
	3	4.8	30	0.991	0.001
	4	3.5	27	0.938	0.01
	5	5.6	33	0.974	0.01
	6	3.8	24	0.982	0.001
	7	3.1	37	0.981	0.001
	Mean	4.1	30.2	0.970	
	± SD	±0.9	±5	±0.02	
During Norepinephrine	1	4.0	23	0.991	0.001
	2	3.8	32	0.954	0.001
	3	4.6	29	0.972	0.01
	4	3.0	28	0.882	0.05
	5	5.2	30	0.974	0.01
	6	3.5	24	0.940	0.001
	7	4.3	37	0.957	0.001
	Mean	4.1	29.1	0.953	
	± SD	±0.7	±5	±0.035	
After Norepinephrine	1	3.9	24	0.999	0.001
	2	4.4	32	0.961	0.01
	3	5.0	31	0.994	0.001
	4	3.1	28	0.908	0.05
	5	4.2	32	0.935	0.01
	6	4.0	23	0.962	0.01
	7	2.8	35	0.966	0.001
	Mean	3.9	29.3	0.961	
	± SD	±0.8	±5	±0.03	

the extrapolated pressure intercept, from 8.1 to 28.3 mm Hg. Both before and after emboli norepinephrine produced significant increases in CO and BP. Also, as seen in previous studies [4] norepinephrine decreased traditionally calculated PVR. However, as illustrated in Table 3, norepinephrine did not alter incremental resistance or outflow pressure. The decrease in calculated PVR as norepinephrine increased CO is explained by an incorrect assumption in the calculation, i.e., that LV filling pressure is the effective outflow pressure. As the data in Table 3 demonstrates, the effective outflow pressure was much higher than the LV end-diastolic pressure and therefore the value for PVR calculated as ([PAP-LA pressure]/flow) becomes flow dependent.

A recent study by Mink et al. [16] investigated pulmonary P-Q characteristics in a canine model of pulmonary emphysema produced by papain injection. Compared to a control group, emphysematous dogs, in both Zone II and Zone III conditions, demonstrated an increase in both incremental resistance and outflow pressure.

Employing another canine model of pulmonary hypertension, Boiteau et al. [23] investigated effects of oleic acid induced pulmonary edema on pulmonary P-Q characteristics. Multiple P-Q coordinates were obtained before and approximately five hours after oleic acid. A second group of six dogs served as time controls. In both dogs, the P-Q plots were well described by a linear relationship, mean r value 0.95. Although there was a marked increase in traditionally calculated PVR following oleic acid (1.9 to 7.0 mm Hg$\cdot$l$^{-1}\cdot$min for oleic acid; 1.9 to 3.5 mm Hg$\cdot$l$^{-1}\cdot$min for controls), in both groups incremental resistance increased equally. On the other hand, effective outflow pressure (intercept pressure) remained constant in controls and almost doubled with oleic acid, from 7 to 12 mm Hg. These findings suggest, in this model, a functional dissociation between outflow pressure and incremental resistance.

The above results indicate that in the absence of frank LV failure, pulmonary hypertension results from increase in both effective outflow pressure and incremental resistance. Accordingly, they indicate that pulmonary hemodynamics may be improved by decreases in one or both of these parameters. For example, in the study of canine pulmonary emboli cited above [18] hydralazine improved hemodynamics predominently by decreasing effective outflow pressure. In another recent study employing the same model, isoproterenol decreased incremental resistance [22]. Conceivably, treatment with isoproterenol and hydralazine could be additive in improving pulmonary hemodynamics and decreasing RV afterload. The concept of combined therapy, where two drugs with different effects on P-Q characteristics are administered requires systematic investigation.

Thrombolytic Therapy

Most investigators believe that thrombolytic therapy is indicated when systemic hypoperfusion complicates acute pulmonary embolism. A previous randomized study demonstrated that compared to heparin, treatment with urokinase or streptokinase was associated with more rapid pulmonary thrombolysis and corresponding hemodynamic improvement [24]. However, protracted thrombolytic therapy is often associated with severe bleeding complications [24].

The availability of tissue plasminogen activator (rtPA) has lead to extensive basic and clinical investigation of thrombolysis [25-28]. A recent clinical study of patients with acute myocardial infarction reported that rtPA was almost twice as effective as streptokinase in inducing coronary thrombolysis [25]. Other clinical and basic studies have confirmed the effectiveness of rtPA in inducing coronary thrombolysis [26-28]. Few studies have previously investigated use of rtPA in pulmonary thromboembolism.

A recent study compared rtPA versus heparin in treatment of acute embolic pulmonary hypertension induced by injection of radioactive autologous blood clots [29]. This study also compared the relative efficacy of rtPA given over 15 minutes versus the same total dose infused over 90 minutes. By continuously

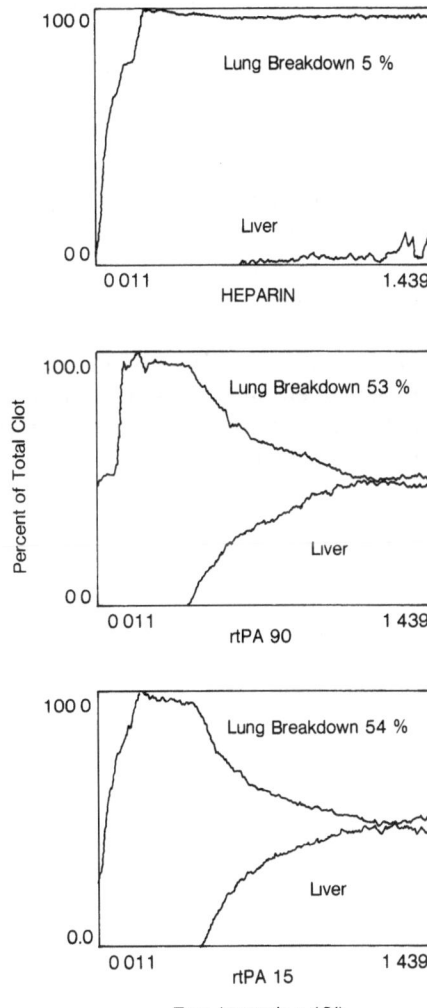

Fig. 1. Plotted are time-activity curves illustrating pulmonary thrombolysis during infusion of heparin and during and after rtPA$_{90}$ and rtPA$_{15}$ infusion. Also illustrated are corresponding hepatic uptake curves

counting radioactivity over both lung fields with a mobile gamma camera, rate
and extent of clot lysis were correlated with corresponding pulmonary hemodynamics. Autologous clot injection increased PAP from 14 to 15 mm Hg
($p < 0.005$) and decreased CO from 3.2 to 2 $1 \cdot min^{-1}$ ($p < 0.001$).

Table 4 depicts mean ($\pm SE$) results and illustrates effects of heparin, rapid
administration of rtPA (1 mg/kg $\cdot$ 15 mins., $rtPA_{15}$) or short-term infusion of rtPA
(1 mg/kg $\cdot$ 90 mins., $rtPA_{90}$) on rate of clot lysis. In dogs given heparin, rate of
lysis was minimal and constant over the three hour treatment interval. In contrast, rtPA markedly increased rate and extent of clot lysis. During infusion, rate
of pulmonary thrombolysis was most rapid with $rtPA_{15}$. Figure 1 plots typical
time-activity curves for each treatment regime. Note the direct relationships between pulmonary thrombolysis and rate of hepatic uptake of circulating radioactive sulfur colloid.

Although the rate of pulmonary thrombolysis was greater with $rtPA_{15}$ versus
$rtPA_{90}$, at 3 hours, for all dogs, the extent of clot lysis was similar, 45% and 42%
respectively. In contrast, in dogs that received heparin total clot lysis was only
7%. Figure 2 compares images obtained over the ten minutes just prior to treatment with the time-decay corrected images obtained over the final ten minutes in
representative dogs from each group. Note that compared to heparin, both rtPA
regimes increased extent of clot lysis. Figure 3 illustrates effects of emboli and
treatment on mean PAP. Corresponding to the rapid rate of thrombolysis during
$rtPA_{15}$ infusion, PAP decreased most rapidly in this group. Ultimately, PAP was
slightly higher in $rtPA_{15}$ compared to $rtPA_{90}$. In two of the $rtPA_{15}$ dogs, an acute
increase in PAP was observed at approximately 70 minutes, corresponding to
clot fragments appearing to migrate from the inferior vena cava to the lungs.
Cardiac output, blood pressure and LV filling pressures were similar between
groups over time. While RVEDP increased in all dogs with embolization, and
remained elevated with heparin, this parameter decreased in both groups given
rtPA. As reflected by the level of circulating fibrinogen, neither rtPA regime
caused a significant systemic fibrinolytic state.

Table 4. Rate of pulmonary thrombolysis

	Clot lysis (%/h) during treatment		
	Heparin	$rtPA_{15}$	$rtPA_{90}$
	1.5	57.6	16.4
	4.8	47.5	27.4
	3.1	52.6	29.9
	2.6	42.1	37.1
	2.6	66.6	21.8
	1.7	70.6	
X $\pm$ SE	2.7 $\pm$ 0.5	56.2 $\pm$ 4.5[a]	26.5 $\pm$ 3.5[b]

[a] Heparin and $rtPA_{90}$, $p < 0.001$;
[b] Heparin, $p < 0.001$

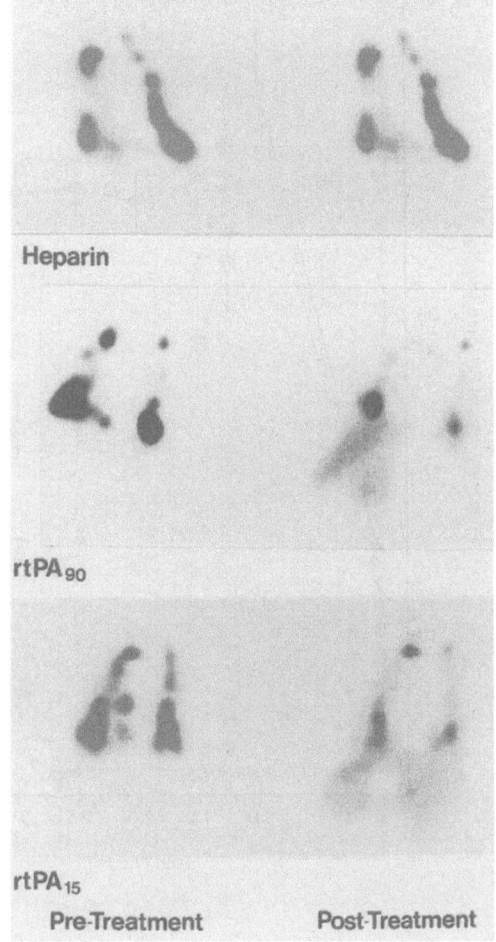

Fig. 2. Illustrated, for the 3 treatment regimes, are images obtained over a 10 min interval prior to treatment and time-decay corrected images obtained over the final 10 min

These results indicate that rtPA may be useful in pulmonary thromboembolism and support further studies designed to optimize dosing regime.

Conclusions

One principle of cardiovascular management of patients with ARDS should be to maintain adequate cardiac output and tissue oxygenation without worsening the degree of pulmonary edema. Because the pulmonary edema is caused by an increase in lung vascular permeability, therapy should be directed towards maintaining a low left ventricular filling pressure, which will tend to decrease the rate of edema formation. If cardiac output is low or falls as a function of therapy (PEEP), flow may be increased with inotropic or vasoactive agents, or both. These agents increase cardiac output and stroke volume so that flow increases

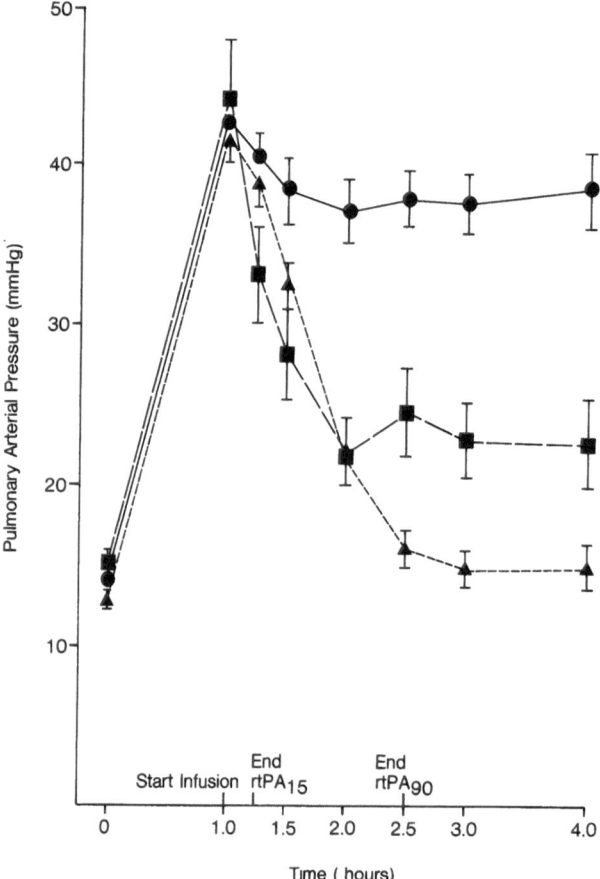

Fig. 3. Illustrates effects of treatment on mean pulmonary artery pressure: ●, ▲ and ■ denotes treatment of heparin, rtPA₉₀ and rtPA₁₅, respectively

despite constant or reduced left ventricular filling pressure. In the setting of low pressure pulmonary edema, drugs which increase cardiac output may reduce arterial oxygen tension. While PEEP increases arterial PO_2, because of potential deleterious effects of PEEP on left ventricular diastolic mechanics, right ventricular afterload, and barotrauma, hypoxemia should be treated with the lowest level of PEEP that provides 95% saturation of the hemoglobin during ventilation with nontoxic inspired oxygen concentrations.

When a marked fall in CO and BP complicated an acute increase in RV afterload, initial therapy should insure adequate RV coronary perfusion pressure. Recent results indicate that norepinephrine, a drug with direct inotropic and pressor effects, may be an excellent drug for a least short-term maintenance of hemodynamic stability. When a moderate decrease in CO complicates an increase in RV afterload, isoproterenol, hydralazine or dobutamine may be used to increase flow. However, since these agents may decrease systemic vascular resistance and BP, careful monitoring is required to insure that an excessive fall in RV coronary perfusion pressure does not occur.

In several canine models of pulmonary hypertension recent studies indicate that changes in both incremental resistance and effective outflow pressure are responsible for the increase in PAP. Accordingly, vasoactive drugs may improve pulmonary hemodynamics and decrease RV afterload via two mechanisms, decreasing incremental resistance and effective outflow pressure, and this approach seems worth clinical trials.

Recent work suggests that rtPA may play an important role in treatment of pulmonary thromboembolism associated with a low output state.

References

1. Zapol WM, Snider MT (1977) Pulmonary hypertension in severe acute respiratory failure. N Engl J Med 296:476–480
2. Laver MB, Strauss WH, Pohost GM (1975) Herbert Shubin Memorial Lecture. Right and left ventricular geometry: adjustments during acute respiratory failure. Crit Care Med 7:509–519
3. Alpert JS, Smith R, Carlson J, Oskene IS, Dexter L, Dalen JE (1976) Mortality in patients treated for pulmonary embolism. JAMA 236:1477–1480
4. Molloy WD, Lee KY, Girling L, Schick U, Prewitt RM (1984) Treatment of shock in a canine model of pulmonary embolism. Am Rev Respir Dis 130:870–974
5. Mathru M, Venus B, Smith RA, Shirakawa Y, Sugiura A (1986) Treatment of low cardiac output complicating acute pulmonary hypertension in normovolemic goats. Crit Care Med 14(2):120–124
6. Ghignone M, Girling L, Prewitt RM (1984) Volume expansion vs noradrenaline in treatment of a low cardiac output complicating an acute increase in right ventricular afterload in dogs. Anesthesiology 60:48–51
7. Molloy, WD, Lee KY, Jones D, Penner B, Prewitt RM (1985) Effects of noradrenaline and isoproterenol on cardiopulmonary function in a canine model of acute pulmonary hypertension. Chest 88:432–435
8. Dantzker DR, Bower JS (1981) Partial reversibility of chronic pulmonary hypertension caused by pulmonary thromboembolic decrease. Am Rev Respir Dis 124:129–131
9. Jardin F, Genevray B, Brun-ney D, Margairaz A (1985) Dobutamine: a hemodynamic evaluation in pulmonary embolism shock. Crit Care Med 13(2):1009–1012
10. Snider MT, Rie MA, Lauer J, Zapol WM (1980) Normoxic pulmonary vasoconstriction in ARDS: detection by sodium nitroprusside (N) and isoproterenol (I) infusions – Massachusetts General Hospital, Boston, Massachusetts. Am Rev Respir Dis (suppl) 121:191
11. Rubin LJ, Handel F, Peter RH (1982) The effects of oral hydralazine on right ventricular end-diastolic pressure in patients with right ventricular failure. Circulation 65:1369–1373
12. Lee KY, Molloy DW, Slykerman L, Prewitt RM (1983) Effects of hydralazine and nitroprusside on cardiopulmonary function when a decrease in cardiac output complicates a short-term increase in pulmonary vascular resistance. Circulation 68:1299–1303
13. Packer M, Greenberg B, Massie B, Dash H (1981) Deleterious effects of hydralazine in patients with pulmonary hypertension. N Engl J Med 306:1326–1331
14. D'Ambra MN, LaRaia PJ, Philbin DM, Watkins WD, Hilgenberg AD, Buckley MJ (1985) Prostaglandin E$_1$. A new therapy for refractory right heart failure and pulmonary hypertension after mitral valve replacement. J Thorac Cardiovasc Surg 89:567–572
15. Mitzner W (1983) Resistance of the pulmonary circulation. Clin Chest Med 4:127
16. Mink SN, Unruh HW, Oppenheimer L (1985) Vascular and interstitial mechanics in canine pulmonary emphysema. J Appl Physiol 59(6):1704–1715
17. Mitzner W, Sylvester JT (1981) Hypoxic vasoconstriction and fluid filtration in pig lungs. J Appl Physiol 51(5):1065–1071
18. Ducas J, Girling L, Shick U, Prewitt RM (1986) Pulmonary vascular effects of hydralazine in a canine model of pulmonary thromboembolism. Circulation 73(5):1050–1057

19. Graham R, Skoog C, Oppenheimer L, Rabson J, Goldberg HS (1982) Critical closure in the canine pulmonary vasculature. Circ Res 50:566-572
20. Permutt S, Riley RL (1963) Hemodynamics of collapsible vessels with tone: The vascular waterfall. J Appl Physiol 18:924
21. Prewitt RM (1987) Pathophysiology and treatment of pulmonary hypertension in acute respiratory failure. J Crit Care 2(3):206-218
22. Ducas J, Duval D, Dasilva H, Boiteau P, Prewit RM (1987) Treatment of canine pulmonary hypertension: effects of norepinephrine and isoproterenol on pulmonary vascular pressure-flow characteristics. Circulation 75:235-242
23. Boiteau P, Ducas J, Schick U, Girling L, Prewitt RM (1986) Pulmonary vascular pressure-flow relationship in canine oleic acid pulmonary edema. Am J Physiol 251 (Heart Circ Physiol 20):H1163-H1170
24. Urokinase Pulmonary Embolism Study Group (1973) Urokinase pulmonary embolism trial. Circulation 47:66-73
25. Chesebro JH, Knatterud G, Roberts R, et al (1987) Thrombolysis in myocardial infarction (TIMI) trial, Phase I: a comparison between intravenous tissue plasminogen activator and intravenous streptokinase. Circulation 76:142-154
26. Verstraete M, Brower RW, Collen D, et al (1985) Double-blind randomized trial of intra-venous tissue-type plasminogen activator versus placebo in acute myocardial infarction. The Lancet Saturday 2, November
27. Van De Werf F, Bergmann SR, Fox KAA, et al (1984) Coronary thrombolysis with intra-venously administered human tissue-type plasminogen activator produced by recombinant DNA technology. Circulation 69(3):605-610
28. Agnelli G, Buchanan MR, Fernandez F, Hirsh J (1985) The thrombolytic and hemorrhagic effects of tissue type plasminogen activator: influence of dosage regimens in rabbits. Thrombosis Research 40:769-777
29. Prewitt RM, Papadimitropoulos R, Hasinoff I, et al (1987) Treatment of embolic pulmonary hypertension: tissue plasminogen activator vs streptokinase (STK) vs heparin. Abstract presented at the Canadian Cardiovascular Society Meeting, October 28-31, Edmonton, Alberta

Right Ventricular Ejection Fraction in Cardiac Surgery Patients

J. Boldt, D. Kling, and G. Hempelmann

The Right Ventricle in Cardiac Patients

A remarkable renewal of interest in the right ventricle has been seen in the last years. Even in disorders that primarily affect the last ventricle, this once-considered passive conduit has proven essential for maintenance of circulatory stability [1, 2]. Because the right ventricle and the left ventricle are in series and mechanically coupled, a perturbation in the mechanical events of one ventricle will influence the behavior of the other ventricle [1, 3].

There is increasing evidence that the traditional methods of monitoring right ventricular (RV) function using central venous pressure (CVP) or right atrial pressure (RAP) may be inadequate for treating cardiac surgery patients [4, 5]. The importance of end-diastolic volume for myocardial function has been pointed out by Frank [6] and Starling. However, the relationship between filling pressure and end-diastolic volume depends on the compliance of the ventricle. The low compliance characteristics of the right ventricle invalidate the use of filling pressure (i.e. CVP) as a guide to right ventricular size. Moreover, especially in cardiac patients, compliance is sometimes markedly altered and is changing under certain conditions. Thus a change in filling pressure may reflect alterations in ventricular volume or compliance or both [2, 7].

Monitoring of Right Ventricular Function in Cardiac Surgery

Diastolic volume, afterload, diastolic compliance, contractile state, and blood supply – all contribute to the overall function of the right ventricle [1, 2, 8]. The method most frequently used to describe the systolic function of the right ventricle is the ejection fraction. Traditionally monitored pressures such as arterial pressure, pulmonary artery pressure, RAP and CVP have failed to explain the deteriorated hemodynamic state of patients undergoing cardiac surgery [9, 10]. Right ventricular performance is difficult to evaluate due to the complex geometry of the right ventricle [11]. Radionuclide or echocardiographic techniques have been applied, but availability and reproducibility are the limiting factors with these methods. Measurement of RV end-systolic volume (RVESV), RV end-diastolic volume (RVEDV), and RV ejection fraction (RVEF) by thermodilution is now possible due to the recently manufacture of rapid-response thermistors which are able to measure beat-to-beat temperature changes in the pulmonary artery [12, 13]. The correlation between this computerized thermodilution method and other techniques such as radionuclide imaging is significant [12].

Factors Influencing Right Ventricular Function in Cardiac Surgery

Impedance of the pulmonary circulation seems to be of major importance for RV function even in patients where cardiopulmonary bypass is used. There is a continuous interplay between the right ventricle and the pulmonary vessels whereby the one influences the other and vice versa. A lot of factors may increase the impedance of pulmonary circulation during cardiac surgery, including constriction of pulmonary vessels mediated by various substances released during extracorporeal circulation, sympathetic reaction, use of catocholamines for pharmacologic support, stiffening of the lungs due to an increase in interstitial fluid accumulation, mechanical ventilation with PEEP and others. Transmission of high airway pressure to the pulmonary circulation by overdistended alveoli, being induced by PEEP ventilation, may increase pulmonary vascular resistance and depress RV function after weaning from cardiopulmonary bypass.

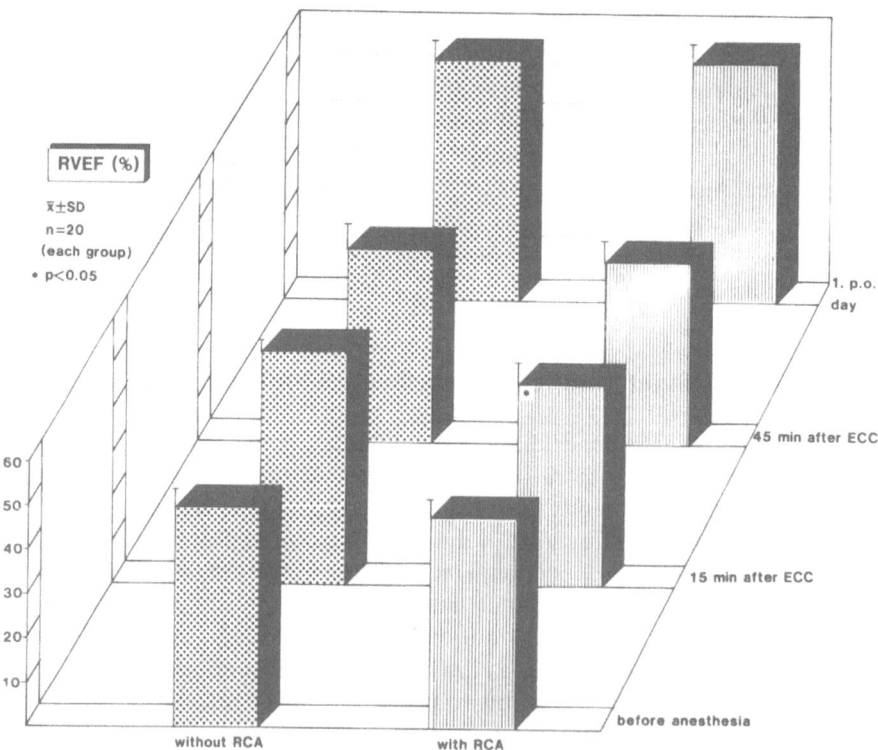

Fig. 1. Change of right ventricular ejection fraction (RVEF) in patients with and without stenosis of right coronary artery (RCA). ECC: extracorporeal circulation

Although resistance in the pulmonary vasculature may be important in the development of RV depression, it does not appear to be the sole determinant. It has been well demonstrated experimentally that the right ventricle can tolerate pulmonary artery constriction if coronary perfusion is improved [7]. A decrease in coronary blood flow, however, may make the right ventricle vulnerable to an increase in RV afterload or to volume application. A right ventricle with normal coronary blood flow is apparently more able to adjust to increase in afterload and volume loading. As pointed out by Martyn et al. [15], the increased oxygen requirement resulting from increased wall stress may not be satisfied when coronary blood flow is decreased and a vicious cycle of RV dilatation and failure may occur. Restoration of an adequate perfusion pressure of the right coronary artery appears to be the prime prerequisite to increase RV contractility and restore cardiac output [16].

Critical depression in RV performance after coronary revascularization may effect the success of the procedure, as well as morbidity, and mortality [17]. In the past we have tended to concentrate on the events at the left side of the heart, but under certain conditions the right ventricle is more vulnerable than the left one. During cardiac surgery the heart is cannulated, made hypothermic, fibrillated and defibrillated, and deprived of normal coronary blood supply – these manipulations may result in a significant impairment in left and right ventricular dysfunction during and immediately after cardiopulmonary bypass. The right ventricle seems very susceptible to injury during cardiac ischemia. In most patients undergoing cardiac operations attention is focused on the protection of the left side of the heart. Hypothermia during ischemia reduces energy consumption, metabolism and thereby myocardial damage. Several investigators have demonstrated, however, that RV hypothermia is more difficult to achieve and maintain, so that the right ventricle seems to be most vulnerable in ischemia [18]. Chiu et al. [19] pointed out that in patients with coronary artery disease, the least protected area of the myocardium was that supplied by stenotic arteries. In an own investigation [9] in 40 patients undergoing aorto-coronary bypass grafting, the influence of concomitant stenosis of the right coronary artery (RCA) on RVEF could be demonstrated in comparison to a group of patients without RCA-stenosis (Fig. 1). Decrease in RVEF (and cardiac output) was significantly more pronounced in patients with RCA-stenosis probably due to an insufficient protection of the right myocardium during cardiopulmonary bypass. Five hours after the end of cardiopulmonary bypass and on the first postoperative day no differences in RVEF between the two groups was no longer demonstrated, and this might be explained as a restoration on RV myocardial performance.

Therapeutical Considerations

Volume expansion may be the appropriate therapy to increase cardiac output when flow is reduced by an increased RV afterload [20, 21]. This therapy, however, would increase RV volume, wall stress and RV oxygen consumption and could result in ischemia leading to deterioration in ventricular performance especially during and immediately after cardiopulmonary bypass. Subendocardial ischemia may then supervene and may result in further depression of RV contractility. Volume loading effects may exceed compensatory mechanism of the right ventricle and RV pump failure may occur. In some critically ill patients during cardiac surgery, failure to respond to volume loading can be explained in part by observations of Calvin et al. [22] who reported that pulmonary capillary pressure (PCP) Does not accurately reflect changes in left ventricular pressure and 80% of the variance in PCP could be explained on the basis of changes in RV end-diastolic volume.

Alternatively, catecholamines could be used to improve RV performance. This, however, may increase RV afterload and RV oxygen consumption compromizing RV O_2 supply/demand ratio and resulting in deterioration of myocardial function.

Conclusion

The theory of the "distensible right ventricle" cannot be supported any longer. Patients who had depressed RV function showed clinical deterioration implicating that RV failure may play a major role in determining the clinical course. In addition to RVEF, RVEDV may give valid information on RV preload and on cardiac contractility. Bedside monitoring of RV function by measuring RVEF allows an earlier therapeutic intervention and may add an important dimension to the care of cardiac patients. This monitoring instrument may prove to be a useful clinical tool in the future for evaluation of myocardial function and therapy.

References

1. Sibbald WS, Drieger AA (1983) Right ventricular function in acute disease states: Pathophysiologic consideration. Crit Care Med 11:339–345
2. Wiedemann HP, Matthey RA (1985) Acute right heart failure. Crit Care Clin 1:631–661
3. Baker BJ, Franciosa KJA (1987) Effect of the left ventricle on the right ventricle. Cardiovasc Clin 17:145–155
4. Rabinovitch MA, Elstein J, Chiu CJ, Rose CP, Arzoumanian A, Burgess JH (1983) Selective right ventricular dysfunction after coronary bypass grafting. J Thorac Cardiovasc Surg 86:444–450
5. Hines R, Barash P (1986) Intraoperative right ventricular dysfunction detected by right ventricular ejection fraction catheter. J Clin Monitoring 2:206–208
6. Frank O (1959) On the dynamics of cardiac muscle. Am Heart J 58:467–478
7. Hoffman MJ, Greenfield LL, Sugerman HJ, Tatum JL (1983) Unsuspected right ventricular dysfunction in shock and sepsis. Nucl Med 198:307–317
8. Suter PM, Neidhart P (1986) Right ventricular dysfunction in severe acute pulmonary failure. In: Vincent JL (ed) Update in Intensive Care and Emergence Medicine, vol 1. Springer, Berlin Heidelberg New York Tokyo, pp 186–190
9. Boldt J, Kling D, Thiel A, Scheld HH, Hempelmann G (1987) Revascularization of the Right Coronary Artery: Influences on thermodilution right ventricular ejection fraction (RVEF). J Cardiothorac Anesth (in press)
10. Baek S, Makabali GG, Bryan-Brown CW (1975) Plasma expansion in surgical patients with high central venous pressure (CVP), the relationship of blood volume to hematocrit, CVP, pulmonary wedge pressure and cardiorespiratory changes. Surgery 78:304–315

11. Foex P (1986) Right ventricular function. In: Vincent JL (ed) Update in Intensive Care and Emergence Medicine, vol 1. Springer, Berlin Heidelberg New York Tokyo, pp 181–185
12. Kay HK, Afshari M, Barash P, Webler W, Iskandrian A, Bemis C, et al (1983) Mundth ED: Measurement of ejection fraction by thermodilution techniques. J Surg Res 34:337–346
13. Jardin F, Gueret P, Dubourg O, Farcot JC, Margairaz A, Bourdarias JP (1985) Right ventricular volumes by thermodilution in the Adult Respiratory Distress Syndrome. Chest 88:34–39
14. Martyn JA, Snider MT, Farago LF, Burke JF (1981) Thermo-dilution right ventricular volume: A novel and better predictor of volume replacement in acute thermal injury. J Trauma 21:619–624
15. Martyn JA, Snider MT, Szyfelbein SK (1980) Right ventricular dysfunction in acute thermal injury. Ann Surg 191:330–335
16. Gaines WE (1987) Perioperative right heart failure: Treatment. Cardiovasc Clin 17:231–238
17. Mangano DT (1985) Biventricular function after myocardial revascularization in humans: Deterioration and recovery patterns during the first 24 hours. Anesthesiology 62:571–577
18. Gonzalez AC, Brandon TA, Fortune RL, Casanno SF, Martin M, Benneson L, et al (1985) Acute right ventricular failure is caused by inadequate right ventricular hypothermia. J Thorac Cardiovasc Surg 89:386–398
19. Chiu RC, Blundell PE, Scott JH, Cain S (1979) The importance of monitoring intramyocardial temperature during hypothermic myocardial protection. Ann Thorac Surg 28:317–322
20. Weber KT, Janicki JS, Shroff SG, Likoff MJ, Sutton MG (1983) The right ventricle: Physiologic and pathophysiologic considerations. Crit Care Med 11:323–328
21. Laver MB, Strauss HN, Pohost GM (1979) Right and left ventricular geometry: adjustments during acute respiratory failure. Crit Care Med 7:509–519
22. Calvin JE, Driedger AA, Sibbald WJ (1981) The hemodynamic effect of rapid fluid infusion in critically ill patients. Surgery 90:71–76

Myocardial Ischemia and Necrosis

Coronary Vasomotor Tone: Implications in Ischemic Heart Disease

G. Berkenboom and P. Unger

Introduction

In the early 1950's, the increase in myocardial oxygen demand was seen as the main mechanism responsible for episodes of angina pectoris [1]. The coronary stenosis was indeed considered as a fixed obstruction on the epicardial vessel, limiting the capacity of the coronary artery to augment coronary flow. Myocardial ischemia was assumed to occur for a given and very reproducible level of myocardial oxygen demands. However, this concept was progressively refuted by the development of coronary angiography. In 1959, Prinzmetal et al. [2] described a group of patients with typical angial pain which was provoked by large vessel coronary spasms, pointed out by coronary angiography. Moreover from angiographic studies [3], even severe atherosclerotic epicardial vessels appear to retain the capacity to dilate and to constrict. Pharmacological studies of isolated human coronary arteries [4] have also shown that severe atherosclerotic segments are not rigid structure.

Effects of Atherosclerosis on Coronary Vasomotor Tone: Pharmacological Aspects

Atherosclerosis seems to modify the responses to various vasoactive agents. These modifications could be partially ascribed to endothelial dysfunction. Endothelium is the major source of prostacyclin which is an endogenous vasodilator with antiaggregating effect on platelets [5]. In addition to this decrease in prostacyclin synthesis, early lesions of atherosclerosis abolish the vasodilating effects of substances released by platelets: adenosine, serotonin, vasopressin and bradykinin [5]. Figure 1 illustrates this alteration in the endothelium-dependent vasodilation, induced by atherosclerosis on isolated human coronary arteries. Although the beta-adrenergic relaxations are endothelium-independent they also seem to be decreased on atherosclerotic segments of human coronary arteries (Fig. 2) [6]. On the other hand, hypersensitivity to vasoconstrictor stimuli has also been described. Localized atherosclerotic lesions have been induced on coronary arteries of dogs by endothelial denudation followed by a high cholesterol diet [7]. These atherosclerotic segments were hypersensitive to specific agonists such as ergonovine and serotonin. Moreover on atherosclerotic segments of coronary arteries isolated from human hearts, a hypersensitivity to vasoconstrictor stimuli of histamine has been demonstrated [4].

In vivo, these alterations in coronary vasomotor tone induced by atherosclerosis have been pointed out by coronary angiography and may present as either a spasm or a more diffuse vasoconstriction.

Coronary Spasm and Variant Angina

The spasm is a localized and intense vasoconstriction, which provokes an almost complete occlusion of one of the 3 main epicardial vessels (rarely more than one main vessel). In an individual patient, episodes of coronary spasm tend to occur always at the same site. The affected segment may be angiographically devoid of atherosclerotic lesion or may exhibit a preexisting stenosis.

The exact pathophysiological mechanisms responsible for this phenomenon are still unknown. However, it has been shown that coronary artery spasm can be induced by at least 3 separate membrane receptors: alpha-adrenergic [8], histaminic [9] and muscarinic [10] receptors. Episodes of coronary spasm are also known to present a circadian distribution with the frequency of ischemic events peaking during early morning [11]. It is likely that during this period, plasma concentrations in vasoactive substance like norepinephrine, epinephrine, acetylcholine and in minerals like calcium, phosphorus, are optimal for episodes of Prinzmetal angina (or also named, variant angina). Although episodes of variant

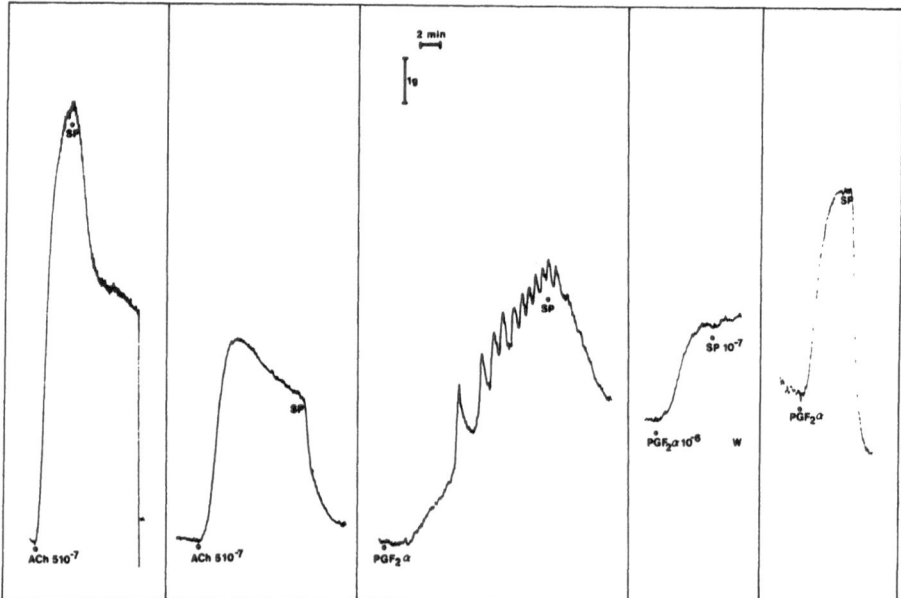

Fig. 1. Substance P (SP, 10^{-7} M) and endothelium-dependent vasodilator caused relaxation of human coronary arteries precontracted with either acetylcholine (Ach 5 10^{-7} M) or prostaglandin $F_{2\alpha}$ (PGF$_{2\alpha}$ 10^{-6} M). The two last examples were obtained from coronary segments isolated from the same heart. The ring with histologically proven atherosclerosis (according to morphological criteria used by Ginsburg et al. [4]) did not relax to substance P

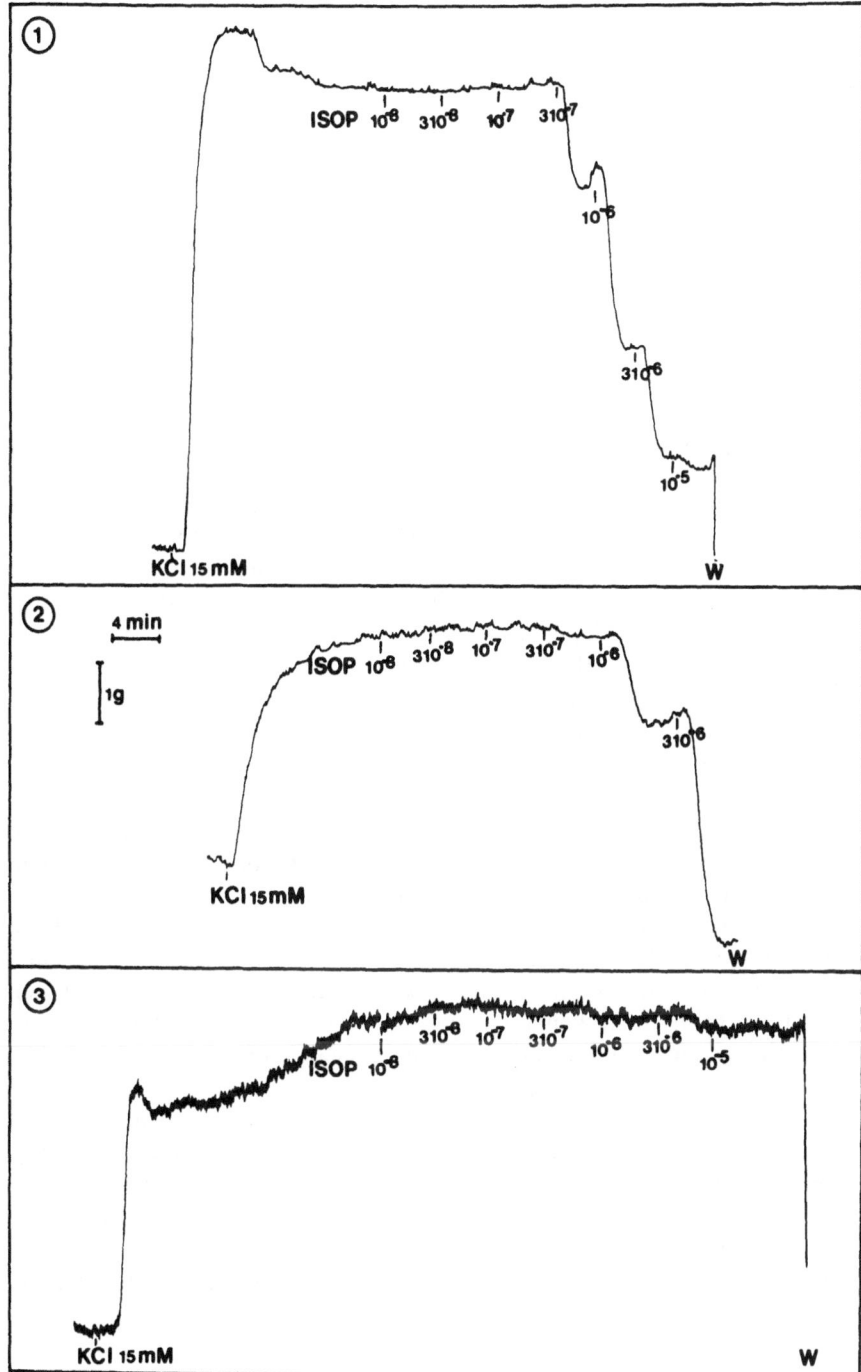

Fig. 2. Isoproterenol (Isop) administered in cumulative doses relaxed human coronary preparations precontracted with KCl (15 mM). The two last examples (2, 3), where isolated from the same heart. On the ring (3) with histologically proven atherosclerosis, the responses to isoproterenol were markedly diminished, which was not the case of the other ring (2), devoid of atherosclerotic lesions

angina most often occur without obvious cause, various stimuli have been identified as triggering factors, including hyperventilation, isometric or dynamic exercise [12]. Nevertheless, the intravenous injection of ergonovine seems to be
the most sensitive and specific test [12].

Diffuse Coronary Vasoconstriction and Chronic Stable Angina

As above mentioned, atherosclerotic coronary arteries are not rigid structures.
Moreover, coronary vessels of patients with chronic stable angina seem to be
hypersensitive to sympathetic vasoconstrictor stimuli like cold pressor testing
[13], isometric [14] or dynamic exercises [15]. Narrowing of coronary stenosis has
been nicely pointed out during these adrenergic stimuli. Intracoronary perfusion
of very small doses of nitroglycerin reverses this vasoconstriction and decreases
the exercise-induced ischemia [14, 15]. Similar results have been reported with
an alpha-blockade relatively selective in the coronary arteries [16]. From these
studies [14, 16] it is tempting to assume on the one hand that constriction of
epicardial stenosis is an important mechanism in the precipitation of transient
myocardial ischemia in patients with chronic stable angina and on the other
hand that this constriction is mediated by alpha-adrenergic stimuli. The pronounced alteration in the beta-adrenergic relaxation observed on isolated atherosclerotic coronary arteries [6] could provide an explanation of these clinical
findings. Indeed, atherosclerosis induced inhibition of beta-adrenergic relaxation could allow the alpha-effect of norepinephrine to predominate on the coronary vessels during these adrenergic stimuli.

Holter monitoring of patients with chronic stable angina has also provided
compelling evidence that alteration in myocardial blood flow is a frequent cause
of ischemic episodes during normal daily life [17].

Indeed, the majority of these episodes occur without increase in heart rate and
blood pressure, the main determinants of myocardial oxygen consumption [17].
Moreover, Deanfield et al. [18] have shown with positron emission tomography
that these transient ischemic episodes correspond to alterations in myocardial
perfusion. Exactly as for variant angina episodes, more than 50% of these episodes are asymptomatic [17].

The mechanisms responsible for these alterations in myocardial blood flow
during normal daily life remain unknown. Although sympathetic coronary vasoconstriction could play a role as during exertion, other mechanisms like vasoactive agents released by the platelets have also been proposed. Indeed, ticlopid-
ine, a potent inhibitor of platelet aggregation has been reported to decrease the
number of ischemic events detected by Holter monitoring in patients with
chronic stable agina [18].

Unstable Angina

As unstable angina encompasses a heterogeneous group of patients its pathophysiology is still less known than for the two other clinical syndromes.

According to Braunwald and Cohn [19], three categories of anginal syndromes can be enumerated under the term "unstable angina":

1. exertion angina with changing pattern; patients with this syndrome have had typical chronic angina which has recently increased in frequency and severity;
2. angina at rest;
3. angina of recent onset, rightaway severe.

Obviously there is an overlap with the Prinzmetal angina syndrome. Indeed, a reduction in regional coronary flow has been demonstrated as the pathophysiological mechanism for the development of angina at rest [20]. However, in a patient with angina at rest and a severe stenosis visualized by coronary angiography, spasm is probably not the etiology of the ischemic episodes. Platelet aggregation at the site of the stenosis associated with thromboxane A_2 and serotonin release could be a more likely explanation. Other mechanisms like atherosclerotic plaque rupture with partially occlusive thrombosis have been also demonstrated in patients with unstable angina [21].

Coronary Vasomotor Tone and Anti-anginal Drugs

The classical anti-anginal drugs can be classified in 3 categories:
- nitrates
- beta-blockers
- calcium antagonists

Nitrates

Over the past 15 years, the mechanism of action of nitrates has been essentially related to a decrease in myocardial demand: by reducing venous tone they allow the blood to sequestrate in the capacitance vessels and entail a decrease in cardiac filling [22].

However recent studies [14, 15] have shown that intracoronary injection of very small doses of nitroglycerin can counteract the coronary vasoconstriction induced by adrenergic stimuli like isometric and dynamic exercises. Therefore, it is likely that nitroglycerin acts on both components to alleviate angina: myocardial demand is decreased and myocardial supply is increased. Efficacy of nitrates has been demonstrated in chronic stable angina and in variant angina. However, attenuation or disappearance of some or all nitrate actions has been pointed out after sustained administration such as intravenous infusion in several well designed studies [23]. This vascular tolerance has been ascribed to oxidation of sulfhydryl groups within the smooth muscle. In fact, nitroglycerin and organic nitrates produce their relaxant effect on the vascular smooth muscle by activation of the cyclic GMP generating enzyme guanylate cyclase. This activation requires preliminary interaction with at least two pools of sulfhydryl groups. Sulfhydryl donors such as N-acetylcysteine have indeed been claimed to restore the vascular responsiveness in tolerant state. This finding was nicely shown by an in vivo study on human coronary arteries [24]. However, the reversal of the vascular responsiveness does not seem to be complete in most of the investigations [23, 25] and further studies are required to assess accurately the mechanism of action of N-acetylcysteine. Other nitrovasodilators such as nitroprusside and molsidomine would directly act on the guanylate cyclase without requiring these sulfhydryl groups and therefore would not exhibit a cross tolerance with nitroglycerin [26].

Beta-blockers

It is currently believed that beta-blockers allow the heart to work "economically". Indeed during exercise, patients with coronary insufficiency, treated with a beta-blocker tolerate higher workloads but the increments in heart rate and blood pressure are smaller than during control exercise [22].

One point which deserves further investigations is their effect on the coronary blood flow. By blocking the beta-adrenergic receptors, they unmask the alpha-receptors and thus promote coronary vasoconstriction. For propranolol this deleterious effect has been demonstrated in patients with variant angina [19]. It is likely that beta-blockers with ancillary properties different from propranolol exhibit the same deleterious effects. Indeed the coronary beta-receptors in humans like in dogs are mainly beta-1 and are unable to translate the weak stimuli induced by the intrinsic sympathetic activity of the drug into a response [27]. However, when the coronary vessels are severely and diffusely atherosclerotic, which is usually not the case in patients with variant angina, the effects of beta-blockers appear beneficial even when the symptoms are mainly rest angina [28]. One explanation to this finding is that on severely atherosclerotic human coronary arteries, the beta-adrenergic responses are almost abolished [6] and therefore the beta-blocker should not unmask the alpha-adrenergic tone. Thus, the more severe and diffuse is the coronary artery disease, the less deleterious should be the effect of a beta-blocking agent on coronary blood flow.

Calcium Antagonists

The three most used calcium antagonists are verapamil, diltiazem and nifedipine. They are potent arterial dilators on peripheral as well as coronary vessels. Their efficacy in variant angina has been well documented [29]. In contrast to nitrates, their coronary dilator effect should not be altered during chronic therapy.

In chronic stable angina, their anti-ischemic effects are probably related both to a decrease in myocardial demand and to an increase in myocardial supply. Indeed verapamil and dilatiazem on the one hand decrease blood pressure and heart rate and on the other hand seem to counteract the coronary vasoconstriction induced by adrenergic stimuli such as during isometric exercise [30]. However nifedipine, which is devoided of inhibitor effect on sino-atrial and atrioventricular functions, is likely to have a prevailing effect on the myocardial supply. According to Specchia et al. [31], this drug increases the coronary blood flow during exercise in about 50% of patients with coronary artery disease, and these patients are the ones who improve their exercise tolerance.

Conclusions

The impairment in coronary blood flow seems to play a dominant role not only in variant angina, unstable angina but also in chonic stable angina. While coronary vasospasm is responsible for the ischemic events in variant angina, platelet plugging and transient thrombosis could play the major role in unstable angina. The exact mechanisms inducing or triggering these clinical manifestations remain unclear.

In patients with chronic stable angina, it is likely that the majority of ischemic events are related to the two components: an increase in myocardial demand and a decrease in myocardial supply. According to the degree of coronary vasomotor tone, ischemic episodes will occur for high or low levels of myocardial oxygen consumption (1 and 3, respectively on Fig. 3). Figure 3 also summarizes how the 3 main anti-anginal drugs act on these components.

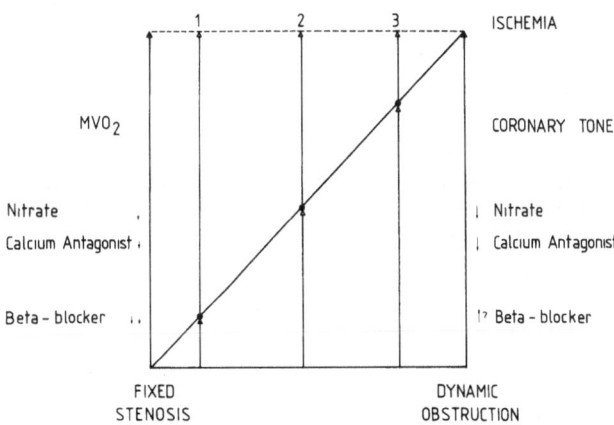

Fig. 3. Hypothetical scheme of the pathophysiology of chronic stable angina. Ischemic episodes (1, 2, 3) occur for progressively lower levels of myocardial oxygen consumption ($M\dot{V}O_2$) when the coronary vasomotor tone increases. Most ischemic episodes in chronic stable angina are probably due to a combination of fixed and dynamic obstructions

References

1. Blumgart HL, Schlesinger MJ, Davis D (1940) Studies on the relation of the clinical manifestations of angina pectoris, coronary thrombosis and myocardial infarction to the pathologic findings. Am Heart J 19:1-91
2. Prinzmetal M, Kenamer R, Merliss R, et al (1959) Angina pectoris I. A variant form of angina pectoris. Am J Med 27:375-388

3. Brown GB, Bolson E, Dodge HT (1984) Dynamic mechanisms in human coronary stenosis. Circulation 70:917–922
4. Ginsburg R, Bristow M, Davis K, Dibiase A, Billingham ME (1984) Quantitative pharmacologic responses of normal and atherosclerotic isolated human epicardial coronary arteries. Circulation 69:430–440
5. Shepherd JT, Vanhoutte PM (1985) Spasm of the coronary arteries: causes and consequences. (The scientist's viewpoint). Mayo Clin Proc 60:33–46
6. Berkenboom G, Depierreux M, Fontaine J (1987) The influence of atherosclerosis on the mechanical responses of isolated human coronary arteries to substance P, isoprenaline and noradrenaline. Br J Pharmacol 92:113–120
7. Kawachi Y, Tomoike H, Maruoka Y, et al (1984) Selective hypercontraction caused by ergonovine in the canine coronary artery under conditions of induced atherosclerosis. Circulation 69:441–450
8. Yasue H, Touyama M, Kato H, Tanaka S, Akiyama F (1976) Prinzmetal's variant form of angina as a manifestation of alpha-adrenergic receptor mediated coronary artery spasm: documentation by coronary arteriography. Am Heart J 91:148–153
9. Ginsburg R, Bristow MR, Kantrowitz N, Baim DS, Harrison DC (1981) Histamine provocation of clinical coronary artery spasm: implications concerning pathogenesis of variant angina pectoris. Am Heart J 109:819–822
10. Yasue H, Horio Y, Nakamura N, et al (1986) Induction of coronary artery spasm by acetylcholine in patients with variant angina: possible role of the parasympathetic nervous system in the pathogenesis of coronary artery spasm. Circulation 74:955–963
11. Hillis LD, Braunwald E (1978) Coronary artery spasm. N Engl J Med 299:695–701
12. Kaski JC, Crea F, Meran DO, et al (1986) Local coronary supersensitivity to diverse vasoconstrictor stimuli in patients with variant angina. Circulation 74:1255–1265
13. Mudge GH, Grossman W, Mills RM, Lesch M, Braunwald E (1976) Reflex increase in coronary vascular resistance in patients with ischemic heart disease. N Engl J Med 295:1333–1337
14. Brown BG, Lee AB, Bolson EL, Dodge HT (1984) Reflex constriction of significant coronary stenosis as a mechanism contributing to ischemic left ventricular dysfunction during isometric exercise. Circulation 70:18–24
15. Gage JE, Hess OM, Murakami T, Ritter M, Grimm J, Kreienbuehl HP (1986) Vasoconstriction of stenotic coronary arteries during dynamic exercise in patients with classic angina pectoris: reversibility by nitroglycerin. Circulation 73:865–876
16. Berkenboom G, Abramowicz M, Vandermoten P, Degre S (1986) Role of alpha-adrenergic coronary tone in exercise – induced angina pectoris. Am J Cardiol 57:195–198
17. Cohn PF (1987) Total ischemic burden: pathophysiology and prognosis. Am J Cardiol 59:3C–6C
18. Fox KM, Jonathan A, Selwyn AP (1982) Effects of platelet inhibition on myocardial ischemia. Lancet 2:727–730
19. Braunwald E, Cohn PF (1984) Unstable angina. In: Maseri A, Goodwin JF (eds) Hammersmith cardiology workshop series, vol 1. Raven Press, New York, pp 161–167
20. Chierchia S, Brunelli C, Simonetti I, Lazzari M, Maseri A (1980) Sequence of events in angina at rest: primary reduction in coronary flow. Circulation 61:759–768
21. Ambrose JA, Winters SL, Stern A, Eng A (1985) Angiographic morphology and the pathogenesis of unstable angina pectoris. J Am Coll Cardiol 5:609–614
22. Simoons ML, Balakumaran K (1981) The effects of drugs on the exercise electrocardiogram. Cardiology (suppl 2) 68:124–132
23. Abrams J (1987) Tolerance to organic nitrates. Circulation 74:1185–1187
24. May DC, Pupma JJ, Black WH, et al (1987) In vivo induction and reversal of nitroglycerin tolerance in human coronary arteries. N Engl J Med 317:805–809
25. Parker JO, Farrell B, Lahey KA, Rose BF (1987) Nitrate tolerance: the lack of effect of N-acetylcysteine. Circulation 76:572–576
26. Kukovetz WR, Holzmann S (1985) Mechanism of vasodilation by molsidomine. Am Heart J 109:637–640

27. Berkenboom G, Fontaine J, De Smet JM, Degre S (1987) Comparison of the effect of beta-adrenergic antagonists with different ancillary properties on isolated canine and human coronary arteries. Cardiovasc Res 21:299–304
28. Glazier J, Chierchia S, Gerosa S, Crean P, Berkenboom G, Maseri A (1986) Atenolol prevents silent and painful ischemia in patients with mixed angina. Circulation 74:II-45 (abst)
29. Stone PH, Antman EM, Muller JE, Braunwald E (1980) Calcium channel blocking agents in the treatment of cardiovascular disorders. Part II: Hemodynamic effects and clinical applications. Ann Int Med 93:886–891
30. Hossak KF, Brown BG, Stewart DK, Dodge HT (1984) Diltiazem-induced blockade of sympathetically mediated constriction of normal and diseased coronary arteries: lack of epicardial coronary dilator effect in humans. Circulation 70:465–471
31. Specchia G, De Servi S, Falcone C, et al (1983) Effects of nifedipine on coronary hemodynamic findings which exercise in patients with stable exertional angina. Circulation 68:1035–1043

Out of Hospital Management of Acute Myocardial Infarction

A. J. McNeill, G. W. N. Dalzell, and A. A. J. Adgey

Early Treatment of Acute Myocardial Infarction

In 1971 we first showed that among those seen early after the onset of acute myocardial infarction and managed out of hospital by a mobile coronary care unit the incidence of cardiogenic shock and hospital mortality was significantly lower in comparison with those seen late (Table 1) [1]. The data concerning these patients managed in 1969 showed a significantly lower incidence of shock and a lower hospital mortality among those seen within the first 3 hours compared with those seen after 3 hours although all were managed in the same way (Table 1). The age range was 30–86 years. There was no significant difference in age, sex or number of patients with previous infarction among the groups indicated. One hundred and sixteen of the 123 patients seen within the first hour were aged 70 or less. The incidence of shock among these patients was 3.5% and the hospital mortality 9%. One hundred and eleven of the 123 patients seen within the first hour survived to leave hospital and 99 (89%) of these patients were alive at the one year follow-up. This was the first time that an overall reduction in hospital mortality and incidence of cardiogenic shock had been shown by the early management of patients with acute myocardial infarction. However, this was in an era when thrombolytic agents were not administered to patients following acute myocardial infarction.

Pump Failure and Left Ventricular Function

It is now well known that pump failure i.e. left ventricular failure and cardiogenic shock are now the major causes of death following myocardial infarction.

Table 1. 447 Patients with acute myocardial infarction (all age groups) managed by the Belfast Mobile Coronary Care Unit (1969)

Initiation of Coronary Care	Within 3 hours	After 3 hours
No. of patients	319	128
Cardiogenic shock[a]	14 (4%) (a)	17 (13%) (b)
Hospital deaths[b]	31 (10%) (a)	24 (19%) (b)

[a] (a) differs significantly from (b), $p < 0.001$.
[b] (a) differs significantly from (b) $0.01 > p > 0.001$.

De Wood et al in 1980 showed that in coronary arteriograms carried out in 126 patients within 4 hours of the onset of symptoms of acute myocardial infarction complete obstruction of the vessel was shown in 87% of cases [2]. The question therefore arose as to how to relieve this obstruction in such a way that overall left ventricular function would be improved.

Lavellee et al in 1985 carried out a series of experiments in conscious dogs where the effect of coronary artery occlusion followed by reperfusion at 1 hour, 2 hours and 3 hours were compared with a permanently occluded group with regard to left ventricular function and regional endocardial function over a 4 week period [3]. They showed that at 1 hour after coronary artery occlusion systolic shortening was depressed by over 100%. In the group of dogs where the vessel remained occluded the systolic shortening remained depressed by 86% when looked at 4 weeks later. However, considerable return of function had occurred in the group of dogs where reperfusion had taken place 1 hour after total occlusion i.e. systolic shortening remained depressed by only 30% when measured at 4 weeks and for the 2 hour group was 58% but for the 3 hour group was 78%. Thus the authors concluded that in the conscious dog coronary artery reperfusion at 1 hour after coronary artery occlusion resulted in substantial return of endocardial function in the most severely ischemic myocardium. However, after 3 hours of coronary artery occlusion little salvage of regional endocardial myocardial function can be induced by acute reperfusion in this model.

Left ventricular ejection fraction correlates only roughly with infarct size, but is a powerful predictor of survival after myocardial infarction. Nevertheless, during the early hours of acute infarction the ejection fraction is an insensitive measure of the severity of hypokinesis in the infarct region because of the influence of compensatory hyperkinesis or other wall motion abnormalities in the non-infarct region. Thus, in many of the initial studies using intracoronary or intravenous streptokinase following acute myocardial infarction there was great difficulty in showing a significant difference between the global left ventricular ejection fraction recorded for the actively treated group and those receiving placebo. One of the earliest studies using intravenous streptokinase in acute myocardial infarction (ISAM) where patients were randomized within 6 hours after the onset of symptoms of acute myocardial infarction to intravenous streptokinase or placebo they showed that of those seen and treated within the first 3 hours of symptoms there was an improvement in left ventricular ejection fraction by 3.4% and in those treated between 3 and 6 hours the improvement in ejection fraction was 2.2% [4].

With the advent of tissue-type plasminogen activator (t-PA) which is normally found at very low concentrations in human blood, and produces thrombus-specific fibrinolysis by activating plasminogen on the surface of fibrin, it has been shown to be essentially devoid of adverse side effects on the hemostatic system. The t-PA has now been produced in adequate quantities by recombinant DNA technology (rt-PA). There are major differences between this agent and streptokinase. Rt-PA is clot specific whereas streptokinase is not. Rt-PA has a very short duration of action and streptokinase is very significantly longer. Rt-PA has specific thrombolytic efficacy whereas streptokinase efficacy in lysis of clots is somewhat less. Reocclusion however has a greater incidence in patients with rt-PA probably due to the short half-life of the agent in comparison with those receiving streptokinase. The bleeding potential is the same for both agents. However, there is an allergic potential for those receiving streptokinase as antibodies can form to the agent but there is no allergic reaction to rt-PA. Thus rt-PA can be repeated at the time of reocclusion whereas streptokinase cannot. The incidence of hypotension following the administration of either agent is minimal.

Recombinant Tissue Plasminogen Activator in Acute Myocardial Infarction: Dose Ranging Study

When we first considered the use of rt-PA in acute myocardial infarction and looked through the published literature for the dosage we found many varying dosages quoted [5]. For the thrombolysis in myocardial infarction (TIMI) trials carried out in the United States between 1984 and 1986 a wide variety of dosages had been used with a marked variation in reperfusion rates at 90 min after the start of the infusion. Thus a dose ranging study using rt-PA in acute myocardial infarction was important to assess the dosage required particularly among patients seen very early after acute myocardial infarction and out of hospital. We studied 50 consecutive patients all aged less than 75 years with pain clinically suspected to be due to acute myocardial infarction. All patients with ST segment elevation on the initial ECG of (a) 0.2 mV in at least 2 of the inferior leads or (b) 0.3 mV in at least 2 of the precordial leads or (c) 0.2 mV in leads 1 and aVL. All patients were seen and treated within 4 hours of the onset of chest pain. The usual exclusion criteria for thrombolytic agents applied. Patients were randomized to either 20 mg, 50 mg or 100 mg rt-PA administered intravenously over a period of 90 min. At 90 min a coronary arteriogram was performed and the reperfusion grade assessed in the infarct related coronary vessel as scored by the TIMI investigators i.e. grade 0 no perfusion, grade 1 penetration with minimal perfusion, grade 2 partial perfusion, and grade 3 complete perfusion. Our results showed that in 14 of 17 (82%) patients receiving 100 mg there was either grade 2 or 3 reperfusion and for those receiving 50 mg 12 of 17 (71%) patients showed similar reperfusion grades. However, in only 8 of 16 (50%) receiving the 20 mg was there reperfusion at that time. It is well known that increasing resistance of thrombi to lysis as they age is not only evident in vivo but also in vitro. The probable explanation for this increasing resistance to lysis is continuing polymerization and cross-linking of the fibrin. The earlier thrombolytic therapy is started the greater the frequency of early reperfusion and thus the greatest potential for salvage of myocardium. Thus when we looked at the 26 patients seen and treated in the first 2 hours of the onset of symptoms we found that 10/10 patients who received 100 mg had grade 2 or 3 reperfusion, 5/5 receiving 50 mg and 6/11 receiving 20 mg. Thus there was no difference between the 50 and 100 mg dosage when patients were seen and treated within the first 2 hours of the onset of symptoms regarding reperfusion grades 2 and 3 at the 90 min angiogram. We also measured the blood clotting factors and found that the percentage fibrinogen remaining at 90 min after the administration was dose related. For 20 mg dosage the percentage fibrinogen remaining was 86%. For 50 mg it was

75% and for 100 mg it was 63%. This is in marked contrast with figures quoted as low as 7% for patients receiving intravenous streptokinase.

At the end of the 90 min infusion in 41 of the patients a further 50 mg rt-PA was infused over 5 hours followed by heparin in order to maintain patency of the vessel. In 7 patients a further 50 mg of rt-PA was infused over 1 hour followed by heparin: these were patients who had shown grade 0 or 1 reperfusion at the 90 min angiogram. The reason for choosing a low dose infusion of rt-PA was an attempt to prevent reocclusion occurring in those vessels that had opened or to help open up vessels that either had very poor perfusion or had remained occluded.

Invasive procedures carried out after the 90 min angiogram depended on the investigator. Three patients had mechanical probing of the infarct related artery. Eight had intracoronary nitrates, 10 had acute percutaneous coronary angioplasty, 2 had elective percutaneous coronary angioplasty and 12 patients required coronary artery bypass grafting – one as an emergency.

Cardiac enzymes were assessed at 4 hourly intervals over a period of 28 hours from the time of administration of rt-PA. For grade 2 or 3 reperfusion at 90 min the mean peak CK-MB was 212 U/1 and for grade 0 or 1 reperfusion the mean peak CK-MB was 290 U/1. Mean peak total CK for those with grade 2 or 3 reperfusion was 2187 U/1 and for the mean peak total CK for grade 0 or 1 reperfusion was 2541 U/1. Thus there appeared to be a reduction in enzyme release for those who had grade 2 or 3 reperfusion. However, these differences were not statistically significant and with the problems of assessment of release of enzymes post reperfusion no firm conclusions can be reached from these data.

Patients who fail to achieve reperfusion or who experience reocclusion of the infarct related artery show no improvement in regional or global left ventricular function. Thus the mean global left ventricular ejection fraction assessed on average 46 hours from the onset of symptoms showed that for grade 2 or 3 reperfusion it was 48% and for grade 0 or 1 reperfusion it was 41%.

However, as other investigators have found, the major difference lies in the infarct related regional third left ventricular ejection fraction. Thus the mean infarct related regional third left ventricular ejection fraction for grade 2 or 3 reperfusion was 46% and for grade 0 or 1 reperfusion it was 35%. These differences were statistically significant ($p < 0.05$).

The incidence of arrhythmias following rt-PA in acute myocardial infarction was no higher than what we would expect from patients seen within the same time frame who did not receive thrombolytic therapy. Four patients developed ventricular fibrillation during the 90 min infusion of rt-PA (1 patient had grade 2 reperfusion of the infarct related artery at the 90 min angiogram and 3 patients had grade 1 reperfusion) and a further 2 patients developed it during the subsequent 5 hours infusion (1 grade 2, 1 grade 3, reperfusion of the infarct related artery). This gives an incidence of 12% which is no higher than expected. No patient in this series had late ventricular fibrillation and pericarditis occurred in only 4 patients (1 had grade 1 reperfusion, 2 had grade 2 reperfusion and 1 had grade 3 reperfusion).

One patient had bleeding into a renal cyst requiring 1 unit of blood, 1 patient had hemoptysis, 1 patient bloody diarrhea, 15 had cutaneous bruising. Reocclusion during hospitalisation occurred in 3 (6%) and the mortality was 8% i.e. 4 patients. All these patients died from cardiogenic shock. No patient died from thrombolytic therapy.

Early Versus Late rt-PA in Acute Myocardial Infarction

In view of these results we thought it imperative to design a trial which was double blind placebo controlled using rt-PA to see whether early reperfusion had a significant effect on left ventricular ejection fraction and enzyme release in comparison with late reperfusion. Thus we randomized patients to an early group i.e. seen and treated on average 119 min (range 38–235 min) or to a late group seen and treated at a mean of 187 min (range 80–285 min). The early group received rt-PA as soon as they were first seen. Those who received the rt-PA late received it in the hospital coronary care unit. Twenty-seven patients were admitted to the early group and 30 to the late group. Angiograms were carried out on average 11 days from the onset of symptoms. Of the 24 patients in the early group who had angiograms assessable at that time period, 19 showed grade 2 or 3 reperfusion whereas of 25 patients with angiograms at the same time period who received late rt-PA, 16 of the 25 showed grade 2 or 3 reperfusion the mean peak total CK was 2690 U/1 whereas for late rt-PA it was 2308 U/1 and for grade 2 and 3 reperfusion mean peak CK-MB was 239 U/1 for early and 208 U/1 for the late group. For those with early rt-PA grade 0 or 1 reperfusion mean peak total CK was 2897 U/1 and 2287 U/1 for late rt-PA and for grade 0 or 1 reperfusion the mean peak CK-MB for early rt-PA was 282 U/1 and 237 for the late rt-PA. There were no statistically significant differences. The mean global left ventricular ejection fraction for grade 2 or 3 reperfusion was 40% for early rt-PA and 37% for late rt-PA whereas the mean infarct related regional third ejection fraction for grade 2 or 3 reperfusion was 42% for early rt-PA and 32% for late rt-PA. The mean global left ventricular ejection fraction with grade 0 or 1 reperfusion for early rt-PA was 40% and for late rt-PA 32%. Mean infarct related regional third ejection fraction for grade 0 or 1 reperfusion for early rt-PA was 26% and for late rt-PA was 24%.

During hospitalisation 2/27 (7%) died in the early group and 3/30 (10%) in the late group. There was a similar rate of reocclusion in the early and late groups i.e. 3/27 for early rt-PA and 4/30 for late rt-PA. There was no significant bleeding.

We conclude from the early results of this study that for those who reperfuse i.e. grade 2 or 3 reperfusion, the regional third left ventricular ejection fractions are improved when rt-PA is administered early in comparison when it is administered late. The question however remains of what to do with the patient at the end of rt-PA. Patients probably fall into 4 groups. In approximately 10% of the total patients as the individual has co-existing severe 3 vessel disease or left main disease coronary artery bypass grafting is imperative. In approximately 20 to 30% of patients the infarct related artery is occluded at the time of study and therefore the question of further therapy for these patients remains. In approximately 10% of patients the infarct related vessel is widely patent i.e. <50% residual lesion and for most of these patients, anticoagulants are indicated. However, in approximately 50–60% of patients the infarct related artery is patent but there is a critical or significant lesion remaining. The question therefore arises should these patients have angioplasty or coronary artery bypass grafting or anticoagulation which will help remould the residual but significant lesion over the subsequent months.

Conclusions

In the 1960's defibrillation revolutionized the treatment of ventricular fibrillation outside hospital. Now, thrombolytic therapy is the second major advance in the management of patients with acute myocardial infarction both from reperfusion of the infarct related vessel and the potential salvage of myocardium. The earlier treatment is started, the easier it is to lyse the clot with resultant greater improvement in the regional third ejection fraction of the left ventricle as it pertains to the infarct area.

References

1. Adgey AAJ, Allen JD, Geedes JS, et al (1971) Acute phase of myocardial infarction. Lancet, 2:501–504
2. De Wood MA, Spores J, Notske R, et al (1980) Prevalence of total coronary occlusion during the early hours of transmural myocardial infarction. N Engl J Med 303:897–902
3. Lavallee M, Cox DA, Vatner SF (1985) Effects of coronary artery reperfusion on recovery of regional myocardial function in conscious dogs. Eur Heart J 6 suppl E 109–116
4. The I.S.A.M. study group (1986) A prospective trial of intravenous streptokinase in acute myocardial infarction (I.S.A.M.): Mortality, morbidity and infarct size at 21 days. N Engl J Med 314:1465–1471
5. Passamani ER (1987) Thrombolysis in myocardial infarction: the NHLBI experience. In: Sobel BE, Collen D, Grossbard EB (eds) Tissue Plasminogen Activator in Thrombolytic Therapy. Marcel Dekker Inc, New York Basel, p 75

Pre-hospital Thrombolytic Intervention in the Treatment of Acute Myocardial Infarction

L. L. Bossaert

Introduction

In an attempt to limit infarct size, the objective of treatment of acute myocardial infarction (AMI) has changed in the past 20 years from limitation of myocardial oxygen consumption (nitrates, beta-blockers, vasodilators) towards improvement of tissue oxygen availability by dissolving the occluding thrombus in the infarct-related coronary artery. Well-designed controlled studies have proven the value of thrombolytic treatment, especially when initiation occurs very early [1–6].

Therefore, optimal treatment of AMI should initiate thrombolytic intervention as soon as possible after onset of symptoms, but without increasing the complications by the thrombolytic treatment itself.

Importance of Time Delay Between Onset of Symptoms and Initiation of Thrombolytic Therapy

Koren et al. [7, 8] found that when intravenous streptokinase (SK) is given less than 1.5 hours after the onset of pain, a significantly higher ejection fraction, infarct-related regional ejection fraction and a lower QRS score were obtained compared to initiation of treatment between 1.5 and 4 hours after the onset of pain. Patients treated even earlier, i.e. "at home", had better preservation of left ventricular function than patients treated later, i.e. in the hospital. The same group found significantly smaller infarct size in patients with anterior AMI treated within 2 hours after onset of chest pain, as compared to patients treated after 2 to 4 hours. In patients with inferior myocardial infarction this critical time-limit was 1.5 hours.

The Dutch Interuniversity Cardiology Institute trial, reported by Simoons et al. [4] revealed that in patients admitted within 1 hour after the onset of symptoms, the reduction of infarct size was 51%; in those admitted between 1–2 hours it was 31%, and in those admitted later than 2 hours it was as low as 13%.

In the ISAM study [9], similar results were obtained: significantly shorter time-to-peak-CK interval, smaller area-under-the-CKMB-curve, and higher global or infarct-related regional ejection fractions were reported in patients treated within 1.5 hrs after onset of chest pain, compared to patients treated 1.5–4 hrs after AMI.

The Italian GISSI study is an important source of data on mortality, and short-term and long-term data on survival, side effects and other events in 10732 patients [5]. The main message of this study was that SK treatment produced at 18% decrease in overall mortality. Patients treated within 3 hours had a reduction in mortality of 23%, while patients treated within 1 hour had the most striking beneficial effect with a mortality reduction of 47%. These trends persisted after a follow-up of one year.

Finally, the first results of the ISIS-2 trial, at the present time including > 16,000 patients, confirmed that in 4800 patients treated early (0–4 hours) there was "proof beyond reasonable doubt" that SK reduced in-hospital mortality from 12 to 8% [6].

Factors Determining Time Delay

The delay between onset of symptoms and initiation of thrombolytic therapy depends on a number of different interrelated factors: the patient ignoring or denying the importance of his chest pain, the speed of response of the physicians and the ambulance to the patients' call, the transportation time and hospital admission procedures, the time required for emergency department and/or CCU evaluation. An important delay between onset of chest pain and treatment has been reported in the ENIM-study (10): the patient delay was 4.4 hours. The combined delay due to the general practitioners (GP) (time to arrival and decision time), the transportation to the hospital, the admission formalities, and the CCU decision time added up to another 5.1 hours.

Patient factors were described in the MILIS study [11]. Paradoxically, high-risk patients (history of congestive heart failure, diabetes mellitus or preexisting systemic hypertension), women and elderly patients as well as those requiring beta blockers and high dosis of nitrates, arrived significantly later in hospital, incurring a higher mortality rate. Patients who were at home at the onset of AMI waited longer before calling for help than those who were at work or on the street.

Equally, a survey by the EMIP (European Myocardial Infarction Project) study group demonstrated that in 8 major cities in Europe, less than 50% of 2571 AMI patients reached the hospital within 4 hours after onset of pain [12].

Pre-hospital Thrombolysis

Pre-hospital thrombolysis was first applied by Koren et al. [7]. These investigators have recently reported their experience in a group of patients successfully treated with intravenous SK by a physician-operated mobile intervention unit [13]. Of the 34 patients, 31 (91%) had clinical or enzymatic evidence of reperfusion; coronary artery patency on coronary angiography at day 4 was found in 25/29 patients (86%). Comparing the pre-hospital treated patients with a group of 84 patients treated in-hospital with SK, the authors found only a minor difference in rapidity of reperfusion after intravenous administration of SK. However, there were significant differences in peak CK, ejection fraction, QRS score and left ventricular (LV) dysfunction index, indicating that the pre-hospital group had a better outcome with a significantly smaller infarct size. There were also striking differences between patients with anterior or inferior infarction: as there is more myocardium at risk, the potential for salvage is greater in anterior than in inferior infarction.

In France, two groups have reported their experiences with prehospital throm bolysis. Villemant et al. [14] have treated 67 patients with 1.5 million units of intravenous SK over 45 minutes, and reported reperfusion in 71% and a time saving of 74 minutes. Castaigne et al. [15] induced thrombolysis by using a bolus injection of 30 units of anisoylated plasminogen streptokinase activator complex (APSAC, Eminase). Twenty-one patients were randomized to at home throm bolysis compared to a control group treated with APSAC after CCU admission. Reperfusion was obtained in 76%, saving 70 minutes of time.

As reported in a recent Editorial, the TEAHAT trial (Thrombolysis Early In Acute Heart Attack Trial) in Sweden studies the effects of tPA given intrave nously in acute heart attack diagnosed exclusively on the history of chest pain without an ECG being performed. In this trial time gain was 46 minutes [16].

In Berlin, Bippus and co-workers randomized at home patients presenting early AMI to treatment with SK (n=21) or heparin (n=20). The control group was treated with SK after arrival in the CCU. No serious side-effects were noted during the pre-hospital phase; two patients died from cardiogenic shock in hos pital [17].

We have studied the possible risk and benefit of pre-hospital initiation of thrombolytic therapy at the patients home in acute myocardial infarction using APSAC [18]. This study was performed in cooperation with a group of 25 gen eral practitioners (GPs), working in an area of 100000 inhabitants. APSAC was selected because intravenous bolus administration is possible due to its long half-life (T/2=110 minutes) [19]. Whenever the diagnosis of recent AMI (≤2 hours) is made by the GP, the medical intervention team of the hospital is acti vated and rapidly transported to the patients home. If diagnosis of AMI is con firmed (history, physical examination, ECG), and contra-indications are ex cluded, a single intravenous bolus of 30 U of APSAC is given, before the patient is transferred to the hospital by a mobile CCU ambulance for follow-up and further treatment. Evaluation of reperfusion and myocardial salvage is based on clinical evolution, serum enzymes, ECG changes, ventriculography and coronary angiography performed the day after admission.

During a 14 month period, 66 patients with suspected acute myocardial infarc tion were evaluated by the GP according to a strict protocol. A total of 45 pa tients were excluded for a number of reasons: 4 patients died before arrival of the GP, 17 were older than 70 years, 14 had chest pain lasting more than 4 hours, 1 had an active peptic ulcer, 5 refused to give their informed consent, 2 were treated with oral anticoagulant drugs and 2 had a history of previous AMI. In 21 cases, the GP alerted the mobile intervention team of our hospital which admin istered APSAC at home in 14/18 patients (Fig. 1). Seven patients did not fulfill the ECG criteria of early AMI (ST-elevation ≥2 mm in ≥2 leads) and did not receive APSAC. In 4 patients, the ECG became positive for AMI in the follow ing hours, and they received thrombolytic treatment after admission. Therefore, the accuracy of GPs in diagnosing AMI on clinical grounds is quite good, since

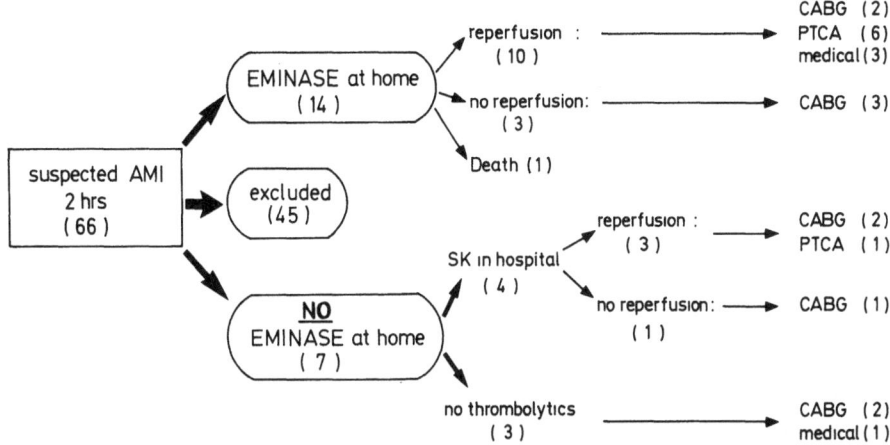

Fig. 1. Clinical course of pre-hospital thrombolysis for acute myocardial infarction (AMI) in a pilot study population. (The number of patients is indicated between parentheses)

the tentative diagnosis of AMI was subsequently confirmed in 86%, and the incorrect diagnosis of unstable angina in three patients can hardly be considered as an error.

Coronary reperfusion was achieved in 13/17 evaluable treated patients (10/13 pre-hospital treated patients, and 3/4 in-hospital treated patient). In two cases reperfusion failure was probably due to circulating antibodies, illustrated by elevated ASL-titers. Reocclusion occurred in one patient.

One patient died with anoxic brain damage after ventricular fibrillation during transportation, requiring prolonged CPR. Except for bradycardia/hypotension following the injection of the thrombolytic drug in 4/14 patients, no major complications were noted during the pre-hospital course.

Subsequent therapy is summarized in Fig. 1: 10/13 reperfused patients underwent an invasive procedure (PTCA, CABG) because of a residual stenosis of ≥75% on the coronary angiogram.

The important time intervals are summarized in Table 1. The estimated time gain by treating the patient at home instead of in the CCU was 44 minutes.

Table 1. Summary of events during pre-hospital course of thrombolytic therapy

Author	#	Treatment	Reperfusion	Time saved	Adverse events
Weiss	34	SK $0.75 \cdot 10^6$ U	91%	55 min	8 (VF 1; H 6; B 1)
Castaigne	21	APSAC 30 U	76%	70 min	6 (VF 1; H 2; B 3)
Villemant	67	SK $1.5 \cdot 10^6$ U	71%	74 min	1 (B 1)
Bossaert	21	APSAC 30 U	77%	44 min	5 (VF 1; H 4)
TEAHAT	ND	rt-PA	ND	46 min	ND
Bippus	21	SK	ND	46 min	ND

ND: No Data; VF: Ventricular Fibrillation; B: Bleeding; H: Hypotension

Importance of Pre-hospital Thrombolysis

Feasibility: All previously cited investigators agree about feasibility of pre-hospital thrombolysis: with minimal effort and with minimal amount of additional equipment, it is possible to administer thrombolytic treatment in the patients home. There are no major logistical obstacles to implement this new treatment mode.

Safety (Table 1): The experience thus far points out that, at least in the privileged context of our teaching hospitals, only minor complications are encountered: minor bleeding, bradycardia/hypotension caused by the thrombolytic drug itself or due to reperfusion. Since the patient is seen earlier in the course of AMI, it is also likely that major rhythm and hemodynamic disturbances will occur in the presence of the intervention team. However it is possible that the results on safety, obtained "on the field", are too optimistic. Indeed, in the EMIP study it was shown that in about 15% of patients, where AMI was clinicaly suspected, the diagnosis of AMI was not confirmed [12]. Using only clinical history as a diagnostic method, it would be possible to encounter life-threatening complications "on the field" due to inappropriate administration of thrombolytic drugs.

Time gain: As summarized in Table 1, an important time gain of at least 44 minutes (44–71 minutes) is possible with pre-hospital thrombolysis. This means earlier reperfusion of ischemic myocardium and less necrosis. Therefore, the long-term prognosis should be better. However, this point needs to be elucidated by large-scale and controlled investigations.

Who May Initiate Thrombolytic Treatment Outside Hospital?

It is well known that the highest mortality of AMI occurs in the first hours after onset, due to ventricular fibrillation or tachycardia, or to hemodynamic collapse. Therefore, the medical personnel initiating at-home thrombolysis will be faced with a higher incidence of potentially lethal complications. The composition of the medical team will differ in function of local possibilities and medical practice. Notwithstanding this, any person treating an AMI victim with thrombolytic drugs in the pre-hospital phase must be experienced in basic and advanced cardiac life support. Mobile coronary care unit should always be available as a back up.

Conclusion

A limited number of pilot studies in Jerusalem, Paris, Berlin, and Antwerp have demonstrated that pre-hospital thrombolytic treatment of AMI is possible and safe, and provides clinically significant time saving of at least 44 minutes. This time saving resulted in a higher reperfusion rate of >70%. However, at the present time, pre-hospital administration of thrombolytic drugs should be considered as clinical investigation, and restricted to study protocols with well-defined criteria. Large-scaled studies are urgently needed to investigate the influence of early thrombolysis on morbidity and mortality of AMI and to measure the cost-benefit ratio of this new and attractive treatment approach.

Pre-hospital thrombolytic therapy should only be started by experienced medical personnel, because of the potentially life-threatening events in the early phase of AMI and the possible adverse events during thrombolytic treatment. Logistical support should be on-hand: medical intervention team, mobile coronary care unit, and hospital-based CCU. We feel that, at least in the Belgian context, the participation of GPs is important for speeding-up the decision-making process.

Thrombolysis at home will be safe, feasible and effective only if all these conditions are met.

References

1. Kennedy J, Ritchie J, Davis, et al (1985) The Western Washington randomized trial of intracoronary streptokinase in Acute Myocardial Infarction. N Engl J Med 312:1073–1078
2. TIMI Study group (1984) The thrombolysis in myocardial infarction trial. N Eng J Med 310:609–613
3. Verstraete M, Bernard R, Bory M, et al (1985) Randomized trial of IV rt-PA versus IV streptokinase in acute myocardial infarction. Lancet i:842–847
4. Simoons M, Serruys P, Brand M vd, et al (1985) Improved survival after early thrombolysis in acute myocardial infarction. Lancet ii:578–582
5. GISSI (1986) Effectiveness of intravenous thrombolytic treatment in acute myocardial infarction. Lancet i:397–402
6. ISIS steering committee (1987) Intravenous streptokinase given within 0–4 hours of onset of myocardial infarction reduced mortality in ISIS-2. Lancet i:502
7. Koren G, Weiss AT, Hasin Y, et al (1985) Prevention of myocardial damage in acute myocardial ischemia by early treatment with intravenous streptokinase. N Engl J Med 313:1384–1389
8. Fine DG, Weiss AT, Sapoznikov D, et al (1986) Importance of early initiation of intravenous streptokinase therapy for acute myocardial infarction. Am J Cardiol 58:411–417
9. The ISAM Study Group (1986) A prospective trial of intravenous streptokinase in acute myocardial infarction (ISAM). N Engl J Med 314:1465–1471
10. Sainsous J, Serradimigni A, Richard JL, Guize L, Leconte T, Tanielian P (1985) How many patients with acute myocardial infarction could be treated in France by intravenous streptokinase? Results of a prospective trial (ENIM 1984). Eur Heart J Suppl 1, 67; (abstract) 197
11. Hartmann JR, McKeever LM, Bufalino VB, et al (1986) Intravenous streptokinase in acute myocardial infarction: experience of community hospitals served by paramedics. Am Heart J 111:1030–1034
12. EMIP subcommittee (1987) Potential time saving with pre-hospital intervention in acute myocardial infarction (submitted).
13. Weiss AT, Fine DG, Appelbaum D, et al (1987) Prehospital coronary thrombolysis. A new strategy in acute myocardial infarction. Chest 92:124–128
14. Villemant D, Barriot P, Bodenan P (1987) Thrombolysis in acute myocardial infarction. A race against time. In: JL Vincent (ed) Update in Intensive Care and Emergency Medicine, vol 3. Springer, Berlin Heidelberg New York London Paris Tokyo, pp 277–286
15. Castaigne AD, Duval AM, Dubois-Rande JL, et al (1987) Prehospital administration of APSAC in acute myocardial infarction. Drugs 33:231–234

16. Editorial (1987) Thrombolytic therapy for acute myocardial infarction. Lancet ii:138–140
17. Bippus PH, Haux R, Schroder R (1987) Prehospital intravenous streptokinase in evolving myocardial infarction: a randomized study about feasibility, safety and time gain. Eur Heart Journal 8, 103
18. Bossaert L, Belgian EMS study group (1987) Safety and tolerance data from the Belgian multicenter study of APSAC versus heparine in acute myocardial infarction. Drugs 33:287–292

Reperfusion Arrhythmias: An Update

J. R. Parratt and C. L. Wainwright

Introduction

Tennant & Wiggers [1] were the first to clearly demonstrate that reperfusion of the ischemic myocardium can be associated with the generation of potentially malignant ventricular arrhythmias. The importance of such arrhythmias has been recognized for many years during surgical reperfusion of the whole heart (e.g. cardiopulmonary bypass with ischemic arrest) but has recently taken on renewed significance because of the interest in thrombolyic therapy for patients with acute myocardial infarction, the establishment of the concept of transient coronary artery spasm with platelet aggregation as one cause of angina pectoris and the evidence suggesting that reperfusion-induced ventricular fibrillation is one cause of sudden cardiac death. The significance of reperfusion arrhythmias in these particular clinical situations has led to a great deal of experimental work to determine precisely under what conditions these potentially lifethreatening arrhythmias arise and how they may be suppressed by drugs. This update attempts to summarize the main factors responsible.

Evidence in Clinical Situations for Arrhythmias Following Reperfusion of the Ischemic Myocardium

There are three main situations where reperfusion arrhythmias may be important. These are in variant and unstable angina where arterial spasm is involved, following recanalization of a coronary artery obstructed by a thrombus and, possibly, in some instances of sudden cardiac death.

Reperfusion Arrhythmias in Patients with Variant and Unstable Angina

In these forms of angina there is a marked coronary artery smooth muscle spasm component, perhaps in areas of endothelial dysfunction. One possible mechanism could be endothelial damage at sites of atherosclerotic coronary obstruction leading to transient platelet adhesion and the release of potentially vasoconstrictor substances such as thromboxane A_2 and serotonine (5-HT). Vanhoutte's group [2] has recently shown that removal of endothelium in isolated canine coronary arteries leads, in the presence of aggregating human platelets, to marked smooth muscle contraction. Since this contraction is inhibited by selective antagonists of thromboxane and 5-HT the suggestion is that these endogenous agents, released from platelets, might induce vessel spasm localized at sites of endothelial injury. Under normal conditions, platelet aggregation and coronary spasm do not occur because of the presence in, and active secretion from, endothelial cells of protective agents such as prostacyclin and endothelium-derived relaxant factor (EDRF). This whole concept, in relation to unstable angina, has been recently reviewed [e.g. 3, 4].

It might be expected that ventricular arrhythmias could occur not only during coronary artery occlusion during spasm (and/or platelet aggregation at the site of a stenosed vessel) but also during the release of spasm (and/or during the breakup of a platelet thrombus and the dispersal of platelet emboli). There is rather limited evidence however that such reperfusion arrhythmias are common. Whilst ventricular tachycardia, fibrillation and complete atrioventricular block are frequently observed during episodes of variant angina (Prinzmetal's disease) and ventricular fibrillation has been actually demonstrated during vasospasm [5] these arrhythmias are apparently rarely seen during reperfusion in these patients. These authors have estimated that reperfusion-induced ventricular tachycardia and fibrillation occur in only about 1% of episodes. A particularly relevant study is that by Kerin et al. [6]. They examined 36 patients with variant angina pectoris and analyzed them using Holter monitoring to determine whether the mechanisms underlying arrhythmias in these patients were related to coronary occlusion or reperfusion (release). Most (80%) of these patients experienced arrhythmias (ventricular premature beats, often progressing to more malignant forms of ventricular arrhythmias such as tachycardia and fibrillation) prior to the acme of ST-segment elevatiton (i.e. during occlusion). Three patients (20%), all of whom had coronary artery obstructive disease, had arrhythmias only following normalisation of the ST-segment, one developing fibrillation from which he could not be resuscitated. A similar arrhythmia time course is also evident from the study of Arnim et al. [7]. In twelve patients with Prinzmetal's variant angina most arrhythmias occurred during the angina episode (i.e. occlusion); in only one patient did arrhythmias commence *after* the episode. Although the patient numbers in these two studies are small, the results suggest that fibrillation is rather more likely to occur following release of spasm (or break-up of a platelet thrombus) than during the occlusion itself. The fact that such reperfusion arrhythmias appear to be relatively uncommon is not surprising in view of the short time (5–10 min) the coronary arteries were occluded in these patients; the relationship of occlusion time to the severity of reperfusion arrhythmias is discussed below.

Reperfusion Arrhythmias in Patients Following Coronary Artery Thrombolysis

One major advance in the treatment of acute myocardial infarction has been attempts to recanalize obstructed coronary arteries particularly using thrombolytic procedures and/or percutaneous transluminal coronary angioplasty (PTCA). In experimental animals reperfusion within the first hours of occlusion results in considerable myocardial salvage [8] whilst in patients with infarction early and successful reperfusion results in improved short term survival [9, 10], improved ventricular function [11] and reduced myocardial ischemic injury [12]. The value and limitations of thrombolytic therapy in early myocardial infarction has been recently reviewed by De Wood and Amsterdam [13]. One potential problem with recanalization, especially if this is attempted early after the occlusive event (i.e. at a time when salvage and recovery of function is optimal) is the occurrence of lifethreatening ventricular arrhythmias. In their review De Wood and Amsterdam [13] discuss five clinical studies in which rhythm disturbances have been examined following reperfusion. These arrhythmias were serious (ventricular tachycardia or fibrillation) in 5–22% of instances where successful recanalization was achieved and reperfusion was believed to be the cause of these rhythm disturbances. Together these studies clearly demonstrate that reperfusion can be associated with rhythm disturbances in man as well as in experimental animals. These arrhythmias are not difficult to control either with standard antiarrhythmic therapy or by cardioversion. One difficulty has been in deciding whether the arrhythmias occurred during occlusion or following recanalization and this can only be determined by immediate coronary angiography. This was done within seconds of the onset of arrhythmias in the study of Goldberg et al. [14]; in all twelve cases that developed arrhythmias during streptokinase infusion (i.e. 80% of those patients who underwent thrombolytic therapy) the use of coronary angiography demonstrated vessel patency. However, in one recent study [15] in which intravenous streptokinase was given early (mean treatment-onset time of 1.7 ± 0.8 hours) to 53 patients with acute myocardial infarction reperfusion arrhythmias were observed (11 instances of ventricular tachycardia; 7 episodes of fibrillation) just as often in those patients in which the coronary artery remained occluded as in those in which the artery became patent and in whom reperfusion was achieved.

In randomized studies [16–18] reperfusion arrhythmias were noted in 20%, 13% and 7%, respectively, of patients who received streptokinase. However, in one study [19] the incidence was as high as 73%. Some could argue that the occurrence of arrhythmias is a marker of successful reperfusion and, because they only occur after reperfusion following relatively short periods of occlusion, indicate that beneficial effects (e.g. salvage) have been achieved. Certainly, in experimental animals, reperfusion after longer periods does not result in either significant salvage or the occurrence of reperfusion arrhythmias.

Many studies using streptokinase, urokinase, anisolylated plasminogen-streptokinase activator complex or which have combined thrombolytic therapy with coronary angioplasty [e.g. 20–22] do not describe arrhythmias following successful recanalization. Whether this is because they did not in fact occur is unclear.

Reperfusion Arrhythmias After Coronary Revascularization

As one might expect, because of the relatively prolonged time interval between the onset of pain (and presumably coronary artery obstruction) and bypass grafting (CABG) this procedure is rarely associated with *new* onset, sustained and recurrent ventricular tachycardia or fibrillation, as opposed to exacerbation of chronic ventricular ectopic activity [23, 24]. In a more recent study [25] novo ventricular tachyarrhythmias occurred in just 12 of 1,675 patients undergoing CABG; one possible mechanism discussed was an increased dispersion of repolarization, secondary to reperfusion, creating a milieu supporting the development of reentrant tachyarrhythmias. These arrhythmias were resistant to lidocaine, quinidine, propranolol and mexiletine, but could be controlled with amiodarone.

Reperfusion Arrhythmias as a Cause of Sudden Cardiac Death

Although the contribution of reperfusion-induced arrhythmias to the incidence of sudden cardiac death is difficult to quantify there seems little doubt that this is one of many causes of lethal venticular arrhythmias in those patients that die suddenly [26].

The failure to demonstrate an occlusive thrombus in many patients who die suddenly and the recent demonstration [27, 28] of platelet emboli downstream from a platelet-fibrin thrombus in a major coronary artery in patients with unstable agina who had died suddenly might suggest reperfusion induced arrhythmias as a cause of death. Such platelet aggregates were found not only in those patients in which the main vessel was completely occluded but also in patients in which the occlusion was not total [28]. *One* explanation for sudden death in these patients is that the artery was occluded in life and that it was the break-up of the thrombus that allowed reperfusion, platelet dispersal and downstream occlusion by emboli of much smaller vessels. The reduction in the incidence of sudden cardiac death in patients with unstable angina given aspirin [29, 30] is also suggestive of an important platelet (and reperfusion?) component as contributing to the pathogenesis of this condition.

Factors Determining the Severity of Reperfusion-induced Arrhythmias

Evidence from experimental studies indicates that a number of factors modify the severity of reperfusion-induced arrhythmias. These are:

Occlusion time: The severity of reperfusion-induced arrhythmias is critically dependent upon the occlusion time, very short or prolonged periods of occlusion do not lead to severe ventricular arrhythmias on reperfusion, whereas intermediate periods do. This is illustrated for different kinds of coronary artery occlusion in anaesthetized rats in Table 1. Very short periods of occlusion (2 min) did not result in arrhythmias either during ischemia or on release. In contrast, five minute occlusions resulted in arrhythmias both during occlusion and especially on release, when the incidence of ventricular fibrillation was 56% and the mortality 44%. Longer periods of occlusion resulted in more severe ischemia (occlusion)-induced arrhythmias but progressively less severe arrhythmias on reperfu-

Table 1. The effect of the duration of coronary artery occlusion on the severity of ventricular arrhythmias occurring during occlusion and reperfusion. (Modified from Kane KA, Parratt JR & Williams FM (1984) Br J Pharmac 82, 349–357)

Duration of occlusion (min)	n	Arrhythmias during occlusion					Arrhythmias on reperfusion				
		Total VEBs	VEBs/min	% VT	% VF	% Mortality	Total VEBs	VEBs/min	% VT	% VF	% Mortality
2	6	0	0	0	0	0	2.4±1.0	–	0	0	0
5	16	159±9	32	56	0	0	591±140	529	100	56	44
15	13	991±213	66	90	54	23	302±120	149	70	50	8
20	9	1543±678	77	79	44	22	87±40	42	14	0	0
30	10	1483±419	49	100	30	10	72±20	70	37.5	0	0

Given are the total number of ventricular ectopic beats (VEBs), the number of VEBs per min, the percentage incidence of ventricular tachycardia (VT), of ventricular fibrillation (VF) and the mortality.

Table 2. Severity of ventricular arrhythmias occurring during the first minute of reperfusion following either a 5 or 15 min coronary artery occlusion: compared with arrhythmias occurring during the corresponding time periods with the occlusion still present. (Modified from Kane KA, Parratt JR & Williams FM (1984) Br J Pharmac 82, 349–357)

Time	n	Mean number of VEB's (over 1 min)	% VT	% VF	Duration of VT
5–6 min occlusion	27	70±24	44	7	3.9±1.5
5–6 min reperfusion	16	359±39[a]	100[a]	56[a]	11.8±4.0
15–16 min occlusion	17	18±8.5	18	6	2.8±2
15–16 min reperfusion	10	156±34[a]	70[a]	50[a]	12.2±4

The table shows the mean number of ventricular ectopic beats (VEB's), the incidence and duration of ventricular tachycardia (VT) and the incidence of ventricular fibrillation (VF) over the 1 min period.
[a] $p < 0.01$

sion. For example, 20 or 30 min periods of occlusion resulted in only a few ectopic beats and some tachycardia on release but no fibrillation (Table 1).

A similar time course is seen in other species. In dogs for example, the highest incidence (80-95%) of fibrillation on reperfusion is seen following 30-40 minutes of coronary artery occlusion [31]. An example of arrhythmias occurring on occlusion and after release is shown in Figure 1.

It is important to emphasize that reperfusion-induced arrhythmias are not simply a continuation of those arrhythmias occurring during the occlusion period itself. This is also clear from Figure 1 (where the dog was in sinus rhythm immediately before the release of the occlusive device) and from Table 2 which compares occlusion and reperfusion arrhythmias at two different times (5-6 and 15-16 minutes). Clearly, reperfusion arrhythmias are more serious than those that occur, over the same period, during ischemia alone. Indeed, in the anesthetized greyhound dog model we have used over many years [e.g. 32] the incidence of ventricular fibrillation was 80-95% on reperfusion following a 40 minute coronary artery occlusion but only 20-25% at any time during the occlusion period itself. The fact that ventricular fibrillation is much more common following reperfusion than during ischemia is both well documented and poorly appreciated.

The relevance of occlusion time to the severity of arrhythmias following reperfusion presumably also applies to the human heart. Such evidence is however difficult to accumulate. The impression is that although early reperfusion (e.g. by thrombolysis in patients with an occlusive thrombus) is more likely to result in arrhythmias than reperfusion many hours after the occlusive event, the time scale must be very different to that in anesthetized rats and dogs. One of the determining factors may well be heart rate and it is possible that inducing bradycardia might be one way of reducing the severity of reperfusion-induced arrhythmias.

Rate of reperfusion – rapid versus gradual: Another reason why reperfusion-induced arrhythmias appear to be less common in the human heart might be that recanalization of an occluded artery is almost certainly more gradual than in the experimental situation where the mechanical occlusive device is suddenly removed. There is recent experimental evidence that sudden reperfusion (i.e. close-chest anesthetized dogs subjected to a three hour intracoronary balloon occlusion) led to a higher frequency of premature ventricular complexes (227 ± 167) than staged reperfusion (partial release followed by balloon deflation and full reperfusion), when the frequency of PVC's was only 14 ± 23 [33]. It seems that more gradual reperfusion in the clinical situation could reduce the persistence of ventricular dysfunction and the incidence of serious reperfusion arrhythmias.

Possible Mechanisms of Reperfusion-induced Arrhythmias in Clinical Situations; Can These Be Prevented by Drugs?

It is not the intention here to deal with the precise electrophysiological mechanisms through which reperfusion-induced arrhythmias arise. Only one highly

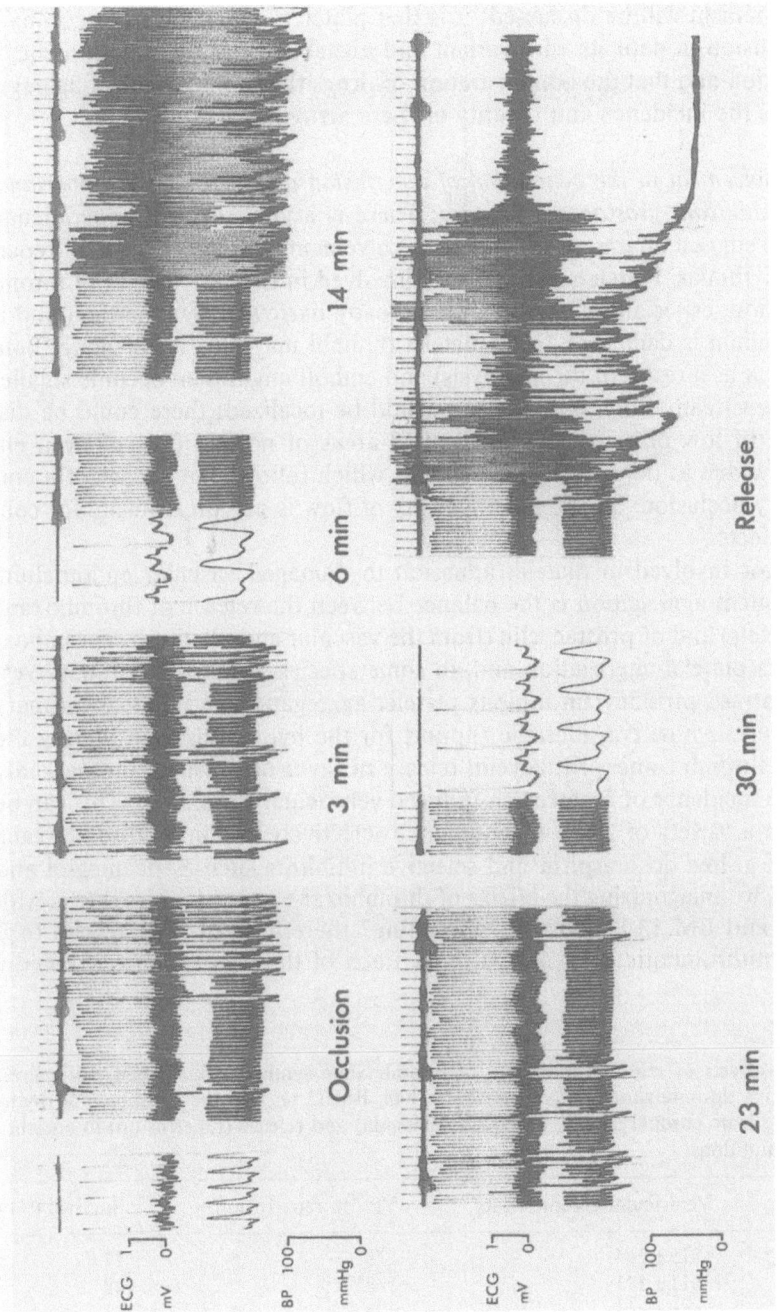

Fig. 1. Arrhythmias occurring at different times during a 40 minute occlusion of the anterior descending branch of the left coronary artery in an anesthetized dog. Ventricular ectopic activity is especially pronounced between 10 and 20 minutes but the dog is in sinus rhythm (although with pronounced ST-segment depression) at 30–40 minutes. Sudden reperfusion at 40 minutes lead to fibrillation within a few seconds of blood flow restoration

likely mechanism will be discussed; it is that platelets are involved in coronary artery occlusion in patients with variant and unstable angina and with myocardial infarction and that the administration of drugs that inhibit platelet aggregation reduce the incidence and severity of these arrhythmias.

Platelet involvement in the generation of reperfusion arrhythmias; the importance of the thromboxane-prostacyclin balance: There is a good deal of experimental evidence to suggest an important platelet involvement in the generation of reperfusion arrhythmias. Platelets are certainly involved in the early stages of thrombus formation, especially if the lumen is already narrowed by atheroma and if the endothelium is damaged. These platelet thrombi may then disintegrate spontaneously (or as a result of thrombolysis) and emboli might then occlude smaller vessels downstream. Such obstructions would be localized; there could be discrete areas of low or zero flow adjacent to areas of normal flow or even enhanced flow due to the hyperemic response which follows the release of a coronary artery occlusion. Such a heterogeneity of flow is one prerequisite for conduction defects.

One factor involved in platelet adhesion to damaged vascular endothelium and subsequent aggregation is the balance between the release of thromboxane (from platelets) and of prostacyclin (from the vascular endothelium). Thromboxane induces platelet aggregation and, in some species, constricts coronary vessels; in contrast, prostacyclin inhibits platelet aggregation and dilates coronary vessels. There is now considerable support for the hypothesis that altering the balance of thromboxane/prostacyclin release in favor of prostacyclin markedly reduces the incidence of reperfusion-induced ventricular fibrillation. This can be achieved in a variety of ways which include selectively inhibiting thromboxane synthesis (e.g. low dose aspirin and selective inhibitors such as dazmegrel and dazoxiben), by antagonizing the effects of thromboxane at receptor level (e.g. with AH 23848 and BM 13.177) or by "promoting" the effects of prostacyclin (e.g. with the antithrombotic drug nafazatrom). Each of these procedures markedly

Table 3. The effects of selective inhibition of thromboxane synthesis (dazoxiben, dazmegrel) and of selective thromboxane antagonists (AH 23848, BM 13.177) on the severity of arrhythmias resulting from coronary artery occlusion (ischemia) and release (reperfusion) in anesthetized greyhound dogs

	Ventricular ectopic beats	VF (on reperfusion)	Survival (%)
Controls	875 ± 264	7/8	12.5
Dazoxiben	511 ± 141	1/8[a]	88[a]
Controls	832 ± 158	7/9	20
Dazmegrel	193 ± 126[a]	2/7[a]	71[a]
Controls	736 ± 155	7/8	11
AH 23848	339 ± 111	2/8	67
Controls	1084 ± 159	6/7	10
BM 13.177	544 ± 179[b]	4/9[c]	50[b]

[a] $p < 0.01$ [b] $p < 0.05$ [c] $p < 0.07$

reduces the incidence of ventricular fibrillation on reperfusion and increases survival from an ischemic reperfusion insult (Table 3). This evidence has been recently reviewed [31, 32] and collectively suggests an important role in the generation of these arrhythmias of platelet/vessel wall interactions. This is further supported by the clinical evidence of a markedly reduced mortality in patients with unstable angina taking normal therapeutic doses of aspirin [29, 30].

References

1. Tennant R, Wiggers CJ (1935) The effect of coronary occlusion on myocardial contraction. Am J Physiol 112:351–361
2. Houston DS, Shepherd JT, Vanhoutte PM (1986) Aggregating human platelets cause direct contraction and endothelium-dependent relaxation of isolated canine coronary arteries. J Clin Invest 78:539–544
3. Maseri A (1984) Spasm and dynamic coronary stenoses. J Cardiovasc Pharmacol 6:S683–S690
4. Parratt JR (1985) Coronary vascular endothelium, spasm and reperfusion arrhythmias; experimental approaches. In: Hugenholtz PG, Goldman BS (eds) Unstable Angina. Schattauer Verlag: Stuttgart pp 19–28
5. Maseri A, Severi S, Marzullo P (1982) Role of coronary arterial spasm in sudden coronary ischemic death. Am NY Acad Sci 382:204–217
6. Kerin NZ, Rubenfire M, Willens HJ, Rao P, Cascade PN (1983) The mechanism of dysrhythmias in variant angina pectoris: occlusive versus reperfusion Am Heart J 106:1332–1340
7. Arnim Th v, Gerbig HW, Erath A (1985) Arrhythmien im Zusammenhang mit transienten ST-Hebungen bei Prinzmetal-Angina: Auslosung durch Okklusion und Reperfusion. Z Kardiol 74:585–589
8. Maroko PR, Libby P, Ginks WR, et al (1972) Coronary artery reperfusion. II Reduction of infarct size at one week after coronary artery occlusion. J Clin Invest 51:2717–2723
9. Kennedy JW, Ritchie JL, Davis KB, Fritz JK (1983) Western Washington randomized trial of intracoronary streptokinase in acute myocardial infarction. N Engl J Med 309:1477–1482
10. Marder VJ, Francis CW (1984) Thrombolytic therapy for acute transmural myocardial infarction; intracoronary versus intravenous. Am J Med 77:921–928
11. Reduto LW, Smalling RW, Freurd GC, Gould KL (1981) Intracoronary infusion of streptokinase in patients with acute myocardial infarction: effects of reperfusion on left ventricular performance. Am J Cardiol 48:403–409
12. Markis JE, Malagold, Parker JA (1981) Myocardial salvage after intracoronary thrombolysis with streptokinase in acute myocardial infarction: assessment by intracoronary thallium-201. N Engl J Med 305:777–782
13. DeWood MA, Amsterdam EA (1985) Value and limitations of thrombolytic therapy in early acute transmural myocardial infarction. Cardiol 72:255–279
14. Goldberg S, Grierspon AJ, Urban PL, et al (1983) Reperfusion arrhythmia: a marker of intracoronary thrombolysis during acute myocardial infarction. Am Heart J 105:26–35
15. Koren G, Weiss AT, Hasin Y, et al (1985) Prevention of myocardial damage in acute myocardial ischemia by early treatment with intravenous streptokinase. N Engl J Med 313:1384–1389
16. Khaja F, Walton JA, Brymer JF, et al (1983) Intracoronary fibrinolytic therapy in acute myocardial infarction. Report of a prospective randomised trial. N Engl J Med 308:1305–1311
17. Anderson JL, Marshall HW, Bray BE, et al (1983) A randomised trial of intracoronary streptokinase in the treatment of acute myocardial infarction. N Engl J Med 308:1312–1318

18. Olson HG, Butman SM, Piters KM, et al (1986) A randomized controlled trial of intravenous streptokinase in evolving acute myocardial infarction. Am Heart J 111:1021-1029

19. Kuck K-H, Jannasch B, Schluter M, Schofer J, Mathey DG (1985) Ineffektive lidocainprophylaxe von reperfusionsarrhythmien bei patienten mit akutem myokardinfarkt. Z Kardiol 74:185-190

20. Marder VJ, Rothbard RL, Fitzpatrick PG, Francis CW (1986) Rapid lysis of coronary artery thrombi with anisoylated plasminogen: streptokinase activator complex. Annals Intern Med 104:304-310

21. Kitazume H, Iwama T, Suzuki A (1986) Combined thrombolytic therapy and coronary angioplasty for acute myocardial infarction. Am Heart J 111:826-832

22. Peterson MB, Machaj V, Block PC, Palacios I, Philbin D, Watkins WD (1986) Thromboxane release during percutaneous transluminal coronary angioplasty. Am Heart J 111:1-6

23. de Soyza N, Therabadu PN, Murphy ML, Kane JJ, Doherty JE (1981) Ventricular arrhythmia before and after orto-coronary bypass surgery. Int J Cardiol 1:123-130

24. Michelson EL, Morganroth J, MacVaugh H (1979) Postoperative arrhythmias after coronary artery and cardiac valvular surgery detected by longterm electrocardiographic monitoring. Am Heart J 97:442-448

25. Topol EJ, Lerman BB, Baughman KL et al (1986) De novo refractory ventricular tachyarrhythmias after coronary revascularization. Am J Cardiol 57:57-59

26. Oliver MF (1982) Sudden cardiac death – an overview. In: Parratt JR (ed) Early arrhythmias resulting from myocardial ischaemia. New York: Oxford University Press, pp 1-13

27. Falk E (1985) Unstable angina with fatal outcome: dynamic coronary thrombosis leading to infarction and/or sudden death. Circulation 71:699-711

28. Davies MJ, Thomas AC, Knapman PA, Hangartner JR (1986) Intramyocardial platelet aggregation in patients with unstable angina suffering sudden ischemic cardiac death. Circulation 73:418-427

29. Lewis HD Jr, Davis JM, Archibald DG, et al (1986) Protective effects of aspirin against acute myocardial infarction and death in men with unstable angina: results of a Veterans Administration cooperative study. N Engl J Med 309:396-403

30. Cairns JA, Gent M, Singer J, et al (1985) Aspirin, Sulfinpyrazone, or both in unstable angina. N Engl J Med 313:1369-1375

31. Parratt JR, Coker SJ, Wainwright CL (1987) Eicosanoids and susceptibility to ventricular arrhythmias during myocardial ischaemia and reperfusion. J Mol Cell Cardiol (in press)

32. Parratt JR, Coker SJ (1985) Arachidonic acid cascade and the generation of ischaemia and reperfusion-induced ventricular arrhythmias. J Cardiovasc Pharmac 7 (Supp 5) 565-570

33. Yamazaki S, Fujibayashi Y, Rajagopalan RE, Meerbaum S, Corday E (1986) Effects of staged versus sudden reperfusion after acute coronary occlusion in the dog. J Am Coll Cardiol 3:564-72

Positron Emission Tomography for the Assessment of Myocardial Viability in Acute Myocardial Infarction

C. Nienaber, M. Schwaiger, and H. R. Schelbert

Introduction

With the emergence of therapeutic modalities to re-establish regional blood flow to jeopardized myocardium in patients with acute myocardial infarction, there is increased interest in the pathophysiology of tissue reperfusion [1–4]. Experimental and clinical studies in humans suggest a transition from reversible ischemic injury to necrosis within 3 to 6 hours which indicates the temporal dependence of beneficial effects of thrombolytic therapy [5–8]. However, early spontaneous recanalization and the individual degree of residual collateral blood flow might significantly influence the time course of infarct development [8]. In addition, energy demand during the acute phase also affects the evolution of tissue infarction [9, 10]. Consequently, the assessment of the extent and stage of the infarction process from the time elapsed from onset of symptoms is difficult but crucial in a given patient [11]. Clinical and histologic evidence indicates the presence of a mixture of necrotic and ischemic but viable myocytes even in late stages. The clinically important task is to identify "incomplete necrosis" which would benefit from therapeutic interventions. Evaluation of blood flow and regional function cannot distinguish between viable but "stunned" from necrotic myocardium. Based on experimental studies that have revealed enhanced glucose utilization relative to blood flow in ischemic but viable tissue [12, 13], the purpose of this study is
a) to assess regional myocardial glucose metabolism in acute myocardial infarction to define the stage of the infarction process, and
b) to compare regional metabolic activity with the outcome of regional function.

Methods

Study Patients

A group of 15 patients (mean age 57 years; 41–80 yrs) with acute myocardial infarction by enzyme and EKG criteria were studied. Ten patients had anterior and five patients had inferior infarctions. The mean CKMB fraction was 63.9 ± 38.1 U/1. The mean interval from admission to the PET study was 5.1 days (2–14 days). Coronary arteriography and left ventriculography was performed in all patients using the femoral approach. Residual stenosis was determined visually by a consensus reading; collateral blood flow in the infarct area was considered when segments of the infarct-related artery was opacified in retrograde.

Positron Emission Tomography (PET)

PET imaging was performed with the ECAT II tomograph (CTI, Knoxville, TN). Regional myocardial blood flow was assessed with N-13 ammonia (20 mCi) and exogenous glucose utilization with F-18 2-deoxyglucose (10 mCi) after an overnight fast as previously described [14]. Cross-sectional imaging following each tracer injection was performed at corresponding levels. The images were analyzed with an operated-interactive program using circumferential profile techniques [14]. Observed normalized counts in each PET scan were compared to the limits established from a normal database.

Regional reductions in N-13 ammonia uptake below 2 SD identified segments of reduced blood flow. Persistence or absence of metabolic activity in these segments were defined by regional F-18 2-deoxyglucose uptake. Scar tissue was defined as concordant segmental reduction of N-13 and F-18 counts of at least 2 SD below normal in two or more adjacent segments. Tissue viability was defined as the F-18/N-13 count ratio greater than 2 SD above normal in two or more adjacent segments [14]. For comparison of regional myocardial N-13 and F-18 counts with regional function, the left ventricle was divided into five segments: anterior, septal, apical, lateral and infero posterior (14), each corresponding to a segment on the PET images. Segmental function was determined at the time of the PET study and followed up at 6.0 ± 4.6 weeks later utilized two-dimensional echocardiography (13 cases) or radionuclide angiography (2 cases). Regional wall motion was graded on a 4 point scale from -1 (dyskinesia) to $+3$ (normal).

Statistics

Mean values and SD are given. Data were compared by paired and unpaired Student's t-test. A probability level of <0.05 was required for statistical significance.

Results

PET was performed at 54 ± 12 hours after acute symptoms and revealed regional blood flow abnormalities in all 15 patients. In 37 segments N-13 ammonia flow was below normal limits. In 20 of these 37 segments there was a decrease in flow as matched by a corresponding decrease in F-18 2-deoxyglucose uptake. These segments are referred to as "PET infarction" (Fig. 1). The cross-sectional left ventricular (LV) tomogram was obtained 42 hours after onset of symptoms in a patient with anterior infarction. Flow images revealed reduced blood flow to

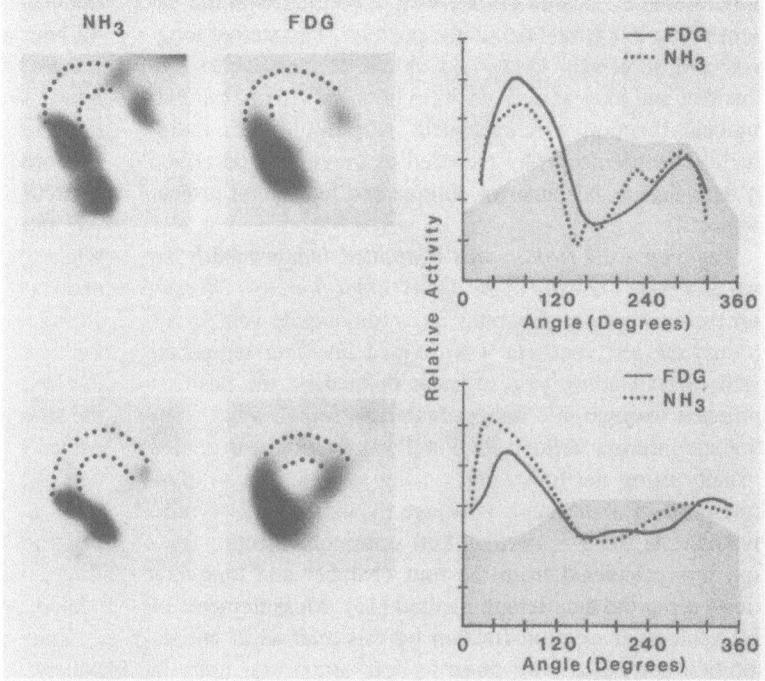

Fig. 1. Patient with anterior "PET infarction" pattern (i.e., matched regional decrease in FDG and NH₃) 42 hours after onset of symptoms. Two planes through the mid- and distal left ventricle are displayed. Uptake of both N-13 ammonia and F-18 deoxyglucose is decreased in anteroseptal segments delineated by the dotted lines. The corresponding circumferential profiles on the right show N-13 and F-18 in both planes as a matched decrease in activity from 160° to 300°. The shaded areas represent the lower limits of normal

the anterior and septal and apical segments. Glucose utilization was concordantly decreased in these segments ("PET infarction"). Regional wall motion ranged from anterior akinesia to apical dyskinesia. In 17 segments, an increase in regional F-18 2-deoxyglucose relative to blood flow was documented. These segments exhibited a regional mismatch of flow and glucose utilization and were referred to as "PET viability". Figure 2 depicts the PET study in a patient four days after acute anterior infarction. Diminished regional perfusion was noted in the anterior and septal segments. In contrast to Figure 1, metabolic imaging with F-18 2-deoxyglucose demonstrated enhanced glucose uptake in the areas of severely reduced flow (i.e., a "mismatch" pattern). Wall motion studies revealed akinesia of compromised but viable anterior and septal segments.

Table 1 summarizes the results in all patients. Ten patients revealed "PET viability" in segments with a mismatch, while five patients exhibited a "PET infarction" pattern. In the 37 LV segments with critically impaired flow, 17 (46%) showed a mismatch pattern indicative of viability. Relative N-13 ammonia uptake was similarly decreased in segments with mismatch versus matching glucose reduction ($48 \pm 16\%$ vs $46 \pm 7.4\%$; NS).

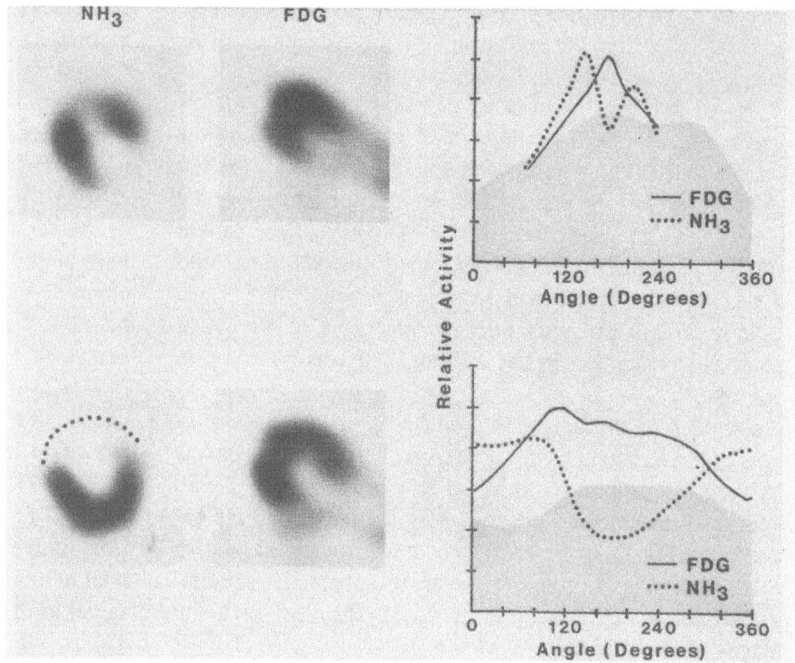

Fig. 2. Example of a study revealing "PET viability" 40 hours after onset of symptoms. There is diminished perfusion (NH₃) in anterior and septal segments in the presence of enhanced FDG uptake (i.e., a mismatch pattern). The corresponding circumferential profiles of relative N-13 and F-18 activity distribution show a mismatch of tracer uptake from 80° to 280° indicative of tissue viability. The shaded area shows the lower limits of normal

Table 1. Summary of PET findings in 15 patients (37 segments) after myocardial infarction

	"PET viable"	PET infarcted
No. of patients	10	5
No. of segments	17 (46%)	20 (54%)
Early data		
Wall motion	0.34±0.84	0.67±0.83
LVEF, %	44.4±15.0	39.0±5.0
Follow-up data		
Wall motion	1.12±1.4[a]	0.69±0.99
LVEF, %	46.7±13.0	44.4±14.0

[a] p<0.01 from early data

Segmental wall motion on the day of the PET study was compared to the follow-up study at 6±4.6 weeks. In the early stage after infarction, myocardial function was impaired in all segments with impaired N-13 ammonia flow with a mean wall motion score of 0.52±0.82. There was no difference between segment in patients with or without F-18 2-deoxyglucose uptake (0.67±0.83 vs

Table 2. Segmental pattern of blood flow (NH₃) and glucose utilization (FDG) in 15 patients with acute myocardial infarction

	Infarct-Related Artery	
	Occlusion (8 patients)	Antegrade Flow (7 patients)
	No. of segments	
Decreased blood flow	20 –	17
Decreased glucose utilization	16 (5)ᵃ	4
Decreased glucose utilization	4 (2)ᵃ	13

ᵃ No. of segments with collateral flow.

0.34±0.84; NS). The LV ejection fraction (EF) averaged 45.4±16% in all patients. There was no difference in LVEF in patients with or without enhanced F-18 2-deoxyglucose uptake (44.4±15% vs 39.0±5%; NS).

The follow-up measurements of segmental LV function revealed no change in wall motion in "PET infarction" segments. In contrast, wall motion improved in "PET viable"egments from the initial to the follow-up study from 0.34±0.84 to 1.12±1.4; p<0.01. However, there was a heterogeneous response. Nine of the 17 segments showed improved regional wall motion as defined by improvement of more than 1 score grade. In the remaining eight segments regional function was unchanged in six and deteriorated in two segments. Subsequently, no significant improvement in global LV function was detected. Of the patients with F-18 2-deoxyglucose/N-13 ammonia mismatch, five individuals had evidence of postinfarction angina. One patient died with "PET infarction" in cardiogenic shock on day 2.

Table 2 summarizes the results of coronary angiography in the study group. The infarct-related vessel was occluded in eight patients and patent in seven patients. Sixteen of the 20 segments related to the territory in the occluded vessel which revealed a matched decrease in flow and metabolism, whereas four segments demonstrated maintained glucose uptake. In contrast, of the 17 segments in the territory of patent infarct-related vessels, 13 segments had evidence of mismatch with maintained or enhanced glucose utilization, while only four demonstrated a matched decrease in flow and metabolism. Significant collateral perfusion was documented in seven segments distal to a complete occlusion. Two of these segments showed a "mismatch pattern" and five had a concordant decrease in flow and metabolism.

Discussion

Results of this clinical trial showed that metabolic imaging with PET identified viable but compromised tissue in the setting of myocardial infarction. Regional wall motion did not improve in any of the myocardial segments with a matched decrease in blood flow and glucose utilization early after infarction. However, patients with a "mismatch", i.e., with decreased blood flow but maintained enhanced regional glucose uptake in the subacute post-infarction period revealed a variable outcome. This suggests a mixture of viable and necrotic myocytes in certain patients. The relative contribution of viable myocardium in the area at risk appears to reflect the severity of the ischemic injury and possibly a regional functional outcome.

Methodological Considerations

A semi-quantitative approach and previously established critera were used to evaluate regional distribution of N-13 ammonia and F-18 2-deoxyglucose [15]. Since the tomograph used in this study had a low temporal (90 seconds) and spatial (1.7 cm) resolution, no quantitative measurements were performed. N-13 ammonia was validated previously as a flow tracer in experimental and clinical studies [16, 17]. F-18 2-deoxyglucose traces transmembraneous glucose transport, phosphorylation and tissue glucose utilization [13, 14, 18]. Comparison of both tracers allows specific identification of scar and viable tissue [14]. The metabolic data were correlated to immediate and follow-up regional wall motion analysis which revealed akinesis in all segments with N-13 ammonia perfusion defects early after infarction. However, factors such as increasing collateralization or spontaneous reperfusion favor the presence of injured but viable tissue in close proximity to necrotic tissue and suggest spatial and temporal heterogeneity of ischemic injury with co-existing tissue islands of different degrees of damage. These segments can be identified by residual or even increased glucose utilization. Contractile function recovers slowly from previous "stunning", while metabolic activity returns earlier and might herald subsequent recovery of function. This observation and documentation in patients without therapeutic interventions is even more important in view of the timing and strategy of revascularization procedures.

Tillisch et al. [17] documented the predictive value of maintained glucose utilization in segments with disturbed flow for functional recovery after bypass surgery, further supporting the concept of local glucose uptake to identify compromised tissue that is potentially salvageable. In contrast, in our patients, no intervention was performed to revascularize and the functional outcome of segments with glucose uptake was variable, despite a significant improvement in mean wall motion score in "PET viable" segments. Thus, the final survival and recovery of function is likely to depend on residual perfusion via collaterals or with spontaneous revascularization. F-18 2-deoxyglucose was found in 12 of 17 segments associated with a patent coronary artery on angiography; two additional segments were supplied in retrograde by collaterals. All segments with a matched decrease in flow and glucose metabolism were situated in the vascular territory of an occluded coronary artery.

The potential reasons for only about 50% of the "PET viable" segments to recover functionally may in some cases be too early to evaluate functional recovery. Moreover, blood flow could have remained severely depressed over a prolonged time period in the absence of recanalization or recruitment of collateral flow. Regional F-18 2-deoxyglucose uptake may thus represent "chronic ischemia" or adaptation of chronic hypoxia as described in postinfarction patients.

Serial metabolic PET studies in a larger number of patients are needed to expose more precisely the time course of ischemic cell death and the predictive ability of PET to identify salvageable myocardium at risk. In addition, quantitative data on blood flow and glucose metabolism may allow more accurate assessment of the degree of ischemia and the quantity of residual viable tissue to better predict the fate of injured myocardium. On the basis of such measurements, guidelines for therapeutic interventions can be developed and patients identified for immediate aggressive therapy [19, 20].

Acknowledgements: The authors would like to thank M. Lee Griswold for preparing and the illustrations and Kerry Engber for her assistance in preparing this manuscript.

References

1. Rentrop P, Blanke H, Karsch KR, Kaiser H, Kostering H, Leitz K (1981) Selective intracoronary thrombolysis in acute myocardial infarction and unstable angina pectoris. Circulation 63:307–317
2. Mathey DG, Kuck KH, Tilsner V, Krebber HJ, Bleifeld W (1981) Nonsurgical coronary artery recanalization in acute transmural myocardial infarction. Circulation 63:489–497
3. Reduto LA, Freund GC, Gaeta JM, Smalling RW, Lewis B, Bould KL (1981) Coronary artery reperfusion in acute myocardial infarction: Beneficial effects of intracoronary streptokinase on left ventricular salvage and performance. Am Heart J 102:1168–1175
4. Ganz W, Buchbinder N, Marcus H, et al (1981) Intracoronary thrombolysis in evolving myocardial infarction. Am Heart J 101:4–15
5. Reimer KA, Lowe JE, Rasmussen MM, Jennings RE (1977) The wavefront phenomenon of ischemic cell death. I. Myocardial infarct size vs duration of coronary occlusion in dogs. Circulation 56:786–794
6. Vokonas PS, Malsky PM, Paul SJ, Robbins SL, Hood WB (1978) Radioautographic studies in experimental myocardial infarction: Profiles of ischemic blood flow and quantification of infarct size of ischemic zone. Am J Cardiol 42:62–72
7. Mathey DG, Sheehan FH, Schofer J, et al (1985) Time from onset of symptoms to thrombolytic therapy: A major determinant of myocardial salvage in patients with acute transmural infarction. J Am Coll Cardiol 6:518–525
8. Nienaber C, Gottwik M, Winkler B, Schaper W (1983) The relationship between the perfusion deficit, infarct size and time after experimental coronary occlusion. Basic Res Cardiol 78:210–216
9. Ong L, Reiser P, Coromilas J, Scherr L, Morrison J (1983) Left ventricular function and rapid release of creatine kinase-MB in acute myocardial infarction – evidence for spontaneous reperfusion. N Engl J Med 309:1–6
10. Nienaber CA, Spielmann RP, Rozza A, Montz R, Bleifeld W, Mathey DG (1985) Prevalence of spontaneous coronary thrombolysis and its relation to left ventricular function. Eur Heart J E6:145–153
11. Sniderman AD, Beaudry JP, Rahal DP (1983) Early recognition of the patient at late high risk: incomplete infarction and vulnerable myocardium. Am J Cardiol 52:669–673
12. Bergmann SR, Lerch RA, Fox KAA, et al (1982) Temporal dependence of beneficial effects of coronary thombolysis characterized by positron tomography. Am J Med 73:573–581
13. Schwaiger M, Schelbert HR, Ellison D, et al (1985) Sustained regional abnormalities in cardiac metabolism after transient ischemia in the chronic dog model. J Am Coll Cardiol 6:336–347

14. Marshall RC, Tillisch JH, Phelps ME, et al (1983) Identification and differentiation of resting myocardial ischemia and infarction in man with positron computed tomography, ^{18}F-labeled fluorodeoxyglucose and N-13 ammonia. Circulation 64:766–778
15. Hoffman EJ, Huang SC, Phelps ME (1979) Quantitation in positron emission computed tomography. I. Effects of object size. J Comput Assist Tomogr 3:299–308
16. Schelbert HR, Phelps ME, Huang SC, et al (1981) N-13 ammonia as an indicator of myocardial blood flow. Circulation 63:1259–1272
17. Tillisch J, Brunken R, Marshal R, Schwaiger M, Phelps M, Schelbert HR (1986) Prediction of the reversibility of cardiac wall motion abnormalities using positron tomography, [18]fluorodeoxyglucose and ^{13}N-ammonia. N Engl J Med 314:884–888
18. Geltman EM, Biello D, Welch MJ, Terr-Pogossian MM, Roberts R, Sobel BE (1982) Characterization of nontransmural myocardial infarction by positron-emission tomography. Circulation 65:747–755
19. Meyer J, Merx W, Schmitz H, et al (1982) Percutaneous transluminal coronary angioplasty immediately after intracoronary streptolysis of transmural myocardial infarction. Circulation 66:905–913
20. DeWood MA, Spores J, Notske RN, et al (1979) Medical and surgical management of myocardial infarction. Am J Cardiol 44:1356–1368

Approaches for the Treatment of Residual Coronary Lesions Following Thrombolysis

P. L. da Luz, A. C. Palandri Chagas, and F. Pileggi

Introduction

Once established that the thrombus responsible for acute myocardial infarction (AMI) can be lysed by thrombolytic agents or even mechanically disrupted, we were left with the problem of the residual coronary lesion observed in most patients. The answer(s) require some considerations concerning the nature of the occlusive phenomenon itself, its time-course as well as other factors that influence the prognosis of the patient. In this chapter, the several ways in which this question has been approached will be examined.

The Nature of the Occlusive Lesion

Occlusive lesions in AMI are formed by a fresh thrombus overlying an atherosclerotic plaque in the large majority of patients. Only a few develop a fresh thrombus in angiographically normal coronaries. As assessed by cineangiography, the magnitude of residual coronary lesions vary significantly; Serruys et al [1], utilizing a computerized system, found a median value of 58%: the 10th percentile value was 37% and the 90th, 74%; less than 50% stenosis were found in 31% of patients and more than 70% was encountered in only 19%. Other authors [2] have found greater degrees of stenosis, mostly in the 75% range. Repeat angiograms within one to two weeks show that the stenosis remain unchanged in most patients but spontaneous reductions have been noticed in a minority of patients; for instance, it was encountered in 14% of cases in the TAMI study [3], to an extent that obviated the need for subsequent angioplasty. This evidently suggest that the thrombus component of the obstruction had not been completely removed by thrombolysis.

Factors that may have precipitated the initial coronary occlusion, namely spasm, endothelial injury, local platelet aggregation and intra-plaque hemorrhage are not removed by thrombolysis, and therefore may continue to promote conditions for repeat occlusions.

Incidence of Re-occlusion and its Significance

Several studies have found that re-occlusion rate amounts to as much as 19% within a week of thrombolysis [4]. The relationship between re-occlusion and the degree of residual stenosis has been examined in different studies. Gold et al. [5]

reported that re-occlusion occurred only in patients with more than 80% residual stenosis who had received intravenous recombinant tissue-plasminogen activator (rt-PA). Harrison et al. [6], using quantitative angiography, reported that arterial lumens of less than 0.4 mm² consistently showed thrombosis, also calling attention to geometric factors in re-stenosis. On the other hand, Nicklas et al. [7] found that the increase in coronary blood flow measured in the great cardiac vein following thrombolysis or angioplasty in patients with acute anterior myocardial infarction was inversely related to the degree of residual stenosis as well as the duration of previous ischemia; increments in flow were highly predictive of functional recovery as assessed by ejection fraction 7 to 10 days later. Improvement in great cardiac vein flow was found only in patients with stenosis of 50% or less. Hence, re-occlusion is primarily related to the degree of the residual lesion as well as the duration of ischemia.

Re-occlusion may induce different physiological consequences, namely nonfatal myocardial infarction, angina without infarction, true silent occlusion and even sudden death. Re-infarction has been examined specifically in some large trials. In the largest populational study of intravenous streptokinase (SK), the GISSI trial [8], non-fatal re-infarction was nearly twice as common among treated patients as among controls by 3 weeks after infarction; the overall incidence was quite low (4.1%) among treated patients, although post-thrombolysis anti-coagulation regimen was not standardized, Schaer et al. [4] recently reviewed extensively this issue. By pooling data of nine SK trials, he found a 8.2% incidence of early re-infarction in 938 treated patients. The incidence of re-infarction ranged from 3.2 to 17.2%. In most trials systemic anticoagulation with heparin was used, while antiplatelet agents were used in fewer. In the three studies using rt-PA the pooled re-infarction rate was 9.4% [9–11]. In the TAMI trial [3], in which only patients with patent coronaries following intravenous rt-PA were examined, the incidence of re-infarction was 12% in 197 patients submitted to either immediate or delayed (7 to 10 days post-AMI) angioplasty. Therefore, re-occlusion rate seems to be slightly higher when only patent vessels are considered than when all patients who receive thrombolytic therapy are included, regardless of whether the infarct-related artery was opened or not. In the TAMI trial cross-over to emergency angioplasty was 16% in the delayed treatment group as compared to only 5% in the immediate angioplasty group.

In the ISAM trial [12], after 21 days treated patients had twice more re-infarctions than controls, although heparin and eventually coumadin had been used. Prevalence of re-infarction was 2.4%. Mortality at 7 months of follow-up was almost identical in SK- and in placebo-treated patient, despite reductions in infarct size and increases in regional ejection fraction in SK treated patients. Furthermore, re-infarction was higher in the SK than in the placebo group. Thus, SK patients behaved as non-Q wave infarctions in that re-occlusion was very frequent and long-term prognosis no different than in transmural AMI.

Recurrent angina is frequent among patients with successful reperfusion. In the extensive review of Schaer et al [4], in five trials there was no difference in the incidence of angina between controls (16.1%) and treated patients (15.7%). Schaer et al. also concluded that recurrent angina had been more frequent in patients with a patent infarct-related artery (34.8%). The interpretation of recurrent angina by itself is difficult because it may be related to lesions in distant arteries as well as re-stenosis of the treated artery.

The incidence of sudden death in patients treated with thrombolytic agents is not really known. In the Western Washington trial [13], 50% of deaths in the year following SK treatment were sudden. Although likely significant, the incidence of sudden death has not been systemically studied in large numbers of patients following thrombolysis, its importance thus awaits more definitive assessment.

Therefore, residual stenosis may limit significantly the efficacy of acute reperfusion and may adversely affect longterm prognosis through re-infarction, angina and death.

The Medical Option

Gold et al. [5] have shown that rt-PA infusion in small dosis (10 mg/hour during 4 hours), following its administration for thrombolysis purposes, greatly reduces the chances of re-stenosis within 10 days. Its long-term effect, however, has not been demonstrated. Anticoagulation with heparin or oral drugs as well as antiplatelet agents have been generally disappointing for prevention of re-occlusions. Hence, medical treatment should probably be reserved for patients with small (< 50%), peripheral lesions involving small areas of myocardium at risk. In addition to anticoagulants, it should include calcium blocking agents, vasodilators and eventually anti-arrhythmic drugs.

Percutaneous Transluminal Coronary Angioplasty (PTCA)

PTCA has been used as single therapy as well as adjunctive and more definitive therapy. Meyer et al. [14] were the first to report on the feasibility of this technique in AMI; they demonstrated a significant reduction in residual stenosis from $90.0 \pm 7.3\%$ to $58.6 \pm 19.5\%$ and 81% success rate in 17 patients previously treated with SK. Hartzler et al. [15] extended these findings by demonstrating striking improvement in global ventricular function and a 86% success rate as well. O'Neill et al. [2–16] randomized 56 patients to immediate PTCA or intracoronary SK. Although reperfusion rate was essentially the same (83 vs 85%), PTCA was associated with smaller residual stenosis, less post-infarction angina and higher ejection fractions. Fung et al. [17], from the same center, submitted 21 patients of the latter trial to exercise thalium scintigraphy and found that SK therapy resulted in 60% incidence of peri-infarct ischemia whereas following PTCA the incidence was only 9% ($p < 0.05$). Erbel et al. [18] randomized 162 patients to SK or PTCA after IV-SK; the PTCA group showed less residual stenosis (47 ± 31 vs $73 \pm 19\%$) and reduced re-occlusion and reperfusion rates as well; further, there was an increment in wall motion with PTCA and no change with SK.

More recently, Rothbaum et al. [19] reported on 151 patients with AMI treated with PTCA as single therapy. Overall success rate was 87%, a higher rate than observed in earlier experiences [4]. Average residual stenosis was 29% but it varied from 0 to 70%. Mortality with successful PTCA was only 5% while it reached 37% when the procedure was unsuccessful. Repeat angiographic study was carried on 70% of 121 patients with successful PTCA; re-stenosis was found in 31% and re-occlusion in 9% all of whom were treated medically. Posthospital mortality was only 2%.

For the specific purpose of defining the ideal time of its application in AMI patients, Topol et al. [3] compared its value in patients who received rt-PA and had patent infarct-related arteries. The results of PTCA performed immediately after rt-PA infusion in 99 patients were compared to delayed PTCA in 98 patients treated 7 to 10 days later. Re-occlusion rate was similar (11 vs 13%), but delayed PTCA was associated with more cross-over to emergency PTCA (16 vs 5%; $p < 0.01$) due to recurrent ischemia. Neither group had improvement in ejection fraction and regional wall motion improved to the same extent in the two groups. Mortality was approximatelly three times higher in the immediate treatment group although the difference was not statistically significant. Thus no clear advantage of immediate PTCA was demonstrated.

Based on the available evidences, it may be concluded that PTCA is the preferred mode of treatment for residual stenosis in single vessel disease or even multi-vessel disease patients with suitable anatomy. Whether it should be performed immediatelly or a week after thrombolysis is not definitely established. However, PTCA presents inherent problems:

1. It requires specialized, expensive facilities and personnel, so that it is not available to everyone;
2. when applied as single mode therapy, it requires 1–2 hours for its application, a precious time during which necrosis steadily progresses (obviously, when used following successful thrombolysis this time is less critical);
3. its long-term efficacy has not been fully established; just as with PTCA for chronic coronary insufficiency, re-occlusion/re-stenosis within 6 months has been found in as much as 18% of initially successful procedures [20];
4. it depends on expertise; results vary widely among different centers depending on how well the technique is applied; this is a most critical factor for the ultimate benefit of the procedure.

Hence, additional studies are still needed to better define its role in the treatment of residual coronary stenosis of AMI.

Surgery

The days of early surgical revascularization following thrombolysis are gone. Surgeons soon found that such an approach was destined to serious complications such as bleeding and thrombosis [21]. However, for patients with multivessel disease and suitable coronary anatomy, it remains an important alternative. Clearly, not all patients are candidates for PTCA. These include severe multivessel disease, left main disease or its equivalent and those with definite ventricular aneurysms. In the recent study of Topol et al. [3] 31.6% of patients with patent arteries following rt-PA were not randomized for PTCA treatment; their mortality was 11% which was more than two times the mortality of randomized patients. They are potential candidates for revascularization surgery. Its appropriate time may vary. While there is consensus that it should be deferred until the systemic effects of thrombolytic agents upon the coagulation system have vaned there uncertainty as to when it should be used thereafter. This decision must be made considering the clinical course of the individual patient and the magnitude of coronary involvement. A particular set of patients is represented by those with established ventricular aneurysms; in those we believe surgery should be delayed for 2–3 months, if at all possible. The reason is that surgical resection of aneurysms is ideally performed at a time when the distinction between scarred tissue and normal myocardium can be clearly made [22].

Conclusions

Prognosis of patients following AMI is mainly determined by the extent of the area of myocardium involved by the obstruction, the presence of distant coronary lesions that may cause additional ischemic events and extent of ventricular dysfunction. Although as mentioned above treatment of residual stenosis is by itself important, it should not be viewed as the only issue. Therefore, treatment must be individualized considering all variables that influence prognosis and peculiarities of each technique. Among all, natural history of patients and local expertise in the applicability of both PTCA and surgery should be considered in selecting therapy.

References

1. Serruys PW, van den Brand M, Ribeiro V, et al (1983) Is transluminal coronary angioplasty mandatory after successful thrombolysis? Quantitative coronary angiographic study. Br Heart J 50:257–265
2. O'Neill WW, Topol EJ, Fung A, et al (1987) Coronary angioplasty as therapy for acute myocardial infarction: University of Michigan experience. Circulation 76:II-79–87
3. Topol EJ, Califf RM, George BS, et al (1987) A randomized trial of immediate versus delayed elective angioplasty after intravenous tissue plasminogen activator in acute myocardial infarction. N Engl J Med 317:581–588
4. Schaer DH, Ross AM, Wasserman AG (1987) Reinfarction, recurrent angina and reocclusion after thrombolytic therapy. Circulation 76:II-57–62
5. Gold HK, Leinbach RC, Garabedian HD, et al (1986) Acute coronary reocclusion after thrombolysis with recombinant human tissue-type plasminogen activator: prevention by a maintenance infusion. Circulation 73:347–352
6. Harrison DG, Ferguson DW, Collins SM, et al (1984) Rethrombosis after reperfusion with streptokinase: importance of geometry of residual lesions. Circulation 69:991–999
7. Nicklas JM, Diltz EA, O'Neill WW, et al (1987) Quantitative measurement of coronary flow during medical revascularization (thrombolysis or angioplasty) in patients with acute infarction. J Am Coll Cardiol 10:284–295
8. Gruppo Italiano per lo Studio Della Streptochinasi Nell' Infarcto Miocardio (GISSI): (1986) Effectiveness of intravenous thrombolytic treatment in acute myocardial infarction. Lancet 1:397–401

9. Verstraete M, Bory M, Collen D, et al (1985) Randomized trial of intravenous recobinant tissue-type plasminogen activator versus intravenous streptokinase in acute myocardial infarction. Lancet 1:842–847

10. The TIMI Study Group (1985) The Thrombolysis in Myocardial Infarction (TIMI) Trial: Phase I findings. N Engl J Med 312:932–937

11. Williams DO, Borer J, Braunwald E, et al (1986) Intravenous recombinant tissue-type plasminogen activator in patients with acute myocardial infarction: a report from the NHLBI Thrombolysis in Myocardial Infarction Trial. Circulation 73:338–346

12. Schroder R, Neuhaus KL, Linderer T, et al (1987) Risk of death from recurrent ischemic events after intravenous streptokinase in acute myocardial infarction: results from the Intravenous Streptokinase in Myocardial Infarction (ISAM) Study. Circulation 76:II-44–51

13. Kennedy JW, Ritchie JL, Davis KB, et al (1985) The Western Washington randomized trial of intracoronary streptokinase in acute myocardial infarction. A 12 month follow-up report. N Engl J Med 312:1073–1080

14. Meyer J, Merx W, Schmitz H, et al (1982) Percutaneous transluminal coronary angioplasty immediately after intracoronary streptolysis of transmural myocardial infarction. Circulation 66:905–913

15. Hartzler BO, Rutherford BD, McConahay DR, et al (1983) Percutaneous transluminal coronary angioplasty with and without thrombolytic therapy for treatment of myocardial infarction. Am Heart J 106:965–973

16. O'Neill W, Timmis GC, Bourdillon PD, et al (1986) A prospective randomized clinical trial of intracoronary versus coronary angioplasty for acute myocardial infarction. N Engl J Med 314:812–818

17. Fung A, Lai P, Juni J, et al (1986) Prevention of subsequent excercise induced peri-infarct ischemia by emergency coronary angioplasty in acute myocardial infarction: comparison with intracoronary streptokinase. J Am Coll Cardiol 8:496–503

18. Erbel R, Pop T, Hendricks K, et al (1986) Percutaneous transluminal coronary angioplasty after thrombolytic therapy: a prospective controlled randomized trial. J Am Coll Cardiol 8:485–495

19. Rothbaum DA, Linnemeier TJ, Landin RJ, et al (1987) Emergency percutaneous transluminal coronary angioplasty in acute myocardial infarction: a 3 year experience. J Am Coll Cardiol 10:264–272

20. Arie S, Bellotti G, Checchi H, et al (1986) Transluminal coronary angioplasty in the acute infarct-related artery. Short and longterm results. J Am Coll Cardiol 7:150A. (Abstract)

21. Andrade JCSA, Buffolo E, Succi JE, et al (1985) Revascularization of acute infarction. Analysis of results with and without previous coronary thrombolysis. The effect of time interval between streptokinase and surgery. Arg Bras Cardiol 44:9–18

22. Jatene A (1985) Ventricular aneurysmectomy: ressection or reconstruction. J Thorac Cardiovasc Surg 87(3):321–331

Right Ventricular Infarction: Pathogenesis of Low Output

K. Chatterjee

Introduction

Right ventricular myocardial infarction (RVMI) is being recognized with increasing frequency because of better understanding of the hemodynamic consequences of RV dysfunction and of the availability of the improved techniques of diagnosis. Isolated RVMI in the absence of left ventricular myocardial infarction is rare, and the incidence is only 3–4% in the autopsy studies [1]. However, the frequency of RVMI in association with left ventricular infarction is more frequent and the incidence in the postmortem hearts of patients dying of acute myocardial infarction ranged from 14 to 44% [2–5]. The clinical incidence of RVMI is high and in patients with inferior wall myocardial infarction, involvement of the free wall of the right ventricle can be documented in up to 40% of patients [6]. Although a proximal right coronary artery occlusion is invariably present, RV necrosis occurs uncommonly in the absence of stenosis of the left anterior descending coronary artery, suggesting that the left to right collaterals play a role in the genesis and extent of RVMI. Preexisting RV hypertrophy and RV systolic hypertension may be associated with a greater extent of RV myocardial necrosis with acute right coronary artery occlusion. Thus, several anatomic and pathophysiologic factors may contribute to the extent of RVMI and the severity of hemodynamic compromise.

Diagnosis

The clinical diagnosis of RVMI depends on the awareness of the fact that RVMI is frequent in patients with anterior wall left ventricular infarction. For all practical purposes, appropriate investigations should be performed in all patients with inferior myocardial infarction for the diagnosis of associated RVMI.

It needs to be recognized that RVMI may be clinically silent without any manifestations of RV failure. Combinations of hypotension, elevated jugular venous pressure and clear lung fields [7] occur only in patients with severe RVMI and these findings may be absent in many patients with a lesser extent of RV necrosis. However, in all patients with suspected RVMI, it is important to search for the clinical features suggestive of RV failure – elevated jugular venous pressure and right ventricular S3 gallop and, if these findings are detected in the absence of overt left ventricular failure, pulmonary edema, and left ventricular S3 gallop, one can assume presence of RVMI. An obvious Kussmaul's sign defined as lack of decrease or an actual increase in the jugular venous pressure during the inspiratory phase of respiration, has been reported to be highly specific for the diagnosis of RVMI [8]. However, Kussmaul's sign may not be appreciated in many patients with RVMI. Although recording of the jugular venous pulse may demonstrate a 'y' descent greater than or equal to the 'x' descent [8–12], such abnormal waveforms are rarely recognized at the bedside. Significant pulsus paradoxus is also a relatively uncommon finding [12]. However, these findings reflect the hemodynamic abnormalities and suggest that the impairment in the ventricular filling characteristics may occur in some patients with RVMI. Tricuspid regurgitation in the absence of clinical evidence for significant pulmonary arterial and RV systolic hypertension, although detected infrequently, indicate severe RVMI.

The electrocardiogram is the most useful, inexpensive noninvasive tool for the diagnosis of acute RVMI. When taken early (within 24 to 48 hours after the onset of chest pain) the V_4R lead demonstrates ST elevation in the vast majority of patients. When the magnitude of ST elevation in the lead V_4R is 0.5 mm, in patients with acute Q wave inferior wall myocardial infarction, a sensitivity of 83% and a specificity of 77% have been reported for the diagnosis of RVMI in patients who had hemodynamic or noninvasive evidence of RV myocardial necrosis [13]. In another study, it was reported that ST segment elevation in lead V_4R within the first 24 hours after the onset of pain, was 100% sensitive and 60% specific for detecting autopsy proven RV necrosis [14]. In patients with acute inferior myocardial infarction, a reciprocal ST segment depression is frequently observed in leads V_1–V_8. If ST elevations occur, one should strongly suspect RVMI [15] and not an associated acute anteroseptal myocardial infarction. In RVMI, the 'r' waves in leads V_1–V_3 are however frequently preserved whereas in anteroseptal myocardial infarctions Q waves develop. When the magnitude of ST segment depression in leads V_1–V_2 is less than 50% of the magnitude of ST segment elevation in leads II, III and AVF, RV dysfunction is frequently observed.

Myocardial scintigraphy with technetium-99m stannous pyrophosphate is an accurate method for the diagnosis of acute RV necrosis and the uptake of the radionuclide in the area of the right ventricle has been reported to occur in approximately 40% of patients with acute inferior wall myocardial infarction [16]. However, technetium-99m pyrophosphate images are not positive before 24 hours of onset of necrosis and thus not very helpful for the differential diagnosis of the low output state which usually occurs soon after the onset of infarction. Furthermore, the positive images may not be detected in many patients with inferior wall myocardial infarction with a hemodynamic profile of RVMI [10, 17].

Assessment of RV and left ventricular systolic function either by radionuclide ventriculography or by echocardiography is more useful not only for the diagnosis of RVMI but also for the understanding of the mechanism and severity of 'low output state' resulting from RVMI. Using either first pass or equilibrium techniques, radionuclide ventriculography demonstrated RV systolic dysfunction in approximately 40% of patients with acute inferior wall myocardial infarction [6, 18–20]. When RV ejection fraction falls below 40% with regional dyskinesis or akinesis, the reported sensitivity and specificity for the diagnosis of hemodynamically significant RVMI were 92%, respectively [17]. Decreased RV ejection fraction, however, may result without RVMI as in patients with acute massive pulmonary embolism; regional wall motion abnormalities, however, are more likely to occur in the presence of RV ischemia or infarction [17, 21].

Two dimensional echocardiography also provides useful information concerning the RV functional derangements in patients with RVMI. M-mode echocardiography however is unreliable in detecting RV enlargement, even in the presence of hemodynamically significant RVMI [22, 23]. Two dimensional echocardiography demonstrates dilatation of the right ventricle and dyskinesis or akinesis of the involved wall segments and when these findings are present, hemodynamically significant RVMI can be diagnosed with a high degree of sensitivity and specificity [24, 25]. However, echocardiography is most useful in the differential diagnosis of cardiac tamponade and RVMI as the altered hemodynamics in RVMI may be similar to those in tamponade.

Hemodynamic abnormalities in RVMI are variable and are related to the extent of RV necrosis, the extent of associated left ventricular ischemia or infarction and the pre-infarction status of right and left ventricular function. The predominant RVMI causes a disproportionate elevation of right atrial pressure compared to the rise in pulmonary capillary wedge pressure and frequently the ratio of right atrial pulmonary capillary wedge pressure is equal to or greater than 0.86. The combined autopsy-hemodynamic study has reported that the presence of right atrial pressure equal to or greater than 10 mmHg and right atrial to pulmonary capillary wedge pressure ratio of approximately 0.86, detected during hemodynamic monitoring prior to death, identified the vast majority of RVMI in the autopsied hearts; the sensitivity and specificity of these hemodynamic abnormalities for the diagnosis of RVMI were 82% and 97%, respectively [5]. This hemodynamic profile however is not universally present and it has been suggested that the volume expansion can unmask the hemodynamics of RVMI [9, 10]. However, aggressive volume loading is not required to establish the diag-

Table 1. Diagnosis of right ventricular myocardial infarction (RVMI)

1. Evidence for associated inferior or inferoposterior myocardial infarction.
2. Evidence for right ventricular failure in patients with mild or no left ventricular failure.
3. Kussmaul's sign in patients with inferior wall myocardial infarction.
4. Electrocardiogram: ST segment elevation in the lead V4R or leads V1–V3 in the presence of electrocardiographic evidence for evolving inferior wall myocardial infarction; ST segment depression in the leads V1–V2 less than 50% of ST segment elevation in leads AVF and III.
5. Radionuclide scintigraphy: Technetium 99 m pyrophosphate uptake by the free walls of the right ventricle; reduced right ventricular ejection fraction (less than 40%) with regional wall motion abnormalities detected by radionuclide ventriculography.
6. Two-dimensional echocardiography: Dilated poorly contracting right ventricle with regional wall motion abnormalities.
7. Hemodynamics: Right atrial pressure equal to or greater than 10 mmHg and right atrial to pulmonary capillary wedge pressure ratio equal to or greater than 0.86.

nosis of RVMI in clinical practice. Furthermore, in the presence of old or recent left ventricular myocardial infarction, the expected relation between right atrial and pulmonary capillary wedge pressure may not be observed and pulmonary capillary wedge pressure may remain significantly higher than the right atrial pressure even in the presence of significant RVMI. It needs to be emphasized also that the hemodynamic abnormalities of RVMI can also occur in other conditions such as restrictive cardiomyopathy, constrictive pericarditis, cardiac tamponade, chronic obstructive lung disease, acute massive pulmonary embolism and severe right heart failure secondary to chronic left heart failure. Thus, the diagnosis of RVMI should not be made by only detecting the hemodynamics, the total clinical profile of the patient and the results of the noninvasive test should be incorporated to establish the diagnosis (Table 1). Indeed, determination of hemodynamics is rarely necessary for the diagnosis of RVMI.

Pathophysiology of Low Cardiac Output in RVMI

Although RV necrosis is common in patients with inferior wall myocardial infarction, only about 10% of patients develop shock or severe low output state. The major determinants for the low output state are the extent of RV ischemia or infarction and the degree of associated left ventricular dysfunction resulting from left ventricular infarction. The proximal occlusion of a dominant right coronary artery can potentially cause necrosis of varying extent of the RV lateral wall and apex, left ventricular posterior wall and posterior one-third of the interventricular septum. In postmortem hearts, a part of left ventricular infero-posterior wall and posterior part of the interventricular septum are almost always involved when obvious RVMI is detected. The extent of the involvement of the free walls of the right ventricle is, however, variable. Grade I – necrosis of less than 50% of the posterior RV wall, Grade II – necrosis limited to, but involving, more than 50% of the posterior wall; Grade III – necrosis of the posterior wall and less than 50% of the anterolateral wall and Grade IV – necrosis of the posterior wall and more than 50% of the anterolateral wall [1]. It is apparent that the low output state is more likely to occur in grades III and IV RVMI. The extent of necrosis of the interventricular septum, as well as of the left ventricular inferoposterior wall, obviously contribute to the severity of hemodynamic compromise and the 'low output state'.

In addition to the extent of RV and left ventricular myocardial necrosis, certain complications may also precipitate systemic hypotension and low systemic output. Loss of timed atrial contraction in patients who develop atrioventricular block may cause hypotension resulting from marked reduction in cardiac output. The incidence of bradyarrhythmias, including complete A-V block appear to be higher in patients with RVMI. Ventricular pacing, even at an adequate heart rate, usually does not increase cardiac output significantly and correct hypotension. Timed atrial systole during atrio-ventricular sequential pacing at the same pacing rate as the ventricular pacing, increases stroke volume and cardiac output significantly [26]. The precise mechanism for the larger stroke volume during atrio-ventricular pacing compared to that during ventricular pacing in patients with RVMI has not been established. However, asynchronous atrial and ventricular diastole during atrio-ventricular sequential pacing, may allow a substantially greater increase in left ventricular preload within the confinement of the pericardium and with a relatively fixed intrapericardial volume.

When hypotension and low cardiac output occur in the absence of bradyarrhythmias, and atrio-ventricular block, decreased left ventricular end-diastolic volume (preload) appears to be the major determinant. In dogs with induced isolated RVMI, left ventricular transmural pressure (left ventricular diastolic pressure – intrapericardial pressure) declines where RV transmural pressure increases. Similarly, left ventricular diastolic volume decreases when RV dimensions increase. It appears that a number of interacting mechanisms contribute to decreased left ventricular preload and hence decreased left ventricular forward stroke volume (Frank Starling mechanism) and decreased systemic output. Following isolated RV infarction in dogs, decreased RV stroke work index is associated with increased RV transmural pressure and volume, suggesting a significant depression of its pump function. Reduced RV stroke output will tend to decrease left ventricular preload as RV stroke volume is the major determinant of the venous return to the left ventricle. Decreased RV stroke volume not only results from the decreased contractile function following infarction, but also from increased RV afterload when there is a significant RV dilatation and/or increase in pulmonary artery pressure. Decreased contractile function results in an increase in RV end-systolic and end-diastolic volumes, increasing its wall stress (afterload). Thus, potential exists for further reduction in RV stroke volume and hence left ventricular preload with progressive dilatation of the right ventricle.

Left ventricular filling may also be compromised due to increased intrapericardial pressure (cardiac tamponade physiology). In experimental isolated RV infarction, the intrapericardial pressure increases along with increased RV and left ventricular end-diastolic pressures. The intrapericardial, RV and left ventricular diastolic pressures also become similar (equalization of diastolic pressures). In patients with RVMI, particularly those who develop hypotension and low cardiac output, equalization of the diastolic pressures occurs rather frequently. The right atrial, RV end-diastolic, pulmonary artery end-diastolic and mean pulmonary capillary wedge pressure become equal (Fig. 1). The mechanism for the

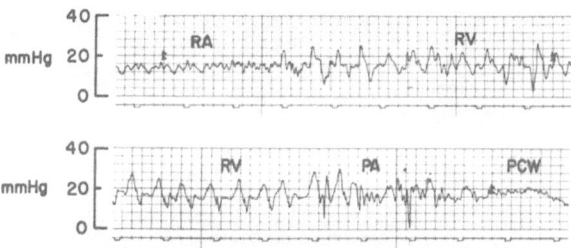

Fig. 1. The hemodynamic abnormalities in acute right ventricular infarction. Right atrial (RAP), right ventricular (RV) enddiastolic, pulmonary artery (PA) end-diastolic and mean pulmonary capillary wedge pressures were initially identical in these patients

equalization of the diastolic pressures is the increase in intrapericardial pressure because, when the pericardium is removed, equalization of the diastolic pressures is no longer present [27]. The findings suggest, therefore, that the increased intrapericardial pressure and relatively nonelastic pericardium exert a constraining effect on ventricular filling and contribute to lower left ventricular preload. Acute RV dilatation encroaches upon the relatively fixed intrapericardial volume, resulting in increased intrapericardial pressure. The lack of stretching of the pericardium acutely and the concomitant increases in RV volume may also alter left ventricular geometry and the orientation of the interventricular septum. During the ventricular filling phase, the interventricular septum normally shifts towards the right ventricle. However, when intrapericardial pressure increases, due to the constraining effect of pericardium, the interventricular septum shifts towards the left ventricle which further decreases left ventricular preload. In experimental RV infarction in dogs, the interventricular septum is considerably flattened, the right ventricle is enlarged and the left ventricular cavity is decreased in size because of a septal shift [28].

Left ventricular diastolic pressure increases despite decreased left ventricular volume and usually decreased transmural pressure. An increase in left ventricular diastolic pressure, however, is associated with an obligatory increase in left atrial, pulmonary artery pressure augments the resistance to left ventricular ejection which causes a further reduction in RV forward stroke volume which, in turn, contributes to decreased left ventricular preload. In patients with RVMI, significant pulmonary arterial hypertension is associated with a more severe low output state and a worse prognosis. It is apparent that a number of interacting functional and hemodynamic abnormalities resulting from RVMI, impair left ventricular filling and decrease systemic output (Fig. 2).

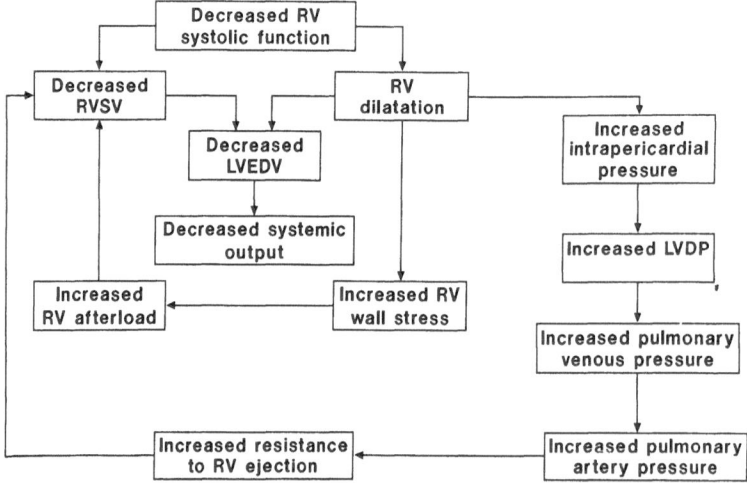

Fig. 2. The interacting pathophysiologic mechanisms for "low output state" in right ventricular (RV) infarction

Therapeutic Approach

The rational therapeutic approach should be directed to increase left ventricular preload to correct 'low output state'. Enhanced left ventricular filling, is expected with the removal of the constraining effect of the pericardium and with increased RV stroke volume. In experimental RV infarction in dogs, following the removal of the pericardium, not only was the equalization of the diastolic pressures absent, but also the left ventricular transmural pressure and volume increased and there was a concurrent increase in left ventricular stroke volume and stroke work [27]. However, in patients with RVMI, pericardial decompression as a therapeutic approach to improve systemic output has not been conformed by any clinical studies.

The physiologic mechanisms that can potentially augment RV stroke volume are

1. increased RV preload or filling pressure (Frank-Starling mechanism);
2. decreased RV afterload; and
3. increased RV contractile function.

In experimental RVMI in dogs, volume loading with intravenous fluid administration, improved RV stroke work which was associated with increased transmural pressure (filling pressure) and diastolic volume [29]. Thus, improvement in RV pump function during volume expansion occurred by the Frank-Starling mechanism. A concomitant increase in left ventricular transmural pressure and volume also occurred along with an increase in left ventricular stroke work. These findings suggested that the improved RV pump function during volume loading augmented left ventricular preload and its stroke output. In patients with RVMI, the response to volume expansion depends on the initial RV and left ventricular filling pressures and the severity of RV systolic dysfunction. When a marked RV dilatation is present and when its transmural pressure is already significantly elevated (right atrial pressure exceeding 15–20 mmHg), a further increase in RV volume and its filling pressure during volume loading is not accompanied by any significant increase in its stroke volume, because, in these circumstances, the right ventricle operates in the relatively flat portion of its function curve. On the other hand, when the RV size is relatively smaller and its transmural pressure lower (RAP less than 10 to 15 mmHg), a fluid challenge may improve RV systolic function and systemic output. In clinical practice, therefore, it is reasonable to administer intravenous fluids in patients with relatively lower RV filling pressures. In patients with markedly elevated right atrial and pulmonary capillary wedge pressures, however, a significant increase in systemic output is not expected with volume expansion [30–32].

A reduction in RV afterload occurs, when RV volume, pulmonary artery pressure and/or pulmonary vascular resistance decline. Vasodilators such as nitroprusside or nitroglycerin can potentially decrease RV and left ventricular afterload and exert a beneficial effect on RV and left ventricular systolic function. In a limited number of patients, nitroprusside therapy was found effective in reversing the low output state resulting from RVMI [7]. However, during vasodilator therapy, intravenous fluid therapy is frequently necessary to maintain adequate

RV preload. It needs to be recognized that vasodilators like nitroprusside and nitroglycerin, not only decrease venous return (venous pooling) but also decreases systemic vascular resistance. Thus, if systemic output does not increase appropriately, severe and unacceptable hypotension may occur.

Positive inotropic agents have been found effective in correcting low output state in patients with RVMI. Dobutamine, a predominantly beta$_1$ adrenergic receptor agonist, causes a substantial increase in RV ejection fraction and systemic output [32]. Dopamine, a dopaminergic receptor agonist and with beta$_1$ and alpha agonist property, also improves cardiac output and systemic hemodynamics in patients with RVMI. However, dopamine can potentially increase pulmonary artery pressure and therefore afterload; thus, the increase in RV stroke volume resulting from its positive inotropic effect, may be curtailed because of the increase in RV ejection impedance. Dopamine, therefore, is the preferred drug in the presence of hypotension. The relative effectiveness of dobutamine and nitroprusside in the management of RVMI has been assessed and dobutamine was reported to be more effective in improving RV and left ventricular pump function. Dobutamine, however, is likely to increase myocardial oxygen consumption and to enhance myocardial ischemia in patients with coronary artery disease. It is apparent that a standard therapeutic approach is unlikely to be beneficial to all patients with RVMI. The therapy should be individualized and also changed if needed, depending on the response to a specific therapy. However, it is reasonable to follow some general principles and guidelines (Table 2) during the management of patients with RVMI.

Table 2. Therapy of right ventricular myocardial infarction

1. Asymptomatic: Observe. Avoid diuretics and venodilators which may induce hypotension and low cardiac output.
2. Symptomatic, low cardiac output:
   (a) *Normotensive with pulmonary capillary wedge (PCWP) or right atrial (RAP) pressures less than 15 mmHg:* Intravenous fluids to increase PCWP and/or RAP to 15–18 mmHg. If cardiac output does not increase with volume expansion, add vasodilator. If cardiac output still remains inadequate add a positive inotropic agent (preferably dobutamine).
   (b) *Normotensive with PCWP or RAP greater than 15 mmHg:* Add vasodilator. If cardiac output still remains inadequate add a positive inotropic agent (preferably dobutamine).
   (c) *Hypotensive with PCWP and/or RAP less than 15 mmHg:* Intravenous fluids initially until PCWP and/or RAP increases to 15–18 mmHg. If remains hypotensive, add a positive inotropic agent (preferably dopamine).
   (d) *Hypotensive with PCWP and/or RAP greater than 15 mmHg.* Add a positive inotropic agent (preferably dopamine).
3. Atrioventricular sequential pacing in the presence of atrioventricular block and subsequent therapy as in number 2.
4. Right ventricular assist or pulmonary artery counterpulsation in selected refractory patients.

References

1. Isner J, Roberts WC (1978) Right ventricular infarction complicating left ventricular infarction secondary to coronary heart disease. Am J Cardiol 42:885–894
2. Myers GB, Klein HA, Hiratzka R (1949) Correlation of electrocardiographic and pathologic findings in infarction of the interventricular septum and right ventricle. Am Heart J 37:720–770
3. Erhardt LR (1974) Clinical and pathological observations in different types of acute myocardial infarction: a study of 84 patients deceased after treatment in a coronary care unit. Acta Med Scand 26 (suppl):7–78
4. Ratliff NB, Hackel DB (1980) Combined right and left ventricular infarction: pathogenesis and clinicopathologic correlations. Am J Cardiol 45:217–221
5. Lopez-Sendon J, Coma-Cannella I, Gamallo C (1981) Sensitivity and specificity of hemodynamic criteria in the diagnosis of acute right ventricular infarction. Circulation 64:515–526
6. Sharpe DN, Botvinick EH, Shames DM, et al (1978) The noninvasive diagnosis of right ventricular infarction. Circulation 57:483–490
7. Cohn JN, Guiha NH, Broder MI, et al (1974) Right ventricular infarction. Am J Cardiol 33:209–214
8. Dell'Italia LJ, Starling MR, O'Rourke RA (1983) Physical examination for exclusion of hemodynamically important right ventricular infarction. Ann Intern Med 99:608–611
9. Coma-Cannella I, Lopez-Sendon J (1980) Ventricular compliance in ischemic right ventricular dysfunction. Am J Cardiol 45:555–561
10. Baigre RS, Hag A, Morgan CD (1983) The spectrum of right ventricular involvement in inferior wall myocardial infarction: a clinical, hemodynamic and noninvasive study. J Am Coll Cardiol 1:1396–1404
11. Cintron GB, Hernandez E, Linares E, et al (1981) Bedside recognition, incidence and clinical course of right ventricular infarction. Am J Cardiol 47:224–227
12. Lorell B, Leinbach RC, Pohost GM, et al (1979) Right ventricular infarction. Clinical diagnosis and differentiation from cardiac tamponade and pericardial constriction. Am J Cardiol 43:465–471
13. Klein HO, Tordjman T, Ninio R, et al (1983) Electrocardiographic diagnosis of right ventricular infarction. Am J Med 70 (6):1175–1180
14. Lopez-Sendon J, Coma-Cannella I, Alcasena S, et al (1985) Electrocardiographic findings in acute right ventricular infarction: sensitivity and specificity of electrocardiographic alterations in right precordial leads V4R, V3R, V1, V2 and V3. J Am Coll Cardiol 6:1273–1279
15. Chou T, Van Der Bel-Kahn J, Allen J, et al (1981) Electrocardiographic diagnosis of right ventricular infarction. Am J Med 70 (6):1175–1180
16. Wackers FJT, Lie KI, Sokole EB, et al (1978) Prevalence of right ventricular involvement in inferior wall infarction assessed with myocardial imaging with thallium-201 and technetium-99m pyrophosphate. Am J Cardiol 42:358–362
17. Dell'Italia LJ, Starling MR, Crawford MH, et al (1984) Right ventricular infarction: identification by hemodynamic measurements before and after volume loading and correlation with noninvasive techniques. J Am Coll Cardiol 4:931–939
18. Rigo P, Murray M, Taylor DR (1978) Right ventricular dysfunction detected by gated scintiphotography in patients with acute inferior myocardial infarction. Circulation 52:268–274
19. Tobinick E, Schelbert HR, Henning H, et al (1978) Right ventricular ejection fraction in patients with acute anterior and inferior myocardial infarction assessed by radionuclide angiography. Circulation 57:1078–1084
20. Reduto LA, Berger HJ, Cohen LS, et al (1978) Sequential radionuclide assessment of left and right ventricular performance after acute transmural myocardial infarction. Ann Intern Med 89:441–447
21. Starling M, Dell'Italia LJ, O'Rourke RA, et al (1984) First transit and equilibrium radionuclide angiography in inferior transmural myocardial infarction patients: Criteria for the diagnosis of associated hemodynamically significant right ventricular infarction. J Am Coll Cardiol 9:15

22. Lopez-Sendon J, Coma-Cannella I, Lombera F, et al (1982) Diagnosis of ischemic right ventricular dysfunction by M-mode echocardiography. Eur Heart J 3:230–237

23. Mikell FL, Asinger RW, Hodges M (1983) Functional consequences of interventricular septal involvement in right ventricular infarction: echocardiographic, clinical, and hemodynamic observations. Am Heart J 105:393–401

24. D'Arcy B, Nanda NC (1982) Two-dimensional echocardiographic features of right ventricular infarction. Circulation 65:167–173

25. Lopez-Sendon J, Garcia-Fernandez MA, Coma-Cannella I, et al (1983) Segmental right ventricular function after acute myocardial infarction: two-dimensional echocardiographic study in 63 patients. Am J Cardiol 51:390–396

26. Topol EJ, Goldschlager N, Ports TA, DiCarlo LA Jr, Schiller NB, Botvinick EH, Chatterjee K (1982) Hemodynamic benefit of atrial pacing in right ventricular myocardial infarction. Ann Intern Med 96:594–597

27. Goldstein JA, Vlahakes GJ, Verrier ED, et al (1982) The role of right ventricular systolic dysfunction and elevated intrapericardial pressure in the genesis of low output in experimental right ventricular infarction. Circulation 65:513–522

28. Sharkey SW, Shelley W, Carlyle PF, et al (1985) M-mode and two-dimensional echocardiographic analysis of the septum in experimental right ventricular infarction: correlation with hemodynamic alterations. Am Heart J 110:1210–1218

29. Goldstein JA, Vlahakes GJ, Verrier ED, et al (1983) Volume loading improves low cardiac output in experimental right ventricular infarction. J Am Coll Cardiol 2:270–278

30. Lopez-Sendon J, Coma-Cannella I, Adanez JV (1981) Volume loading in patients with ischemic right ventricular dysfunction. Eur Heart J 2:321–338

31. Shah PK, Maddahi J, Berman DS, et al (1985) Scintigraphically detected predominant right ventricular dysfunction in acute myocardial infarction: Clinical and hemodynamic correlates and implications for therapy and prognosis. J Am Coll Cardiol 6:1264–1272

32. Dell'Italia LJ, Starling MR, Blumhardt R, et al (1985) Comparative effects of volume loading, dobutamine and nitroprusside in patients with predominant right ventricular infarction. Annu Rev Med 34:377–390

Management of Cardiac Crisis

New Inotropic Agents in the ICU

J. F. Dhainaut

Introduction

Acute myocardial insult results in substantial loss of ventricular contractility and hence cardiac performance. The treatment of heart failure has traditionally centered on the combination of diuretics and cardiac glycosides. The digitalis glycosides have been extensively reviewed recently [1] and will not be discussed here. New therapeutic interventions may be directed at reducing ventricular loading conditions with vasodilating drugs or increasing ventricular contractility with positive inotropic agents. Considerable effort devoted to the search for such pharmacologic agents capable of augmenting cardiac contractility has led to a growing number of these promising new agents, many apparently acting by new mechanisms. Most positive inotropes may increase contractility by altering intracellular calcium kinetics.

The biochemical basis of myocardial contraction involve the release, utilization, and sequestration of intracellular calcium, regulated by calcium channels, enzymes and the sarcoplasmic reticulum [2–3]. Cardiotonic agents can augment contractility:

1. by increasing cAMP due to activation of adenylcyclase, thereby resulting in increased transcellular calcium influx through slow calcium channels in response to depolarization as β-adrenergic agonists,
2. by blocking the breackdown of cAMP due to inhibition of phosphodiesterase: bipyridine (amrinone, milrinone) or imidazolone (fenoximone, piroximone ...) derivatives,
3. by using other mechanisms: inhibition of re-uptake of calcium by the sarcoplasmic reticulum (caffeine), direct increase of calcium influx (dihydropyridine), improvement of the sensitivity of the contractile proteins for calcium (sulmazole) or
4. by the combination of several mechanisms [3].

This review focuses primarily on the new positive inotropic agents that have been used for short-term administration in critically ill patients with severe and acute heart failure.

Catecholamines

Cathecholamines have in common positive inotropic action, but otherwise differ considerably by receptor activation. The most frequently employed new catecholamines are dopamine, dobutamine and dopexamine.

Dopamine

The effects of this endogenous precursor of norepinephrine are due to the combination of its actions on alpha, beta, and dopamine receptors as well as release of endogenous norepinephrine. Infusions of dopamine therefore elicit a dose-related triphasic hemodynamic response. At low doses (<5 $\mu \cdot kg^{-1} \cdot min^{-1}$), stimulation of renal dopaminergic receptors increases renal blood flow, glomerular filtration rate, and sodium clearance [4]. At higher doses, dopamine's positive inotropic effects are due principally to stimulation of cardiac β-adrenergic receptors. Doses higher than 10 $\mu \cdot kg^{-1} \cdot min^{-1}$ cause both stimulation of alpha$_1$-adrenergic receptors and release of norepinephrine from nerve endings, resulting in increased systemic arterial and venous pressures. Such effects often become indistinguishable from those of norepinephrine.

Except for the clinical use of low doses of dopamine to improve renal function in a variety of conditions (low renal perfusion, hepato-renal syndrome ...), this drug, with its combined positive inotropic and vasoconstricting properties, has been widely employed to improve and stabilize the hemodynamic status of patients with conditions causing both cardiac failure and marked hypotension [5]. As an example, in cardiogenic shock with low systemic blood pressure, the infusion of dopamine should be initially directed at increasing systemic blood pressure to an adequate coronary perfusion pressure ($\geqslant 55$ mmHg). At this point, another agent as vasodilator or dobutamine can be added to both further improve organ-tissue perfusion and decrease myocardial oxygen consumption [6]. Dopamine is also the first-line drug for primarily noncardiogenic shock states, characterized by combined vasodilation and myocardial depression, as some poisonings (carbamates, calcium channel-blockers, β-blockers ...) and septic shock [7].

In this clinical setting, infusions of dopamine is followed by an increase in cardiac output, stroke volume and systemic blood pressure. Ventricular filling pressure remains the same, then increases at doses higher than 6 $\mu \cdot kg^{-1} \cdot min^{-1}$ Potentially deleterious effects of dopamine include tachycardia, arrhythmias and myocardial oxygen demand [4]. Dysrhythmias, especially atrial fibrillation, usually appear at doses higher than 8 $\mu \cdot kg^{-1} \cdot min^{-1}$, except for patients with hypovolemia and pre-existing dysrhythmias [7]. Local tissue necrosis may occur at the infusion site and local injection of phentolamine may be effective to avoid tissue necrosis. Digital necrosis have been reported with prolonged and high dose infusions [5], especially in patients with pre-existing vascular disease or fulminans purpura.

Dobutamine

This synthetic sympathomimetic amine has a potent positive inotropic action as a selective β1-agonist, with little effect on vascular tone and is not accompanied by significant positive chronotropy and dysrhythmias than the other catecholamines, resulting in a slight increase in myocardial oxygen consumption. There is strong evidence that the beneficial hemodynamic effects of dobutamine may be due to a more complex action with alpha and β-adrenergic receptors in both the heart and peripheral vasculature, leading to additional preload and afterload-reducing properties [8]. Unlike dopamine, dobutamine neither stimulate renal dopamine receptors nor release endogenous norepinephrine.

In the clinical setting, dobutamine infusions are followed by an increase in cardiac output, stroke volume, and, to a lesser extent, systemic blood pressure, while ventricular filling pressures decrease. Optimal dosages usually range between 7.5 and 15 $\mu \cdot kg^{-1} \cdot min^{-1}$. The hemodynamic effects are achieved by 2 minutes after infusion and the maximal effects are observed 10 minutes later. The short half-life of dobutamine, as the other catecholamines, is a favorable feature in the treatment of clinically instable patients in whom the management of undesirable effects is facilitated by rapid elimination [5].

However, the development of desensitization of myocardial β-adrenergic receptors which leads to a progressive unresponsiveness to β-adrenergic agonists over time, represents a major limitation to the long therm use of catecholamines. After 4 days of continuous infusion, 43 percent of the initial hemodynamic effect of dobutamine is lost. Such a tolerance also develops during administration of other synthetic sympathomimetic agents (pirbuterol, or prenalterol) [3]. A possible exception may be the oral agent levodopa, which is converted to dopamine in situ.

Positive inotropic action increases myocardial oxygen consumption. Dobutamine may concomitantly elicit changes which tend to decrease myocardial oxygen consumption. With dobutamine, the decrease in end-diastolic and end-systolic volumes reduces wall stress, whereas the concomitant increase in diastolic systemic blood pressure associated with a fall in left ventricular filling pressure leads to a increase in coronary perfusion pressure without causing an increase in heart rate. Dobutamine thus increases coronary blood flow and oxygen delivery equal to or greater than the increase in myocardial oxygen consumption in patients with non-ischemic heart failure. In patients with heart failure secondary to coronary artery disease, Bendersky et al. [9] demonstrated that dobutamine infusion improves cardiac function, including contractility of ischemic segments. Few patients elicit myocardial lactate production, indicating a reduction of cellular oxygenation in one or more regions with dobutamine. This phenomenon appears related to the degree of tachycardia and/or a more heterogeneous myocardial blood flow pattern.

In the postoperative period after cardiac surgery, optimal doses of dobutamine elicit less tachycardia and reduced ventricular filling pressure more than comparable doses of dopamine. Fowler et al. [10] showed that dobutamine and dopamine altered hemodynamics similarly, but only dobutamine increased coronary blood flow commensurate with the increase in myocardial oxygen consumption.

The combination of dobutamine and dopamine is recommended in two clinical settings:

1. to improve renal blood flow, glomerular filtration rate and sodium clearance by dopaminergic-receptor stimulation, and

2. to increase systemic vascular resistance and hence coronary perfusion pressure during cardiogenic shock associated with marked hypotension [6, 11] and during septic shock [12].

Dhainaut et al. [13] demonstrated that the combination of dobutamine and dopamine was followed by an increase in coronary perfusion pressure and coronary sinus blood flow, while coronary vascular resistance decreased. Before inotropic support, despite marked coronary vasodilation in all 40 patients, only six patients with both low cardiac output and perfusion pressure developed myocardial hypoxia, defined as myocardial lactate production. Despite high levels of positive inotropic drugs myocardial hypoxia vanishes, because the increase in myocardial oxygen supply is higher than the increase in myocardial oxygen demand.

Clinical and hemodynamic monitoring (via pulmonary artery thermodilution catheter and/or echocardiography) provides proper adjustment of the dobutamine infusion rate and fluid administration to maintain adequate ventricular preload.

Dopexamine

This dopamine analogue stimulates dopaminergic and β-adrenergic receptors but not alpha-adrenergic receptors, causing increase in renal blood flow and myocardial contractility associated with systemic vasodilation [14].

The Oldest Catecholamines

Despite their potent inotropic actions, the clinical use of norepinephrine, epinephrine and isoproterenol has been limited by their positive chronotropic actions, their tendency to exacerbate cardiac arrhythmias and their too powerful vasoactive effects. As mentioned in the sections discussing dopamine and dobutamine, norepinephrine may occasionally have to be used to re-establish and maintain adequate coronary perfusion pressure in case of severe hypotension as during septic shock [15] or pulmonary embolism [11].

Phosphodiesterase Inhibitors

Inhibition of phosphodiesterase increases cardiac contractility by decreasing cAMP breakdown. In fact, the phosphodiesterase inhibitors that are in widespread clinical use such as methylxanthines (theophylline, caffeine), have several other pharmacologic actions; inhibition of calcium re-uptake by the sarcoplasmic reticulum, increase in the sensitivity of the contractile proteins for calcium [2], stimulation of the synthesis and release of endogenous catecholamines, potentiation of the effects of β-agonists ... [3]. Although methylxanthines (theophylline, caffeine) have been shown to have a positive inotropic effect, they have not been of great therapeutic benefit. High doses, needed to obtain a meaningful effect on myocardial contractility, are accompanied by undesirable neurologic and gastro instestinal side effects and marked positive chronotropy and arrhythmogenic effects. Recently, new phosphodiesterase inhibitors appear to have both potent positive inotropic and vasodilatory effects.

Bipyridine Derivatives

The first of this group is *amrinone*. Despite extensive experimental evaluation, the precise mechanism of this drug remains elusive. Only intravenous infusion was approved by the Food and Drug Administration in 1984 for the short-term treatment of refractory heart failure [3]. The relative contributions of vasodilation and inotropic effect to the improvement of hemodynamic state with amrinone remains controversial. Hermiller et al. [16] have found no evidence for a positive inotropic effect in patients with heart failure.

The initial intravenous dose is usually 0.75 mg·kg^{-1} with a maintenance infusion of 5 to 10 μ·kg^{-1}·min^{-1}. The infusion of amrinone usually leads to a reduction in systemic and pulmonary vascular resistances and ventricular filling pressure without changing heart rate. Cardiac output increases secondary to afterload, and this response appears similar or higher to the response noted with vasodilators. Higher infusion rates may occasionally be necessary, but at such doses careful monitoring is advisable to avoid excessive hypotension.

The use of amrinone as first-line positive inotropic intervention in critically ill patients must be questioned [5]. The reasons for this are the following.

1. Amrinone induces a systemic vasodilation, not always appropriate in patients with severe hypotension or shock.
2. Modest unpredictable inotropic properties often lead to use high levels of this drug in severely ill cardiac patients, increasing the frequency of side effects.
3. Compared to catecholamines, the elimination half-life of amrinone is long (>2 hours) and, in patients with heart failure, it may exceed 12 hours [3]. This is a serious disadvantage if undesirable effects occur [5].

Milrinone, closely related to amrinone, is 15 times more potent and much better tolerated than amrinone. Colucci et al. [3] have shown that this drug had an effect intermediate between those of nitroprusside and dobutamine. Milrinone may also cause an improvement of myocardial relaxation and no increase in myocardial oxygen consumption. This drug has a half-life of two hours, excreted unchanged in the urine.

Imidazolone Derivatives

Enoximone has pharmacologic and hemodynamic effects that are very similar to those of bipyridines [17]. Although enoximone is rapidly metabolized, hemodynamic effects persist for 8 hours, because its metabolite is effective.
Piroximone is another imidazolone derivative. Some preliminary studies suggested that its inotropic effects is higher than enoximone.

Among this extensive class of drugs, sulmazole has been reported to increase the sensitivity of cardiac myofibrils to calcium.

Conclusion

β-adrenergic agonists are the first-line drug for acute cardio-circulatory failure, phosphodiesterase inhibitors should probably be used as a second-line drug in instances in which β-agonists become ineffective, or reserved for patients with chronic congestive heart failure, more especially as only long-term therapy with oral phosphodiesterase inhibitors appears to affect functional class favorably.

References

1. Lewis RP (1986) Digitalis. In: Leier CV (ed) Cardiotonic drugs. Basic and Clinical Cardiology. Marcel Dekker Inc; New York, pp 85–150
2. Fabiato A, Fabiato F (1979) Calcium and cardiac excitation-contraction coupling. Annu Rev Physiol 41:473–484
3. Colucci WS, Wright RF, Braunwald E (1986) New positive inotropic agents in the treatment of congestive heart failure. N Engl J Med 310:290–299 and 349–358
4. Goldberg LI (1974) Dopamine-clinical uses of an endogenous catecholamine. N Engl J Med 291:707–710
5. Leier CV (1986) Acute inotropic support. In: Leier CV (ed) Cardiotonic drugs. Basic and Clinical Cardiology. Marcel Dekker Inc; New York, pp 49–84
6. Richard C, Ricome JL. Rimailho A, Bottineau G, Auzepy P (1983) Combined hemodynamic effects of dopamine and dobutamine in cardiogenic shock. Circulation 67:620–624
7. Regnier B, Safran D, Carlet J, Teisseire B (1979) Comparative hemodynamic effects of dopamine and dobutamine in septic shock. Intensive Care Med 5:115–120
8. Ruffolo RR Jr, Spradlin TA, Pollock GD, Waddell JE, Murphy RT (1981) Alpha and beta adrenergic effects of the stereoisomers of dobutamine. J Pharmacol Exp Ther 219:447–452
9. Bendersky R, Chatterjee K, Parmley WW, Brundage BH, Ports TA (1981) Dobutamine in chronic ischemic heart failure: Alterations in left ventricular function and coronary hemodynamics. Am J Cardiol 48:554–561
10. Fowler MBF, Alderman EL, Oesterle SN, et al (1984) Dobutamine and dopamine after cardiac surgery: greater augmentation of myocardial blood flow with dobutamine. Circulation 70 (suppl I):103–111
11. Molloy WD, Lee KY, Jones D, Penner B, Prewitt RM (1984) Treatment of shock in a canine model of pulmonary embolism. Am Rev Respir Dis 130:870–874
12. Dhainaut JF, Huyghebaert MF, Monsallier JF, et al (1987) Coronary hemodynamics and myocardial metabolism of lactate, free fatty acids, glucose, and ketones in patients with septic shock. Circulation 75:533–541
13. Dhainaut JF (1986) Effects of the combination of dobutamine and dopamine on hemodynamics and coronary circulation in human septic shock. Br J Clin Practice 40 (suppl 45):59–62
14. Brown RA, Farmer JB, Hall JC, Humphries RG, O'Connor SE, Smith GW (1985) The effects of dopexamine on the cardiovascular system of the dog. Br J Pharmacol 85:609–619
15. Desjars P, Pinaud M, Potel G, Tasseau F, Touze MD (1987) Reappraisal of norepinephrine therapy in human septic shock. Crit Care Med 15:134–137
16. Hermiller JB, Leithe ME, Magorien RD, Unverferth DV, Leier CV (1984) Amrinone in severe congestive heart failure: Another look at an intriguing new cardioactive drug. J Pharmacol Exp Ther 228:319–325
17. Strain J, Grose R, Maskin CS, LeJemtel TH (1985) Effects of a new cardiotonic agent, MDL-17,043, on myocadial contractility and left ventricular performance in congestive heart failure. Am Heart J 110:91–96

Treatment of Serious Cardiac Arrhythmias

R. W. F. Campbell

Introduction

Cardiac arrhythmias may be a mere cosmetic blemish, may cause symptoms, may be hemodynamically significant or may be of prognostic significance. Those arrhythmias which have an immediate hemodymanic effect are serious and may threaten life. Examples include rapid tachyarrhythmias, asystole and complete heart block. Initial management in the presence of a sustained event must be to restore a normal rhythm or to reduce the hemodynamic consequences of the abnormal rhythm. When the acute situation has resolved, continuing management may be necessary as a protection against repetitive events. As in all areas of medical endeavour, treatment should be profiled for efficacy and safety. In the management of life-threatening cardiac arrhythmias a moderate incidence of unwanted effects and perhaps even quite serious risks of therapy may be acceptable as the price to pay for protection.

Immediate treatment of serious cardiac arrhythmias may be either medical or electrical.

Acute Management

Medical Treatment

Drug formulation: The armamentarium of antiarrhytmic drugs has enlarged greatly in the last decade but most agents have been introduced for the chronic management of relatively stable ventricular arrhythmias. Few antiarrhythmic medications have been developed specially for rapid parenteral administration for acute arrhythmia control, although a parenteral form of most is available.

Narrow QRS tachycardias: A small proportion of narrow QRS tachycardias will revert with vagotonic manoeuvers. The majority, by the time they present for medical attention, will persist unless treatment is given. Numerous studies have demonstrated that verapamil given intravenously can terminate a majority of narrow QRS tachycardias regardless of their basic pathophysiology [1]. This eficacy depends upon the fact that the AV node is involved in the three main types of narrow QRS tachycardia – 'true' atrial tachycardia, intra AV nodal re-entry tachycardia (IAVNRT) and the reciprocating tachycardias (RT) associated with accessory pathways. The cells of the AV node are calcium dependent and the calcium antagonists of which verapamil is one example, slow impulse transmission in this structure sufficient to interrupt or modify re-entrant arrhythmias using this conduction route (IAVNRT and RT). True atrial tachycardia does not require the AV node for its maintenance and the effect of verapamil administration during this arrhythmia is usually to slow ventricular response.

Atrial flutter and fibrillation: Paroxysmal atrial flutter and fibrillation may seriously compromise patients if the ventricular response rate is very rapid. Acutely administered antiarrhythmic drugs are disappointing in this situation. Digoxin, calcium antagonists and beta-blockers have all been recommended but have the deficiencies of relative inefficacy, delay before their onset of action or a short half-life. Intravenous amiodarone offers the combination effects of ventricular rate control by an action on the AV node and a high success rate for medical cardioversion with restoration of sinus rhythm [2]. The clinical value and risks of this intervention remain to be established as studies to date have been relatively small. However, short term acute intravenous amiodarone therapy would not be expected to cause the important adverse effects associated with the chronic oral use of this drug.

Atrial fibrillation and pre-excitation: Atrial fibrillation developing in the presence of an accessory pathway with anterograde conduction capability may cause extremely rapid ventricular response rates resulting in ventricular fibrillation [3]. The arrhythmia is not common but should be recognized by its characteristic electrocardiographic pattern of an irregular polymorphic tachycardia with a high proportion of broad QRS complexes. The QRS polymorphism reflects conduction over the AV node, accessory pathway or both. Caution is advised in managing this arrhythmia. Patients may be hypotensive and may not tolerate acute intravenous antiarrhythmic therapy. If there is serious hemodynamic compromise, cardioversion is probably indicated, but if the situation is less urgent, medical therapy is appropriate. Any antiarrhythmic drug which depresses the AV node may paradoxically accelerate the ventricular response rate as atrioventricular conduction will be "forced" through the accessory pathway. This arrhythmogenic response might be expected with drugs such as the calcium antagonists [4] but can occur with many other agents including amiodarone [5]. The ideal is to administer an antiarrhythmic agent with predominant effects on the accessory pathway. The Vaughan Williams Class Ic drugs (flecainide, encainide, propafenone, lorcainide etc) are appropriate but their capacity to depress myocardial function may be relevant in this situation and they should be administered in modest doses and slowly.

Ventricular tachycardia: Ventricular tachycardia is common arrhythmia if the definition embraces brief salvos of consecutive ventricular ectopic beats. Sustained ventricular tachycardia (more than 30 seconds or requiring resuscitation) is more unusual and is associated with serious underlying cardiovascular disease. As sustained ventricular tachycardia is often rapid, the arrhythmia may be very badly tolerated and may degenerate to ventricular fibrillation. Lidocaine is reasonably effective in stopping ventricular tachycardia and probably prevents recurrences [6], Adverse reactions are remarkably infrequent. In the event of failure of lidocaine, it is questionable whether any other antiarrhythmic drug should be given as there is increasing danger of electrophysiological or hemodynamic deterioration with polypharmacy. If a second antiarrhythmic agent is to be used, parenteral amiodarone or the Vaughan Williams class Ic drugs are logical choices. Parenteral mexiletine and tocainide have been recommended in this context and they have the advantage of minimal cardiovascular toxicity. However, their electrophysiological profiles are so similar to lidocaine that their efficacy following lidocaine might merely indicate inadequate lidocaine dosing. Cardioversion should be considered at all stages of management and is indicated for those patients in hemodynamic crisis and when medical therapy has failed.

It is important to diagnose ventricular tachycardia correctly. Misdiagnosis of this broad QRS rhythm as supraventricular tachycardia with the consequent administration of verapamil has resulted in disaster [7, 8]. Supraventricular tachycardia with abberation is very rare. All tachycardias with broad QRS complexes should be diagnosed and treated as ventricular tachycardia until proven otherwise.

Electrical Treatment

Bradyarrhythmias – asystole and heart block: Pacing is the treatment of choice to manage asystole and complete heart block. Endocardial pacing is optimal but may not be immediately available. Emergency transthoracic pacing, transesophageal and "stab" intracardiac pacing systems can be useful temporary procedures to maintain life while arrangements are made for more reliable support.

Tachyarrhythmias – ventricular fibrillation: DC defibrillation is required to revert ventricular fibrillation. The successful restoration of a perfusing rhythm depends upon a variety of factors including the etiological basis of the arrhythmia and the time delay from the onset of ventricular fibrillation to life support. Success rates range from nearly 100% in electrocution victims seen early after the event and in patients with so-called "primary" ventricular fibrillation complicating acute myocardial infarction to rates of less than 30% when ventricular fibrillation complicates shock and/or heart failure. Nonelectrical defibrillation (spontaneous [9] or drug induced [10]) does occur but is rare and at present has little if any implication for the emergency management of this arrhythmia.

Tachyarrhythmias – SVT and VT: There is surprisingly little awareness of the value of electrical treatment for management of acute supraventricular (narrow QRS) and ventricular tachycardias. The majority of these arrhythmias being reentrant, can be terminated by programed stimulation techniques [11]. Using an electrode catheter positioned in the right ventricle, standard stimulation sequences (underdrive, overdrive, 1, 2 or 3 critically timed extra stimuli) and sophisticated automatic stimulation programs (auto decremental, concertina, scanning etc) can be delivered during the arrhythmia. Almost all narrow QRS tachycardias and the vast majority of ventricular tachycardias can be terminated by these techniques. Electrical management of these arrhythmias offers the advantage that arrhythmia diagnosis can be confirmed from the endocardial electrophysiology and more importantly, arrhythmia reversion is accomplished without recourse to potentially hazardous antiarrhythmic drugs or to general anesthesia. Electrophysiological management of this type does demand easy access to fluoroscopy facilities for catheter placement and is therefore restricted in availability. However, the stimulation sequences need not be sophisticated and most arrhythmias will respond to the pulse trains available from standard external pacing boxes. Electrical management of tachycardias is particularly relevant for hospitalized patients subject to frequent repetitive arrhythmic events.

Long Term Management

Long term arrhythmia prophylaxis may be necessary following acute arrhythmia control. Some arrhythmias such as ventricular fibrillation complicating acute stage myocardial infarction need only a short period of prophylactic therapy before antiarrhythmic medication can be withdrawn. This strategy is tenable only because the electrophysiological milieu that supported the arrhythmia has disappeared with maturation of the myocardial infarction. Most other arrhythmias pose a continuing risk. Those secondary to a definable and correctable abnormality are managed by attention to the primary problem. Repetitive ventricular tachycardia provoked by exercise induced ischemia will disappear with myocardial revascularization procedures [12]. Similar arrhythmia "cures" are possible with surgical or catheter destruction of accessory pathways [13], with electrophysiologically guided resection procedures for ventricular tachycardia and ventricular fibrillation [14, 15] and perhaps more crudely with cardiac transplantation. There is growing recognition of the cost benefit of surgery in Wolff-Parkinson-White patients with life-threatening responses to artrial fibrillation. Only marginally less accepted is the offer of surgery to those whose quality of life is markedly impaired by repetitive reciprocating tachycardia or by the adverse effects of therapy used to control arrhythmic events. Results for medical prophylaxis of sustained ventricular tachycardia post infarction are poor [16]. Whilst antiarrhythmic surgery in these patients carries an appreciable operative mortality, longer term survival figures now favor surgical management.

When long term medical antiarrhythmic prophylaxis is considered the best option, the choice of agent poses difficulties. Safety, compliance and efficacy are the essential elements but each may be compromised by the other. Selecting the optimal drug for long therm prophylaxis is difficult but generalizations are relevant. Optimal cost benefit ratios are achieved if the least toxic therapies are tried first. They may not offer particular efficacy but in the few patients who are protected an excellent management strategy will have been identified. Potentially toxic agents (amiodarone, procainamide etc) or agents with adverse effects which may encourage non-compliance (mexiletine, tocainide, disopyramide, quinidine) generally should be tried only when other agents have failed. Predicting that a chosen drug will be effective for long term arrhythmia prevention is not easy and may be seriously unreliable. Invasive electrophysiological tests, if applicable to the index arrhythmia (supraventricular tachycardia, sustained ventricular tachycardia) can be used. Drugs when given acutely and which prevent the electrophysiological induction of the arrhythmia are highly likely to provide effective long term prophylaxis when given orally [17]. For a time it was considered that amiodarone could not be assessed in this way but evidence now suggests otherwise [18, 19].

All patients taking chronic antiarrhythmic therapy for arrhythmia prophylaxis should be seen regularly and consideration given as to whether continued therapy really is required. If the arrhythmia does not threaten life then periodic drug withdrawal, as an out patient, will answer the question. When the arrhythmia is potentially lethal then this approach is unacceptable. As a minimum, hospitalization would be necessary but, depending upon the frequency of the arrhythmia and the half-life of the medication, many months might need to be spent under surveillance. In practice, the decision is usually to continue therapy unless adverse reactions dictate reappraisal of the situation. The arrhythmias most likely to modulate with time include the reciprocating tachycardias related to accessory pathways, intra AV nodal re-entry tachycardia and arguably late post infarction ventricular fibrillation.

The role of the automatic implantable cardioverter defibrillator (AICD): The development of the AICD is a remarkable technological achievement which has far reaching implications for our management of patients at risk of lethal ventricular arrhythmias [20]. At present the relatively high cost of the unit has confined its use both in terms of patient populations and in implanting institutions. The device offers the ultimate safety net in the event that prophylactic therapy should fail. Ventricular tachycardia or fibrillation is automatically detected and electrically corrected by internal delivery of a DC shock. Limitations of AICD systems include the extensive implantation procedure, inappropriate shock delivery, limited life span and psychological disturbances in device recipients. Further development will improve the device technology and will permit better prediction of its place in our therapeutic armamentarium.

Conclusions

Management of serious cardiac arrhythmias is difficult. So many factors need consideration if optimal immediate and long term treatment is to be identified. Too often the commendable efforts in controlling a serious acute arrhythmic event are wasted by inadequate attention to prevention of recurrences. Successful, immediate and long term management of these arrhythmias requires a wide knowledge of cardiovascular pathophysiology and perhaps more importantly, consideration of the cost benefit ratio of each and every possible treatment strategy.

References

1. Waxman HL, Myerburg RJ, Appel R, Sung RJ (1981) Verapamil for control of ventricular rate in paroxysmal supraventricular tachycardia and atrial fibrillation or flutter. Ann Intern Med 94:1-6
2. Cowan JC, Gardiner P, Reid DS, Newell DJ, Campbell RWF (1986) A comparison of amiodarone and digoxin in the tratment of atrial fibrillation complicating suspected acute myocardial infarction. J Cardiovasc Pharmacol 8:252-256
3. Campbell RWF, Smith RA, Gallagher JJ, Pritchett ELC, Wallace AG (1977) Atrial fibrillation in the pre-excitation syndrome. Am J Cardiol 40:514-520
4. Gulamhusein S, Ko P, Klein GJ (1983) Ventricular fibrillation following verapamil in the Wolff-Parkinson-White syndrome. Am Heart J 106:145-147
5. Scheinman BD, Evans T (1982) Acceleration of ventricular rate by fibrillation associated with the Wolff-Parkinson-White syndroma. Br Med J 285:999-1000
6. Koster RW, Dunning AJ (1985) Intramuscular lidocaine for prevention of lethal arrhythmias in the prehospitalisation phase of acute myocardial infarction. N Engl J Med 313:1105-1110
7. Buxton AE, Marchlinski FE, Doherty JU, Flores B, Josephson ME (1987) Hazards of intravenous verapamil for sustained ventricular tachycardia. Am J Cardiol 59:1107-1110
8. Rankin AC, Rae AP, Cobbe SM (1987) Inappropriate use of intravenous verapamil in patients with ventricular tachycardia. Br Heart J 57:591-595
9. Moskowitz RM, Schwartz AB (1987) Spontaneous termination of prolonged ventricular fibrillation after acute myocardial infarction. Arch Int Med 147:171-172
10. Sanna G, Arcidicacono R (1973) Chemical ventricular defibrillation of the human heart with bretylium tosylate. Am J Cardiol 32:982-987
11. Wellens HJJ, Bar F, Gorgels AP, Farre L (1978) Electrical management of arrhythmias with emphasis on the tachycardias. Am J Cardiol 41:1025-1034
12. Rasmussen K, Lunde PI, Lie M (1987) Coronary bypass surgery in exercise induced ventricular tachycardia. Eur Heart J 8:444-448
13. Gallagher, Sealy WC, Cox JL, Kasell JH, German LD (1983) Anatomic substrates of the Wolff-Parkinson-White syndrome. In: Elizari MV, Rosenbaum MB, (eds) Frontiers of Cardiac Electrophysiology. Martinus Nijhoff Boston, pp 689-701
14. Bourke JP, Tansuphaswadikul S, Cowan JC, Hilton CJ, Campbell RWF (1987) Role of surgical therapy for sustained ventricular tachycardia and fibrillation early after myocardial infarction. In: Breithardt G, Borggrefe M, Zipes DP (eds) Non Pharmacological Therapy of Tachyarrhythmias. New York, Futura
15. DiMarco JP, Lerman BB, Kron IL, Sellers TD (1985) Sustained ventricular tachyarrhythmias within two months of acute myocardial infarction; results of medical and surgical therapy in patients resuscitated from the initial episode. J Am Coll Cardiol 6:759-768
16. Wellens HJJ, Bar FWHM, Vanagt EJDM, Brugada P (1982) Medical treatment of ventricular tachycardia: Considerations in the selection of patients for surgical treatment. Am J Cardiol 49:186-193
17. Horowitz LN, Josephson ME, Koster JA (1980) Intracardiac electrophysiological study as a method of optimization of drug therapy in chronic VT. Prog Cardiovasc Res 2:381-389
18. Horowitz LN, Greenspan AM, Spielman SR, et al (1985) Usefulness of electrophysiologic testing in evaluation of amiodarone therapy for sustained ventricular tachyarrhythmias associated with coronary heart disease. Am J Cardiol 55:367-371
19. Naccarelli GV, Fineberg NS, Zipes DP, Heger JJ, Duncan G, Prystowsky EN (1985) Amiodarone: risk factors for recurrence of symptomatic ventricular tachycardia identified at electrophysiologic study. J Am Coll Cardiol 6:814-821
20. Gabry MD, Brodman R, Johnston D, et al (1987) Automatic implantable cardioverter - defibrillation: Patient survival battery depletion and shock delivery analysis. J Am Coll Cardiol 9:1349-1356

Interest of Calcium Channel Blockers During the Perioperative Period

P. Coriat, M. D. Rossignon, and L. S. Montejo

The incidence of perioperative myocardial ischemia and hypertension is high in patients suffering from coronary artery disease (CAD) who are scheduled for non-cardiac surgery. Increases in myocardial oxygen consumption need to be minimized by controlling heart rate and/or blood pressure during stress resulting from anesthesia, surgery or recovery [8]. Although the narcotic anesthetic techniques often used in these patients prevent myocardial depression, they are unfortunately associated with a high incidence of perioperative myocardial ischemia and hypertension.

Since the beneficial effects of calcium channel blockers during the perioperative management of hypertension and/or CAD are well known [10], and further, since the efficacy of these drugs in attenuating the ischemic manifestations induced by pacing or exercice in patients with fixed coronary artery stenosis have been well established [4], calcium channel blockers would appear to be useful drugs in the anesthesiologist's armamentarium.

The choice of a calcium channel blocking drug during the perioperative period should depend on its cardiovascular effects and the pathophysiology of the hemodynamic changes which are specific during the operative period. Accordingly, calcium channel blockers might be given pre-, intra- and postoperatively for the following purposes:

- treatment or prevention of perioperative myocardial ischemia;
- control of perioperative hypertensive episodes;
- control of perioperative supra-ventricular arrhythmias.

Preoperative Administration of Calcium Channel Blockers

It is well established that both antihypertensive and antianginal medications should be continued up until the night before surgery and given in the morning of the surgical procedure [12]. When considering calcium channel blockers, this attitude is particularly useful since the interactions of these drugs with both anesthetic agents and the hemodynamic response to stressful situations during the operative period are much more beneficial than detrimental.

The hemodynamic response to anesthesia in patients with CAD receiving oral diltiazem or nifedipine just before surgery shows that the effects of diltiazem and anesthetic agents on cardiac function and peripheral vasculature are almost additive [3]. The arterial dilating effects of the two drugs are dependent on the basal level of vascular resistances. Therefore they can be given preoperatively in normo-tensive patients without provoking a significant decrease in blood pressure.

We studied the interactions between diltiazem given intravenously at a dose of 3 mcg·kg^{-1}·min^{-1} with fentanyl-N$_2$O anesthesia in CAD patients undergoing vascular non cardiac surgery [8]. In this study diltiazem plasma blood levels var-ied at induction between 50 et 200 ng/ml. A pre-anesthesia diltiazem infusion lead to a 10% decrease in mean arterial pressure and heart rate without changes in cardiac index and pulmonary capillary wedge pressure. However, during an-esthesia no significant differences was found between the hemodynamic param-eters of patients receiving diltiazem and patients receiving placebo. Since in con-trast to patients receiving the placebo, no significant increase in heart rate and/or arterial pressure was observed at incision, during the surgical procedure and at recovery, diltiazem appeared as potentially useful in controlling these hemo-dynamic parameters during such stressful situations. Obviously such interactions of diltiazem with intraoperative hemodynamic changes are beneficial since in-traoperative increases in myocardial oxygen demand can lead to intraoperative myocardial ischemia.

The effects of dihydropyridine calcium channel blockers in awake patients com-bine direct negative inotropism and vasodilatation together with reflex sympathetic activation. In a recent study we investigated whether reflex sympathetic activation exists when dihydropyridine calcium channel blockers are given during fentanyl-benzodiazepine anesthesia, and if it does whether it influences intraoperative he-modynamic parameters. In this double blind study, patients received (vs placebo) an intravenous continuous infusion of nisoldipine, a calcium channel blocker very similar to nifedipine. Twenty patients scheduled for carotid endarterectomy were studied with a history of chronic hypertension which was adequately controlled prior to surgery. Norepinephrine plasma levels and heart rate significantly de-creased under anesthesia only in the placebo group. These levels are significantly higher in patients receiving nisoldipine, this suggesting that reflex sympathetic ac-tivation in response to nisoldipine infusion exists under fentanyl-N$_2$O anesthesia. Interestingly, mean arterial pressure was similar in both groups at the time of in-duction and incision. No hypertension and a lower incidence of hypertensive epi-sodes were observed intraoperatively in the patients receiving nisoldipine. Thus the drug interaction between dihydropyridine calcium channel blockers and fentanyl-benzodiazepine anesthesia is far from being deleterious, and appears beneficial. The reflex sympathetic activation observed intraoperatively in patients receiving nisoldipine, may have played a role in the differences demonstrated between the two groups in cardiac index and heart rate.

Thus both diltiazem or nifedipine, when chronically taken by the cardiac pa-tients must be given orally one hour before induction of anesthesia.

Treatment or Prevention of Intraoperative Myocardial Ischemia Using Calcium Channel Blockers

Calcium channel blockers exert their beneficial anti-ischemic effects not only by decreasing myocardial oxygen demand by afterload reduction (without increasing the heart rate for diltiazem) but also by improving myocardial oxygen supply through direct coronary vasodilatation or prevention of coronary vasoconstriction.

When considering the pathophysiology of perioperative myocardial oxygen imbalance, the anti-ischemic effects of calcium channel blockers appear to be particularly well suited for prevention or treatment of perioperative ischemic episodes which deleterious effects have been well established.

Deleterious Effects of Perioperative Myocardial Ischemia

Myocardial ischemic episodes may result in ventricular arrhythmias. The acute left ventricular dysfunction that appears within seconds of the onset of ischemia may lead to a threatening decrease in cardiac output under anesthesia or to an acute pulmonary edema in the postoperative period. The development of transesophageal echocardiography to monitor left ventricular wall motion during surgical procedures has pointed to the intraoperaitve occurrence of new segmental wall motion abnormalities indicating ischemia in patients with CAD undergoing surgery [11].

Several studies, using transesophageal echocardiography or radionuclide techniques demonstrate that regional left ventricular dysfunction caused by intraoperative myocardial ischemia may be prolonged and persists in the postoperative period. This is not surprising since the unconscious patient is unable to stop the stressful situation which led to myocardial oxygen inbalance, which often provokes a "stunning" of the myocardium. Furthermore, when considering the results of several studies it appears that intraoperative myocardial ischemia might lead to postoperative myocardial infarction.

Treatment of Perioperative Myocardial Ischemia
Using Calcium Channel Blockers

Narcotic anesthesia is a very popular technique for patients with CAD. Under such approach, myocardial ischemia is associated with hemodynamic changes and results from an increased myocardial oxygen demand. In most cases, deepening of anesthesia using volatile agents is adequate to control intraoperative increase in heart rate or blood pressure.

However at recovery from anesthesia several factors tend to increase global oxygen consumption and preload and afterload stress. At this time, the intravenous administration of diltiazem is particularly effective to limit heart rate and blood pressure responses to recovery and restore a favorable myocardial oxygen balance without impairing the hemodynamic function. In this instance, diltiazem can be given as a bolus of 0.5 mg/kg, this resulting in a therapeutically active plasma concentration.

Although myocardial ischemia due to hemodynamic changes is the most common, recent studies have pointed out that the incidence of intraoperative myocardial ischemia not associated with hemodynamic changes is far from negligible. The treatment of ST-segment depression, which occurs without hemodynamic changes must call for drugs which can increase the anginal threshold such as calcium channel blockers. Humphay and Blanck [9] reported ichemic episodes occurring during anesthesia for coronary artery surgery, which persisted despite nitroglycerin infusion and which regressed after intravenous boluses of verapamil 2.5 mg.

In some cases, actual coronary artery spasm has been documented during anesthesia. Obviously, intravenous diltiazem or intranasal nifedipine represents an adapted treatment for treatment and prevention of such events.

Prevention of Intraoperative Myocardial Ischemia Using Calcium Channel Blockers

The two following arguments lead us to attempt to prevent intraoperative myocardial ischemia with anti-ischemic agents in patients with disabling CAD undergoing non-cardiac surgery:

1. Diagnosis of intraopertive ischemic type segment depression is not always easy since a high incidence of ischemia occurred without hemodynamic changes. Moreover, wall motion studies have confirmed that intraoperative ST-segment depression is a late and inconsistent sign of ischemia [11].
2. The incidence of myocardial ischemia remains high whathever the anesthetic protocol used, in patients with disabling CAD.

The prevention of intraoperative myocardial ischemia using continuous infusion of anti-ischemic agents should be considered only in patients particularly prone to developing intraoperative myocardial ischemia or in patients with disabling angina. Nitroglycerin can be used to prevent myocardial ischemia during non-cardiac surgical procedures. However, the marked decrease in venous return and the reflex tachycardia limit the use of this agent for this purpose, leading one to undertake large volume infusions to avoid falls in blood pressure, tachycardia and a decrease in cardiac output. Diltiazem, which can be given intravenously, has none of such limitations since it does not affect preload, and it decreases heart rate. In a double blind study (vs placebo) [8] we found that intravenous diltiazem at a dose giving serum levels varying from 50 to 300 ng/ml. (0.15 mg/kg as a bolus followed by a continuous infusion of 3 mcg $\cdot$ kg^{-1} $\cdot$ min^{-1}) could be safely used with fentanyl-N$_2$O anesthesia in patients with angina pectoris undergoing non-cardiac surgery. This study demonstrated that intravenous diltiazem is a potentially useful drug in decreasing the incidence of intraoperative myocardial ischemia during non cardiac surgery. During the surgical procedure and at recovery fewer patients in the diltiazem group showed an increase in systolic arterial blood pressure and/or heart rate of more than 20% in relation to the pressure or heart rate noted at preoperative control time. This reduction in blood pressure and heart rate associated with the use of diltiazem suggests that a reduction in myocardial oxygen demand was the mechanism by which diltiazem acts in ischemia induced by surgical stress. However, other potential mechanisms of action of diltiazem (increased myocardial blood flow of the ischemic zone) may have played a part in the beneficial perioperative anti-ischemic effect of this drug.

The lack of increases in arterial blood pressure at recovery in patients receiving diltiazem, which is particularly beneficial after carotid endarterectomy, is not surprising because during exercise testing in CAD patients a significant reduction in arterial blood pressure is observed following a single oral administration of diltiazem. In hypertensive patients this effect is particularly evident [13].

Treatment of Supraventricular Arrhythmias

The occurrence of intraoperative or postoperative supraventricular arrhythmias is not rare in cardiac patients. Such events must be rapidly treated since they deteriorate the hemodynamic status, and compromize myocardial oxygen balance. Because their interaction with anesthetic agents are not deleterious, verapamil and diltiazem appear to be the treatment of choice for supraventricular arrhythmias occurring in the perioperative period. In our experience a bolus dose of 0.5 mg/kg of diltiazem is effective and safe to slow heart rate during a supraventricular arrhythmia. The effects of such a bolus last about 45 minutes.

Treatment of Postoperative Hypertension

The postoperative period mainly during recovery from anesthesia is the most stressful time of the perioperative period for both hypertensive and CAD patients [6].

Recovery from general anesthesia is associated with increased sympathetic nervous system discharge and increases in heart rate, blood pressure, and global oxygen consumption. The factors responsible for these changes are rewarming stress, hypoxia, emergence excitement, and postoperative pain. Patients suffering from chronic hypertension or CAD and patients who underwent vascular surgery are particularly prone to develop postoperative hypertensive episodes. Because of their preferential vasodilatator properties, dihydropyridine calcium channel blockers are particularly interesting drugs in this instance.

Intranasal or sublingual nifedipine, or nicardipine (which may be given intravenously since it is photoresistant and water soluble), are widely used in our department to treat postoperative hypertension in vascular surgery. To better understand the site of action of calcium channel blockers in the control of blood pressure, we compared the effects of nicardipine and nitroglycerin on hemodynamics and left ventricular function assessed by 2D-transesophageal echocardiography when these agents are used intravenously for the treatment of postoperative hypertension [1]. Transesophageal 2D-echocardiography provides the opportunity for continuous monitoring of myocardial function in patients under mechanical ventilation. Ejection fraction area obtained by this technique closely correlates with ejection fraction determined with gated radionuclide angiography [5]. Both drugs were efficacious in the rapid treatment of post abdominal aortic surgery hypertension, and both ameliorated left ventricular function by allowing a better emptying of the left ventricle. In addition, the results of this study emphasized that the effects on capacitance vessels of these two drugs are readily apparent in the treatment of postoperative hypertension. A significant decrease in pulmonary wedge pressure and end-diastolic area was observed only in patients treated with nitroglycerin. Such differences in preload explain the lower stroke index in these patients.

Cardiac index increased only in the nicardipine group as a result of the lack of decrease in venous return while the arterial vasodilatation led to a better emptying of the left ventricle. The lack of effect of calcium channel blockers on capacitance vessels is a very important advantage when considering the postoperative administration of such agents, since postoperatively both volume and tone of capacitance vessels are experiencing wide changes. These hemodynamic characteristics explain why dihydropyridine calcium channel blockers, when used to control hypertension at recovery from general anesthesia, improve the adaptation of cardiac output to the increased postoperative oxygen needs of the organism.

Using mixed venous oxygen saturation ($S\bar{v}O_2$) monitoring, we demonstrated that postoperative hypertension may be associated with decreased $S\bar{v}O_2$ although cardiac index increased [7]. Thus such an increase in cardiac index does not compensate for the increased $\dot{V}O_2$ which characterized the postoperative period. In this study the treatment of postoperative hypertension with intranasal nifedipine raised cardiac index and notably improved $S\bar{v}O_2$ [7].

Thus dihydropyridine calcium channel blockers can be considered as the treatment of choice for hypertension in the postoperative period, since in addition to their beneficial anti-ischemic effects, they permit a better adaptation of the cardiac output to the marked postoperative increases in the oxygen needs of the surgical patients.

Following dihydropyridine calcium channel blockers both vasodilatation and direct or reflex sympathetic activation lead to an increased heart rate. Since recovery from general anesthesia is associated with increased sympathetic nervous system discharge, postoperative heart rate is often high. Therefore, it may be interesting to consider the antihypertensive effects of intravenous diltiazem which reduces afterload without increasing the heart rate. Accordingly, we designed a study to assess the efficacy of intravenous diltiazem in treatment of postoperative hypertension and to determine its effects on hemodynamics and left ventricular function assessed using transesophageal 2D-echocardiography.

After surgery, when systolic blood pressure increased above 165 mmHg still under mechanical ventilation, patients were treated with intravenous diltiazem, administered in boluses (15 ng/ml every 30 seconds) to achieve the same systolic blood pressure as before induction. This was followed 15 minutes later by another single bolus of 15 ng/ml. In the 8 patients studied, intravenous diltiazem restored preinduction systolic blood pressure. Hemodynamic data recorded during postoperative hypertension and after treatment are presented in Table 1.

Intravenous diltiazem bolus administration, when used to control postoperative hypertension, is associated with a better emptying of the left ventricle while preload is maintained. This explains the increased stroke index and the improvement in ejection fraction. Simultaneously heart rate is lower, which is largely

Table 1. Hemodynamic and transesophageal echocardiographic data during hypertension and 15 minutes after treatment with intravenous diltiazem 25 to 50 mg, to restore preinduction blood pressure

	Baseline	After diltiazem
Heart rate, b/min	90±9	76±5
Mean arterial pressure, mmHg	129±8	90±4[a]
Pulmonary artery wedge pressure, mmHg	12±2	14±2
Cardiac output, l/min	6.5±0.4	7.0±0.4
Stroke volume, ml	72±4	92±5[a]
End-systolic area, cm^2	6.0±0.3	5.4±0.4[a]
End-diastolic area, cm^2	12±1	13±1
Ejection fraction area, %	50±4	58±3[a]

[a] $p < 0.05$ vs baseline

beneficial for myocardial oxygen balance. These data suggest that the decrease in afterload helped to compensate for the myocardial depression when diltiazem is used to control hypertensive episodes.

Prevention of Postoperative Hypertension

After some types of surgical procedure, the deleterious effects and high incidence of postoperative hypertension have been well documented. Particularly, after carotid endarterectomy control of hypertension is essential to minimize the risk of hematoma, neurologic deficit and cardiac events. The arterial dilating effects of dihydropyridine calcium channel blockers are dependent on the basal level of vascular resistances.

Therefore they can be given to normotensive patients for prevention of hypertensive episodes. When given at the end of surgery intranasal nifedipine, intravenous diltiazem or nisoldipine significantly decrease the incidence of postendarterectomy hypertension. When diltiazem is used in the prevention of postoperative hypertension, fewer patients showed at recovery an increase in heart rate in relation to the control value [8]. When dihydropyridine calcium channel blockers such as intravenous nisoldipine are given in the prevention of postoperative hypertension, such a beneficial effect occurs in spite of large increases in catecholamine levels found at the time of extubation, while cardiac index increased by 45% and heart rate by 25% from preinduction values [2]. Thus the beneficial postoperative antihypertensive effects of dihydropyridine calcium channel blockers do not seem to stem from a decrease in catecholamine synthesis or secretion, but rather to a direct effect on resistance vessels. We can speculate that an alpha-2 presympathic antagonism, which has been suggested under such category of calcium channel blockers, has played a part in the increased postoperative plasma catecholamine levels noted in patients receiving a nisoldipine infusion.

In conclusion, calcium channel blockers may be used to optimize myocardial oxygenation and minimize the risk of intraoperative myocardial ischemia during the perioperative period. Since heart rate changes are so important determinants of myocardial oxygen consumption in CAD, the main benefit from diltiazem given intravenously appears in the control of increased heart rate often seen in response to perioperative noxious stimuli.

The treatment of postoperative hypertension should be efficient and rapidly acting, it should improve myocardial perfusion, and it should not decrease blood pressure more than needed or compromize left ventricular function and cardiac output. With regards to these aims intranasal nifedipine, intravenous diltiazem or nicardipine seem ideal to control postoperative hypertension.

References

1. Ben Ammar M, Coriat P, Houissa M, et al (1987) Nicardipine vs trinitrine for treatment of postoperative hypertension: effects on hemodynamics and left ventricular function. Anesthesiology 67: A139
2. Braz J, Coriat P, Bertrand M, et al (1987) Prevention of post-carotid endarterectomy hypertension with iv nisoldipine: hemodynamic and hyperadrenergic response to recovery. Anesthesiology 67: A140
3. Britt BA (1985) Diltiazem (review article). Can Anaesth Soc J 32:30–44
4. Braunwald E (1982) Mechanism of action of calcium channel blocking agents. N Engl J Med 307:1618–1627
5. Bruère D, Coriat P, Philip I et al (1986) Transesophageal 2D-echocardiography ejection fraction area: correlation with gated radionuclide angiography. Anesthesiology 67: A177
6. Coriat P, Fauchet M, Bousseau D, Mundler O, Echter E, Viars P (1986) Response of left ventricular ejection function to recovery from general anesthesia: measurements by gated radionuclide angiography. Anesth Analg (Clev) 65:593–600
7. Godet G, Coriat P, Samama M et al (1986) Treatment of post-carotid endarterectomy hypertension with nifedipine: effects on hemodynamics and mixed venous oxygen saturation. Anesthesiology 65: A75
8. Godet G, Coriat P, Baron JF (1987) Prevention of intra-operative myocardial ischemia during non cardiac surgery with intravenous diltiazem: a randomized trial versus placebo. Anesthesiology 66:241–245
9. Humphrey LS, Blanck TJJ (1985) Intraoperative use of verapamil for nitroglycerin refractory myocardial ischemia. Anesth Analg 64:68–71
10. Reves JG, Kissin I, Lellw A, Tosone S (1983) Calcium entry blockers: uses and implications for anesthesiologists. Anesthesiology 57:504–510
11. Smith JS, Caholan MK, Nyrd BP et al (1985) Intraoperative detection of myocardial ischemia in high risk patients: electrocardiography versus two-dimensional transesophageal echocardiography. Circulation 72:1015–1021
12. Waller JL, Kaplan JA (1981) Anaesthesia for patients with coronary artery disease. Br J Anaesth 757–765
13. Yamakado T, Norysohi O, Kondo S, Nojiri A, Nakado T, Takejawa H (1983) Effects of diltiazem on cardiovascular responses during exercise in systemic hypertension and comparison with propranolol. Am J Cardiol 52:1023–1027

Hemodynamic and Metabolic Response After Cardiopulmonary Bypass: Continuous Monitoring of CO_2 Production*

P. Giomarelli, O. Chiara, and R. Rosi

Introduction

The increase in metabolic rate after cardiopulmonary bypass (CPBP) represents a critical factor in patients with reduced oxygen availability due to hypovolemia or unstable cardiac function [1, 2]. Raison et al. [2] demonstrated an increased oxygen consumption ($\dot{V}O_2$) in postoperative open heart surgery patients. The effects of oxygen debt repayment, mechanical ventilation, and shivering were proposed as possible explanations for changes in metabolic rate [3, 4]. Rodriguez et al. [4] observed an increase in energy requirements in patients after major surgical procedures complicated by intraoperative hypothermia.

In a previous study [5] we demonstrated a role of body temperature changes in the increases in $\dot{V}O_2$ and CO_2 production ($\dot{V}CO_2$) after surgery. A peak change in metabolic needs was recorded at a time when the spontaneous rewarming was maximum. This period lasted about 6 hours postoperatively. By calculating energy requirements (REE) it was possible to observe that the increase in REE during the first postoperative hours reached levels comparable to that of hypermetabolic septic patients [5]. However, the state of myocardial function is of extreme importance in the management of patients after CPBP. Postoperative course may be considered as normal when the cardiac output is adequate for the metabolic needs. Temporary depression (without permanent structural or biochemical damage), myocardial edema and particularly myocardial necrosis may affect myocardial performance postoperatively.

Patients with coronary artery disease but preserved left ventricular function usually show an hyperdynamic response to pain and stress, while those with poor function usually show evidence of left ventricular failure. During transient or ongoing myocardial ischemia any patient may develop transient ventricular failure [6].

In patients with valvular diseases, a decreased preoperative myocardial reserve, as suggested from a high NYHA functional class, appears to reduce the safe time limits of cardioplegic arrest [7]. Preoperative myocardial reserve, surgical damage and ischemic arrest, hypovolemia and transient or ongoing myocardial ischemia may all affect myocardial performance postoperatively. On the other hand, surgical stress by raising metabolic needs, requires adequate cardiac output. The probability of death in fact is strongly dependent of cardiac index [8].

---

* This study was supported, in part, by the CNR, NCRG (Grant 8202155), and M.P.I. 40%.

The most frequent method used for measuring cardiac output is the thermo-dilution technique, utilizing a pulmonary artery catheter. This method is rapid and simple but expensive, subjected to sometimes severe complications and not suitable for on-line monitoring of flow [9]. Moreover, after CPBP changes in hemoglobin, lung function, temperature and cardiac output can all occur inde-pendently and rapidly, so that it is probably safer and more reliable to monitor variables which reflect changes in cardiac performance [10].

From $\dot{V}CO_2$ and $\dot{V}O_2$ it is possible to assess the variations in energy require-ments and indirectly the metabolic stress during the first postoperative hours. Many problems may be imposed in the measurement of metabolic rate by means of exhaled gases during mechanical ventilation by changes in temperature, hu-midity, atmospheric pressure, and instrument calibration. Many open circuit methods and closed circuit techniques have been developed but all may be sub-jected to a number of errors [11–14]. The most important source of errors seems to be the difficulty to maintain a stable FiO_2 during mechanical ventilation [15, 16]. On the contrary, the analysis of $\dot{V}CO_2$ is not affected by FiO_2 fluctuations, so that it can represent a more accurate measurement [17]. In a previous work of our institution performed in 16 adult patients undergoing open heart surgery, continuous $\dot{V}CO_2$ monitoring was suggested as a reliable clinical method in the early detection of the metabolic changes in postoperative mechanically venti-lated patients [5]. After this initial experience this method was routinely applied in our ICU.

On-line Monitoring System

We considered a series of 200 consecutive patients after hypothermic CPBP for coronary or valvular disease. All patients were monitored by an on-line monitor-ing device managed by a "patient data management system" (Hewlett Packard 1000, Coppertino, California). The monitoring system includes the instantenous acquisition every 30 seconds of following data: heart rate (HR), mean arterial pressure (MAP), pulmonary artery pressure (PAP), right (RAP) and left atrial pressure (LAP), minute ventilation ($\dot{V}_E$), respiratory rate (RR), peak inspiratory pressure (PPK), plateau pressure (PPL), end tidal CO_2) ($ETCO_2$), minute CO_2 production ($\dot{V}CO_2$). The last six data are derived from a Servo Ventilator (900C Siemens Elema) connected with a capnometer (930 Siemens Elema) which de-rives $\dot{V}CO_2$ from expiratory CO_2 and flow (Fig. 1): this method has shown a good correlation ($r=0.991$) with mass spectrometry $\dot{V}CO_2$ and $ETCO_2$ measure-ments [18].

From manual entry it is possible to insert into the data-base various other information like blood flow measurements by thermodilution, therapy, medical observations, nursing notes, etc. The monitoring system has been also connected with a gas analyzer (ABL4 Radiometer) with the acquisition of blood pH, PCO_2, PO_2, HCO_3^-, hemoglobin saturation (SO_2), and oxygen content (CO_2) acquired on-line may be controlled with O_2 contents measured with a Lex-O_2-CON (Lex-ington Instruments). A good correlation between the two methods has been proved ($r=0.99$, $p<0.001$). Each time gas analysis are acquired, the system au-

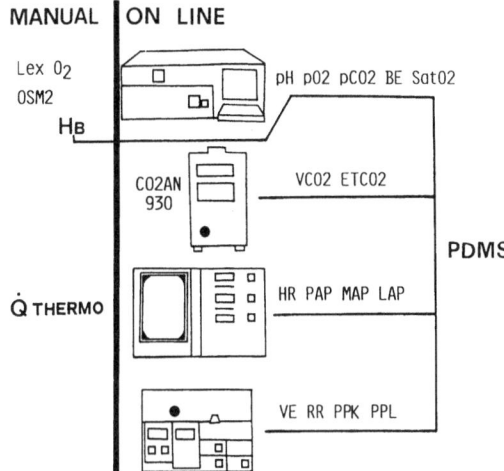

Fig. 1. Schematic diagram of the on-line monitoring system

tomatically records hemodynamic and ventilatory parameters which are filled for data retrieval and statistical analysis.

Blood Flow Measurement

To obtain measurement of cardiac output using the system previously described we applied the Fick principle by using $\dot{V}CO_2$ and arteriovenous O_2 difference (avO_2D). In a series of 70 patients the respiratory quotient (RQ) was derived from $\dot{V}CO_2$ measured by means of capnometry and $\dot{V}O_2$ calculated from thermodilution cardiac output and avO_2D. The mean postoperative RQ was 0.90 ± 0.11. Assuming this mean RQ as constant it is possible to calculate cardiac output from the Fick equation $= \dot{V}CO_2/(avO_2D \times 0.9)$.

This parameter has been controlled in 70 cardiac outputs obtained by thermodilution with a good correlation (0.94, angular coefficient 1.13, $p < 0.001$).

Clinical Applications of On-line Monitoring

The system previously described permits a continuous evaluation of physiologic trends. Figure 2 represents an on-line plotting of two variables, $\dot{V}CO_2$ and $ETCO_2$ during the first postoperative hours of a cardiac patient. The monitoring shows a marked increase of $\dot{V}CO_2$ and $ETCO_2$ during the first three hours. If this variation was not promptly corrected with adequate increase in mechanical ventilation, respiratory acidosis could occur. To optimize ventilatory needs to increased demand, a normal $ETCO_2$ value may be used as the optimal clinical goal. Continuous monitoring has not only the utility to demonstrate an emergency but also to retrieve the record of the episode in order to control efficiency of medical and nursing staff. A more sophisticated approach is to individualize

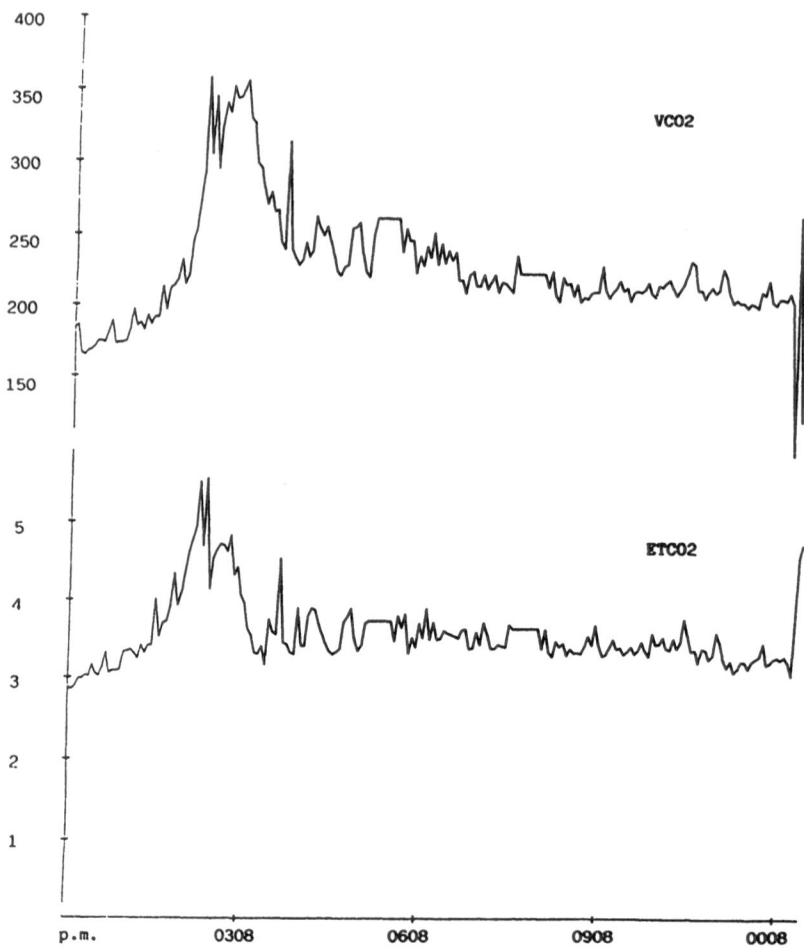

Fig. 2. On-line plot of V̇CO₂ and ETCO₂ in a postoperative patient (see text for explanations)

Table 1. Collection and analysis of data

Variables used for statistical evaluation

Temperature: T (°C)	*Observation at:*
Hemoglobin: Hb (gr/dl)	T0: arrival in ICU
Base excess in arterial blood: BE (mEq/l)	T1: three hours after arrival in ICU
Partial pressure of O_2 in mixed venous blood: $P\bar{v}O_2$ (torr)	T2: six hours after arrival in ICU
Arterio-venous O_2 difference: avO_2D (vol%)	
Heart rate: HR (b/min.)	*Statistical evaluations:*
Left atrial pressure: LAP (mmHg)	– multivariate analysis using stand-
Mean arterial pressure: MAP (mmHg)	ardized variables
Minute CO_2 production index: VCO_2I (ml·min/m²)	– Cluster analysis
Cardiac index: (l·min/m²)	– Fischer and Student's *t* tests
Left ventricular stroke work index: LVSWI (gr·m/m²)	
Ventricular function: VF (rad)	

physiologic states using the retrospective analysis of data. An example is presented in Table 1.

From the analysis of the 12 variables summarized, we found that the variation in $\dot{V}CO_2$ and avO_2D during the first three postoperative hours (T1) were the main explanation (first principal component) of the response to postoperative stress. Applying a cluster analysis on these variables it was possible to identify three groups of patients, according to the physiologic adaptation to stress [19, 20].

Cluster analysis was performed on patients at all periods of observation (T0, T1, T2) and three groups (CG1, CG2, CG3) were identified. Statistical analysis using Fischer and Student's t tests was also applied to evaluate variance into each group and between observations. No differences between groups were found for hemoglobin, base excess, MAP and LAP. The variables are presented in Table 2. Temperature showed an increase from T0 to T2 which was more marked in Cluster groups 1 and 2 (CGI, CG2). $\dot{V}CO_2$ and cardiac index (CI) increased with temperature in CG1 and CG2, but showed only minor changes in CG3. Ventricular function (VF) was stable with time, but was lower in CG1 and CG3 than in CG2. Finally, $P\bar{v}O_2$ was generally unchanged in various moments, but was usually lower in CG1 and CG3 than in CG2.

The cluster groups that have been identified in this manner may by physiologically defined (Fig. 3):

Cluster Group 1: patients with normal to elevated $\dot{V}CO_2$ and venous arterial CO_2 difference ($vaCO_2D = avO_2x0.9$). These patients have increased metabolic needs in this time of observation.

Table 2. Comparison of hemodynamic and metabolic parameters of cluster groups 1-2-3 at moments T0, T1 and T2 (mean values $\pm$ SD)

		T0	T1	T2
T°	CG1	37.7± 0.8	36.1± 0.9[a]	37.2± 1
(°C)	CG2	35.8± 0.9	37.1± 0.7[a, b]	37.4± 0.6
	CG3	35.5± 0.8	36.5± 0.8[a]	36.5± 0.9
$\dot{V}CO_2$	CG1	137 ±24	182 ± 4[a]	154 ±16
(ml·min/m²)	CG2	117 ±15[b]	142 ±18[a, b]	129 ±10[b]
	CG3	95 ±10	118 ±16[a]	110 ±13
PvO_2	CG1	26 ± 4	27 ± 4[a]	30 ± 4
(torr)	CG2	34 ± 5[b]	35 ± 5[b]	35 ± 4[b]
	CG3	28 ± 3	28 ± 3	29 ± 4
Cardiac index	CG1	2.2± 0.7	2.9± 1[a]	3.3± 1.1
(l·min/m²)	CG2	3.2± 0.8[b]	3.7± 1[a, b]	3.5± 0.7[b]
	CG3	1.8± 0.3	2.2± 0.3[a]	2.2± 0.2
Ventricular function	CG1	6.5± 2.4	6.6± 1.8	7.4± 1.7
(rad)	CG2	7.7± 2[b]	8.2± 2[b]	7.8± 1.8[b]
	CG3	6.1± 1	6.5± 2	5.7± 1

[a] $p < 0.01$, T1 versus T0 & T2
[b] $p < 0.01$, CG2 versus CG1 & CG3

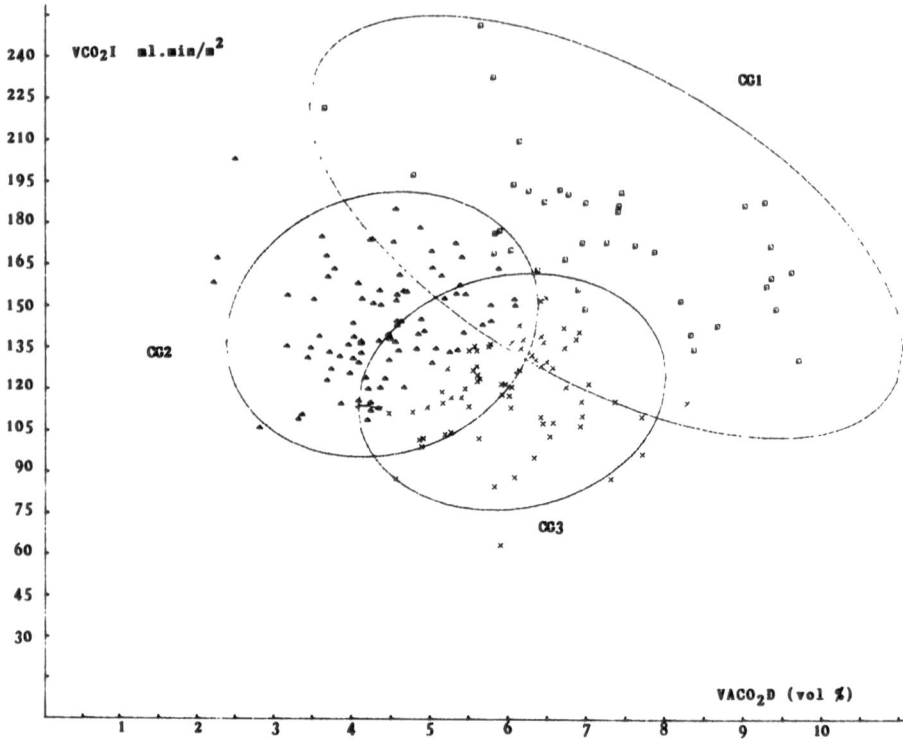

Fig. 3. Representation of the three groups (CG1, CG2, CG3) identified using the cluster analysis at T0

- Cluster Group 2: patients with normal to elevated $\dot{V}CO_2$ and with a lower vaCO$_2$D than CG1.
- Cluster Group 3: patients with reduced $\dot{V}CO_2$ and increased vaCO$_2$D with respect to metabolic needs.

The CG1 may be seen as patients in which to an increased $\dot{V}CO_2$ corresponds a physiologic response with rise in cardiac performance and in peripheral extraction. The CG2 includes patients in which the increased in $\dot{V}CO_2$ is lower with respect to CG1 and metabolic needs are supported only by a rise in cardiac performance without changes in peripheral extraction. The patients of CG3 show a lower $\dot{V}CO_2$ with an enlarged vaCO$_2$D indicating a decreased cardiac performance with respect to metabolic needs.

Conclusion

The continuous recording of physiologic variables is an useful tool into an intensive care unit especially when a high risk of physiologic derangement exists, as in cardiac patients immediately after hypothermic cardiopulmonary bypass. First, $\dot{V}CO_2$ is primarily a metabolic parameter which describes the energy requirements at any moment and thus defines the needs of cardiac performance, ventilation and peripheral extraction. Second, into an integrated analysis of data, $\dot{V}CO_2$ may indicate the adequacy of physiologic response to stress. In fact, in presence of an increase of $\dot{V}CO_2$ (i.e. of metabolic needs) the cardiovascular adaptation may use two physiologic responses: the increase in cardiac performance and blood flow or the increase in peripheral oxygen extraction. To an increased $\dot{V}CO_2$, a marked widening of $vaCO_2D$ corresponds to a reduction of cardiac functional reserve which impairs the rise in blood flow. Otherwise, if cardiac function is normal, in presence of a rise in metabolic requirement the $vaCO_2D$ is stable or shows only minor changes.

With the cluster analysis previously presented, it has been possible to identify three groups of patients which represent three different models of physiologic adaptation to stress. Movement a patient from a group to another may be a helpful aid to early therapeutic intervention.

References

1. Ade T (1974) Influence of cardiac surgery using cardiopulmonary bypass on metabolic regulation. Jap Circ J 38:13-18
2. Raison JCA, Osborn JJ, Beaumont JD (1969) Oxygen comsumption after open heart surgery measured by a digital computer system. Ann Surg 171:471-484
3. Kirklin JW, Kirklin JK, Cell WA (1983) Cardiopulmonary by-pass for cardiac surgery. In: Sabiston DC, Spencer FC (eds), Gibbon's, Surgery of the Chest, 4th ed, Philadelphia, WB Saunders Co pp 909-925
4. Rodriguez J, Weisman C, Damask MC (1983) Physiological requirements during rewarming: Suppresion of the shivering response. Crit Care Med 11:490-497
5. Chiara O, Giomarelli P, Biagioli B, Rosi R, Gattinoni L (1987) Hypermetabolic response after hypothermic cardiopulmonary by-pass. Crit Care Med 15:1071-1075
6. Waller JL, Kaplan JA (1981) Anaesthesia for patients with coronary artery disease. Br J Anaesth 53:757-765
7. Chambers DJ, Darracott-Cenkovic S, Brainbridge MV (1983) Clinical and quantitative birefringence of 100 patients with aortic clamping periods in excess of 120 minutes and hypothermic cardioplegic arrest. Ann Thorac Surg 36:320-326
8. Appelbaum A, Kouchoukos NT, Blackstone EH, Kirklin JW (1976) Early risks of open heart surgery for initial valve disease. Am J Cardiol 37:201-205
9. Mackenzie JD, Haites NE, Rawles JM (1986) Method of assessing the reproducibility of blood flow measurement: factors influencing the performance of thermodilution cardiac output computers. Br Heart J 55:14-24
10. Schmidt CR, Frank LD, Estafanous FG (1983) Continuous pulmonary artery oximetry. An early warning monitor in cardiac surgery patients. Anesthesiology 59 (suppl) A 139 (Abstract)
11. Webb P, Trautman SJ (1970) An instrument for the continuous measurements for oxygen consumption. J Appl Physiol 26:867-871
12. Lister G, Hoffman JE, Rudolph AM (1974) Oxygen uptake in infants and children. A simple method for measurement. Pediatrics 53:656-662
13. Engstrom CG, Herzog P, Norlander P (1961) A method for the continuous measurement of oxygen consumption. Acta Anaesth Scand 5:115-128
14. Hankelin K, Michelsen H, Kuliak V, et al (1985) Continuous on line real time measurement of cardiac output and derived cardiorespiratory variables in the critically ill. Crit Care Med 13:1071-1073
15. Fairley HB, Britt BA (1964) The adequacy of the air mix control ventilators operated from an oxygen source. Can Med Assoc J 90:1394-1396

16. Browing JA, Lindberg SE, Turney SF, et al (1982) The effects of fluctuating FiO2 on metabolic measurements in mechanically ventilated patients. Crit Care Med 10:82–85
17. Damask MC, Weisman C, Askanazi J, et al (1982) A systematic method for validation of gas exchange measurements. Anesthesiology 57:213–218
18. Olsson SG, Fletcher R, Jonson B, et al (1980) Clinical studies of gas exchange during ventilatory support – A method using the Siemens Elema CO_2 analyzer. Br J Anaesth 52:491–498
19. Fukunaga CK, Koonts WLG (1970) Application of the Karhunen-Loeve Expansion to Feature Selection and Ordering. IEEE Trans Computers C-19 311–318
20. Anderberg RM (1973) Cluster analysis for applications. Academic Press, New York, pp 324–355

Heart Transplantation at the Free University of Brussels

J. P. Goldstein and G. Primo

Introduction

After the first human heart transplantation (HTX) performed by Barnard in 1967 [1], disappointing results maintained this procedure for desperate cases. However, during the last decade, considerable advances have been made, prompting a resurgence of interest in HTX.

One of the main improvements in survival rate was the significant reduction in acute rejection achieved with cyclosporine, introduced in our country in 1982. Moreover, other factors were also involved, such as a more critical selection of recipients, the use of new immunosuppressive regimens, improvements in myocardial preservation methods, and early detection of rejection by repeated endomyocardial biopsies.

From March 1982 until November 1987, 102 HTX were performed in 101 patients. We report the result of our experience and review the current trend in HTX.

Patient Selection

All patients were in New York Heart Association (NYHA) Class IV with end-stage cardiac disease and were evaluated for one week in our hospital. Recent degradation in cardiac symptoms with a life expectancy no more than six months were present in every patient. Age criteria have been modified, stimulated by the early good results. The upper limit has now been extended from 50 to 65 years. Of the 101 patients, 95 were male and 6 were female. The mean age was 47 years (range, 5 to 64). The diagnosis was ischemic heart disease in 51, cardiomyopathy in 44, valvular heart disease in 4, toxic myocarditis in 2, and chronic rejection in 1. Eighteen patients had previous cardiac operation (mainly bypass grafting and valve replacement).

Patients with fixed pulmonary vascular resistance greater than 6 Wood units were excluded, so as to avoid graft failure resulting from acute right heart dysfunction in the early postoperative period. Other contraindication criteria were searched, such as recent infection, malignancy, irreversible hepatic or renal disease, or recent pulmonary infarction. Finally, psychosocial status should be evaluated carefully. Patients with alcohol or drug dependency and those with poor psychosocial support should not be accepted.

All candidates for HTX were enlisted on the Eurotransplant waiting list. The mean waiting time was 35±4 days, but with a wide range from 1 day to 6 months.

Donor Criteria and Organ Procurement

Because of the high incidence of undetected coronary disease, male donors should not exceed 40 years, or female donors 45 years. Potential donors with severe chest trauma, cardiac abnormality, or transferable disease were excluded. The donor should be hemodynamically stable, without dependency of high doses of pressor agents (dopamine infusion less than 10 μ/kg/min).

ABO blood group compatibility and relative organ size matching (±20%) were the main requirements before HTX. HLA tissue matching and lymphocytes crossmatching were performed retrospectively.

Removal of the donor heart was performed using the standard techniques, usually in coordination with the harvesting of the liver and the kidneys [2, 3]. The heart was than packed in iced saline solution and stored in a container filled with ice.

Twenty-five hearts came from our institution, 50 others from Belgium, and 25 from Europe (mainly West Germany and The Netherlands). The mean ischemic time was 121 min, ranging from 50 to 225 min.

Orthotopic cardiac transplantation was performed using the standard technique described by Lower and Shumway [4] in 1960.

Immunosuppression

Since the beginning of the cyclosporine program in 1982, the preoperative loading dose of this drug has been largely reduced to limit renal toxicity. Currently, our therapy includes a loading dose of cyclosporine (5 mg/kg) and azathioprine (3 mg/kg), given orally. Methylprednisolone (500 mg) is infused at the end of cardiopulmonary bypass.

Starting the first postoperative day (POD), oral cyclosporine is administered targeting a serum through level around 150–250 ng/ml. Azathioprine is progressively tapered to around 1–1.5 mg/kg/d at the end of the first month with a regular control of WBC counts (>5000/mm^3). During the first POD, methylprednisolone is infused at a dose of 125 mg three times a day. Thereafter, oral prednisone is given at 1 mg/kg/d and gradually tapered to 0.15 mg/kg/d at 1 month. To avoid early cyclosporine nephrotoxicity in high risk patients, OKT 3 antibodies have been recently used instead of cyclosporine as preventive therapy during the first 14 POD (4 patients).

Endomyocardial biopsy is weekly performed during the hospital stay. The frequency is than reduced to one biopsy 2, 4, and 6 months after HTX. Rejection was diagnosed according to the Billingham [5] criteria.

Results

Early Mortality

All patients came off cardiopulmonary bypass with some inotropic and chrono-tropic support (low doses of dopamine and isoproterenol infusion). The mean stay in the intensive care unit was 4 days.

In-hospital mortality included 13 patients. Sepsis was responsible for 6 deaths. Right heart failure, early after HTX, was responsible for 3 deaths, despite inten-sive therapy to reduce right heart afterload. In the early experience with higher doses of cyclosporine, 3 patients died from severe cerebral hemorrhage, asso-ciated with acute renal failure and systemic hypertension. One patient died from acute vascular rejection (18th POD). Eighty-nine patients were discharged from the hospital in good condition.

Early Morbidity

Infection: As expected in immunosuppressed patients, 35 septic episodes (mainly pneumonia and mediastinitis) required vigorous treatment. In 7 patients, Legionella pneumophila was responsible for a servere pneumonia, successfully treated with erythromycin.

Acute renal failure: Transient renal insufficiency (serum creatinine > 3 mg/dl) was observed in 17 patients, mainly at the beginning of the program. Nine early patients required transient hemodialysis.

Rejection: 51 rejection episodes were diagnosed during the first month in 48 pa-tients. Rejection episodes are treated firstly with methylprednisolone pulse ther-apy (1g IV for 3 days). If reversibility is not obtained, anti-lymphocytes globulines (ALG) are infused for 7 to 10 days.

OKT3 (Ortho Corporation) murine monoclonal antibodies are used as rescue therapy when the other drugs fail or in case of rejection with acute myocardial failure (2 patients).

Systemic hypertension: Hypertension was observed in 20 patients and required varied combinations of vasodilating agents, diuretics, beta-blockers, and anti-converting enzyme drugs.

Late Mortality and Morbidity

With a mean follow-up of 15 months and a range of 0 to 66 months, 11 patients died from rejection (8) hypoglycemia (1) or unknown cause (2). The actuarial survival was 78% and 70% at 1 and 2 years, respectively. One patient, who died from chronic rejection after 9 months, suffered also from cutaneous Kaposi sar-coma, diagnosed 3 months after HTX. One patient developed pulmonary tuberculosis 3 years after HTX, and was successfully cured with triple antibiotherapy.

Coronary angiogram is performed annually, during a one-week in-hospital evaluation. Moderate coronary artery disease was seen in 2 patients.

Comments

Our current experience with HTX is in line with several other reports [6, 7], which demonstrate that HTX represents today an effective therapy for selected patients with end-stage cardiac disease. However, the diagnosis and the treatment of long-term complications, such as chronic rejection with coronaropathy, or lymphoproliferative disorders, remain challenging and could jeopardize the early good results.

New immunosuppressive medication has certainly increased the survival and the better quality of life after HTX. Using a triple "low dose" therapy, rejection episodes are more easily treated and severe infections are decreased. However, the long-term effects of cyclosporine therapy are not known. Hypertension and chronic renal dysfunction are worrisome.

Despite an annual increase in HTX performed at our hospital (11 in 1985, 30 in 1986, 50 in 1987), still 10% to 15% of our patients die while waiting for HTX. Moreover, following the alterations in the early rigid selection criteria, a larger excess of recipients may be expected in the near future. This, in turn, may necessitate a revision of the currently required criteria for organ donation, which could for instance lead to accept older donors.

References

1. Barnard CN (1967) A human cardiac transplantation. An interim report of a successful operation performed at Groot Schuur Hospital, Cape Town. S Afr Med J 41:1271–1274
2. Hardesty RL, Griffith BP, Deeb GM, Bahnson HT, Stanzl TE (1983) Improved cardiac function using cardioplegia during procurement and transplantation. Transpl Proc 15:1253–1255
3. Rosenthal JT, Shaw BW, Hardesty RL, Griffith BP, Starzl TE, Hakal TR (1983) Principles of multiple organ procurement from cadaver donors. Ann Surg 198:617–621
4. Lower RR, Shumway NE (1960) Studies on orthotopic homotransplantation of the canine heart. Surg Forum 11:18–19
5. Billingham ME (1981) Diagnosis of cardiac rejection by endomyocardial biopsy. Heart Transpl 1:25–30
6. Baumgartner WA, Augustine S, Borkon AM, Gardner TJ, Reitz BA (1987) Present expectations in cardiac transplantation. Ann Thorac Surg 43:585–590
7. Slater AD, Klein JB, Gray LA (1987) Clinical orthotopic cardiac transplantation. Am J Surg 153:582–593

Acute Renal Failure Following Heart and Heart-Lung Transplantations

M. E. Rogerson and G. H. Neild

Introduction

The last five years have been a period of enormous expansion in the provision of heart and heart-lung transplantation. The outcome of these procedures improved dramatically following the introduction of cyclosporin as the major immunosuppressive agent [1]. One-year survival is now expected at 80% and 85% of long-term survivors are fully rehabilitated [2]. As more successful outcomes have been achieved, patient selection cirteria have become less stringent. Older patients, those with concurrent medical problems or multisystem disorders are now being considered suitable recipients.

There have also been major advances in the management of both donor and recipient contributing to the reduction in morbidity and mortality and even allowing the transplantation of the heart of combined heart-lung recipients into a third patient, (living, non-related heart transplantation) [3]. Nevertheless transplantation is still a last resort. By this stage recipients are often chronically unwell. They are malnourished, even cachectic and their prolonged low-output state with or without hypoxia may have lead to secondary organ damage, principally seen in the liver and kidneys. In such patients the stress of the transplant procedure and its associated fluid and metabolic changes, with the added risks of immunosuppression predispose to several complications including infection and renal failure.

Cyclosporin has been shown to be an effective immunosuppressant in all forms of transplantation with a reduction in long-term complications, particularly of infection, when compared with earlier regimes. However, it is nephrotoxic, both acutely and chronically, in patients with normal or abnormal renal function as well as renal allograft recipients [4]. Other unwanted effects include hypertrichosis, gingival hyperplasia [5], tremor and more rarely other neurological syndromes (coma, convulsions, ataxia, cerebellar syndrome) [6]. Acute nephrotoxicity is reversible and dose-dependent, however there is a wide variation in patient susceptibility to the drug and in pharmacokinetics making the definition of a precise therapeutic range difficult [7]. Most units therefore undertake frequent drug level monitoring but this may not avoid toxicity. Chronic nephrotoxicity is characterized by interstitial fibrosis which is irreversible and may rarely progress to end-stage renal failure.

The incidence of acute renal failure in the transplant population is around 12% (Harefield Hospital 1986), some of these patients are too unwell to transfer and others are managed by hemofiltration in the transplant centre.

Table 1. Indications for transplantation

Heart (n = 8)
  – Cardiomyopathy (5)
  – Ischemic heart disease (3)

Heart-Lung (n = 7)
  – Right-to-left shunt (5)
    – Patent ductus arteriosus (1)
    – Ventricular septal defect (2)
    – Single ventricle/transposition (1)
    – Unknown (1)
  – Alpha$_1$-antitrypsin deficiency (1)
  – Idiopathic pulmonary hypertension (1)

Between November 1984 and November 1987 we have managed 15 patients with acute renal failure following heart (8) or heart-lung (7) transplantation, including one heterotopic heart and two "live-donor" heart transplants. There were eight males and seven females, with a mean age of 36 (range 20–60) years. Indications for their operations are shown in Table 1.

Renal Failure

Renal failure developed 2–60 days (mean 13) following transplantation. The recipient of the heterotopic heart experienced immediate hemodynamic instability and oliguria, three patients were initially non-oliguric, one becoming anuric later. Five patients were treated with intermittent hemodialysis, daily or on alternate days, three patients received high-volume hemofiltration because of cardiac instability, and in the remaining patients, low volume hemofiltration was used with intermittent hemodialysis. One patient did not require renal replacement therapy.

Vascular access was by double-lumen subclavian or left internal jugular catheter in the first instance in each case, these were replaced as necessary and arterio-venous shunts were substituted in eight cases. Renal biopsy was contraindicated by thrombocytopenia in the early part of the illness. In one case prolonged anuria, despite good progress in other respects, lead to renal biopsy. This patient had required intra-aortic balloon pumping, high dose adrenaline support, and peritoneal dialysis pre-operatively. The biopsy showed acute tubular necrosis and the patient recovered renal function after a period of 50 days. The other patient requiring peritoneal dialysis pre-operatively was shown to have cortical necrosis at post-mortem. Other post-mortem renal histology was unhelpful.

Cardio-respiratory Support

Five patients required inotropes at the time of transfer. These were discontinued in four cases within 48 hours of arrival. Support was reintroduced in one and was continued throughout his course (60 days). Five patients were artificially ventilated on arrival and seven more became hypoxic at a later stage. This was due to infection in six and graft rejection in one. Only one of these patients subsequently regained spontaneous ventilation.

Immunosuppression

Immediately following the operation patients commenced azathioprine 75–125 mg daily and cyclosporin 5–10 mg/kg/day. Cyclosporin levels, at Harefield Hospital, were monitored daily by radio-immunoassay (RIA) of plasma samples taken pre-dose and doses were adjusted according to daily levels and renal function. Graft rejection was diagnosed clinically with the help of external cardiac monitoring, daily ECG recordings and weekly endocardial biopsies. The highest plasma level recorded in each patient was in the range 154–1463 ng/ml, mean 648 ng/ml (therapeutic range 150–300 ng/ml). Whole blood cyclosporin levels were measured in our unit and at the time of arrival, the mean pre-dose level (RIA) was 537 ng/ml, range 75–2000 (therapeutic range 200–800 ng/ml). The drug had already been withdrawn in 6 patients and was stopped in one more, nevertheless, in each case the cyclosporin level remained greater than 200 ng/ml for more than seven days.

Azathioprine was continued at a dose dictated by the white blood cell count and prednisolone was introduced in those patients who were no longer receiving cyclosporin. In the 5 patients in whom the drug was continued, the level was maintained in the range 200–400 ng/ml, mean dose 4.9 mg/kg/day (range 2.5–10).

Rejection was diagnosed on 7 occasions in six patients (3 heart, 3 heart-lung) by clinical criteria (pulmonary infiltrates or dysrhythmia) in four cases and after endocardial biopsy in three. All resolved satisfactorily by histological criteria. Treatment was with pulses of methylprednisolone with or without anti-thymocyte globulin.

Nutrition

Three patients remained well enough throughout to continue oral feeding. The majority however required intensive support with nasogastric feeds in four and full parenteral regimes with appropriate dialysis/filtration schedules in the others.

Microbiology

Routine specimens were taken regularly to isolate pathogens and establish sensitivity patterns early where possible. Infection became evident in all patients at some stage who had fever or hemodynamic instability. Pathogens were:

1. Pseudomonas species commonly, colonizing 7 patients in either chest or peritoneum,
2. other Gram negative organisms,
3. Candida was a significant infection in three and probably non invasive in three others.

The two former cases succumbed despite anti-fungal treatment and were found at post-mortem to have disseminated cytomegalovirus (CMV) infection. The third also died. Serological evidence of CMV reactivation was found in one patient who survived. Staphylococci were not isolated.

Neurology

The level of consciousness deteriorated in nine patients to the point of coma. Three patients convulsed, one who was in respiratory failure when he was thrombocytopenic, and with evidence of hepatocellular dysfunction. This patient's plasma cyclosporin level was 55 ng/ml, at the time of fitting. The other two patients fitted at a time of high whole blood cyclosporin levels (680 and 500 ng/ml 3 days after stopping the drug), hyponatremia (around 120 mmol/l) and abnormal clotting tests. There were no localizing neurological signs. CT-scans and EEGs were not performed in the majority of cases. Convulsions were readily controlled by conservative measures and benzodiazepines.

Laboratory Data

Pre-operative

Pre-operative assessment revealed renal impairment in eight patients. Mean plasma creatinine was 190 μmol/l (range 134–300 μmol/l), and urea 16 (range 10.2–24) mmol/l (data for one patient unavailable). Two patients already required peritoneal dialysis. Hepatic dysfunction was documented in six patients with mean plasma bilirubin of 76 mmol/l (range 16–159), alkaline phosphatase of 213 IU/l (range 75–537), and AST of 35 IU/l (range 16–52).

Post-operative

Hyponatremia occurred in the post-operative phase in 12 of the patients. The lowest plasma sodium level recorded ranged from 118 to 134 mmol/l (mean 126.7) and was noted within the first week in eight of these, in four it occurred later at the time of development of renal impairment. Six patients remained hyponatremic on arrival with a mean Na of 130.8 mmol/l (119–142).

Abnormalities of liver function tests were noted in all patients at some time. On arrival, mean bilirubin level was 173 μmol/l (range 42–427 μmol/l) AST 45

IU/l (range 8–104) and alkaline phosphatase 371 IU/l (range 200–556). All of these parameters deteriorated.

Eight patients had abnormal hemostasis on arrival (prothrombin time greater than 18 sec and/or APTT greater than 42 sec). This also deteriorated to a maximum mean PT of 21.5 secs (16–35), APPT 58 sec (35–114), thrombin time 15 sec (12–24). Mean platelet count on arrival was $144 \cdot 10^3$/l (range 32–412) and was less than $100 \cdot 10^3$ in 6 patients).

Outcome

All patients deteriorated initially, despite full support. Five patients survived (33%). Mean age of the survivors was 29 years and mean time on dialysis was 21 days (2–50) compared with 28 days (1–90) in the non-survivors. Four of the survivors had normal pre-operative renal function and only one required inotropic support after the immediate post-surgical period. Only one of the five patients who was ventilated at the time of transfer survived and only one of those who required later respiratory support survived. Coma was a poor prognostic sign since seven of the ten affected subsequently died. However, two of the three patients who fitted lived despite the other concurrent metabolic abnormalities described above.

Liver function tests were more abnormal in the non-survivors with prominent intra-hepatic cholestasis (Table 2).

Cause of death was established by post-mortem examination in seven cases. Two patients were transferred to their country of origin, one whilst still on dialysis but died shortly afterwards, and a second without further examination. Autopsy was refused in one case.

Graft failure was the major cause of death in three patients: one (heterotopic heart recipient) had early pump failure, one overwhelming rejection – predominantly evident in the lungs and a third had intractable dysrhythmias. Two patients had bronchopneumonia and hepatic failure and were found at post-mortem to have widespread CMV intracellular inclusions in several organs. Sepsis and hepatic failure were prominent in four other cases. Cyclosporin was probably a significant contributory factor in two cases but may have influenced the development of renal impairment in others.

Table 2. Worst liver enzyme measurements (mean) in relation to survival

	Bilirubin µmol/l	Alkaline Phosphatase IU/l	AST IU/l
Survived	122	479	145
Died	338	936	72

Conclusions

Acute renal failure in the recipients of heart and heart-lung transplantation is multifactorial. Pre-renal factors are prominent as in other "surgical" causes of acute renal failure. However, cyclosporin is nephrotoxic and may potentiate other, particularly ischemic, causes of renal impairment in these patients. Cyclosporin may also contribute to coma and convulsions and to a syndrome similar to thrombotic thrombocytopenic purpura [7]. The outcome for patients who develop acute renal failure is poor, but may be more favorable in the younger recipients without pre-existing multi-system impairment.

In order to minimize cyclosporin toxicity care should be taken to monitor renal function and urine electrolytes carefully. Episodes of hypotension, the concomitant use of other nephrotoxic drugs and hepatic dysfunction will all increase the likelihood of acute renal failure. The dose of cyclosporin should be reduced when either blood levels are high or when creatinine rises. However, renal failure requiring dialysis is not a contra-indication to cardiac transplantation.

References

1. Oyer PE, Stinson EB, Jamieson SW, et al (1983) Cyclosporin A in cardiac allografting. Transplant Proc 15:1247–1252
2. Schroeder JS, Hunt SA (1986) Cardiac transplantation: Where are we? N Engl J Med 315:961–963
3. The Sunday Times (1987) Times Newspapers, London, 3rd. May 1987
4. Yee GC, Kennedy MS, Deeg HJ, Leonard TM, Thomas ED, Storb R (1985) Cyclosporin associated renal dysfunction in marrow transplant recipients. Transplantation Proceedings 17 (suppl 1)):196–201
5. Myers BD, Ross J, Newton L, Leutscher J, Perloth M (1984) Cyclosporin-associated chronic nephropathy. N Engl J Med 311:699–705
6. Beaman M, Parvin S, Veitch PS, Walls J (1984) Convulsions associated with Cyclosporin A in renal transplant recipients. Br Med J 290:139–140
7. Rogerson ME, Marsden JT, Reid KE, Bewick M, Holt DW (1986) Cyclosporin blood concentrations in the management of renal transplant recipients. Transplantation 41:276–278
8. Shulman N, Striker G, Deeg HJ, Kennedy M, Storb R, Thomas ED (1981) Nephrotoxicity of cyclosporin A after allogeneic marrow transplantation: glomerular thromboses and tubular injury. N Engl J Med 305:1392–1395

Monitoring of the Critically Ill:
Invasive and Non-Invasive

Physiological Meaning of Intravascular Pressure

A. Versprille

Introduction

Changes in pressure result from changes in density of molecules which are so small for fluid that volume changes in a fluid can be neglected for all pressure changes within a physiological range. When we take a breath and dive to ten meters below water surface ambient pressure will be doubled to two atmospheres. This increase in pressure will not change the volume of our body except for the gas volumes of our lungs and intestine. These cavities will decrease to half their normal value according to the law of Boyle Gay Lussac: PV/T is constant, where P is pressure, V is volume and T is absolute temperature.

In this chapter intravascular pressures and their meaning for the circulation of blood will be considered for workers in the field of intensive care medicine and anesthesiology.

Zero Blood Pressure

Pressures in our body follow the changes in ambient air pressure to the same extent. To eliminate such nonphysiological changes ambient air pressure is reset to zero, and pressures are given as their differences from ambient air pressure. Then, zero pressure in the circulation has to be defined as the actual ambient pressure. However, this definition of zero pressure is not satisfactory, because we are dealing with a system of three dimensional character implying also differences in height. Height causes pressure due to the weight of the fluid column, which is called hydrostatic pressure.

To assess the condition of the circulation for medical reasons we are usually less interested in hydrostatic pressure differences. Then, we prefer to know the pressure differences necessary to maintain flow in the system, i.e. hydrodynamic pressures.

Hydrodynamic and Hydrostatic Pressure

I will use a simple physical model of a pump and a circular tube to explain the driving hydrodynamic pressures and the effect of hydrostatic pressure. With use of this model we will explain the elimination of hydrostatic pressure from physiological and clinical measurements.

In Figure 1a, a pump delivers a flow which causes a pressure of 10 cmH$_2$O at the entrance of a horizontally situated circular tube. At the end of the tube, i.e. at the entrance of the pump, the pressure is 0. Thus, pressure fall is 10 cmH$_2$O. The diameter of the tube is constant, the wall is rigid, and the circular width is 20 cm. Half way pressure will be 5 cmH$_2$O. The pressure fall of 10 cmH$_2$O in this system is necessary to overcome flow resistance in the system. The system will behave according to the general hydrodynamic law: $\Delta P = \dot{Q} \cdot R$, where ΔP is pressure fall, $\dot{Q}$ is flow and R is flow resistance. This law is similar to Ohm's law for electricity $E = i \cdot r$, where E is voltage (V), i is electrical current (A) and r is resistance (Ω). Pressure and flow are measured variables, flow resistance is calculated and therefore a derived variable depending on the model behind the calculation.

The pressure necessary to maintain flow against a flow resistance is a hydrodynamic pressure, i.e. a pressure necessary for the functional behavior of the system.

Now the tube is placed in vertical position (Fig. 1b) with the pump at the highest position. The same flow will be delivered and therefore the same dynamic pressure fall will govern flow along the tube. However, actual pressures in the system are changed. Half way the tube a dynamic pressure of 5 cmH$_2$O will exist, which can easily be understood from Fig. 1a. But actual pressure at this point in the vertical position will be 25 $(5+20)$ cmH$_2$O, because the point is 20 cm below the level of the pump, where we have zero pressure.

When the tube is in a vertical position with the pump at the lowest point of the circle (Fig. 1c), actual pressure half way the tube will be -15 cmH$_2$O $(+5-20)$. This fluid flows from a point with an actual pressure of -15 cmH$_2$O to a point with an actual pressure of 0, which looks as an uphill flow. However, this flow is also driven by a height difference of 20 cmH$_2$O, and therefore the driving pressure is $20-15=5$ cmH$_2$O, which is the same value in the driving pressure from half way the circle in horizontal position.

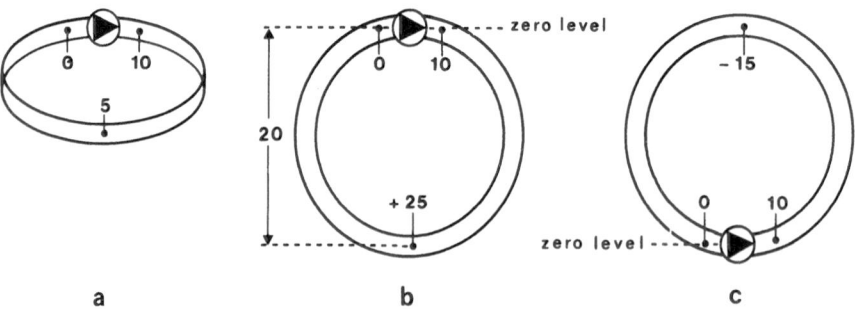

a   b   c

Fig. 1a–c. A circulation model in horizontal and two vertical positions to illustrate the effect of height differences on actual pressure. The circular diameter is 20 cm. Pressures in the tube are given in cmH$_2$O. Actual pressures are the sum of hydrodynamic pressure and hydrostatic pressure and have been given outside the tube in numbers. *a* hydrostatic pressure is zero, therefore all numbers indicate hydrodynamic pressures depending on $\Delta P = \dot{Q} \cdot R$. *b* hydrostatic pressure acts positively on actual pressure and in *c* it acts negatively. Further explanations are given in the text

Elimination of Hydrostatic Pressure

For assessment of the hydrodynamic conditions in the model of Figures 1b and 1c we have to eliminate the differences in hydrostatic pressure. Most pressure measurements are performed with use of pressure transducers, which measure blood pressure on one side of a membrane against ambient air pressure on the other side. Displacement of the membrane is linearly transformed in an electrical signal.

Blood pressure will be zero when it causes the same pressure on the membrane as ambient air pressure. Let us suppose a catheter is filled with saline and connected to the transducer. Pressure will be zero when the tip of the catheter is at the same height as the membrane of the transducer. When we lift the tip to a level 10 cm above the membrane, a pressure of 10 cmH_2O will be measured due to the weight of the water column pressing on the membrane.

Actual pressure is the sum of hydrostatic and hydrodynamic pressures. To measure actual pressure at a point in a system, not only the tip of the catheter has to be in that point but also the transducer has to be positioned at the same height, otherwise the weight of the water column in the catheter will affect the measured value.

To measure only hydrodynamic pressure the transducer has to be balanced to zero via a side way of the stopcock connecting catheter and transducers, and the opening of the side way has to be at the correct zero level of the system. This is the input side of the pump in Figure 1. When the tip of the transducer is kept at the level of the lowest point of the tube in Fig. 1c, but outside the tube, the tip is 20 cm below the zero level of the transducer. Then, a water column of 20 cmH_2O pulls on the membrane causing a pressure measurement of -20 cmH_2O. When now the catheter is inserted into the tube at its lowest point an actual pressure of $+25$ cmH_2O acts on the tip. Thus, a pressure of $-20+25=5$ cmH_2O will be measured, which is the hydrodynamic pressure at this point, as given in Figure 1a.

The same can be reasoned for the situation of Figure 1b. The transducer will measure zero when the tip is at the level of the 0-pressure in the system, the level of the input of the pump. At the highest point in the vertical model the fluid column in the catheter will cause a pressure of $+20$ cmH_2O on the membrane. Connected to the tube it comes into an environment where a pressure of -15 cmH_2O exists, resulting in a pressure measurement of $+5$ cmH_2O.

Thus, when a transducer is balanced to zero at a certain level, in preference a level in the circulatory system where actual pressure is zero, and when pressure elsewhere in the system is measured with the use of a fluid filled catheter, differences in hydrostatic pressure in the circulatory system are compensated for by the opposite effect of the same hydrostatic pressure differences in the catheter leading to the measurement of hydrodynamic pressure only. When using a fluid filled catheter for measurements of pressure in a three dimensional circulatory system all height differences are eliminated, resulting in a system of vessels positioned in a horizontal plane through the zero-level.

The definition of zero pressure has to be extended now:

Zero pressure in the circulation is the pressure equal to ambient air pressure when the pressure transducer is balanced against a fluid surface at a chosen height.

For the human circulation the best zero level is taken at the level of the tricuspid valve in the heart, where pressure is lowest in the system.

Additional Remarks

In clinical practice pressure transducers are usually placed at the same bedside level, and the side outlet of the stopcock is used as the zero level to balance the transducers to zero. On itself such a condition of the same height of transducers is not necessary. The only important condition for an accurate zero level is the height of a fluid surface where the transducers are connected to when balanced to zero level. In our experimental laboratory a reference bottle partly filled with saline is used for that reason. The fluid level is adjustable to the level of the manubrium of the pig in supine position. All transducers are zero-balanced to this level.

It has to be emphasized that even such precautions do not guarantee the same zero levels for all individual experiments. The manubrium is an external reference level of the animal. The heart of each individual animal will not necessarily be at the same level with respect to this point. In supine position the chosen zero level might have differences from the real zero level of about 1 cmH$_2$O in positive or negative direction.

In patients this usually will be less accurate. When comparing venous or low intracardiac pressures in groups of patients such differences in zero level might cause relatively large errors. Therefore, in patient studies an accurate estimation of the level of the tricuspid valve should be done to establish an accurate zero level.

Hemodynamic Pressures

Pressure Fall

The function of the heart is to maintain the difference in pressure between aorta and caval veins in the systemic circulation and between pulmonary artery and the pulmonary veins in the pulmonary circulation. These pressure differences are necessary to maintain flow through both circulations. Thus, the function of the heart is to pump blood at low pressure up to blood at high pressure. This investment of potential energy in the blood is lost again as frictional heat due to flow resistances in the peripheral circulation. Such energy dissipation mainly occurs by movement of blood layers along each other in the vessels. In the circulation of blood hydrodynamic pressures are usually called hemodynamic pressures.

When arterial to venous pressure difference ($\Delta P = P_a - P_v$) is large at normal flow ($\dot{Q}$) flow resistance (R) will be large. We have to keep in mind that such pressure difference mainly depends on arterial pressure. Venous pressure is usually maintained close to zero level when heart function is normal.

Consideration of arterial to venous pressure difference in clinical practice usually implies consideration of difference in mean pressures. Mean pressure can be taken over a cardiac cycle, it can also be calculated over a longer period. For reasons of a pressure-flow-relationship mean pressure should be restricted to a cardiac cycle and if necessary followed beat to beat. However, in medical care flow is usually determined by methods which take several seconds up to a minute, therefore also mean pressures will be taken over the same time period.

The thermodilution method will take 5–10 s for passage of indicator, which is represented by the time period of the dilution curve. The Fick method takes about 20–40 s when blood is sampled adequately. Therefore, an analysis in patients extending only one full cardiac cycle is usually not possible except during open heart surgery when a flow probe can be placed around the pulmonary artery or the ascending arch of the aorta.

Vascular Resistance of the Systemic Circulation

To calculate arterial vascular resistance of the systemic circulation arterial and venous pressures will be taken over the same time period as necessary for the measurement of flow. Total vascular resistance will be found from $\Delta P/\dot{Q}$. When this value increases we usually conclude to vasoconstriction and when it decreases we conclude to vasodilatation. These conclusions are well known and well accepted. Such conclusions can only be correct when $R = \Delta P/\dot{Q}$ is applicable to the circulation.

The hemodynamic law $\Delta P = \dot{Q} \cdot R$ depends on the conditions of continuous open vessels and laminar flow. Laminar flow means a movement of blood in cylindrical layers along each other with the largest velocity in the axial cylinder and a lower velocity the more a cylindrical layer is away from the axis. The velocity profile is parabolic.

Vascular Resistance of the Pulmonary Circulation

It is not allowed from a theoretical point of view to apply the same theory to the pulmonary circulation. In the pulmonary circulation the conditions of the hemodynamic law $\Delta P = \dot{Q} \cdot R$ are not fulfilled in all parts of the system. Under circumstances of spontaneous breathing lung perfusion is subdivided in zones of no flow (zone 1), flow through Starling resistors, i.e. flow alike a waterfall (zone 2), and flow according to the conditions of the hemodynamic law (zones 3 and 4). Under circumstances of mechanical ventilation zone 2 is enlarged due to the compression of capillaries in the alveolar system by increased alveolar pressure.

Flow through a Starling resistor will increase without much change in arterial to venous pressure difference (Fig. 2) as flow over the Niagara falls will increase without much change in the water level (pressure) before and behind the rim.

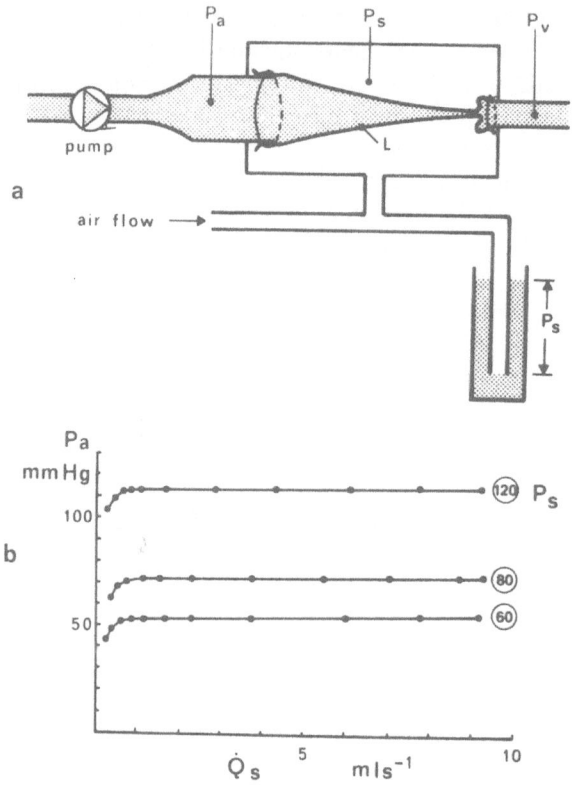

Fig. 2a, b. Model of the functional behavior of a Starling resistor. *a* The model is constructed as a latex tube (L) in a rigid chamber. The latex tube is fixed between two perpex tubes. Fluid is pumped through these tubes. Before and after the latex tube pressures are equal to P_a and P_v respectively. P_s is the pressure surrounding the latex tube, which is controlled by an air flow through a water valve. *b* The diagram gives the relationship between P_a and flow $\dot{Q}_s$. Over a large range of flow P_a is independent of flow, because as soon as P_a becomes larger than P_s the valve will open widely. Then an increased flow through the Starling resistor will decrease blood volume before the resistor and will recover P_a to the value close to P_s. When P_a is smaller than P_s the valve will be closed completely and no flow through the Starling resistor will occur, resulting in an increase of blood volume before the resistor until P_a is high enough to open the latex valve again.

This model will function only as a Starling resistor when P_v is lower than P_s, otherwise the tube will be open from its backside and P_a will be higher than P_s as well to maintain flow.

Another analogy of a Starling resistor is a waterfall, where downstream water level has no effect on the water flow over the rim as long as it is lower than the rim (otherwise it is no waterfall) and where water level before the rim depends on the height of the rim.

(With permission of Intensive Care Med 1984, vol. 10, 51–53)

Moreover, the water level downstream the fall does not affect flow over the rim. In analogy venous pressure does not affect flow through a Starling resistor, which implies that arterial to venous pressure difference (ΔP) has no meaning for the pressure-flow relationship. Thus, application of $R = \Delta P / \dot{Q}$ in a circulation where flow is partially governed by Starling resistors leads to wrong conclusions with respect to changes in flow resistance.

It has to be emphasized that flow resistance cannot be measured. Flow resistance is a derived variable based on a model. When the conditions of the model are not fulfilled the derived variable cannot be correctly estimated. Under such circumstances it is wise to assess circulatory changes only by considering changes in pressure and flow.

When flow is changed without any change in driving pressure a real chance will exist that the circulation is mainly characterized by Starling resistors. When during constant ventilatory conditions by some reasons pulmonary arterial pressure is increased and venous pressure and cardiac output are constant, we will conclude for an increased flow resistance in the muscular arteries due to vasoconstriction.

However, the calculation of the flow resistance before and after the vasoconstriction will lead to false values:

Calculation of flow resistance in the pulmonary circulation will lead to a meaningless value.

Mean Systemic Filling Pressure

Mean systemic filling pressure could certainly be classified under hemodynamic blood pressures. Because of its virtual character in some sense and its real existence as a venous pressure at certain sites in the small veins in another, this concept needs a separate paragraph.

The Concept

When the output of the left ventricle is stopped suddenly arterial pressure will fall by loss of arterial blood volume into the venous system, where pressure will rise. The resulting pressure at equilibrium is the filling pressure of the systemic circulation and has been called mean systemic filling pressure (P_{sf}). P_{sf} is dependent on the tightness of the circulatory system around the blood volume. Either increase of blood volume or increase of smooth muscular tone of the vessels will increase P_{sf}. The venous system has a larger volume and capacity function, i.e. change in volume per unit of pressure change, than the arterial system. Therefore, mean systemic filling pressure depends predominantly on the tightness of the venous system.

During normal circulation arterial to venous pressure gradient is about 100 mmHg. Somewhere in the roots of the peripheral veins pressure will be equal to P_{sf}, which has a value of 7–10 mmHg in mammals. When left ventricular output suddenly stops, upstream of the site where blood pressure is equal to P_{sf} pressure will fall and downstream pressure will rise. Thus, blood will be lost from the arteries and capillaries and it will be accumulated in the venous system downstream from sites in the vessels where venous pressure is equal to P_{sf}.

The same processes will occur when initially venous pressure is raised, e.g. by insufflation of the lungs during mechanical ventilation. Insufflation will increase intrathoracic pressure (P_{th}) and central venous pressure (P_{cv}). Such a rise of P_{cv} causes an accumulation of blood in the venous system. Right ventricular output is decreased and therefore also left ventricular output with a delay of a few heart beats. The decreased input into the arterial system causes a fall in arterial pressure (P_a). When insufflation is followed by an inspiratory hold a new equilibrium will be established at a lower level of cardiac output (and venous return) an increased P_{cv} and a decreased P_a. When a larger volume is insufflated into the lungs the rise of P_{cv} is also larger as well as the fall in venous return, cardiac output and P_a.

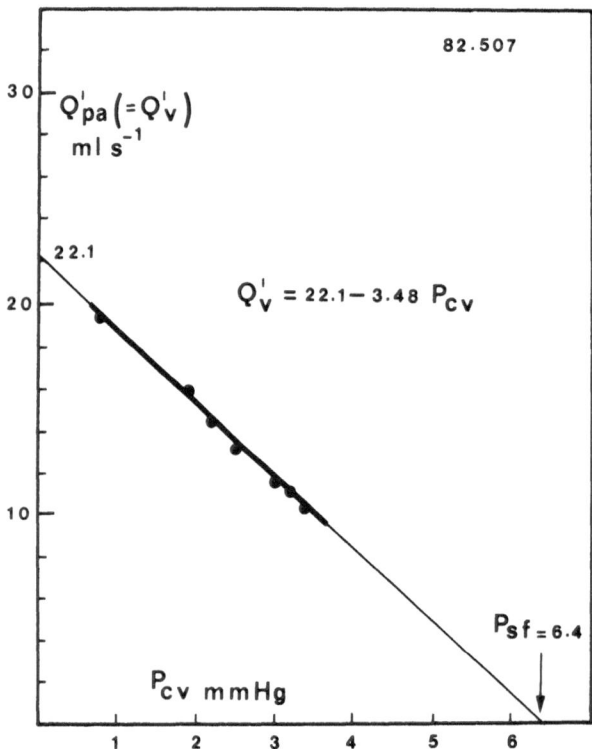

Fig. 3. Relationship between venous return ($\dot{Q}_{pa}$) and central venous pressure (P_{cv}) during inspiratory hold procedures as demonstrated in Fig. 7. During stationary conditions $\dot{Q}_{pa} = \dot{Q}_v \cdot P_{cv}$ values were obtained by inflation of different tidal volumes. When $P_{cv} = 0$ flow is 22.1 ml·s^{-1}. When $P_{cv} = P_{sf}$ flow is zero. In general the formula can be written $\dot{Q}_v = a - bP_{cv}$. For flow is zero $a = bP_{cv}$, giving $P_{sf} = a/b$. The slope b of the line is equal to $\dot{Q}_v/(P_{sf}-P_{cv})$, thus $1/b = (P_{sf}-P_{cv})/\dot{Q}_v$, which is resistance R_{sf}. (From [3] with permission)

Venous Return

Guyton and coworkers [1, 2] observed a linear relationship between the rise in P_{cv} and the decrease in venous return in dogs under circumstances of open chest and right to left bypass. We confirmed their theory on venous return in pigs with intact circulation and closed chest condition. In Figure 3 an individual example of the relationship between P_{cv} and venous return is shown. The method of such experiments is published elsewhere [3] in detail, but Figure 7 gives an example of the procedure to increase P_{cv} by insufflation and to measure flow during the stationary phase of the inspiratory pause. Such an increase of P_{cv} could be chosen to different levels by insufflation of different volumes.

For a certain circulatory condition P_{sf} has a certain value. The venous pressure equal to P_{sf} is at a constant location in the venous roots for a given circulatory condition. When this site is characteristic for a given hemodynamic condition it will imply that an increase in P_{cv} will cause a linear fall in $P_{sf}-P_{cv}$. This fall in pressure gradient over a given venous flow resistance will cause a linear fall in venous flow after a transient phase of additional filling of the venous capacities due to venous pressure rise. In Figures 4 and 5 this hemodynamic behavior is

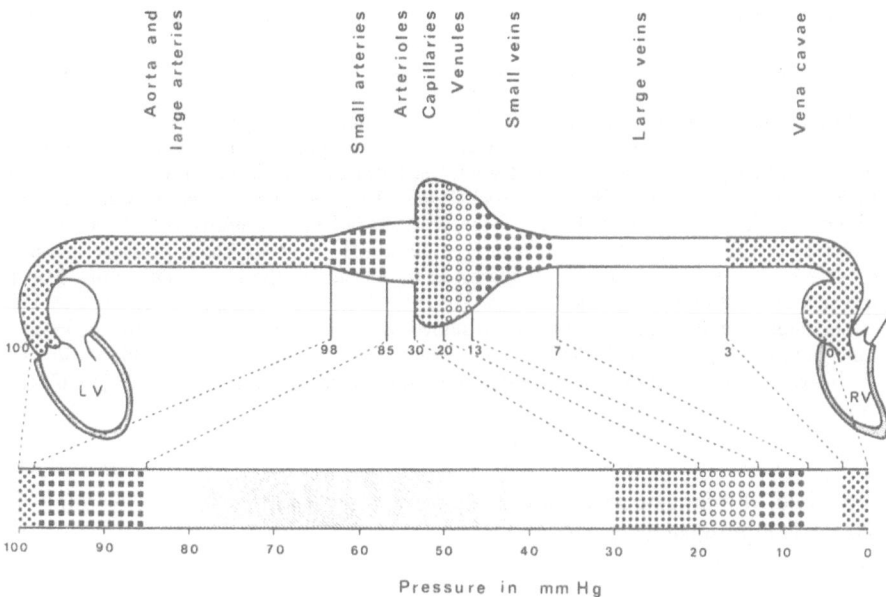

Fig. 4. The systemic circulation modelled as a tube of constant diameter. The numbers give the pressures at the characteristic points of the circulation. They also represent the percentage of total flow resistance over the downstream part of the system. Note that the anatomical projection on the tube is nonlinear. Long wide arteries and veins are represented by small parts of the tube due to their low flow resistance, whereas the short and narrow arterioles take more than half the length of the tube. (From [3] with permission)

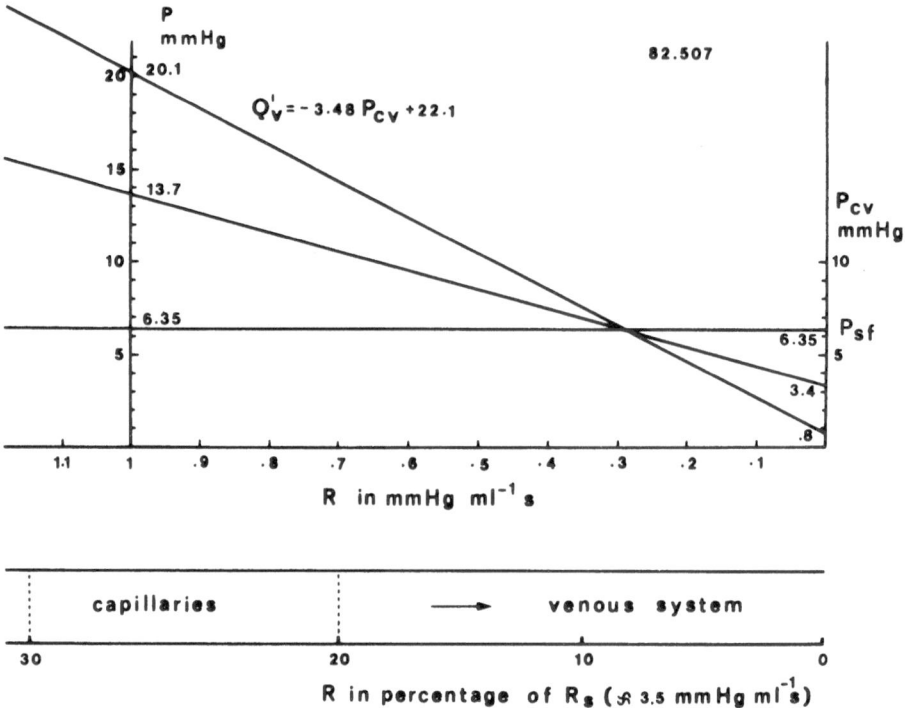

Fig. 5. A physical and graphical model of venous return. The tube is the capillary and venous part of the model in Figure 4. The diagram gives the changes in pressure fall in the tube when P_{cv} is increased. The data are taken from the relationship in Figure 3. In this experiment total vascular flow resistance (R_s) was 3.5 mmHg ml^{-1} s.

In the graphical model the X-axis is given in resistance units in upstream direction starting at the end of the system where P_{cv} exists. Here a Y-axis is positioned. A second Y-axis was set upstream at a flow resistance of 1 mmHg ml^{-1} s. This position was taken for reasons of convenience. When $P_{cv}=0.8$ mmHg, $\dot{Q}_v=22.1-3.48 \cdot 0.8 = 19.3$ jl s^{-1} (see regression equation in Fig. 3). Over a resistance of 1 mmHg ml^{-1} s a pressure fall of 19.3 mmHg will be necessary to maintain this flow ($\Delta P=\dot{Q}\cdot R$). Because $P_{cv}=0.8$ mmHg at $R=1$ blood pressure is equal to $0.8+19.3=21.3$ mmHg. When P_{cv} is increased to 3.4 mmHg the same calculations lead to a pressure at $R=1$ of 13.7 mmHg.

This model predicts P_{sf} at a constant distance from the right atrium in terms of resistance units during an increase of P_{cv}. This is a consequence of the linear decrease in blood flow when P_{cv} increases and stationary hemodynamic conditions are attained again. (From [3] with permission)

modelled. It might be an example of future analyses in patients. This analysis is extensively published elsewhere [3].

Effects of Changing Hemodynamic Conditions

It has to be emphasized that the linear decrease of venous return during an increase of P_{cv}, obtained by an increase of P_{th}, only counts for hemodynamic stationary pressure and flow conditions and a constant circulatory status, i.e. no changes in neurogenic and humoral control. Such conditions will be fulfilled during the first five seconds of an inspiratory hold procedure.

When circulatory control mechanisms are changed in their activity several functions of the circulatory system will be changed.

When the venous smooth muscles are relaxed the tightness of the system around the blood volume will be decreased and therefore P_{sf} will decrease. This includes a decrease of $P_{sf}-P_{cv}$ and also a fall in cardiac output. When venous smooth muscular tone increases the opposite effect will occur. An increased tightness also can be obtained by a G-suit, which also has a positive effect on cardiac output [4]. An increase in blood volume has a similar effect on P_{sf} compared with an increased venous muscular tone.

We could describe the effect of both variables on P_{sf} in a slightly different way. P_{sf} results from the ratio between the volume of blood and the nonstressed volume of the venous system. When the nonstressed volume of the venous system is small with respect to blood volume the veins will be stretched markedly and P_{sf} will be large. When the nonstressed volume is equal to blood volume in the veins P_{sf} is zero and no venous return will be possible.

Changes in R_{sf} Without Changes in P_{sf}

When the arterioles are dilated P_{sf} will be hardly changed, because the volume in the arterioles hardly contributes to the volume of the systemic circulation. The total systemic flow resistance will decreased, which implies a larger pressure gradient in the venous system. Vasodilation will firstly increase venous return at the expense of arterial blood volume. A fall in arterial pressure will follow. With delay of a few heart beats left ventricular output is increased and arterial pressure will be recovered partly. In Figure 6 the effect of decreased peripheral resistance is shown on R_{sf} and on the site where blood pressure is equal to P_{sf}.

When cardiac output, and thus venous return, are increased and venous flow resistance has not been changed a larger pressure fall over the venous system is obligatory. Thus, the site in the venous system where pressure is equal to P_{sf} is shifted downstream, the same $P_{sf}-P_{cv}$ will drive flow over a smaller resistance, which is in accordance with a larger flow. This flow resistance between the sites in the venous roots where P_{sf} exists and the heart is part of the total venous flow resistance. It has been symbolized as R_{sf}. During a given hemodynamic condition the equation $R_{sf}=(P_{sf}-P_{cv})/\dot{Q}$ can be used to calculate R_{sf}. For the same $P_{sf}-P_{cv}$ and a larger $\dot{Q}$ R_{sf} will have been decreased, which is accomplished by a downstream shift of the site where $P_v=P_{sf}$. Thus, vasodilatation of the arterioles also decreases R_{sf}.

Hemodynamic Changes Without Changes in P_{sf} and R_{sf}

An example will be presented in which neither R_{sf} nor P_{sf} nor cardiac output are changed, whereas large changes in hemodynamic conditions occured. This example is given for better understanding the way we will have to look at these variables to assess circulatory conditions.

In Figure 6a a simple systemic circulation is given. $\dot{Q}_v$ is cardiac output and ΔP total pressure gradient. Somewhere in the system pressure is equal to P_{sf}. We assume $P_{cv} = 0$. Then $R_{sf} = P_{sf}/\dot{Q}_v$. We will now apply a conceptual change of the system which hardly can be realized. The systemic circulation is doubled by a parallel circuit between the aortic arch and the right atrium (Fig. 6b). The additional circuit is filled up to the same extent and its tightness is similar to the original circuit. Thus, P_{sf} will not be changed. We assume a constant cardiac output $\dot{Q}_v$. Then R_{sf} for the double system will be the same as R_{sf} of only the original system.

However, total flow resistance becomes half its original value when the circuit is doubled, according to $1/R = 1/R_1 + 1/R_2$, where R_1 and R_2 are equal and represent flow resistances of the original and the additional circuit respectively. For the same flow only half the pressure gradient is necessary. Moreover, only half this flow will pass now the original circuit and in this circuit $P_{sf} - P_{cv} = \frac{1}{2}\dot{Q}_v \cdot R_{sf}$, where P_{sf} is constant and P_{cv} is 0. Thus, R_{sf} of the original system will have to be doubled. This was fulfilled by an upstream shift of the venous site where pressure is equal to P_{sf}. Then the length of the venous system between the site of venous pressure equal to P_{sf} and the right atrium is increased.

The upstream shift of P_{sf} can also be reasoned from the point of view on the pressure gradient. When the pressure gradient over a system decreases to half its value the blood pressure equal to P_{sf} will be found upstream.

This experiment was hypothetical. P_{sf} was the same whereas blood volume was doubled, which only could occur by doubling the frame. P_{sf} on itself cannot

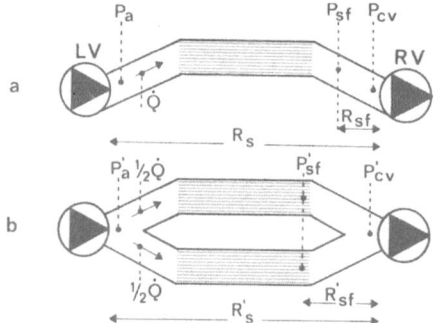

Fig. 6a, b. Doubling of the systemic circulation at constant cardiac output ($\dot{Q}$). *a* In this single system vascular flow resistance $R_s = (P_a - P_{cv})/\dot{Q}$ and $P_{sf} - P_{cv} = \dot{Q} \cdot R_{sf}$. LV, left ventricle; RV, right ventricle. *b* In the double system $R_s' = (P_a - P_{cv})/\dot{Q}$. Because $R_s' = 1/2R_s$ pressure gradient will be half its original value, and because P_{cv} is zero $P_a' = 1/2P_a \cdot P_{sf}' = P_{sf}$, see text, and $R_{sf}' = (P_{sf} - P_{cv})/\dot{Q}$. Thus, $R_{sf}' = R_{sf}$. The flow resistance downstream from the point where blood pressure is equal to P_{sf} in one limb of the doubled system is increased, according to $(P_{sf}' - P_{cv})/1/2\dot{Q}$. Thus, P_{sf} shifted upsteam. This also can be concluded from a constant R_{sf}' and a fall in R_s, which implies a larger part of circulation between P_{sf} and the right atrium.

The same reasoning counts for a constant frame as in 6a and a flow, which is decreased to half its value. In that case $R_{sf}' = 2 R_{sf}$

give us full information about the conditions of the circulation. Its value will give us an indication of the ratio between blood volume and the tightness of the system around it. When blood volume is large as measured by an independent method and P_{sf} is low we could conclude for a large relaxation of predominantly the venous system. To be more extensively informed about the hemodynamic conditions we also need to be informed about R_{sf}, but this variable was also constant. Another important variable, however, changed in our hypothetical experiment. R_{sf} the overall flow resistance decreased to half its value. R_{sf} for the double system was the same as for the original system. Therefore, R_{sf}/R_s increased, indicating an upstream shift of the site where blood pressure is equal to P_{sf}.

This example illustrates that the fall in pressure gradient over the systemic circulation could not be explained by a vasodilation at constant flow, because then P_{sf} would have been shifted downstream which has been explained on page 379. Doubling the circulatory system causes half the value of blood flow through the original system. Therefore, the same changes, except for a double value of overall R_{sf} will be found, when changing cardiac output to half its value in the original system. Such a single change is also a hypothetical example, but it enhances the understanding of its hemodynamic effects.

Mechanical Ventilation

During insufflation of air into the lungs an increase of P_{cv} occurs due to the increase of intrathoracic pressure. The rise in P_{cv} during insufflation is illustrated by Figure 7. When peak insufflation was attained a plateau phase in P_{cv} followed. However, the concomitant decrease in right ventricular output due to the decreased venous return recovered partly during the plateau of constant P_{cv}.

When P_{sf} is constant and located at specific sites in the small veins as explained on pages 375 to 378, $P_{sf}-P_{cv}$ gradually decreased during insufflation. The minimal value of this difference will be reached at peak insufflation when P_{cv} attained its highest value. The characteristic flow value is attained within a few seconds after peak insufflation. However, during the rise in P_{cv}, venous return ($\dot{Q}_v$) fell below its characteristic value given by $\dot{Q}_v = (P_{sf}-P_{cv})/R_{sf}$. The extra fall in flow during the rise of P_{cv}, i.e. the fall of $P_{sf}-P_{cv}$, can be attributed to the capacity function of the venous system. During the rise of P_{cv} venous pressure will rise gradually over the whole venous system downstream of the site where $P_v = P_{sf}$. Such a rise depends on the stretch of the vessel wall by an increase of the volume. The investment of volume will be done at the expense of the output of the venous system, which is venous return into the right heart.

This behavior is simulated with use of a physical model (Fig. 8). This model consists of a tube of constant diameter representing the lumped venous system between the small veins where $P_v = P_{sf}$ and the right atrium. The tube has a flow resistance R_{sf}, subdivided in three resistances R_1, R_2 and R_3. Although the real venous system has a capacity function over the whole length the model is stiff and provided with two capacities at the points P_{v1} and P_{v2}, respectively. This simplification is done for reasons of understanding. Below the physical model

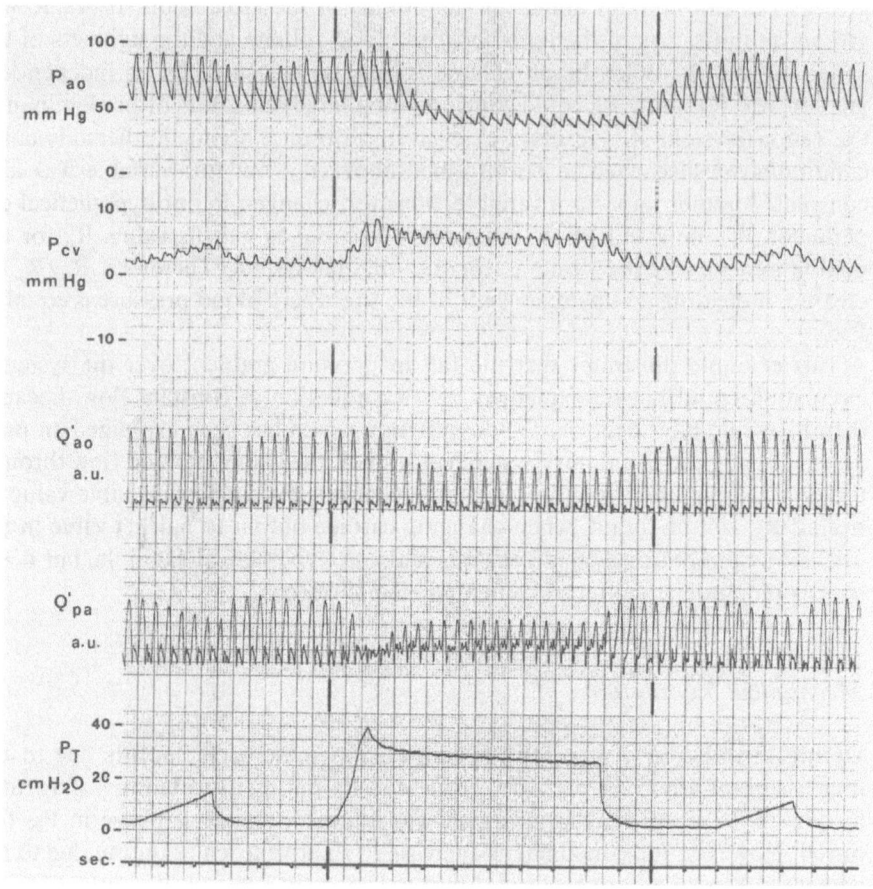

Fig. 7. Recording of arterial pressure (P_{ao}), central venous pressure (P_{cv}), flow in the ascending aorta ($\dot{Q}_{ao}$) and the pulmonary artery ($\dot{Q}_{pa}$), and airway pressure (P_T). Time is marked at the bottom of the recording. First a normal ventilatory cycle is seen, which is followed by an insufflation of larger volume in half the time and next by an inspiratory hold of 7.2 s. (From [3])

the behavior of the system during insufflation is graphically represented. The X-axis of the diagram represents flow resistance. At both endings of this axis a Y-axis is placed, one for P_{sf} and the other for P_{cv}. P_{sf} is taken constant at 10 mmHg and P_{cv} is assumed to be zero at end expiration. The line connecting $P_{sf} = 10$ and $P_{cv} = 0$ has a $\alpha tg = (P_{sf} - P_{cv})/R_{sf}$, which is equal to flow ($\dot{Q}_v$), see page 373. At end expiration $\dot{Q}_1 = \dot{Q}_2 = \dot{Q}_3$.

We assume a rise of P_{cv} during insufflation from 0 to 5 mmHg. During this rise also upstream pressure P_{v2} will rise. However, as soon as P_{v2} increases its capacity will be filled up to a higher level. Such filling takes time and therefore the rise of P_{v2} will be retarded. As a consequence $P_{v2} - P_{cv}$ will stay temporarily smaller than at its new equlibrium after full rise of P_{cv}. The tangent or slope of the flow line connecting P_{v2} to P_{cv} over R_3 is less steep than the slope of the line

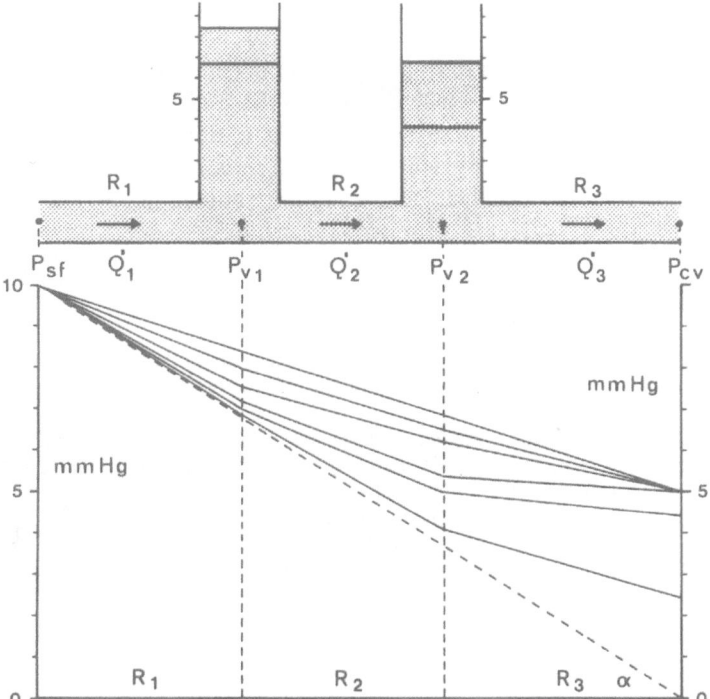

Fig. 8. Model of the venous system downstream of the site where blood pressure is equal to P_{sf}. The upper, physical, model is composed of a stiff tube and two capacities. The lower model is a graphical description of the physical model. At end expiration P_{cv} is taken zero. The X-axis between the two Y-axes at P_{sf} and P_{cv} is equal to R_{sf}, and subdivided in three resistances by two capacities at P_{v1} and P_{v2}. The slope of the dashed line ($tg\alpha$) gives the amount of flow. This slope, and therefore flow, becomes half its value when P_{cv} increases from 0 to 5 mmHg, and when stationary conditions are attained again. During increase of P_{cv} from 0 to 5 mmHg the capacities at P_{v1} and P_{v2} are filled up as explained in the text. The flow lines have temporarily a lower slope compared with the line when the new stady state is reached

after the new equilibrium is reached. The same reasoning counts for the rise in P_{v1} as a result of the rise in P_{v2}. Following this reasoning again less steep flow lines are found over R_2, and also over R_1, compared with the line at equilibrium after full insufflation. When full insufflation is reached P_{cv} is at its highest level and the equilibrium will be settled soon.

During rise of P_{cv} (insufflation) the flow lines attain less steep slopes, explaining the fall in venous return. Recovery of equilibrium implies recovery of steepness of the flow lines to the new characteristic value, which is the slope between $P_{sf} = 10$ mmHg and $P_{cv} = 5$ mmHg. This slope is smaller than the initial value when P_{cv} was 0 mmHg. The new equilibrium is again fully dependent on the equation $\dot{Q}_v = (P_{sf} - P_{cv})/R_{sf}$. This new stationary flow fulfils the linear relationship with P_{cv} as long as the neurogenic and humoral control mechanisms are not changed in activity. This will not occur within the short time period of a ventilatory cycle, even when a short inspiratory pause is involved. Time constants of these control processes are much longer than the duration of a ventilatory cycle.

When after insufflation expiration occurs the capacities empty again and venous return is transiently larger than the stationary value at end expiration. Also this behaviour can be observed in Fig. 6, not only after a ventilation with inspiratory pause but also when insufflation is immediately followed by expiration, thus even when the capacities are not yet completely filled up.

References

The references serve as 'porte d'entrée' to literature and more detailed studies on circulation in general and mean systemic filling pressure in particular.

1. Guyton AC (1981) Textbook of Medical Physiology, 6th ed. Saunders, Philadelphia
2. Guyton AC, Jones CE, Coleman TG (1973) Circulatory Physiology: Cardiac output and its Regulation. Saunders, Philadelphia
3. Versprille A, Jansen JRC (1985) Mean systemic filling pressure as a characteristic pressure for venous return. Pflügers Arch 405:226-233
4. Payen DM, Carli PA, Brun-Buisson CJL, et al (1985) Lower body positive pressure vs dopamine during PEEP in humans. J Appl Physiol 58:77-82

Technological Advances in Pressure Monitoring

B. W. Atwater, J. W. Parker, and R. T. Chilcoat

Introduction

Fast, accurate determination of a patient's status is an indispensable element of patient care. Intermittent sampling of such crucial parameters as blood pressure and blood gas levels has serious limitations, yielding only periodic knowledge of the status of cardio-respiratory function. Not only is it well known that large variations in blood pressure and dissolved gas concentration can occur within minutes (Fig. 1), but also the dynamics of such parameters may be indicative of a patient's status. Continuous monitoring is essential in the management of the critically ill.

Pressure measurements, both blood pressure and partial pressure of dissolved gases, are among the earliest and most important indicators of serious problems with a patient. Continuous monitoring of blood pressure, including identification of the wave form, reflects how well the heart is functioning. Knowledge of the partial pressure of oxygen (PO_2) and carbon dioxide (PCO_2) are needed to evaluate the effectiveness of gas exchange at the lungs and the systemic tissue.

New technologies are furnishing increasingly reliable pressure sensors. Similarly, older technologies such as pressure transducers and electrochemical sen-

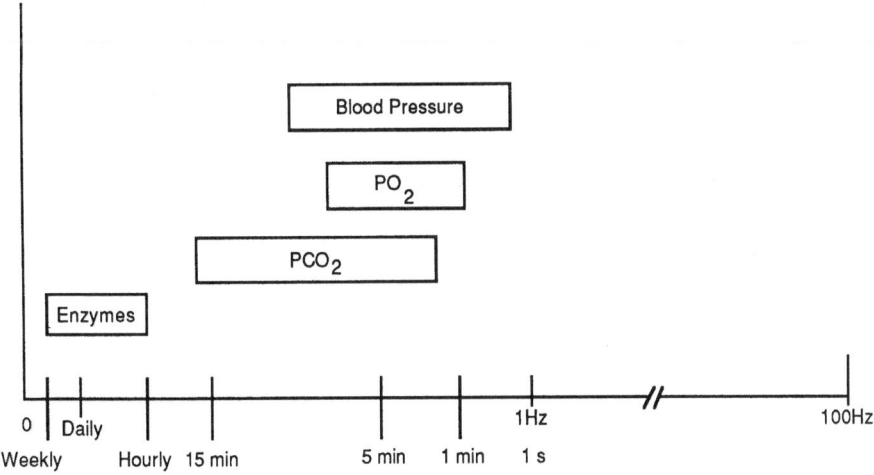

Fig. 1. Typical time constants for clinical monitoring

sors are progressing, providing small and accurate continuous pressure monitors. Recent advances in fiber optics offer novel new technologies for sensors. The small size and lack of electrical interference of fiber optic sensors make this technology uniquely suited for medical applications. This paper, while discussing some older measurement techniques, will focus on current developments of fiber optic sensors for continuous monitoring of blood pressure and the partial pressure of carbon dioxide and oxygen.

Fiber Optic Sensors

Fiber optics is one of the most rapidly growing technologies associated with medical monitoring. Flexible optical fibers transmit light over long distances with little loss. Typical fibers consist of a cylindrical core, through which light travels, surrounded by a material with a lower index of refraction. When encountering a medium with a lower index of refraction, light traveling through a medium with a higher index of refraction will exhibit total internal reflection if the angle between the plane of the surface and the light propagation axis is shallow enough. Thus, light that is launched into the fiber in the appropriate angle will remain in the fiber. Light conduction in an optical fiber is illustrated in Figure 2.

The concept of a fiber optic sensor is simple: light from a source travels through an optical fiber to a sensing element (sometimes the fiber itself) where the light is somehow altered before traveling via the fiber to a detector. Fiber optic sensors can be either single or double ended, as shown in Figure 3.

Physical fiber optic sensors are based either on the application of a micro-transducer that converts physical signals to optical signals or on direct variation of the optical characteristics within the fiber in response to changes in physical parameters. Changes in birefringence, polarization, and reflectometry are the principal techniques used in physical fiber optic sensors; such techniques are well suited for blood pressure monitoring.

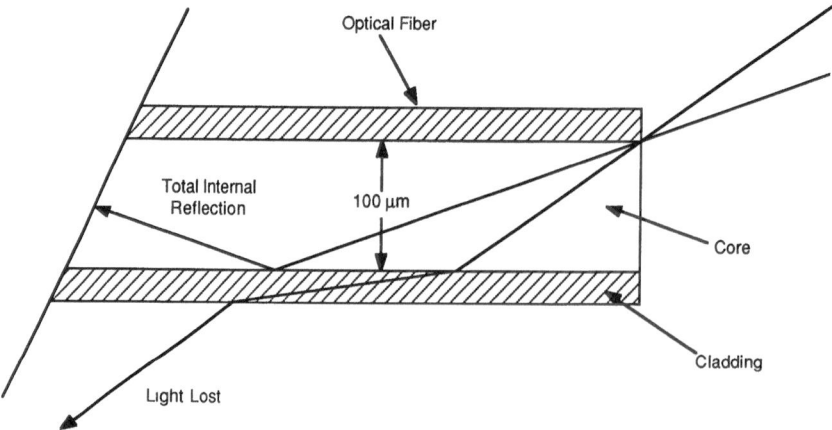

Fig. 2. Schematic illustrating light conduction in an optical fiber

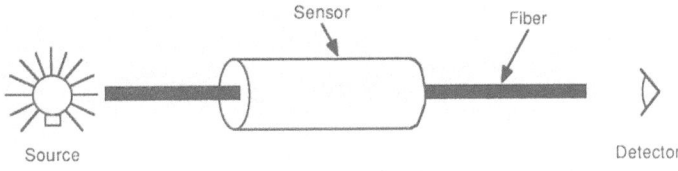

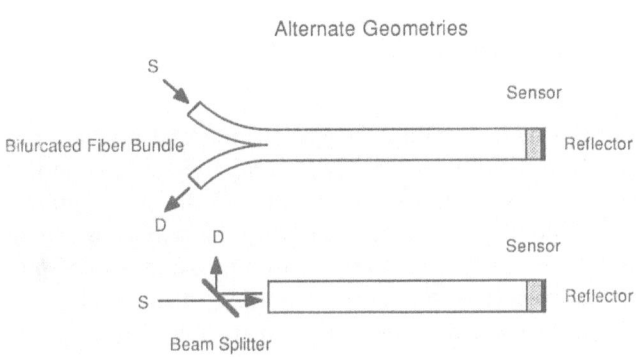

Fig. 3. Schematic diagram of the basic components of fiber optic sensors

Many fiber optic chemical sensors rely on immobilized indicator systems bound to the fiber. This arrangement allows commonly used indicator reagent chemistry to be adapted to fiber optic sensors. Reversible fluorimetric or colorimetric (absorption) measurements are the most common techniques being applied in the chemical fiber optic sensors under development today.

Invasive Pressure Monitoring

The most recent advances in pressure monitoring have come in the area of fiber-optic methods. Several of these fiber optic pressure transducers have been commercialized, with mixed success.

Fiber optic pressure transduction can be divided into those in which the intensity of the light is modulated, and those in which some other variable of the light, such as color (wavelength) or polarization, is modulated. Generally, an intensity-modulated signal is the easiest to achieve, and the majority of fiber optic pressure sensors fall into this category.

Figure 4 illustrates a simple method of making an intensity modulated pressure transducer. In this scheme, pressure applied to the diaphragm causes movement of one of the fibers, resulting in a reduction in the amount of light coupled between the fibers. In this way, a change in applied pressure will result in a change in the intensity of light appearing at the output of the second fiber. This design is complicated and would be difficult to manufacture in quantity. A number of simple designs, all operating by altering the amount of light transmitted or reflected into an output fiber, have been described.

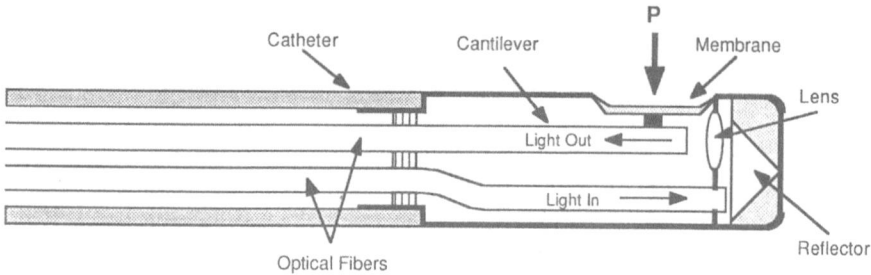

Fig. 4. Diagram of intensity based fiber optic blood pressure sensor

Figure 5 is a typical example of such a practical pressure transducer. This design, patented by Knute and Bailey [1], and assigned to Camino Laboratories of San Diego, California, utilizes a miniature bellows is mounted at the tip of a catheter. The blood pressure interacts with the interior of the bellows, causing it to vary in length with pressure. The closed proximal end of the bellows incorporates a reflective surface that sends a portion of the light from one optical fiber into a second. Movement of the end of the bellows causes proportional variation in this reflected light resulting in an intensity-modulated pressure signal in the second fiber.

A major difficulty with intensity-modulated fiber optic sensors is that any other variable light loss, such as occurs from bending of the fibers, is interpreted as a change in the measured variable. Because of this, many intensity-modulated sensors incorporate compensating mechanisms. For example, the sensor in Figure 5 includes a second fiber pair that are optically linked by a fixed reflective coupler. Since losses due to bending of the catheter will occur approximately equally in all fibers in the catheter, the second pair serves as a reference.

A different configuration for an intensity based fiber optic pressure transducer is shown in Figure 6. In this device [2] the pressure-sensitive diaphragm is mounted on the side of the catheter and includes a cantilever that carries a small reflector. This reflector moves relative to the input and output fibers in a small bundle, and varies the optical coupling between them. A compensation for bending is not included in this device, but it does contain a second fiber bundle for *in-vivo* monitoring of hemoglobin oxygen saturation.

Yet another configuration is shown in Figure 7. This transducer, which em-

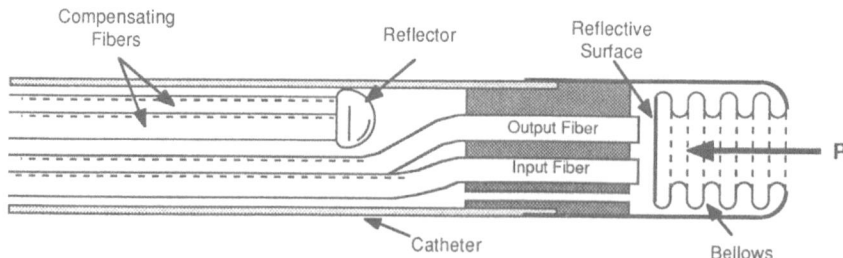

Fig. 5. Schematic of pressure transducer patented by Knute and Bailey

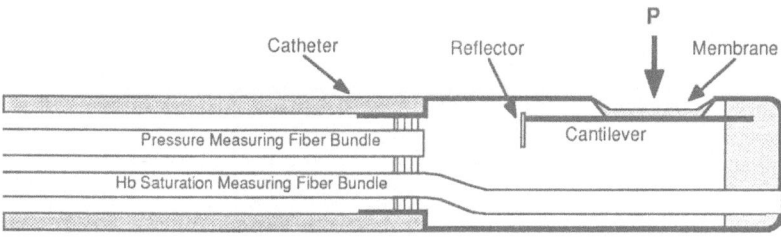

Fig. 6. Blood pressure sensor that utilizes a cantilever for pressure monitoring

ploys a bifurcated fiber bundle with the individual fiber randomly distributed at the distal end was described by Hansen [3], and commercialized by AME, Horten, Norway. A reflective, pressure sensitive diaphragm is spaced a small distance from the ends of the combined bundle. As the diaphragm is distorted by changes in pressure, the reflective coupling between the two sets of fibers varies and results in a change in light intensity in the output fibers.

Lieberman, Blonder and Tighe [4] reported the fiber-tip pressure transducer illustrated in Figure 8. In this device a cavity is formed by photolithography in a small disk of elastic material. The bottom of this cavity is aluminized to make it reflective. The complete assembly is bonded to the end of an optical fiber that has been coated with a semitransparent layer of chromium. The assembly forms an optical interference cavity with an optical path length that changes with pres-

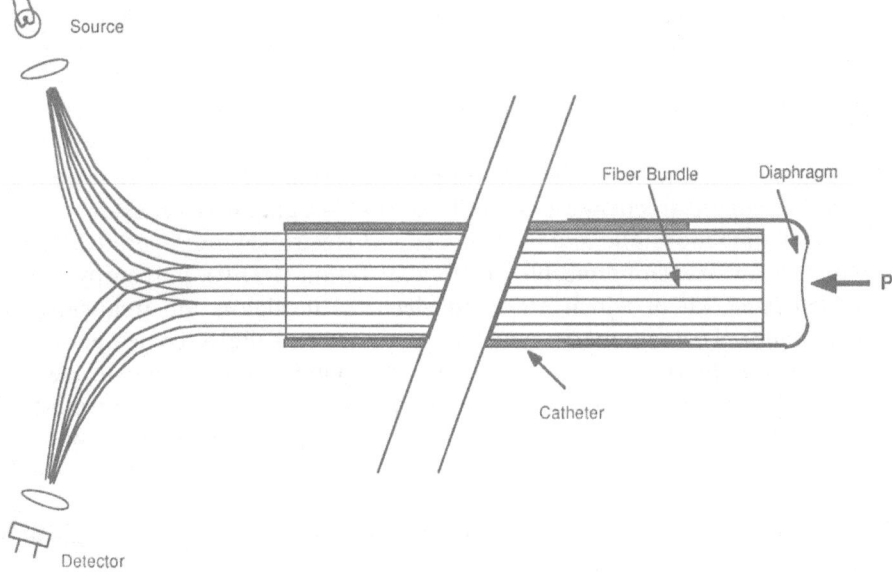

Fig. 7. Diagram of pressure sensor designed by Hansen that employs a pressure sensitive diaphragm

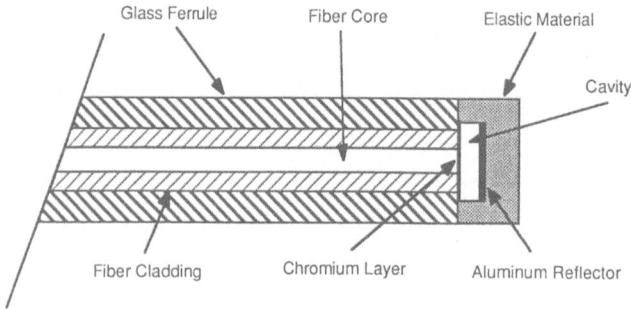

Fig. 8. Interferometric pressure sensor designed by Lieberman et al.

sure. The intensity of the ligth reflected back into the fiber, I_r, is approximately given by the equation governing Fabry-Perot interferometers:

$$I_r = I_o \; \lambda \; \sin2(\iota/2)$$

where, I_o is the incident light intensity, λ is its wavelength, and ι is the optical path length.

Improvements in the design of this interferometric pressure transducer are described by Lieberman and Blonder [5]. In these variations both front and back surfaces of the interferometer are formed from layers of glass, bonded together with a thin layer of silicon. A cavity is etched either into the layer of silicon or into the lower glass layer. A well is etched into the outside surface of the upper glass layer, reducing its thickness over the optical cavity. Pressure applied to this glass membrane varies the path length of the underlying interferometric cavity, resulting in a linear change in light intensity.

Partial Pressure Measurement

The most common techniques for measuring partial pressure of dissolved gases in blood are electrochemical. The Clark [6] polarographic electrode is used for PO_2 determination. The anode, cathode, and electrolyte are separated from the blood by an oxygen permeable membrane. Teflon (PTFE), polypropylene, and polyethylene, all of which are good electrical insulators are frequently used membranes. The cathode is generally platinum and the reference electrode is silver/silver chloride. The electrolyte usually contains potassium chloride and is buffered to a pH around 7 [7]. As the oxygen diffuses through the membrane, it is reduced at the cathode to hydroxide anions by the following reaction:

$$O_2 + 2H_2O + 4e^- \rightarrow 4OH^-$$

These ions are buffered by the electrolyte. The anions are oxidized at the anode and so a constant potential with respect to the solution is maintained. At the reference electrode the reaction is:

$$Ag \rightarrow Ag^+ + e^-$$

Finally, the silver ions generated at the reference electrode react with chloride ions in the electrolyte to form silver chloride. The resulting steady flow of charge between the cathode and the anode provides a current that is a function of the oxygen diffusion through the membrane. As with most electrochemical devices the Clark electrode is subject to drift, requires frequent calibration and recharging of the electrolyte.

Currently, all sensors for measuring PCO_2 are based on pH measurements. The Stow-Servinghaus [8] electrode, the most commonly used device for measuring carbon dioxide in the blood, is no exception. The pH of a thin film of distilled water or bicarbonate solution [9] surrounding the glass pH electrode is measured. The aqueous solution is separated from the blood by a thin rubber membrane. Rubber is permeable to carbon dioxide, but not hydrogen or bicarbonate ions or water. The CO_2 molecules diffuse through the rubber and change the pH of the aqueous solution surrounding the pH electrode as a result of the following reversible reactions:

$$CO_2 + H_2O \rightleftharpoons H_2CO_3 \rightleftharpoons H^+ + HCO_3^-$$

The pH is measured as a change in voltage between the pH electrode and a reference electrode. As indicated by the above reaction, the Stow-Sevringhaus electrode is an equilibrium device, and so the layer of aqueous solution between the rubber membrane and the glass electrode must be kept very thin in order to achieve an adequate response time [7].

Progress in electrochemical determination of PO_2 and PCO_2 has resulted primarily from advances in materials, alternative geometries, and miniaturization. Such advances are examplified in the carbon dioxide catheter recently developed by Opdycke and Meyerhoff [10]. In this sensor a unique geometry is developed by using a tubular polymer pH electrode inside a gas-permeable silicone rubber catheter. The classical glass pH electrode has been replaced by a polymeric pH electrode [11] containing an polymeric pH sensitive membrane. This membrane is located on the side of the pH electrode, rather than the tip, to minimize damage during catheter insertion or removal. As in call carbon dioxide sensors, the pH electrode is surrounded by an aqueous solution. This PCO_2 sensor exhibits relatively good reliability and stability over the short term (6 to 20 hours).

Although electrochemical sensors are commonly used for blood gas measurements, fiber optic sensors offer distinct advantages. Optical devices are not susceptible to electrical interference and require less frequent, if any, calibration. Colorimetric and fluorescent analysis provide the foundation for most optic measurements of dissolved CO_2 and O_2 in the blood.

The attenuation of fluorescence intensity as a function of an analyte is the basis of fluorescence sensors. Fluorescent sensors can have a large dynamic range. For example, with the correct choice of fluorophore, attenuation of emission intensities of up to 80% can be seen in the physiological PO_2 range. As with the pressure sensors discussed above, the disadvantage to intensity-based optical sensors is that light losses in the optical system will change the intensity reaching the detector; thus compensation must be provided. Colorimetric sensors utilize the different absorption properties of two species in equilibrium. By monitoring the ratio of the two absorption maxima of compounds whose equilibrium concentrations change as a function of pH, a self-compensating sensor is obtained. If both of the equilibrium forms fluoresce, then the two fluorescence maxima can be monitored thus using the best features of both sensors.

Both colorimetric and fluorescent sensors have been developed to monitor oxygen partial pressure. Zhujun and Seitz [12] report a colorimetric sensor using hemoglobin. The positions of maximal absorption for oxy- and deoxyhemoglobin immobilized on an ion exchange resin are 405 nm and 435 nm, respectively. Light from a tungsten halogen lamp filtered through either a 405 nm or 435 nm band-pass filter is transmitted through a bifurcated optical fiber bundle to a 0.500 mm layer of immobilized hemoglobin with a reflective coating underneath the protein. Some of the filtered ligth is absorbed by the hemoglobin. A ratio of the reflected intensities, $I_{405\,nm}/I_{435\,nm}$, is sigmoidal in a shape that mimics the saturation curve of oxygen binding to hemoglobin. The partial pressure of oxygen in a buffered solution, $pH = 7.20$, can be measured between 20 and 100 torr with 4% accuracy. The immobilized hemoglobin is, however, susceptible to oxidation and this reduced the shelf life of the sensor to seven days at 4°C. Although an invasive sensor was not prepared, this colorimetric technology has significant advantages over fluorescent sensors. Absorption properties of a compound are affected less by impurities than are emission properties. Moreover, by taking a ratio of the two absorption maxima, or one of the maxima and the isobestic point, a self-referencing sensor is produced eliminating errors due to light losses in the optical hardware.

More commonly, fluorescence quenching by oxygen of a suitable fluorophore is used as a sensor. For example, Cox and Dunn [13] used 9,10-diphenylanthracene trapped in polydimethylsiloxane to measure oxygen concentrations. In a pure oxygen atmosphere, 50% of the fluorescence from 9,10-diphenylanthracene was quenched. This large amount of quenching results from both the high diffusivity of oxygen in PDMS, $3.5 \cdot 10^{-5}$ cm^2/sec and high solubility, $1.2 \cdot 10^{-2}$ M at 25°C and $PO_2 = 760$ torr. This design can be readily adapted to fiber optics by binding the polymer matrix to the fiber tip.

A fluorescence sensor was also used by Gehrich et al. [14] in conjunction with CDI, Irvine, California to develop an oxygen sensor as part of an intravascular blood gas monitoring system (see Fig. 9). The overall four parameter probe is

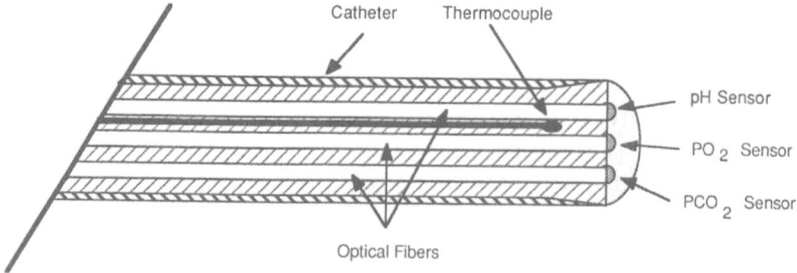

Fig. 9. Fiber optic chemical sensor for measuring PO_2, PCO_2, pH and temperature as developed by CDI, Irvine CA

smaller than 0.600 mm in diameter so that it can fit through a 20 gauge catheter. The fluorophore and polymer matrix used in the device are not disclosed. The fluorophore absorbs light at 385 nm and emits at 515 nm. The sensor can respond between 20 and 200 torr with an error of 3.3 torr. A comparision of *in vivo* and *in vitro* measurements shows little discrepancy up to 200 torr. At pressures greater than 200 torr, the *in vivo* measurements underestimate values obtained *in vitro* which were judged to be more accurate [15]. The response time of the measurements is 0.7 minutes and the deviation over a twelve hour period is 5 torr.

Another blood gas of clinical interest is carbon dioxide. As with all carbon dioxide sensors the optical sensors devised for this gas measure the pH of a bicarbonate buffer into which CO_2 can freely diffuse; the pH is a function of the carbonic acid which is formed as CO_2 enters an aqueous solution.

The CO_2 sensor developed by CDI [14] incorporates a fluorescent pH sensitive dye, hydroxypyrene trisulfonic acid with a pKa of 7.0, covalently bound to a cellulose matrix. Both the acid and base forms, which absorb light at 410 nm and 460 nm, respectively, fluoresce at 520 nm. The ratio of the emission intensities from the dye excited at the two absorption wavelengths is a relative measure of the acid/base equilibirum. This PCO_2 sensor responds from 10–100 torr with a standard deviation of 3.2 torr. The response time is 0.9 minutes and the deviation over twelve hours is 2.8 torr. The probe includes a thermocouple which measures the temperature at which the measurements are made. These values are then corrected to a standard 37°C at which all blood gas measurements are reported.

An imaginative approach to pH sensors has been taken by Jordan, Walt, and Milanovich [16] who use a method based on nonradiative energy transfer. A molecule in an excited singlet state (energy donor) can transfer its energy through space to another molecule (energy acceptor). The rate of energy transfer depends on the spectral overlap of the donor and the acceptor; the fluorescence spectrum of the donor must overlap the absorption spectrum of the acceptor. Eosin was chosen as the energy donor since its emission is independent of pH. Phenol red was selected as the acceptor. The base form of the dye absorbs light in the region where eosin emits. The protonated form of phenol red absorbs at shorter wavelengths than the base form, where eosin does not emit, and spectral overlap is diminished. Consequently, acidification of the sensor results in less energy transferred from eosin. Energy transfer and fluorescence are competing modes of decay from the excited singlet state of a molecule. The rate of energy transfer is much greater than the rate of fluorescence. Thus, it follows that an increase in energy transfer results in a decrease in the fluorescence emission. Eosin and phenol red were chemically bound to the distal end of a 0.200 mm fiber. Light from an argon-ion laser (488 nm or 514.5 nm) was focused into the fiber. The returning emission was monitored at 546 nm. The sensor responds within the pH range of 5 to 8 with better than 0.01 unit accuracy. The response time was 10 seconds.

The sensors discussed previously were all attached to the tip of an optical fiber. Attridge, Leaver, and Cozens [17] have developed a pH sensor where the refraction index of the fiber cladding changes with pH. Refractive index is a function of the light scattering property which is the complement of light absorbance; these two properties have been related by the KramersKroning equation. As the light absorbance ability of a medium increases, the refractive index of that medium changes. An interesting fiber design is used for this sensor. The fiber core contains two coaxial fibers separated by glass of a lower index of refraction (see Fig. 10). The cladding incorporates a pH sensitive dye. Light is efficiently coupled from the central fiber to the outside fiber when their phases are matched. The change in the index of refraction of the cladding as the form of phenol red is changed from acid to base is 0.005 at 633 nm. This is sufficient to couple 80% of the light between the two fibers at the point of matched phases. A pH fiber optic sensor was not tested but the authors estimate that this technology can be used to construct a sensor with 1% accuracy in the physiological range.

The response of many dyes to pH is dependent on the ionic strength of the solution being measured. This could be a problem in blood where the concentration of electrolytes is high. If the dye is not ion strength independent then the response must be corrected. A solution activity sensor has been devised which uses two pH sensors, one of which is ionic strength independent [18].

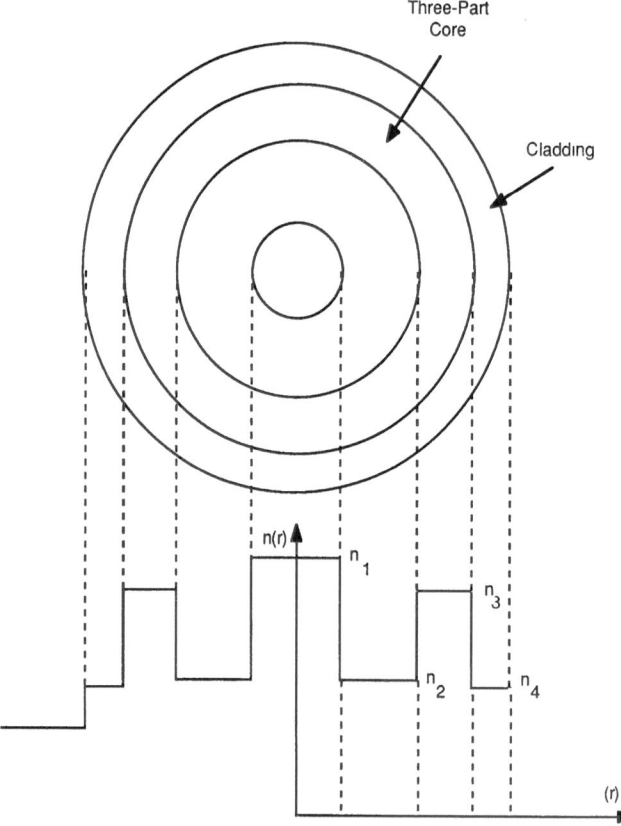

Fig. 10. Schematic illustrating the core of the fiber used for pH sensor described by Attridge et al. based on pH sensitive cladding where $n(r)$ is the index of refraction as a function of the radius, r

References

1. Knute WL, Bailey WH (1984) Fiber-optic transducer apparatus. European Patent application 0127476
2. Matsumoto H, Saegusa M, Saito K, Mizoi K (1978) The development of a fiber optic catheter tip pressure transducer. J Med Eng Tech 2:239–242
3. Hansen T-E (1983) A fiberoptic micro-tip pressure transducer for medical applications. Sensors and Actuators 4:545–554
4. Lieberman RA, Blonder GE, Tighe S (1987) A single-fiber pressure sensor for biomedical applications. Tech Digest, Optical Fibers Communication Conference, U.S.A., paper TUI6
5. Lieberman RA, Blonder GE (in press) An improved interferometric pressure optrode. Fiber Optic & Laser Sensors V, SPIE Proceedings (in press)
6. Clark LC (1956) Monitoring and control of blood and tissue oxygen. Trans Am Soc Artif Intern Organs 2:41–48
7. Parker D (1987) Sensors for monitoring blood gases in intensive care. J Phys E: Sci Instrum 20:1103–1112
8. Stow RW, Baer RF, Randall B (1957) Rapid measurements of the tension of carbon dioxide in blood. Arch Phys Med Rehabil 38:646–650
9. Servinghaus JW, Bradley AF (1958) Electrodes for blood PO_2 and PCO_2 determination. J Appl Physiol 13:515–520
10. Opdycke WN, Meyerhoff ME (1986) Development and analytical performance of tubular polymer membrane electrode based carbon dioxde catheters. Anal Chem 58:950–956
11. Schulthess P, Shijo Y, Pham HV, Pretsch E, Ammann D, Simon W (1981) Anal Chim Acta 131:111–116
12. Zhujun Z, Seitz WR (1986) Optical sensor for oxygen based on immobilized hemoglobin. Anal Chem 58:220–222
13. Cox ME, Dunn B (1985) The use of fluorescence quenching to measure oxygen concentration. SPIE Vol. 576 Optical Fibers in Medicine and Biology:60–65
14. Gehrich JL, Luebbers DW, Opitz N, Hansmann DR, Miller WW, Tusa JK, Yafuso M (1986) Optical fluorescence and its application to an intravascular blood gas monitoring system. IEEE Trans Biomed Engin BME-33:117–132
15. Reader GD, Hood AG (1983) Accuracy of oxygen partial pressure measurements: an *in vitro* study. J Extracorporeal Tech 15:89–95
16. Jordan DM, Walt DR, Milanovich FP (1987) Physiological pH fiber-optic chemical sensor based on energy transfer. Anal Chem 59:437–439
17. Attridge JW, Leaver KD, Cozens JR (1987) Design of a fiber-optic pH sensor with rapid response. J Phys E: Sci Instrum 20:548–553
18. Wolfbeis OS, Offenbacher H (1986) Fluorescence sensor for monitoring ionic strength and physiological pH values. Sensors and Actuators 9:85–91

Systolic Pressure-Dimension Relationship in the Assessment of Left Ventricular Function

H. Heinrich

Introduction

The endsystolic pressure-volume relationship (ESPVR) is a preload insensitive and afterload incorporating parameter of left ventricular contractility [1]. The slope of the linear relationship between endsystolic volumes (X-Axis) and end-systolic pressures (Y-Axis) is directly related to changes in the myocardial contractile state. The maximal slope at endsystole is called E_{max} (elastance). Basically, the ESPVR is the linear approximation of Frank's maxima curves within the physiological limits of left ventricular volumes and pressures [2].

In contrast to Frank [2] and others [3] who described different curves for iso-volumetric, isotonic and auxotonic beats, the ESPVR assumes a single curve for the above 3 different types of left ventricular contraction [1, 4]. In fact there are different curves [3] but for clinical purposes the use of only one curve has proven to be justified because the differences between the 3 curves are small.

Determination of the Endsystolic Pressure-Volume Relationship

Because the regression line between left ventricular pressures and volumes does not pass the origin of the pressure-volume diagram at least two different pressures and volumes are required for determination of the slope. This requires transient load manipulation.

For manipulation of ventricular pressures and volumes, preload changes [5] or combination of preload and afterload changes [6, 7] has been used. Considering these requirements, difficulties in contractility measurements during clinical routine are obvious. Two major problems have to be considered:

1. Transient changes of left ventricular pressures and volumes activate homeometric autoregulation which in turn may change contractility during the period of measurements [8];
2. Determination of ventricular volumes and ventricular pressures is not practicable for routine clinical use.

The problem of the homeometric autoregulatory response to contractility can be solved by autonomic blockade. Besides this possible solution one can determine the ESPVR without autonomic blockade if only a transient decrease of arterial pressure is performed. The response of the autonomic nervous system to a pressure decrease is only sympathetic activation. Because of the relatively slow re-

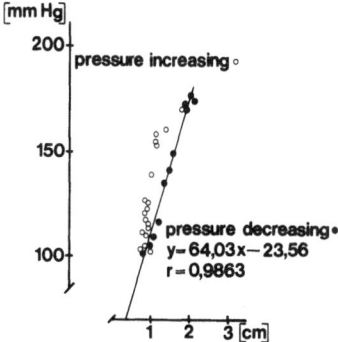

Fig. 1. Determination of the systolic pressure-diameter relationship. For transient manipulation of arterial pressure a bolus of 0,2 mg nitroglycerin was injected. Systolic pressures and end-systolic diameters during the pressure decrease after nitroglycerin show a close linear relationship. In contrast, values taken during normalization of arterial pressure are shifted leftwards indicating increased contractility. This increased contractility is caused by sympathetic stimulation due to the baroreceptor reflex

sponse of the sympathetic nerve, ESPVR is unchanged by homeometric autoregulation if pressures and volumes are used only during the first seconds of a decrease in ventricular pressure [9]. Rapid changes in arterial pressures and early determination of ventricular pressures and volumes is the precondition for determination of the ESPVR without autonomic blockade [9]. This precondition excludes steady state techniques in the manipulation of arterial pressure if no autonomic blockade is present.

Furthermore, it has been shown that instead of ventricular volumes and pressures also peripherally measured peak systolic pressures and left ventricular diameters can be used. This peak-systolic pressure endsystolic diameter relationship is also linear and responds in the slope to contractility changes as the original ESPVR does [10, 11] (Fig. 1).

Thus, the use of echocardiography for the measurement of left ventricular diameters and cuff for the measurement of peak systolic pressures enables complete noninvasive determination of this load-insensitive parameter of left ventricular contractility.

Simplifications of the ESPVR – The Endsystolic Quotient

In order to avoid transient pressure manipulation the simple quotient between endsystolic pressure and volume has been proposed [12, 14]. Because the quotient assumes that ESPVR is passing through the origin of the pressure-volume diagram (which is not the case) the simple quotient is afterload sensitive: It changes with contractility and also with afterload. An increase in afterload increases the quotient and a decrease in afterload decreases it.

Other authors propose to use the quotient between endsystolic wall stress and endsystolic volume, because endsystolic wall stress is considered to be a better parameter of afterload than systolic ventricular pressures [15, 16]. In spite of the afterload sensitivity of the endsystolic quotient, this parameter has proven more sensitive to changes in the contractile state than to loading conditions. The quotient has been shown to be more reliable than traditional parameters of left ventricular contractility, e.g. ejection fraction [12, 15, 16].

Also the simple quotient between peak systolic pressure and endsystolic diameter of the left ventricle was found to be more sensitive to the contractile state than to the afterload and superior to the fractional shortening (which is an equivalent of the ejection fraction) [17].

Systolic Pressure Diameter Relationships as a New Concept for Monitoring of Left Ventricular Function

The determinants of left ventricular pumping are preload, afterload and contractility. A new concept, based on transesophageal echocardiography has been described, which uses enddiastolic diameters (preload) and systolic pressure-diameter relationship (contractility) of the left ventricle for monitoring of left ventricular function [18]. Afterload is represented by the peak systolic pressure (Fig. 2)

The use of this concept promises to improve left ventricular monitoring, because it realizes essential parts of the original pressure-volume diagram in a clinically practicable way, and it is non-invasive. In presence of hemodynamic instability, the physician can easily answer the following questions:

Is there a need for fluid therapy (Decreased enddiastolic diameter)?
Is there a need for inotropic therapy (Decreased slope of the systolic pressure-diameter relationship)?

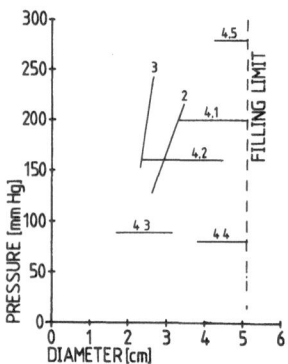

Fig. 2. The systolic pressure-diameter relationship in combination with the enddiastolic diameter in a new concept of left ventricular monitoring.
    Preload limit means an arbitrarily determined limit for diastolic filling.
    2: lower contractility; *3:* higher contractility; *4:* diameter-equivalents of stroke volume; *4.1:* low contractility, no preload reserve; *4.2:* high contractility, preload reserve; *4.3:* hypovolemia, high contractility; *4.4:* low contractility, low afterload; *4.5:* low contractility, increased afterload

Is there a need for increasing afterload (Systolic pressure decreased, normal end-diastolic diameter, normal slope of the systolic pressure-diameter relationship)?

Even if no quantitative measurements are done but the concept kept in mind immediate therapeutic interventions can be started.

Limitations of the Systolic Pressure-Diameter Relationship

There are limitations of the systolic pressure-diameter relationship which are partly related to the simplifications from the original ESPVR. In presence of segmental wall motion abnormalities a single "ice pick" diameter is no longer representing left ventricular volume. In these cases cross section areas of the left ventricle rather than diameters are better reflecting left ventricular volumes. Peripherally measured peaksystolic pressures are reflecting left ventricular peak pressures only if no stenosis of the conducting system is present. In presence of valvular aortic stenosis, peripherally measured peaksystolic pressure does not reflect the developed ventricular pressure, so that other methods must be used for the determination of left ventricular pressures and volumes such as the conductance catheter system [9].

Another major limitation of the systolic pressure-diameter relationship as well as of the ESPVR is the unavailability of practicable normalization of the slope. (What is a "normal" slope of the relationship?) Presently we are able only to measure intraindividual changes or to compare slopes between groups of patients. Attempts for normalization have been made [19, 20] but the problem is still uncompletely solved.

References

1. Suga H, Sagawa K, Shoukas AA (1973) Load independence of the instantaneous pressure-volume ratio of the left ventricle and effects of epinephrine and heart rate on the ratio. Circ Res 32:314–322
2. Frank O (1897) Die Wirkung von Digitalis (Helleborein) auf das Herz. Sitzungsberichte der Gesellschaft für Morphologie und Physiologie zu München H2:14–43
3. Jacob R, Weigand KH (1966) Die endsystolischen Druck-Volumenbeziehungen als Grundlage einer Beurteilung der Kontraktilität des linken Ventrikels in situ. Pflügers Archiv 289:37–49
4. Holt JP (1857) Regulation of the degree of emptying of the left ventricle by the force of ventricular contraction. Circ Res 5:281–287
5. Little WC, Freeman GL, O'Rourke RA (1985) Simultaneous determination of left ventricular end-systolic pressure-volume and pressure-dimension relationships in closed-chest dogs. Circulation 71:1301–1308
6. Grossman W, Braunwald E, Mann T, McLaurin LP, Green LH (1977) Contractile state of the left ventricle in man as evaluated from end-systolic pressure-volume relations. Circulation 56:845–852
7. Mehmel HC, Stockins B, Ruffmann K, von Olshausen K, Schuler G, Kübler W (1981) The linearity of the endsystolic pressure-volume relationship in man and its sensitivity for assessment of left ventricular function. Circulation 63:1216–1222

8. Sarnoff SJ, Mitchell JH, Gilmore JP, Remensnyder JP (1960) Homeometric autoregulation of the heart. Circ Res 8:1077–1091

9. Kass DA, Yamazaki T, Burkhoff D, Maughan WL, Sagawa K (1986) Determination of left ventricular end-systolic pressure-volume relationships by the conductance (volume) catheter technique. Circulation 73:586–595

10. Heinrich H, Fösel TH, Fontaine L, Silker D, Winter H, Ahnefeld FW (1987) Assessment of contractility changes in humans by transoesophageal echocardiography-reliability of the peak-systolic pressure end-systolic diameter relationship (PSPESDRS). Int J Clin Mon Comput 4:243–248

11. Marsh JD, Green LH, Wynne J, Cohn PF, Grossman W (1979) Left ventricular end-systolic pressure-dimension and stress-length relations in normal human subjects. Am J Cardiol 44:1311–1317

12. Ramanathan K, Erwin SW, Sullivan JM (1984) Relationship of peak-systolic pressure/end-systolic volume ratio to standard ejection phase indices and ventricular function curves in coronary artery disease. Am J Med Sc 288:162–168

13. Watkins J, Slutsky R, Tubau J, Karliner J (1982) Scintigraphic study of relation between left ventricular peak systolic pressure and end-systolic volume in patients with coronary artery disease and normal subjects. Br Heart J 48:39–47

14. Dehmer GJ, Lewis SE, Hillis LD, Corbett J, Parkey RW, Willerson JT (1981) Exercise-induced alterations in left ventricular volumes and the pressure-volume relationship: a sensitive indicator of left ventricular dysfunction in patients with coronary artery disease. Circulation 63:1008–1018

15. Gash AK, Carabello BA, Cepin D, Spann JF (1983) Left ventricular ejection performance and systolic muscle function in patients with mitral stenosis. Circulation 67:148–154

16. Carabello BA, Nolan SP, MsGuire LB (1981) Assessment of preoperative left ventricular function in patients with mitral regurgitation: value of the endsystolic wall stress- end-systolic volume ratio. Circulation 64:1212–1217

17. Heinrich H, Fontaine L, Wilder-Smith O, Winter H, Ahnefeld FW (1987) Usefulness of the endsystolic quotient and of fractional shortening for assessment of contractility changes under different loading conditions. Anesthesiology 67 (Suppl): A109

18. Fontaine L, Heinrich H, Winter H, Spilker D, Binner L (1986) Patient monitoring using ventricular systolic and diastolic pressure-dimension relationships. A concept based on transesophageal echocardiography. Int J Clin Mon Comput 2:222

19. Suga H, Hisano R, Goto Y, Yamada O (1984) Normalization of end-systolic pressure-volume relation and E_{max} of different sized hearts. Jap Circ J 48:136–143

20. Suga H, Yamada O, Goto Y, Igarashi Y, Yasumura Y, Nozawa T (1986) Reconsideration of normalization of E_{max} for heart size. Heart and Vessels 2:67–73

Quantitative Evaluation of Left Ventricular Function by Doppler Echocardiography

D. Bruère and P. Viars

Introduction

It may be difficult to accuratly assess left ventricular (LV) function in patients with acute cardiac and/or respiratory failure since data obtained from pulmonary artery catheters do not always allow to define the level and the type of LV dysfunction [1].

The use of ultrasound in cardiology markedly improved both diagnosis and therapeutic decisions in cardiac patients. The Doppler echocardiography is a particularly suitable technique to evaluate LV function in critical care patients, since it is non-invasive and can be used at the bedside. It is the only method allowing to assess in real time all the heart structures which might be involved in the cardiac failure. It also permits to determine LV dimensions. Finally the Doppler method has recently given the opportunity to assess intracardiac flows. Technical advances led to a new wave of both very high performance Doppler echo equipment and esophageal probes with several funtions: M mode and to dimensional (2D)-echocardiography, pulsed Doppler and color flow mapping. Such probes have several advantages including high quality images in most of the patients (85%), even those under mechanical ventilation; and a better signal to noise in Doppler mode. Transesophageal Doppler echocardiography could lead to a better assessment of hemodynamic status in critically ill patients. 2D-echocardiography and Doppler echocardiography are complementary techniques to study both filling and ejection flows of the LV. The analysis of the flow data permits measurement of cardiac output and accurate assessment of LV systolic performance and diastolic function.

Doppler Echocardiography – General Principles

The general principles have been reported in detail elsewhere [2]. So that only the basic principles are briefly reviewed here (Fig. 1.).

When an ultrasound beam with a frequency Fe emitted by a stationary transducer meets moving red blood cells, the ultrasound signal is reflected back to the transducer with a modified frequency FR. Blood flow velocity V is obtained by the Doppler equation:

$$V = \frac{C}{2Fe} \cdot \frac{Fd}{\cos \theta} \quad \text{(Fig. 1)}$$

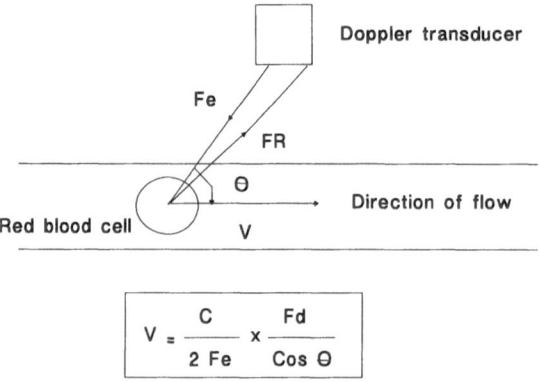

Fig. 1. General principle of Doppler echocardiography.
Fd: Doppler shift (=FR–Fe); *Fe:* Frequency of emitted ultrasound; *FR:* Frequency of refleted ultrasound; *V:* Velocity of blood; *θ:* Angle between direction of flow and direction of ultrasonic signal; *C:* Velocity of sounds in tissues (1540 m/s)

For accurate measurements of velocity, the θ angle must be as low as possible (less than 20°).

In modern equipment, the reflected signal is analyzed in real time by spectral analysis. This spectral analysis of the velocities is displayed on the ordinate over time on the abcissa. By convention, blood flow toward the transducer is above the baseline and conversely. One advantage of combining 2D-echocardiography with Doppler is the opportunity to align the Doppler beam with the blood flow. This is easy to perform since the direction of the Doppler beam is displayed on the 2-D echo image as a line.

At present, four types of Doppler mode can be used to record flow velocity.

Pulsed Wave Doppler (PWD)

The piezo-electric crystal acts both as emitter and receiver. A short burst of ultrasounds is emitted during a period t1, then after a t2 period the reception of the reflected signal and lasts a t3 period. The t3 period reflects the sample volume size and the t2 period determines the depth at which the velocity is measured. The main advantage of the PWD is its ability to measure velocity at very specific locations (within the sample volume). The main disadvantage is its limited ability to measure high velocities. However, this limitation is unimportant for both cardiac output measurement and evaluation of LV funtion.

The High Pulse Repetition Frequency Pulsed Doppler (HPRF)

This Doppler method allows measurements of high velocities with a good quality of recording (narrow band of frequencies).

The Continuous Wave Doppler (CWD)

Two separate crystals are used to transmit and receive the ultrasounds. Although this techniques allow measurement of high velocities, it does not permit to select the location of the measurements.

Real Time Color Flow Mapping

With such a technique, on the 2D image the flows are displayed in a color scale according to their velocities and directions. This allows a better spatial orientation of flow within the cardiac structure and permits to adequately position the sample volume in PWD mode. In addition, this method can determine the functional diameters of the cardiac valves.

Cardiac Output Measurements

The thermodilution method is invasive and provides no information about the instantaneous blood flow or the pattern of the LV ejection flow. Non-invasive assessment of cardiac output is one of the applications of the Doppler echocardiography. Stroke volume (SV) is obtained by the formula:

$$SV \ (cm^3) = A \ (cm^2) \cdot VTI \ (cm)$$

where A is the area of the valvular orifice and VTI is the velocity time integral (area under the time velocity curve).

Measurements of aortic or mitral area are derived from the determination of their diameter. This is the reason why even minor inaccuracies in diameter determination will lead to significant errors in SV.

The planimetry of the time velocity curve needs high quality recordings which in most cases can only be obtained using PWD mode (narrow band of frequencies). In addition, the velocity has to be measured in a site where the velocity profile is flat. It is well documented that velocity profile is flat at the level of the valves thus allowing to consider the velocity measured in the sample volume as representative of all the velocities within the valve.

A close relationship has been found between SV measured either by thermodilution or Fick oximetry and by Doppler echocardiography performed either on the mitral [3-5] or the aortic valve [6, 7].

Quantitative Assessment of Systolic LV Function
Using Doppler Echocardiography

In an experimental study performed in dogs and published in 1966, Noble et al [8] first established that maximal acceleration of the aortic flow is a reliable index of LV function influenced by inotropism but not by preload. In this study, the flow velocity was measured using an electromagnetic flowmeter, and this invasive technique is difficult to use for clinical investigation. These velocity indices are increasingly used to assess LV funtion since ejection velocity can be accurately determined using Doppler techniques. Figure 2 shows an example of the ascending aortic blood flow obtained in PWD mode with a non-imaging transducer held in the supra-sternal notch.

In a clinical study, Bennet et al. [9] found data similar to those of Noble using Doppler echocardiography to assess maximal flow acceleration and SV. These two studies and the one from Wallmeyer et al. [10] strongly suggest that aortic flow acceleration is a reliable and reproducible index of LV performance mainly affected by inotropism and independent of preload. Moreover, a close correlation has been found between velocity indices measured using Doppler and those obtained from electromagnetic flowmeter which can be considered as a reference method [10]. At present, whether or not maximal aortic flow acceleration is afterload-independent has not been definitely established. Although few investigators have studied this, an inverse correlation between afterload and maximal acceleration might exist [11]. An accurate assessment of maximal acceleration is difficult. Indeed, Noble's studies [7, 12] clearly show that acceleration is maximal about 30 ms after the start of the ejection and remains at this value during only 5 ms. Only high quality recordings with an optimal signal to noise ratio allow a reliable assessment of this parameter. Moreover, when using a high pass filter frequency, the initial part of the aortic flow, where the acceleration is maximal, is not displayed. These methodologic difficulties lead to propose other indices easier to obtain such as the peak velocity, the mean acceleration and the

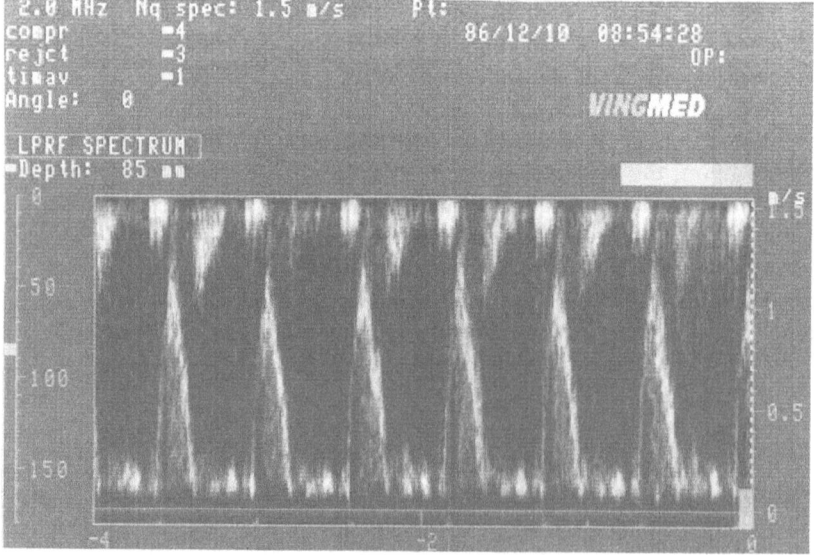

Fig. 2. Ascending aortic blood flow obtained in PWD mode with the transducer held in the supra-sternal notch

ejection force. These indices of LV performance have been used for non-invasive quantification of LV dysfunction in a large population of patients. Accordingly, Sabbah et al. [13] found a close correlation between maximal acceleration and ejection fraction but there was some overlap between patients with normal and abnormal ejection fraction. The index proposed by Isaaz et al. [14] seems more discriminant. This index allows a continuous beat-to-beat assessment of LV function, and is particularly useful to determine the efficiency of the treatment in acute cardiac failure.

Quantitative Assessment of LV Diastolic Function Using Doppler Echocardiography

The different methods used to assess diastolic LV function (invasive LV pressure assessment, cineangiography, radionuclide angiography) are obviously difficult to use in ICU patients. Echocardiography has also been proposed to assess diastolic LV function. Using this technique Jardin et al. [15, 16] clearly evidenced that acute right ventricular dilatation, resulting from an increase in right ventricular afterload, decreases LV compliance.

Doppler echo permits to analyze transmitral flow thus allowing a beat-to-beat assessment of the dynamics of the LV filling. The studies from Yellin's group [17, 18] clearly demonstrated that the LV filling pattern depends on left atrial pressure (LAP), LV afterload, LV compliance and relaxation and atrial systole. The pattern of transmitral flow reflects changes in instantaneous pressure gradient between the left atrium and the left ventricle [17]. The diastolic period includes three phases which depend upon several factors (Fig. 3). The rapid filling phase is affected by LAP and LV relaxation and compliance. The passive filling is affected by LV compliance. The influence of the atrial systole on LV filling depends upon the quality of left atrial systolic function, which is a parameter not well understood yet.

The rapid filling of the LV is an important part of the LV filling. Ishida et al. [18] clearly demonstrated that the ratio of the amount of blood entering the LV until the peak early filling rate (PEFR) and the total transmitral volume remains constant even when the LV loading conditions change. These findings emphasized that the LV filling pattern determined using Doppler-echo allows an

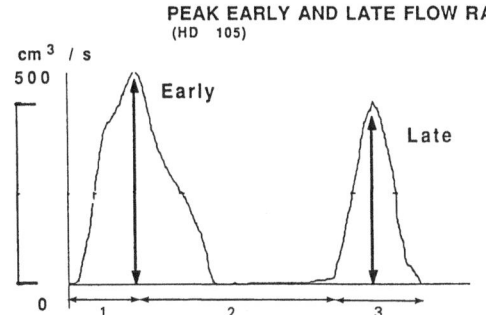

Fig. 3. The 3 phases of the diastolic period.
1: Rapid filling phase; *2:* Passive filling; *3:* Atrial systole

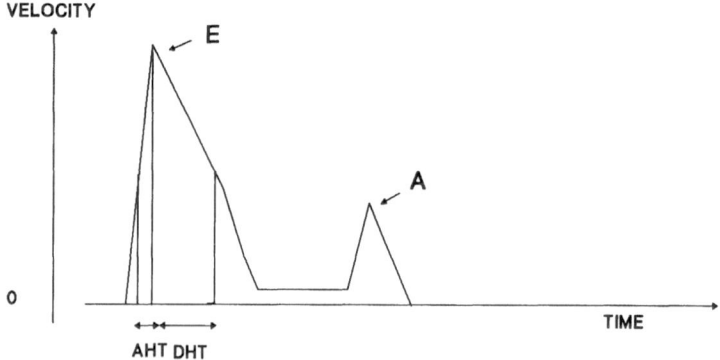

Fig. 4. Velocity indices of LV diastolic function (pulsed Doppler technique).
E: Peak early velocity ⎫
 ⎬ → > E/A ratio;
A: Peak late velocity ⎭
AHT: Acceleration half-time; DHT: Deceleration half-time

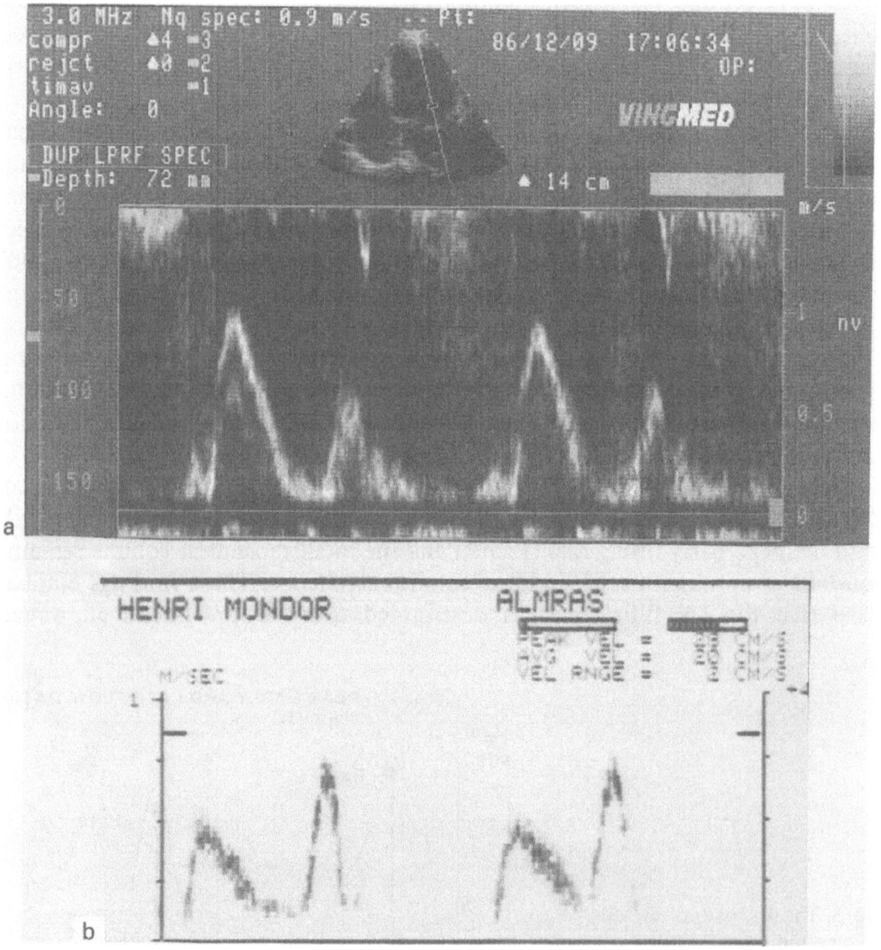

Fig. 5a, b. Transmitral flow velocities. A: normal (E/A ratio > 1); B: abnormal (E/A ratio < 1)

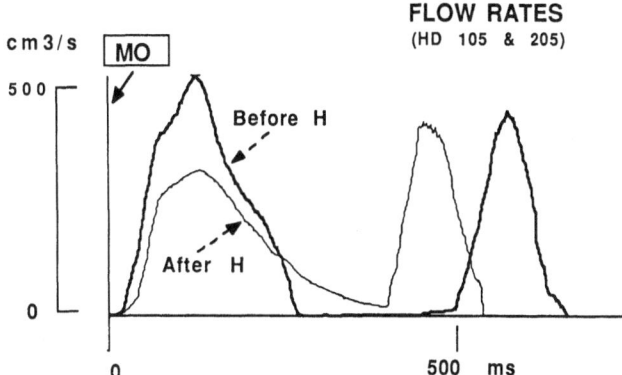

Fig. 6. Flow rates before and after hemodialysis (H) (one patient), showing that PEFR decreases after hemodialysis

accurate assessment of LV diastolic function. Accordingly, several velocity indices have been proposed to assess LV diastolic function (Fig. 4). In Figure 5 are shown a normal transmitral flow velocity profile (A) and an abnormal one (B). In addition, other indices taking into account transmitral flow rate (PEFR, peak late filling rate, filling volume to PEFR and filling volume related to atrial systole) can be used to assess LV diastolic function.

Several studies validated some of these indices [19–21]. However, at present no Doppler index can accurately determine either LV compliance or LV diastolic pressure. The value of peak early velocity (E) or the PEFR give an accurate assessment of the quality of relaxation, but are largely affected by LAP [18]. Consequently, transmitral blood flow analysis is particularly useful to better understand the LV filling pattern and to study its changes in front of myocardial ischemic episodes [22] or right ventricular dilatation [23] for example.

We recently analyzed LV filling pattern changes induced by hemodialysis in patients with chronic renal failure [24]. An example is given in Figure 6.

In conclusion, the pulsed Doppler analysis of transmitral flow provides reliable beat-to-beat informations about LV filling dynamics. The opportunity to assess transmitral flow velocity with transesophageal pulsed Doppler may be of great interest in mechanically ventilated patients experiencing acute cardiac events.

References

1. Raper R, Sibbald WJ (1986) Misled by the wedge? The Swan-Ganz catheter and left ventricular preload. Chest 89:427–434
2. Hatle L, Hangelsen B (1985) Doppler ultrasound in Cardiology. Physical principles and clinical applications (ed 2). Philadelphia, Lea & Febiger
3. Fisher DC, Sahn DJ, Friedman MJ, et al (1983) The mitral valve orifice method for non-invasive two-dimensional echo-Doppler determination of cardiac output. Circulation 67:872–877
4. Lewis JF, Kuo LC, Nelson JG, Limacher MC, Quinones MA (1984) Pulsed Doppler echocardiographic determination of stroke volume and cardiac output: clinical validation of two new methods using the apical window. Circulation 70:425–431

5. De Zuttere D, Touche T, Saumon G, Nitemberg S, Prasquier R (1988) Doppler echocardiographic measurement of mitral volume flow: validation of a new method in adult patient. J Am Coll Cardiol (in press)
6. Ihlen H, Amlie JP, Dale J, et al (1984) Determination of cardiac output by Doppler echocardiography. Br Heart J 51:54-60
7. Christie J, Sheldahl LM, Tristani FE, Sagar KB, Ptacin MJ, Wann S (1987) Determination of stroke volume and cardiac output during exercice: comparison of two-dimensional and Doppler echocardiography. Fick oximetry and thermodilution. Circulation 76:539-547
8. Noble MIM, Trenchard D, Guz A (1966) Left ventricular ejection in conscious dogs: I. Measurement and significance of the maximum acceleration of blood from the left ventricle. Circ Res 139-147
9. Bennet ED, Barclay SA, Davis AL, Mannering D, Mehta N (1984) Ascending aortic blood velocity and acceleration using Doppler ultrasound in the assessment of left ventricular function. Cardiovasc Res 18:632-638
10. Wallmeyer K, Wann S, Sagar KB, Kalbfleisch J, Klopfenstein HS (1986) The influence of preload and heart rate on Doppler echocardiographic indexes of left ventricular performance: comparison with invasive indexes in experimental preparation. Circulation 74:181-186
11. van den Bos GC, Elzinga G, Westerhof N, Noble MIM (1973) Problems in the use of indexes of myocardial contractility. Cardiovasc Res 7:834-848
12. Innes JA, Mills CJ, Noble MIM, et al (1987)Validation of beat by beat pulsed Doppler measurements of ascending aortic blood velocity in man. Cardiovasc Res 21:72-80
13. Sabbah HN, Khaja F, Brymer JF, et al (1986) Noninvasive evaluation of left ventricular performance based on peak aortic blood acceleration measured with a continuous-wave Doppler velocity meter. Circulation 74:323-329
14. Isaaz K, Cloez JL, Thompson A, Pernot C (1986) Assessment of ventricular ejection dynamics by Doppler using a new method in congestive cardiomyopathy. Circulation 74 (II):50
15. Jardin F, Farcot JC, Boisante L, Curien N, Margairaz A, Bourdarias JP (1981) Influence of positive end-expiratory pressure on left ventricular performance. N Engl J Med 304:397-392
16. Jardin F, Farcot JC, Boisante L, Prost JF, Gueret P, Bourdarias JP (1982) Mechanism of paradoxic pulse in bronchial asthma. Circulation 66:887-894
17. Yellin EL, Sonnenblick EH, Frater RWM (1980) Dynamic determinants of left ventricular filling: an overview. In: Baan J, Arntzenius AC, Yellin EL (eds) Cardiac dynamics. Martinus Nijhoff, The Hague, pp 145-158
18. Ishida Y, Meisner JS, Tsujioka K, et al (1986) Left ventricular filling dynamics: influence of left ventricular relaxation and left atrial pressure. Circulation 74:187-196
19. Rokey R, Kuo LC, Zoghbi WA, Limacher MC, Quinones MA (1985) Determination of parameters of left ventricular diastolic filling with pulsed Doppler echocardiography: comparison with cineangiography. Circulation 71:543-550
20. Spirito P, Maron BJ, Bonow RO (1986) Noninvasive assessment of left ventricular diastolic function: comparative analysis of Doppler echocardiographic and radionuclide angiographic techniques. J Am Coll Cardiol 7:518-526
21. Friedman BJ, Drinkovic BN, Miles H, Shih WJ, Mazzoleni A, deMaria AN (1986) Assessment of left ventricular diastolic function: comparison of Doppler echocardiography and gated blood pool scintigraphy. J Am Coll Cardiol 8:1348-1354
22. Labovitz AJ, Lewen M, Kern M, Vandormael M, Habermehl K (1986) Temporal relationship of left ventricular systolic and diastolic dysfunction during percutaneous transluminal coronary angioplasty. Circulation 74 (II):358
23. Louie EK, Rich S, Brundage BH (1986) Doppler echocardiographic assessment of impaired left ventricular filling in patients with right ventricular pressure overload due to primary hypertension. J Am Coll Cardiol 8:1298-1306
24. Bruere D, Benmaadi A, Buisson C, Malak J, Cordier A, Brun P (1987) Changes in left ventricular filling pattern induced by hemodialysis. Abstract presented at 3rd International Congress of Cardiac Doppler, Köln

Strategy for Arterial Catheterization

C. Martin, P. Saux, and F. Gouin

Introduction

Arterial catheterization is a technique widely used by anesthetists and intensivists because it has numerous advantages. First it provides much more reliable measurements of intravascular arterial pressure than indirect methods with the exception of automatic oscillometry. Second arterial catheters allow repeated sampling for blood gas analysis without repeated punctures. Lastly it enables measurement of cardiac output by colorimetric methods after injection of a dye through a central vein catheter. As early as 1960, Barr and Soila [1] proposed radial artery catheterization using Teflon catheters and this technique has been almost universally adopted. The purpose of this study is to review the advantages and disadvantages of the different routes of arterial catheterization. The complications of arterial catheterization are discussed accessorily. For further details the reader is referred to previous publications devoted specifically to complications [2–4].

The Radial Artery

The most common route of arterial catheterization in both adults and children mainly is the radial artery because it is superficial and thus easily accessible. The major risk during catheterization is thrombosis which can occur at any time even in the very first hours. Given this danger, an essential precaution is to test collateral circulation in the ulnar artery which in case of thrombosis of the radial artery can supply blood to the hand via the superficial palmar arch and to a lesser degree the deep palmar arch. The superficial palmar arch and the ulnar artery, which feeds it in most cases, are thus crucial to supplying blood to the hand [5]. This network is complete in 80% of cases according to the necroscopic data of Coleman and Anson [5]. In subjects studied during anesthesia or in vigil, circulatory function testing of the hand showed that 95 to 98% of subjects have adequate collateral circulation and that 0.4 to 1.2% are at risk of developing acute ischemia of the hand after thrombosis of the radial artery as a result of an indwelling catheter [6].

In practice, *ulnar collateral flow* can be evaluated using several bedside techniques. The Allen test consists in having the patient raise his hands to face level and close his fists tight for one minute in order to force blood out. Next the examining physician compresses the radial artery with the thumb leaving the ulnar artery open and the patient opens his fingers. The test is considered to be normal if normal skin color is rapidly restored. The time necessary for restoration of skin color was not precisely defined by Allen. This test has been modified by several practitioners and notably by Richard [7] and by Kamienski and Barnes [8]. Both the radial and cubital arteries are closed off by the physician and the patient is instructed to open and close his hand several times in rapid succession and then to leave it open. At this time the ulnar artery is freed. If collateral circulation is normal, pallor should subside completely within 6 seconds [8] or 15 seconds [9]. The patient is considered to have failed the test if color is not restored to any part of the hand within this time and puncture of the radial artery is contraindicated. According to Oh and Davis [10], ulnar collateral circulation can be graded as follows: 1) complete restoration of skin color within 7 seconds; 2) color restored completely but poorly within 8 to 14 seconds; 3) incomplete and slow restoration of color in over 15 seconds. The patient must be instructed not to stretch his fingers or wrist out since this result in false negative tests in 70% of cases. The value of the modified Allen test can be demonstrated by comparison with more sophisticated methods such as Doppler flow measurement [8] or measurement of systolic arterial pressure in the thumb. Using the latter method, Husum and Berthelsen showed that in 99.2% of cases the Allen test allowed correct assessment of vicarious circulation [11].

In comatose or uncooperative patients, the method described by Barber et al. [12] can be used. The radial pulse is located before placing the Esmarch's bandage on the patient's forearm to exsanguinate the limb. A blood pressure cuff is placed above the elbow and inflated to a systolic pressure higher than the patient's. The bandage is removed (the member should appear livid), the radial artery is compressed at the level of the marker and the blood pressure cuff is taken off. Hyperhemia appears and if collateral circulation is adequate, hand color is totally restored.

Ramanathan et al. [13] suggested another simple method whose reliability was demonstrated by comparison with Doppler data. This technique which does not require patient cooperation consists in compressing the proximal part of the artery with his index finger. With his middle finger, one should feel a pulse resulting from backfilling of the distal part of the radial artery if collateral flow is adequate. To double check patency of the palmar arch, the ulnar artery is closed off with the other hand, and this should normally stop backfilling.

Although the Allen test is a safe and reliable test, its findings do not constitute an absolute guarantee of the success or failure of catheterization. In a series of 1699 catheterizations without ischemic complication, Slogoff et al. [14] performed this test in only 411 cases and even cannulated 16 patients in spite of negative results. On the other hand, some cases of gangrene have been reported despite the use of the Allen test or similar maneuvers. Moreover, these tests cannot predict cutaneous necrosis at the site of puncture. Indeed the deep and superficial layer located up to 10 cm from the base of the metacarpus are supplied by fine end branches of the radial artery and these vessels can be occluded by thrombus from the radial artery or by the presence of the catheter itself. With regard to thrombotic complications, it must be underlined that in the vast majority of cases they are discovered during routine investigation (Doppler, arteriography) and have no clinical consequences. In a series of 107 catheterizations, we found subclinical thrombosis in 85% of cases [4]. In their series of 1699 catheterizations, Slogoff et al. reported an incidence of thrombosis of 25% with no clinical manifestations.

On balance, if only for medico-legal reasons, performance of the Allen test is advisable. When patient cooperation cannot be obtained, the methods of Barber et al [13] or Ramanathan et al [14] can be used. Obviously the purpose of these tests is to prevent ischemia of the hand or fingers, a complication regularly reported in the literature which can lead to necrosis and amputation if normal circulation does not resume after removal of the catheter.

Radial artery catheterization is now a well codified technique. The hand is placed palm side up on a hard surface; a roll of tape or paper towels can be useful in dorsiflexing the wrist. The artery is palpated along several centimeters above the wrist. If the patient is conscious, local anesthesia is advisable. The optimal angle of puncture is between 30 and 45 degrees. When thin, needle-mounted catheters are used, a small cutaneous incision can be made to facilitate entry. The Seldinger technique is also frequently used. Another method consists in intentionally transfixing the vessel then after removing the stylet slowly withdrawing the catheter until blood is seen and at that time advancing the catheter up the arterial lumen. Obviously, cannulation must be performed under strictly sterile conditions (disinfection of the site, scrubbed hands, gown, gloves, cap, mask, and drapes). After placement, the catheter should be sutured to the skin. A stopcock for sample taking is installed and an occlusive bandage must be applied to the site as a precaution against infection. One advantage of the radial artery route is the low risk of infection. Although bacterial cultures from the extremities are positive in 20 to 25% of cases [4, 15, 16] after prolonged catheterization, the incidence of clinical infection or septicemia is lower than 5%. In many series, no infectious complications were recorded [15, 16]. A crucial factor in preventing infection is to maintain sterility especially when taking blood samples.

Catheterization of the dorsal arch of the radial artery is an alternative. At the level of the wrist the course of the radial artery passes over the lower end of the radius from front to back. On the outer side of the carpus it arrives at the upper edge of the first interosseous space which it crosses from back to front before reaching the palm of the hand where it forms the deep parmar arch. It is possible to catheterize the radial artery on the back of the hand as it emerges from the "tabatière anatomique" (anatomic snuffbox). The artery is palpated on the back of the hand between the bases of the first and second metacarpal bones. Puncture is made when blood is seen the catheter is advanced up the arterial lumen. This technique is successful in 80% of cases. The advantage of this site is that the contribution of the radial artery to the superficial arch (the main collateral) occurs proximal to the "tabatière anatomique". Puncture of the dorsal arch of the radial artery is the distal to beginning of the anastomosis. The only precaution is not to enter the catheter more than 3 cm in order not to encroach on the commencement of the anastomosis. This site can be used for short or long term catheterizations in adults as well as children [17].

The radial artery is the most convenient site of arterial catheterization because access is direct, placement is rapid, compression is easy at the time of withdrawal, and the rist of infection is low. However, this site may be unavailable due to an unpalpable radial pulse on both sides, extensive burns or trauma, septic areas in the wrist area, and absence of the radial ulnar anastomosis. Moreover decannulation from the radial artery may be necessary because of inflammation or ischemia. In these cases an alternative site must be chosen.

The Dorsalis Pedis Artery

The dorsalis pedis artery is a suitable aternative site [18]. Blood is supplied to the foot by the dorsalis pedis artery, the posterior tibial artery and to a lesser degree the peroneal artery and maleolar network. The dorsalis pedis artery is palpable in 85 to 98% of subjects. It is the main blood supplier to the toes and particular to the big toe in 20 to 50% of subjects. The incidence of deficient collateral circulation varies from 2 to 20% and seems to increase with age [19]. Theoretically, in case of thrombosis, the risk of skin or toe necrosis is low and to our knowledge only one such case has been reported in the literature. Sporel et al. published a series of 100 catheterizations without complication. We have used this site in more than 200 patients without a single case of clinical ischemia. Husum et al. [19] recommend measurement of arterial pressure in the big toe (by plethysmography) before and while the dorsalis pedis artery is compressed. When the value recorded is less than 40 mmHg, catheterization is considered to be contraindicated. This happended in 20% of the patients studied.

Table 1. Comparison of puncture of the radial artery and dorsalis pedis artery

	Dorsalis pedis artery	Radial artery
N	38	50
Age, years	57±2	55±2
Men	60%	74%
Right side	42%	52%
Vessel transfixed	27%	53%
Success rate	79%	86%
Success after 1 or 2 punctures	55%	80%
Hematoma after failure	5%	0%
Duration of insertion	13±2 min (range 3–20 min)	9±1 min (range 1–45 min)
Duration of catheterization	13.1±1.5 days (range 1–39 days)	13,8±2.0 days (range 2–41 days)
Catheterizations longer than 7 days	74%	84%
Ischemic complications	0%	0%
Positive catheter culture	14%	20%

Catheterization of the dorsalis pedis artery is very easy. The success rates reported in various series ranges from 80 to 87%. Table 1 lists the results of our experience with this technique during a controlled prospective study including 38 cases. The artery is palpated on the dorsal side of the foot in the first intermetatarsal space and puncture is performed with the foot slightly extended. The artery passes obliquely from the front to the inner side.

The risk of thrombosis of the dorsalis pedis artery after catheterization varies from 7 to 25% (Doppler, plethysmography) [19, 20]. After decannulation, full reestablishment of the flow in a thrombotic vessel can be long as suggested by Husum et al. [19] who detected deficiencies as late as 3 to 5 months after removal of the catheter. The risk of infection seems to be low although little study has been made in this regard. In our experience, bacterial cultures of catheters were positive in 14% of cases but no case of septicemia was recorded. Thus the dorsalis pedis artery appears to be a site to consider for arterial catheterization. It should however be remembered that in elderly patients circulation in the foot may be impaired by atherosclerosis and thus this site should not be used unless bedside tests prove that the collateral flow is adequate.

The Superficial Temporal Artery

The superficial temporal artery is another alternative site for arterial catheterization. It is the outer and superficial branch of the external carotid artery. It is palpable as it emerges from behind the parotid gland at the level of the line running between the upper edge of the auditory canal and the middle part of the upper edge of the orbit. It then passes in front of the tragus and behind the temporomaxillary joint. The catheter is inserted via cutdown. The incision is made either horizontally over 1 cm at the upper edge of the helis or vertically over 3 cm between the helix and the targus [21]. Humphrey and Stone [21] reported no complication in a series of 23 catheterizations performed on patients between 10 and 69 years of age for period lasting from 1 to 27 days (mean duration 7 days).

Large Arteries: The Femoral Artery and the Axillary Artery

In view of the high incidence of thrombosis associated with catheterization of small arteries (usually the radial artery), several authors have proposed the femoral artery and the axillary arteries as alternative routes [22-24]. The rationale behind this choice is that with a larger vessel thrombosis should be limited and thus complete occlusion of the vessel less likely. Another advantage is their easy cannulation in case of peripheral vasoconstriction or arterial hypotension.

On the basis of a series of 350 prolonged catheterizations (6.3 days, 30% longer than a week) without noteworthy complication, Gurman and Kriemerman [23] claimed that these large arteries are sites of choice for arterial catheterizations. Importantly no case of clinical ischemia was recorded, a finding which was confirmed by others in axillary artery catheterizations.

The incidence of septic complications is also very low. Only 7.6 and 11.1% of catheters have positive bacterial cultures after axillary and femoral puncture, respectively. Catheter-induced septicemia was recorded in 2.2% of cases. The low risk of infection using the femoral site was confirmed by Thomas et al. [16] who reported that, though 25% of catheters cultured positive, no catheter infection was recorded in a series of 73 catheterizations. Thus these two sites can be considered as interesting alternatives for prolonged catheterization if no other site is available.

With regard to the use of axillary artery, a word of caution is needed. It sometimes happens that during washout air bubbles are trapped in the system. A gas emboli can thus be formed and migrate against stream to the cerebral vessels. This complication which has now been well documented is rare when the radial artery is used. It is particularly dangerous when the axillary arteries are used because of their proximity to the cerebral bound arteries.

Newborns and Infants

From 0 to 5 days the umbilical artery can be used. With this site the main risk is mycotic arterial aneurysm that can require surgery. The superficial temporal artery was successfully used after arteriotomy in 17 children by MacGovern and Baker [25]. The use of the femoral artery is no recommended in newborn and infants because there is a major risk of necrosis and gangrene of the lower extremity. In fact, the radial is the most widely used site of catheterization even in newborns weighing as little as 1.1 kg, according to Jodres [26]. For obvious reasons, a small catheter must be used and to facilitate percutaneous puncture, transillumination should be used with the light of a fiberscope or a Doppler system. Under these conditions catheterization is usually successful after one or two attempts in 80 to 85% of cases. Furman et al. [27] published a series of 500 radial artery punctures without a single complication. In their report, these authors also pointed out that the dorsalis pedis artery can be easily used.

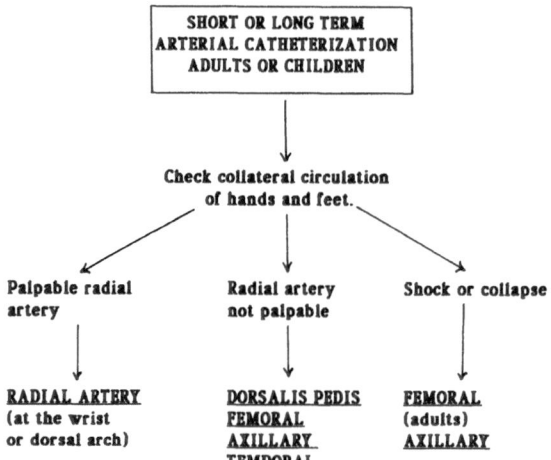

Fig. 1. Strategy for arterial catheterization (humeral artery should never be used)

Conclusion

Thus several sites are available for arterial catheterization. In the vast majority of critically ill patients, the radial artery is a satisfactory site. In some special cases however, other sites must be used. Figure 1 gives site selection criteria for almost all situations.

References

1. Barr PO, Soila P (1960) Introduction of soft cannula into artery by direct percutaneous puncture. Angiology 2:168–172
2. Bedford RF, Wollman H (1973) Complications of percutaneous radial artery cannulation: an objective prospective study in man. Anesthesiology 38:228–236
3. Marcillon M, Marcotte C, Merot S, et al (1986) Le cathétérisme de l'artère radiale en anesthésie-réanimation. Ann Fr Anesth Réanim 5:48–57
4. Martin C, Crama P, Courjaret P, Auffray JP, Hemon Y (1984): Le cathétérisme prolongé de l'artère radiale. Evaluation prospective du risque thrombogène et infectieux. Ann Fr Anesth Réanim 3:435–439
5. Coleman JS, Anson BJ (1961) Arterial patterns in the hand based upon a study of 650 specimens. Surg Gynecol Obstet 113:409–424
6. Mozersky OJ, Buckley CJ, Hagood CO (1973) Ultrasonic evaluation of the palma circulation. Am J Surg 126:810–812
7. Richard RL (1970) Peripheral arterial disease, a physician's approach. Livingstone London p 47
8. Kamienski RW, Barnes RW (1976) Critique of the Allen test for continuity of the palmar arch assessed by Doppler ultrasound. Surg Gynecol Obstet 142:861–864
9. Greenhow DE (1972) Incorrect performance of Allen's test. Ulnar-artery flow erroneously presumed inadequate. Anesthesiology 37:356–357
10. Oh TE, Davis NJ (1975) Radial artery cannulation. Anaesth Intens Care 3:12–18
11. Husum B, Berthelsen P (1981) Allen's test and systolic arterial pressure in the thumb. Br J Anaesth 53:635–637
12. Barber JD, Wright DJ, Ellis RH (1973) Radial artery puncture. A simple screening test of the ulnar anastomotic circulation. Anaesthesia 28:291–292
13. Ramanathan S, Chalon J, Turndorf H (1975) Determinating patency of palmar arches by retrograde radial pulsation. Anesthesiology 42:756–758
14. Slogoff S, Keats AS, Arlund C (1983) On the safety of radial artery cannulation. Anesthesiology 59:42–47
15. Band JD, Maki DG (1979) Infections caused by arterial catheters used for hemodynamic monitoring. Am J Med 67:735–741
16. Thomas F, Burke JP, Parker J, et al (1983): The risk of infection related to radial vs femoral sites for arterial catheterization. Crit Care Med 11:807–812
17. Amato JJ, Solod E, Cleveland RJ (1977) A "second" radial artery for monitoring the perioperative pediatric cardiac patient. J Pediatr Surg 12:715–717
18. Johnstone RE, Greenhow DF (1973) Catheterization of the dorsalis pedis artery. Anesthesiology 39:654–656
19. Husum B, Palm T, Eriksen J (1979) Percutaneous cannulation of the dorsalis pedis artery. A prospective study. Br J Anaesth 51:1055–1058
20. Youngberg JA, Miller ED (1976) Evaluation of percutaneous cannulation of the dorsalis pedis artery. Anaesthesiology 41:80–82
21. Humphrey CP, Stone NH (1970) Technique of chronic catheterization of the superficial temporal artery for obtaining multiple arterial samples. J Trauma 10:699–701.
22. Brown M, Gordon LH, Brown OW, Brown EM (1985) Intravascular monitoring via the axillary artery. Anaesth Intens Care 13:38–40

23. Gurman GM, Kriemerman S (1985) Cannulation of big arteries in critically ill patients. Crit Care Med 13:217–220
24. Ersoz CY, Hedden M, Lain L (1970) Prolonged femoral arterial catheterization for intensive care. Anesth Analg Curr Res 49:160–166
25. McGovern B, Baker AR (1968) Temporal artery catheterization for the monitoring of blood gases in infants. Surg Gynecol Obstet 127:600–603
26. Jodres ID, Rogers MI, Shannon DL, Moylan FMB (1975) Percutaneous catheterization of the radial artery in the critically ill neonate. J Pediatr 87:273–275
27. Furman EB, Hairabet JK, Roman DG (1972) The use of indwelling radial artery needles in pediatric anesthesia. Br J Anaesth 44:531–532

New Developments in PaO$_2$ Monitoring

G. J. Shortland, I. Scott, and E. R. Verrier Jones

Present Methods of Oxygen Monitoring in Neonatal Critical Care

The measurement of arterial oxygen tension in the neonate is essential for those requiring supplementary oxygen and ventilatory support. This measurement should be standard care to avoid the development of hypoxia with low oxygen tensions and subsequent acidemia, decreased surfactant production and persistent fetal circulation. Also in the premature infant high oxygen tensions are a cause of retinopathy of prematurity and possible blindness [1].

Neonates require added oxygen and ventilatory support for a number of different indications. These include respiratory distress syndrome, meconium aspiration, perinatal asphyxia, pneumonia and congenital malformations such as diaphragmatic hernia. Exact limits between which the PaO$_2$ should be kept will vary according to the clinical situation, but commonly will be maintained between 60–90 mmHg to minimize the complications already mentioned previously. Therefore frequent arterial blood gas analyses are required. Associated with this is the requirement for minimal handling of sick neonates, as any invasive procedure may cause the neonate to cry and develop irregular respiratory patterns which cause a drop in PaO$_2$. Minimal handling also reduces problems of temperature regulation and infection spread from person to baby. Therefore a number of different ways for monitoring PaO$_2$ have been developed to satisfy the above mentioned points.

These methods include intermittent peripheral arterial puncture of radial, ulnar, brachial and posterior tibial arteries. This involves considerable handling and after frequent use the arteries are quickly unusable. Therefore this method can only be used for occasional samples and not frequent sampling from sick, fragile neonates requiring more than 30% to 40% oxygen supplementation. As an extension of this technique, arterial cannulation of the radial, ulnar and posterior tibial arteries using fine gauge cannulae may be performed. These cannulae are then irrigated with a heparinized solution continuously. Whilst handling of the neonate is greatly reduced, these lines are prone to blockage and there is risk of thrombosis distal to the cannula.

Alternatively the most widely used technique for neonates requiring frequent sampling is the insertion of a catheter FG 3.5 or 5 into the umbilical artery. The indications for placement of umbilical artery catheters varies from nursery to nursery but would generally include infants who require mechanical ventilation or an inspired oxygen concentration of greater than 50%. This facilitates easy blood sampling, the possibility of blood pressure monitoring and the route as a method

Table 1. Complications of umbilical arterial catheters

Accidental hemorrhage
Blanching or cyanosis of extremities
Catheter clotted
Hypertension
Necrotizing enterocolitis
Vessel thrombosis
Sepsis

---

of infusion of fluids. The tip of the catheter is positioned via the umbilical artery and into the aorta to lie either above the celiac axis (T12–L1) or below the inferior mesenteric artery (L3–L4).

This is to minimize the complication of thrombosis from the catheter. There is evidence to suggest that placement of the catheter in the higher position results in less complications [2]. The catheter is constantly infused with heparinized saline and its position is checked radiographically. Reported complications arising from these catheters are given in Table 1.

Because the oxygen requirements of a sick neonate may change very rapidly, frequent samples would be required. In a neonate this would entail unacceptable blood loss. Therefore this method can be used in collaboration with a transcutaneous PO_2 monitor. These rely on measuring arterilized capillary PO_2 by warming the skin. The PO_2 of the skin rises to a value close to the arterial PO_2 and is measured on the skin by a modified Clark electrode. This has the advantage of being continuous and non-invasive. However, the need to avoid air trapping under the monitor, variation with peripheral perfusion and temperature, and the risk of skin burns to the neonate means that this method is not without its drawbacks. Calibration against arterial blood samples are also required when the site of the transcutaneous monitor is changed, usually every four hours.

The last technique is a combination of an umbilical catheter with a PO_2 sensor mounted in the catheter. The advantage is that it both provides access for blood sampling and a continuous true measurement of PaO_2. The effects of nursing and clinical procedures and changes in an infant's condition can be seen within a few seconds and management can be quickly optimized. The drawbacks are those as previously mentioned for umbilical arterial catheters and the need for an accurate PO_2 sensor. A variation of this method is the use of a fibre-optic catheter device for continuous oxygen saturation measurement [3]. This does not, however, provide a sensitive guide to changes of blood oxygenation above a PO_2 of about 100 mmHg and it is therefore not useful in guarding against hyperoxemia.

Method of Oxygen Measurement

The most common method of measuring dissolved oxygen tension is the polargraphic cell. This technology in modified forms is used in blood gas measuring machines, for transcutenous oxygen monitors and the intra-arterial oxygen sensors we are using in our trial. The beginning of modern blood oxygen measurement started in 1956 when Clark [4] first used a polargraphic oxygen electrode to measure the PO$_2$ of whole blood. The technique consisted of applying a voltage between two wires in an electrolyte solution. The negative wire was platinum (cathode) and the positive wire (anode) was silver. Oxygen is reduced at the cathode and chloride ions oxidized at the anode to produce silver chloride. The wires and electrolyte were separated from the medium to be measured by a membrane permeable to oxygen but impermeable to water, proteins, blood cells and ions. The current which flowed in the external circuit was proportional to the oxygen tension (Fig. 1).

The most commonly used invasive PO$_2$ sensor was first developed and results published by Parker and Soutter in 1975 [5]. The cathode and anode are silver and a modified polystyrene membrane is dip coated over the tip. Prior to this, KCl crystals are applied to the cathode (reference) surface to provide an electrolyte once hydrated.

A large review of clinical experience over four years, using commercially produced catheters (G. D. Searle and Company), raised a number of interesting points [6]. Twenty five per cent of the catheters did not measure PO$_2$ satisfactorily. A further 9% had temporary malfunctions for a variety of reasons including clotting on the tip of the catheter. Another 9% stopped recording when they were still clinically required for reasons thought to be due to clotting on the tip. There was a general impression the incidence of thrombosis in arteries and of electrode failure could probably be reduced in the future if materials with very smooth surfaces that resisted thrombogenesis were used in the construction of the electrode catheters. Other authors further report the impression that the output from these catheters gradually falls over several days as the electrode deteriorates [7].

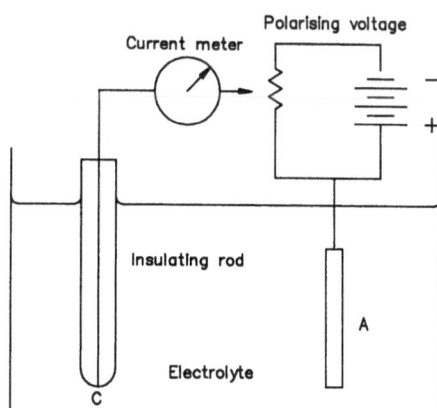

Fig. 1. The basic outline of a polarographic oxygen cell, showing the cathode wire (C) in a glass insulating rod, the reference anode (A), and the polarising circuit

New Developments in Catheter Technology

Because of the disadvantages of previous oxygen sensors with drift and clot formation on the tip, efforts have been made to improve the catheters by using alternative materials with polyurethane for the catheter tubing. Polyurethane catheters avoid many troublesome complications such as catheter kink, bend and deformation often encountered with other catheters. Also they have been shown to have a lower thrombogenicity than other types of catheter [8]. As well as thrombo-resistance of the catheter, stiffness may be of crucial importance as studies in newborn animals suggest that the thrombogenicity of catheters in prolonged use is related to damage of the endothelium and subsequent clot formation at the site of the vessel injury rather than clot formation on the catheter [9]. The coating of the sensor is with a membrane specially formulated to reduce following of the sensor by blood (Fig. 2). The sensor is mounted on a size 3.5 F gauge catheter. This catheter has been developed by British Viggo Laboratory and animal testing has demonstrated that this sensor is safe, has a fast, accurate response and is not subject to excessive drift over extended periods (unpublished data). The sensor has a similar sensitivity to the conventional sensor whilst having a cathode of thirteen times smaller area. This reduction in diffusion barrier leads to a significant increase in response time from about one minute for previous sensors to about one second for the new device.

Therefore a clinical trial was formulated to test the hypothesis that the new catheters would improve the monitoring of PaO_2 in the neonate without increas-

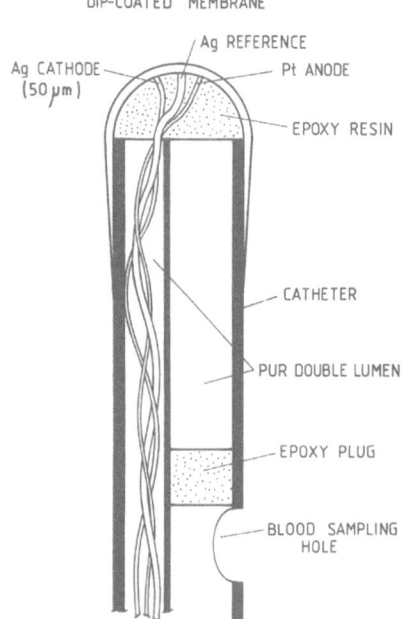

Fig. 2. DIP-coated membrane

ing the acknowledged complication rates of these catheters. An outline of the trial and preliminary results are shown below.

Trial and Results

This was to assess the in vivo performance of the Viggo catheter in terms of complications in vivo drift and duration of effective function. The Viggo oxygen sensing umbilical artery catheter was inserted generally into those babies requiring greater than 40% supplemental oxygen and very premature babies requiring frequent blood sampling. The oxygen sensor readings were compared with ABL blood gas recordings and transcutaneous oxygen monitors.

The membrane of the catheter was hydrated prior to use. On catheter had a failed insertion because of difficulty with passing the catheter along the umbilical artery. This was a full term infant weighing 3.5 kg and provision of the oxygen sensor on a size 5 French guage catheter would have facilitated the insertion of the catheter in this infant. One other catheter also had a failed insertion but it was not possible to insert other alternative catheters by the umbilical artery either.

Seven catheters successfully inserted have caused no significant problem with difficulty with insertion.

All these catheters were monotoring following insertion. the duration for which it has been possible to sample through the catheters has been between 8 hours and 120 hours for individual catheters. Monitoring of arterial PO$_2$ was successful between a range of 4 hours and 99 hours (Table 2).

Two catheters were removed because of clotting in the line. The other six catheters were used for sampling until clinically not required. One neonate died whilst the catheter was in situ. All the catheter tips were sent for bacteriological culture and these were all sterile. There was no evidence of any umbilical sepsis during the time the catheters were in place. With two catheters there was transitory blueness of a distal limb when they were initially inserted, and which

Table 2

Catheter	Time used for sampling	Time successful PO$_2$ monitoring	Comments
1	120 hrs	8 hrs	Child transferred at 8 hrs (unable to continue monitoring)
2	72 hrs	12 hrs	Catheter blocked
3	16 hrs	16 hrs	Catheter blocked
4	48 hrs	16 hrs	Neonate died
5	48 hrs	12 hrs	Catheter withdrawn for clinical reasons
6	92 hrs	12 hrs	Catheter withdrawn for clinical reasons
7	99 hrs	99 hrs	Catheter withdrawn for clinical reasons

quickly resolved on re-positioning of the catheter. There was no permanent evidence of ischemia. Necrotizing enterocolitis did not occur as a complication with any catheters.

Conclusion

We have described the importance of arterial PO_2 monitoring as a standard procedure for care of the sick neonate. We further propose the use of a new catheter with new materials to improve the monitoring performance and reduce complication rates. Some preliminary results are described and further user experience of this catheter and comparison with alternatives is currently being evaluated. Further trials to assess the accuracy of the monitor and response time in the clinical situation are required. Further improvements could include the use of multiparameter intra-arterial probes including pH and PCO_2 measurements.

References

1. Baum JD, Tizard JPM (1970) Retrolental fibroplasia: management of oxygen therapy. Br Med Bull 26:171–173
2. Mokrolisky MD (1978) Low positioning of umbilical artery catheters increases associated complications in newborn infants. N Engl J Med 299:561–564
3. Wilkinson AR et al (1979) Continuous in-vivo oxygen saturation in newborn infants with pulmonary disease. Crit Care Med 7:232–236
4. Clark LC (1956) Monitoring and control of blood and tissue oxygen tensions. Trans Am Soc Artif Intern Organs 2:41–45
5. Soutter, Conway, Parker (1975) A system for monitoring arterial oxygen tension in sick newborn babies. Biomed Engineering 257–261
6. Pollitzer MJ, Soutter, Reynolds (1980) Continuous monitoring of arterial oxygen tension in infants. Four years experience with an intravascular oxygen electrode. Pediatrics 66:31–36
7. Roberton NRC (1986) A manual of neonatal intensive care (2nd ed). Arnold (Publishers) Ltd., London, pp 101–102
8. Lar-Erik Lauder et al (1984) Material thrombogenicity in central venous catheterisation: A comparison between soft, antebrachial catheters of silicone elastomer and polyurethane. JPEN 8:399–406
9. Chidi CC, King DR, Boles JR (1983) An ultrastructural study of the internal injury induced by an indwelling umbilical artery catheter. J Ped Surg 18:109–115

Conjunctival Oxygen Tension Monitoring

E. Abraham

The adequacy of tissue oxygenation in any anatomic region is dependent both on the perfusion and the oxygen content of the blood perfusing that site. These two variables are integrated in the calculation of oxygen delivery (DO_2), which represents the product of arterial oxygen content ($CaO_2 = [1.36 \cdot Hgb \cdot SaO_2] + [0.003 \cdot PaO_2]$) and cardiac index (CI). In addition, oxygen concentration in peripheral tissues will be dependent on regional metabolic activity and oxygen consumption, as well as local differences in vascular resistance and blood flow.

Direct, non-invasive and continuous measurement of peripheral tissue oxygenation was made possible by the development of miniaturized polarographic oxygen electrodes [1]. These oxygen electrodes are similar to those utilized in standard blood gas machines and consist of a silver chloride anode and a platinum cathode. If a drop of arterial blood is placed directly on these miniaturized oxygen sensors, an accurate measurement of PaO_2 will be obtained. Placement of the electrode on a surface such as skin or the palpebral conjunctiva permits measurement of the oxygen tension in the tissues underlying the sensor.

The initial sensors developed were transcutaneous oxygen monitors, which were placed on the skin of the upper arms or chest [2]. The transcutaneous monitors require a heating element in order to measure tissue oxygen tension. The stratum corneum of the skin acts as an effective barrier to diffusion of oxygen from the subcutaneous layer to the surface oxygen sensor. Heating the skin surface to 43° C causes liquification of the stratum corneum and permits the surface oxygen electrode to measure underlying tissue oxygen tension. This requirement for heating results in capillary dilation, increased tissue metabolism, and a rightward shift of the oxyhemoglobin disassociation curve on the area beneath the transcutaneous sensor. These alterations in localized oxygen delivery and utilization, which occur as a result of heating and are necessary for monitoring of tissue oxygenation at subcutaneous sites, mean that the readings obtained with the transcutaneous sensor, while reflecting trends in underlying tissue oxygen tension, do not necessarily measure the actual level of oxygen tension which would exist if heating had not been applied [3].

The conjunctival oxygen sensor uses a polymethylmethacrylate ocular conformer to position a miniaturized oxygen electrode against the lateral aspect of the superior palpebral conjunctiva. The anatomic advantage of this location is its lack of a keratinized layer, permitting placement of the oxygen electrode within 30 μ of the underlying capillary bed [4]. Because no stratum corneum is present, there is no requirement for heating and no artifactual changes in tissue oxygen tension, such as those seen with the transcutaneous oxygen sensor, are produced.

The conjunctival conformer does not cover the cornea, so minimal discomfort is present after insertion. Usually, in the alert patient a drop of topical anesthetic, such as 0.5% tetracaine, is administered into the eye before placement of the conjunctival sensor. Once the sensor is inserted, the patient can maintain the eye open, with full ocular movements, without disturbing the continuity or quality of tissue oxygen tension measurements. The conjunctival sensor can be left in the eye for as long as 24 hours, even though most monitoring periods are 8 hours or less.

Both the transcutaneous and conjunctival sensors require calibration before use. The partial pressure of oxygen in the atmosphere generally is used for this calibration step. At sea level, the partial pressure of oxygen is approximately 157 torr, so the oxygen sensor is adjusted to this value while exposed to air, before insertion. The conjunctival electrode is quite stable, and drift during the usual monitoring period (<8 hours) is insignificant.

The conjunctival oxygen sensor as well as the transcutaneous oxygen electrode originally were developed with the hope that these modalities could provide a continuous non-invasive measure of arterial oxygen tension (PaO_2). In the hemodynamically stable patient, with normal cardiac output and no abnormalities in peripheral perfusion, the conjunctival oxygen electrode closely follows PaO_2 [5, 6]. Under these conditions, the $PcjO_2$ to PaO_2 ratio is approximately 0.6 to 0.7.

In the critically ill patient with decreased cardiac output, intense peripheral vasoconstriction often is present, potentiating the fall in oxygen delivery to peripheral sites. Cellular metabolic needs usually are increased in critical illness, and the combination of diminished supply and increased demand for oxygen can result in markedly decreased peripheral tissue oxygen tension even though PaO_2 is normal. Tissue oxygen delivery and utilization are the primary determinants of $PcjO_2$, and in states associated with diminished peripheral perfusion, such as hemorrhagic or cardiogenic shock, $PcjO_2$ may become completely disassociated from PaO_2 [6, 7]. The lack of association between $PcjO_2$ and PaO_2 was initially thought to preclude any use of this non-invasive sensor in unstable patients. However, further experience with the conjunctival sensor has shown that measured values of $PcjO_2$ in the critically ill patient reflect important physiologic alterations at an earlier point than do standard non-invasive parameters, such as vital signs. In particular, values obtained with the conjunctival oxygen tension index ($PcjO_2$ Index $= PcjO_2/PaO_2$) can be used to detect physiologic instability associated with abnormalities in blood volume, cardiac output and peripheral perfusion before hypotension develops [5]. In addition, conjunctival oxygen monitoring is useful in determining the effects and endpoints of therapeutic interventions aimed at achieving hemodynamic stability in critically ill patients.

Because heating of the conjunctival sensor is unnecessary, oxygen tension in the tissue beneath the electrode can be measured accurately without the artifacts inherent in transcutaneous monitoring. Relevant measurements with the conjunctival sensor are achieved within 60 seconds of insertion. The rapid stabilization of the conjunctival sensor makes it particularly useful in the initial management of critically ill patients both in the prehospital and emergency department areas. Analysis of the relationship between the conjunctival oxygen sensor and the capillary bed approximately 30 μ beneath it indicates that the measured oxygen tension is 5 to 10 mmHg less than that present in the capillary blood [4].

Blunt trauma can produce occult blood loss from intraabdominal sources such as a ruptured spleen or lacerated liver. In previously healthy persons, blood pressure often is well maintained until blood loss exceeds 30 per cent of total blood volume. If blood pressure is normal, adequate volume resuscitation for hemorrhage may not be accomplished until the patient's clinical condition further deteriorates and the magnitude of the blood loss is recognized.

Conjunctival oxygen monitoring has been shown to be particularly useful in the detection and treatment of significant hemorrhagic hypovolemia [5]. Hemorrhage produces abnormal tissue perfusion and oxygen delivery before any alteration in blood pressure is apparent, and these physiologic abnormalities can be easily detected with the conjunctival sensor [7].

Experimental studies on hemorrhage have shown that the $PcjO_2/PaO_2$ ratio falls below 0.5 after loss of approximately 18% of the calculated blood volume [7]. Blood pressure does not show substantial, clinically detectable decreases until over 35% of the blood volume has been lost. Similarly, during resuscitation of animals bled to a blood pressure of 40 mm Hg, blood pressure returns to normal values after 70% of the blood volume has been restored [8]. In contrast, $PcjO_2$ and the $PcjO_2/PaO_2$ ratio do not return to baseline until the blood volume is more than 90% of normal. These results suggest that blood pressure is an inadequate parameter in assessing volume status of critically ill patients with significant blood loss. In contrast, $PcjO_2$ appeared to be a much more sensitive indicator for detecting and treating hemorrhagic hypovolemia.

Clinical studies have substantiated the utility of conjunctival monitoring in detecting and treating blood loss in critically ill patients. In one series [3] examining 16 normotensive emergency department patients with histories consistent with significant blood loss and no history of cardiac disease, every patient with a $PcjO_2/PaO_2$ ratio less than 0.50 had a deficit of at least 15% in measured blood volume. Similarly, in a prospective series [9] of patients presenting to an emergency department, 16 of 44 multiple trauma patients had a $PcjO_2/PaO_2$ ratio < 0.50, and all of these patients had an estimated blood loss of greater than 1000 ml. Only 2 of the 16 patients with $PcjO_2/PaO_2$ ratio < 0.50 were hypotensive, again demonstrating the relative sensitivity of $PcjO_2$ in detecting blood loss.

In addition to rapid detection of hemorrhagic hypovolemia in multiple trauma patients, conjunctival oxygen monitoring also is capable of guiding fluid resuscitation in these patients. Normalization of the relationship between $PcjO_2$ and PaO_2 (i.e. to a $PcjO_2/PaO_2$ value > 0.50) in patients with baseline normal cardiac function indicates that a near normal blood volume has been achieved [5].

In critically ill patients with normal volume status, conjunctival oxygen monitoring is useful in detecting alterations in ventilatory and hemodynamic condition [6, 9]. Low values for $PcjO_2$ will be found with hypoxemia as well as in conditions associated with decreased cardiac output and tissue oxygen delivery. Although both hypoxemia and decreased cardiac output result in diminished $PcjO_2$, these conditions can be differentiated by drawing an arterial blood gas and calculating the $PcjO_2/PaO_2$ ratio. With ventilatory compromise, the PaO_2 will be low and the $PcjO_2/PaO_2$ ratio maintained at >0.50. In contrast, with circulatory impairment accompanying decreased cardiac output, the $PcjO_2/PaO_2$ ratio will be less than 0.50. In patients with combined circulatory and ventilatory abnormalities, the decrease in peripheral perfusion and oxygen delivery appears to be predominant in determining $PcjO_2$, so even if PaO_2 is restored to normal levels through the use of therapies such as intubation or the administration of supplemental oxygen, $PcjO_2$ will remain low until cardiac output is returned to normal levels.

Initial studies with the conjunctival oxygen monitor showed that this modality would reflect changes in PaO_2 accurately and rapidly in patients with normal cardiac output. Assessment of the adequacy of ventilatory interventions (e. g. intubation or the administration of bronchodilating agents to the severely asthmatic patient) could be made in a continuous manner. Worsening hypoxemia in the patient with respiratory failure could be detected as it occurred. Additionally, measurement of conjunctival oxygen tension was capable of detecting a fall in cardiac output due to myocardial ischemia or arrhythmias before there was any change in blood pressure.

In patients with cardiac arrest, $PcjO_2$ showed changes in a patient's physiologic condition as early or earlier than standard non-invasive parameters, such as blood pressure, palpation of pulses, or assessment of skin blanching [9]. A fall in $PcjO_2$ from previously stable values in the setting of myocardial ischemia often presaged the development of a cardiac arrest [10]. A rise in $PcjO_2$ frequently was found to be the first indication of improvement in cardiac function after defibrillation, cardioversion or administration of cardioactive pharmacologic agents for treatment of cardiac arrest [9]. Changes in $PcjO_2$ also may occur during cardiopulmonary resuscitation (CPR), reflecting the relative efficacy of the external chest compressions in achieving even minimal levels of cardiac output. This observation suggests that $PcjO_2$ may be a useful way of monitoring the consistency and adequacy of CPR during a cardiac arrest.

Aeromedical transport of critically ill patients from the scene of accidents to the emergency department or from one hospital to another is becoming increasingly common. Helicopters often are used, and present unique problems in patient monitoring because of noise and vibration. It is frequently impossible to auscultate or even palpate blood pressure or pulse in this environment, and patient stability is determined by observation alone.

The conjunctival oxygen sensor has been utilized in monitoring critically ill patients during helicopter transport, and was found to detect abnormalities in ventilatory and circulatory condition which otherwise would not have been apparent during the flight [11]. One series [11] found that a third of the patients transported had cardiorespiratory abnormalities which were inapparent by standard monitoring methods, but could be detected and corrected during transport through the use of conjunctival oxygen monitoring.

The blood supply to the palpebral conjunctiva is derived largely from the ophthalmic artery, which branches from the internal carotid. Because of this unique blood supply, several investigators have proposed that monitoring of conjunctival oxygen tension may provide some indication of the state of cerebral oxygenation [12]. During carotid endarterectomy, clamping of the carotid produces immediate and profound decreases in PcjO$_2$. Restoration of carotid flow after placement of a graft or relief of obstruction results in return of PcjO$_2$ to normal values [13].

Complications with the conjunctival oxygen sensor are rare. Placement of the conjunctival conformer may produce a corneal abrasion if foreign material such as glass or dirt is on the ocular surface and is wiped onto the cornea. Prolonged use (i.e. >6 hours) of the conjunctival sensor may result in a punctate keratopathy; this complication is particularly likely to occur during anesthesia or in the unresponsive patient, in whom drying of the ocular surface results from the lack of closure of the eyelids. Patching of the eye for 24 to 48 hours achieves resolution of this condition. Chemosis of the conjunctiva may occur with use of the conjunctival sensor. This complication occurs most frequently with maxillofacial trauma and usually resolves within 48 hours of removal of the conjunctival conformer.

References

1. Abraham E (1986) Noninvasive measurement of cardiorespiratory parameters. Emerg Med Clin North Am 4:791–807
2. Tremper KK, Shoemaker WC (1981) Transcutaneous oxygen monitoring of critically ill adults, with and without low flow shock. Crit Care Med 9:706–709
3. Tremper KK, Waxman K, Shoemaker WC (1979) Effects of hypoxia and shock on transcutaneous PO$_2$ values in dogs. Crit Care Med 7:526–531
4. Fatt I, Deutsch FA (1983) The relaltionship of conjunctival PO$_2$ to capillary bed PO$_2$. Crit Care Med 11:445–448
5. Abraham E, Oye RK, Smith M (1985) Detection of blood volume deficits through conjunctival oxygen tension monitoring. Crit Care Med 12:931–934
6. Abraham E, Smith M, Silver L (1984) Continuous monitoring of critically ill patients with transcutaneous oxygen and carbon dioxide and conjunctival oxygen sensors. Ann Emerg Med 13:1021–1026
7. Smith M, Abraham E (1986) Conjunctival oxygen tension monitoring during hemorrhage. J Trauma 26:217–224
8. Abraham E, Fink S (1986) Cardiorespiratory and conjunctival oxygen tension monitoring during resuscitation from hemorrhage. Crit Care Med 14:1004–1009
9. Abraham E, Fink S (1988) Conjunctival oxygen tension monitoring in emergency department patients. Am J Emerg Med (In press)
10. Abraham E, Smith M, Silver L (1984) Conjunctival and transcutaneous oxygen monitoring during cardiac arrest and CPR. Crit Care Med 12:419–421
11. Abraham E, Lee G, Morgan MT (1986) Conjunctival oxygen tension monitoring during helicopter transport of critically ill patients. Ann Emerg Med 15:782–786
12. Isenberg SJ, Shoemaker WC (1983) The transconjunctival oxygen monitor. Am J Ophthalmol 95:803–806
13. Shoemaker WC, Lawner PM (1983) Method for continuous conjunctival oxygen monitoring during carotid artery surgery. Crit Care Med 11:946–947

Indications and Limitations of $S\bar{v}O_2$ and $ScvO_2$ Monitoring

K. Reinhart, M. Schäfer, and M. Specht

Introduction

Recent clinical reports on the possibility of continuous measurement of mixed venous oxygen saturation ($S\bar{v}O_2$) have prompted a resurgence of interest in the value of this parameter as indicator of cardiorespiratory function [1–3].

The primary aim of our therapy of cardiorespiratory insufficiency is not to increase systemic blood pressure or wedge pressure but to improve the transport of oxygen and other substrates to the tissues [4]. Despite this, we are still blood-pressure-oriented because pressure is much easier to measure than blood flow. The introduction of ECG and systemic blood pressure measurement into clinical medicine almost 100 years ago was a big step forward in patient monitoring. However, these parameters, that are still the cornerstones of hemodynamic monitoring today, only poorly reflect oxygen transport. Figure 1 shows the poor correlation between the mean arterial pressure (MAP) and convective O_2-transport

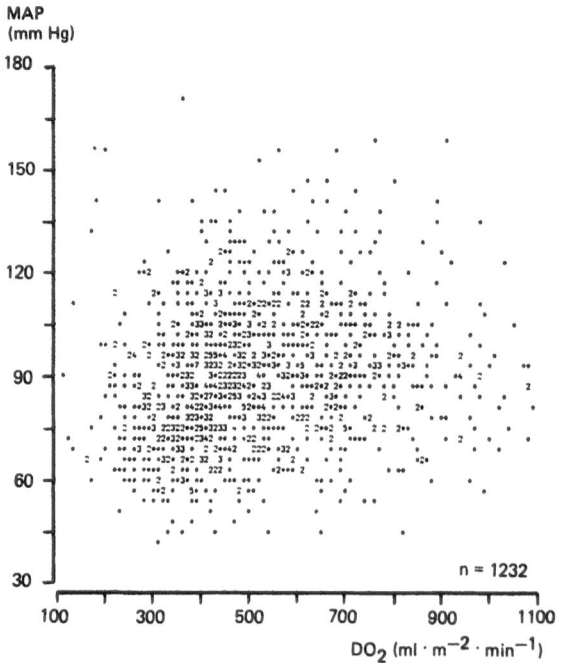

Fig. 1. Correlation between mean arterial pressure (MAP) and O_2-delivery (DO_2) in patients with aorto-bifemoral bypass grafting

in the vascular beds (DO_2). The amount of oxygen transported to the tissues in the vascular bed (DO_2) is calculated as the product of the arterial oxygen content (CaO_2) and cardiac output (CO):

$$DO_2 = CaO_2 \cdot CO$$

Organ function is always the best indicator of the adequacy of tissue oxygenation. Of course, the generation of blood pressure and the number of heart beats are expressions of cardiac function, but heart rate is only one of the four major determinants of cardiac output and blood pressure depends on five different factors, usually unknown: cardiac output, systematic vascular resistance, blood volume, blood viscosity, and elasticity of the vessels. Performing therapy on the basis of blood pressure alone means to be directed by a parameter that has five unknown determinants.

Urine production is a very good indicator of adequate circulation, but the time course of a decrease of urine output may be too long in circulatory failure. What is warranted in critically ill patients, is an early warning system for imbalance of O_2-supply-to-O_2-demand-ratio before organ dysfunction occurs.

According to the Fick's principle [5], an increase in oxygen consumption ($\dot{V}O_2$) can be met by an augmentation of cardiac output and/or a rise in arterial venous oxygen content difference. In healthy exercizing men, both compensatory mechanisms work to accommodate the increased tissue demands for oxygen. There is a more than threefold increase in cardiac output as well as in arteriovenous O_2 difference [6]. In patients with severe heart disease, who often already have an increased oxygen extraction at rest, an increased oxygen consumption during exercise is accompanied by an only small increase of cardiac output, and almost exclusively a widening of arterio-venous O_2 difference [7].

When DO_2 is decreased by a reduction of cardiac output, $\dot{V}O_2$ can only be maintained by an increase in arterio-venous oxygen difference. A fall in DO_2 due to a decreased arterial oxygen content can only be compensated by increasing cardiac output and/or lowering mixed venous oxygen content. Arterio-venous oxygen difference and SⅴO₂ are linked with DO_2 and $\dot{V}O_2$, and reflect changes of the oxygen supply-to-demand ratio. That is why they indicate to what extent the major compensatory mechanisms of the organism either are used or fail [8].

In several clinical studies, a persistant decrease of SⅴO₂ below 50% or of PⅴO₂ below 27 mmHg was accompanied by signs of anaerobic metabolism and poor outcome [9, 10–12]. On the other hand, reports indicate that patients with severe chronic heart failure of chronic pulmonary insufficiency can live with SⅴO₂ around 30% without signs of anaerobic metabolism [13]. This can be explained by adaptive processes such as a right shift of the oxygen dissociation curve, which facilitates O_2-release, and an increase in the capillary density, which shortens the distance between capillaries and the cells.

If SⅴO₂ falls, we know that oxygen supply-to-demand ratio has changed, because either DO_2 decreased or $\dot{V}O_2$ increased (Fig. 2). Unfortunately, we do not know which one of the determinants has changed, but we are warned and can look for the possible causes. The effects of therapeutic measures on O_2-supply-to-O_2-demand ratio can also be judged.

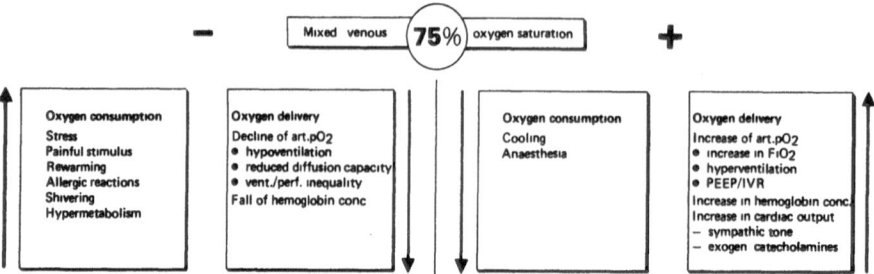

Oxygen consumption	**Oxygen delivery**	**Oxygen consumption**	**Oxygen delivery**
Stress	Decline of art.pO2	Cooling	Increase of art.pO2
Painful stimulus	• hypoventilation	Anaesthesia	• increase in FiO2
Rewarming	• reduced diffusion capacity		• hyperventilation
Allergic reactions	• vent./perf. inequality		• PEEP/IVR
Shivering	Fall of hemoglobin conc		Increase in hemoglobin conc.
Hypermetabolism			Increase in cardiac output
			− sympathic tone
			− exogen catecholamines

Fig. 2. Determinants of total body O_2-balance

SvO2 was suggested as a good indicator of changes in cardiac output, and linear correlations were calculated between these two parameters [14–16]. This is mathematically incorrect because first, according to the Fick's principle, the correlation between SvO2 and cardiac output is not linear but curvilinear, and second, this correlation exists only if $\dot{V}O_2$ does not change. Besides cardiac output, both $\dot{V}O_2$ and arterial oxygen content can change over a wide range, so that the

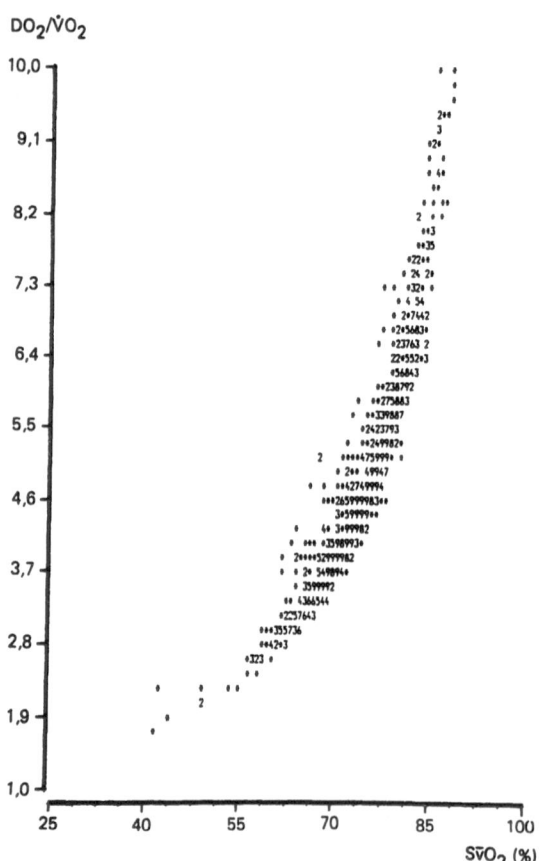

Fig. 3. Mixed venous O_2-saturation (SvO2) compared to O_2-supply-to-demand ratio ($DO_2/\dot{V}O_2$) in patients with aorto-bifemoral bypass grafting during the perioperative period

relationship between Sv̄O$_2$ and cardiac output is usually poor. We found it also perioperatively in patients undergoing aorto-bifemoral bypass surgery (unpublished data).

It is of much greater interest to the clinician to know to what extent a measured cardiac output meets the oxygen requirements of tissues by measurement of Sv̄O$_2$ and V̇O$_2$ at the bedside. The poor relationship between Sv̄O$_2$ and cardiac output does not limit the clinical usefulness of Sv̄O$_2$ monitoring. Figure 3 shows the close relation of DO$_2$/V̇O$_2$ to Sv̄O$_2$ over a wide range. In contrast to V̇O$_2$ and DO$_2$, Sv̄O$_2$ can now be easily measured continuously at the bedside [1, 2, 8, 14, 16, 17] to obtain continuous real-time information on changes of DO$_2$ in relation to V̇O$_2$.

Limitations of Sv̄O₂-Monitoring

Sv̄O$_2$ only reflects the global oxygen reserve of the whole body. Already under normal conditions, O$_2$-reserve and O$_2$-extraction are different in the various organs (Fig. 4). O$_2$ reserves are very limited for the heart which has an oxygen

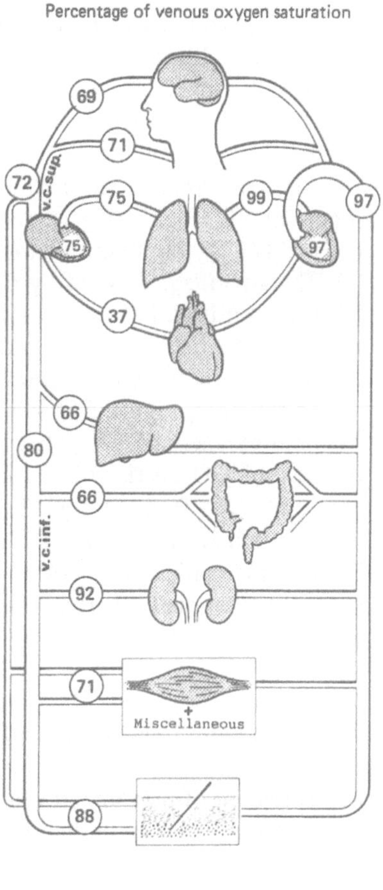

Fig. 4. Oxygen extraction in various organs

extraction of more than 60% already under normal conditions at rest, but higher in kidney and skin, which have a low O_2-extraction. This means that in situation-with limited oxygen delivery or increased O_2-demand, blood flow can be redistributed away from skin and kidneys to heart and brain to meet oxygen demand in these organs, while oxygen consumption can still be maintained in the kidneys and skin with limited blood flow but higher O_2 extraction [18]. These physiological differences in $DO_2/\dot{V}O_2$ between the various organs can further change in acute situations with limited DO_2 or sharp increases of $\dot{V}O_2$.

There are several disease states that limit the interpretation of the absolute values of $S\bar{v}O_2$ as indicators of tissue oxygenation [19]. In patients with sepsis or hepatic failure, normal or high $S\bar{v}O_2$ values can be accompanied by tissue hypoxia [20–22]. This also holds true for disturbed unloading of hemoglobin due to left shift of the oxygen dissociation curve [3] or blockage of the enzymes of the respiratory chain of the mitochondrias as in cyanide poisoning and sepsis [23–25].

Continuous Measurement of $S\bar{v}O_2$

In vivo measurements of oxygen saturation by reflection spectrophotometry using modern commercially available $S\bar{v}O_2$-monitoring systems consist of optical modules and fiberoptics incorporated in conventional flow-directed thermal dilution pulmonary artery catheters [1, 2, 8, 14, 16]. Older devices were complicated by catheter stiffness, large drift and calibration problems, which have prevented their wide clinical use [26–28].

We found similar correlation between in vivo and in vitro control measurements of $S\bar{v}O_2$ with two currently available systems: Opticath, Oximetric Inc ($r = 0.88$) and Swan Ganz Oximetry TD catheter, Edwards Laboratories ($r = 0.87$) [3]. The advantage offered by continuous monitoring systems is their ability to indicate trends and abrupt changes in the oxygen-supply-to-demand ratio immediately at the bedside. Determinations of cardiac output and arterial blood gas analysis can be limited to situations with larger changes in $S\bar{v}O_2$.

For example, Figure 5 shows reduced $S\bar{v}O_2$ due to a tension pneumothorax. The improvement of $S\bar{v}O_2$ after the application of a chest tube was caused by an increase of DO_2, a rise of cardiac index from 4.1 to 10.2 $1/min/m^2$ and an increase of PaO_2 from 11.4 to 13.5 kPa. Mean arterial pressure (MAP) rised from 85 to 90 mmHg and heart rate from 105 to 115 beats/min. In some situations, $S\bar{v}O_2$ yields earlier and better information on changes in O_2 supply-to-demand ratio of the whole body than the other usually measured hemodynamic parameters [17].

Mixed Venous Versus Central Venous O_2-Saturation

Measurement of true mixed venous O_2-saturation requires pulmonary artery catheterization which is limited by its invasiveness and high costs to high-risk patients. We were interested in the question as to what extent the measurement of

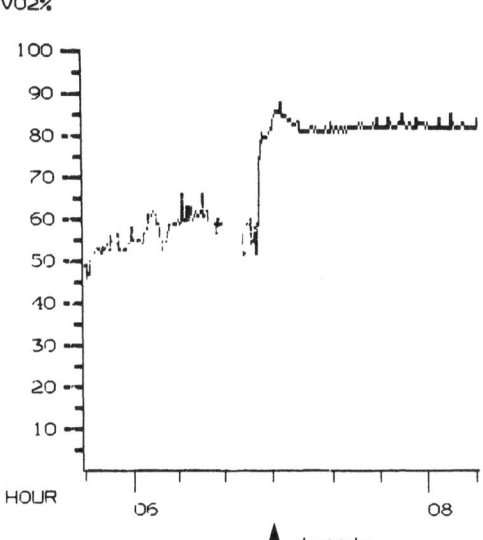

Fig. 5. Example of a patient with acute respiratory failure, where a reduced Sv̄O$_2$ was due to tension pneumothorax. Immediate improvement of Sv̄O$_2$ was noted after placement of a chest tube

central venous O$_2$-saturation (ScvO$_2$) can replace that of mixed venous saturation. During aorto-bifemoral bypass surgery, changes in O$_2$-supply-to-demand ratio were paralleled by changes in central venous O$_2$-saturation [29]. The difference between ScvO$_2$ and Sv̄O$_2$ was increased by the specific influence of the anesthetics on regional blood flow and regional O$_2$-consumption. With halothane, the difference between these two parameters increased: ScvO$_2$ was up to 6% higher than Sv̄O$_2$. It is known that inhalational anesthetics increase cerebral blood flow and decrease cerebral O$_2$-consumption, resulting in higher O$_2$-saturation in the superior cava vein.

Redistribution of blood flow is also known to occur in shock, where blood flow to the vital organs, heart and brain, is increased relative to the kidneys, gut, muscle and skin [12]. Most of the latter organs are drained into the inferior vena cava, which has a lower O$_2$-saturation than the superior vena cava. Therefore, the difference between ScvO$_2$ and Sv̄O$_2$ increases. In septic shock, we observed a widening of the difference between ScvO$_2$ and Sv̄O$_2$. The changes of the two parameters were consistent, however, in each observation (Fig. 6).

Central venous catheterization with multilumen central-venous catheters is routinely used in many ICU patients. Continuous control of O$_2$-supply-to-demand ratio via fiberoptic fibers incorporated in a central venous catheter would yield important additional information on the adequate function of the patient's cardiorespiratory system. Although absolute values of ScvO$_2$ cannot be trusted, changes of O$_2$-supply-to-demand ratio are indicated by changes of both ScvO$_2$ and Sv̄O$_2$. The effects of the ongoing therapy on O$_2$-balance can also be followed by this method. Without any increased invasiveness and with only some limitations, the advantages of on-line Sv̄O$_2$ monitoring can be extended to critically ill patients who do not need Swan-Ganz catheterization.

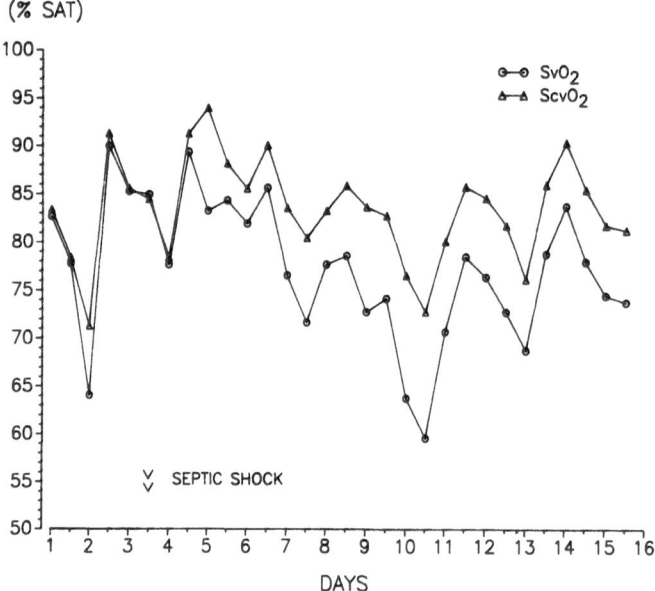

Fig. 6. Changes of ScvO$_2$ and S$\bar{v}$O$_2$ in the course of sepsis and septic shock in a 48 years old patient with sepsis after total hip replacement

Continuous S$\bar{v}$O$_2$ monitoring either in the pulmonary artery or via a central-venous catheter offers new and often better insight into the rapidly changing biological processes of critically ill patients than most of the usually monitored cardiorespiratory variables.

References

1. Beale PL, McMichan JC, Marsh MB, Sill JC, Sourther PY (1982) Continuous monitoring of mixed venous saturation in critically ill patients. Anesth Analg 61:513–517
2. Fahey PJ, Harris K, Vanderwarf C (1984) Clinical experience with continuous monitoring of mixed venous oxygen saturation in respiratory failure. Chest 5:748–752
3. Reinhart K, Moser N, Rudolph T, Gramm HJ, Goecke J (1987) Comparison of two mixed-venous saturation catheters in critically ill patients. Anesthesiology (Abst)
4. Shoemaker WC, Czer LSC (1979) Evaluation of the biologic importance of various hemo-dynamic and oxygen transport variables. Crit Care Med 7:237–245
5. Fick A (1870) Über die Messung des Blutquantums in den Herzventrikeln. Sitzungsber. Phys Med Ges Würburg Bd II: XVI
6. Bishop JM, Donald KW, Wade OL (1954) Minute to minute changes in cardiac output by the direct Fick method in normal subjects during exercise and recovery. J Physiol 123:12–56
7. Bishop JM, Wade OL, Donald KW (1958) Changes in jugular and renal arterio-venous oxygen content difference during exercise in heart disease. Clin Sci 611–627
8. Reinhart K (1988) Zum Monitoring des Sauerstofftransportsystems. Anaesthesist (in press)
9. Boyd AD, Tremblay RE, Spencer FC, Behnson HT (1959) Estimation of cardiac output soon after intracardiac surgery with cardiopulmonary bypass. Ann Surg 150:613–626

10. Kasnitz P, Druger GL, Frederick Y, Simmons DH (1976) Mixed venous oxygen tension and hyperlactatemia: Survival in severe Cardiopulmonary disease. JAMA 236:570-577
11. Kawakami Y, Kishi F, Yamamato H, Miyamoto K (1983) Relation of oxygen delivery mixed venous oxygenation and pulmonary hemodynamics to prognosis in chronic obstructive pulmonary disease. N Engl J Med 308:1045-1051
12. Patt GVS, Blackstone EH, Kirklin JW (1974) Cardiac performance and mortality early after intracardiac surgery in infants and children. Circulation 51:867-873
13. Schlichting R, Cowden VL, Chaitman BR (1986) Tolerance of unusually low mixed venous oxygen saturation adaptations in the chronic low cardiac output syndrome. Am J Med 80:813-818
14. Jamieson WRE, Turnbull KW, Larrieu AJ, Dodds WA, Allison JC, Tyers GFO (1982) Continuous monitoring of mixed venous oxygen saturation in cardiac surgery. Canad Surg 25:538-543
15. Muir AL, Kirby BJ, King AJ, Miller HC (1971) Mixed venous oxygen saturation in relation to cardiac output in myocardial infarction. Brit Med J 4:276-278
16. Waller JL, Kaplan JA, Bauman DI, Craver JM (1982) Clinical evaluation of a new fiberoptic catheter oximetry during cardiac surgery. Anesth Analg 61:676-679
17. Reinhart K, Gramm HJ, Specht M, Föhring U, Mayr O, Schäfer M, Dennhardt R (1986) Physiologische Grundlagen und klinische Erfahrungen mit der kontinuierlichen In vivo-Registrierung der gemischtvenösen Sauerstoffsättigung bei Risikopatienten. Intensivmed 23:346-352
18. Forsyth RP, Hoffbrand BM, Melmon KL (1970) Redistribution of cardiac output during hemorrhage in the unanaesthetized monkey. Circ Res 27:311-320
19. Aghdami A, Ellis R (1985) High oxygen saturation does not always indicate arterial placement of catheter during internal jugular venous cannulation. Anesthesiology 62:372-373
20. Bihari D, Grimson A, Waterson M, Williams R (1984) Tissue hypoxia during fulminant hepatic failure. Crit Care Med 12:233-241
21. Finley RJ, Duff JH, Holliday RL, Jones D, Marchuk JB (1975) Capillary muscle blood flow in human sepsis. Surgery 78:87-92
22. McLean LD, Mulligan WG, McLean APH, Duff JH (1967) Patterns of septic shock in man. Ann Surg 166:543-562
23. Conn JN, Buurk LP (1979) Nitroprusside. Ann Intern Med 91:752-765
24. Moss GS, Erve PP, Schumer W (1969) Effect of endotoxin on mitochondrial respiration. Surg Forum 20:24-36
25. Tinker JH, Michenfelder JD (1982) Cardiac cyanide toxicity induced by nitroprusside in the dog: potential for reversal. Anesthesiology 49:109-114
26. Cole JS, Martin WE, Cheung PW, Johnson CC (1972) Clinical studies with a solid state fiberoptic oximeter. Am J Cardiol 29:383-388
27. Gamble WJ, Hugenholtz PG, Monroe RG, Polanyi M (1965) The use of fiberoptics in clinical cardiac catheterization. Circulation 31:328-343
28. Polanyi ML, Hehir RM (1962) In vivo oximeter with fast dynamic response. Rev Sc Instr 33:1050-1054
29. Reinhrt K, Kersting K, Föhrung U, Schäfer M (1986) Can central-venous replace mixed-venous oxygen saturation measurements during anesthesia. In: Longmuir S (ed) Oxygen transport to tissue, vol 8. Plenum Press, New-York, pp 67-72

Dual Oximetry

J. Räsänen

Introduction

As critical care medicine has developed, patient monitoring capability has become increasingly complex. Variables relevant to the patient's disease process preferably should be monitored continuously in an on-line fashion, to allow repeated assessment and rapid adjustments of ongoing therapy. Monitoring should not subject the patient to a significant risk of complications, and cost should be proportional to the value of the information provided. The ability of the observer, physician or nurse, to process information is easily overwhelmed when the patient's vital functions are fragmented into a simultaneous display of multiple variables. Therefore, an ideal monitoring system should combine and analyze data automatically, and present it to the observer in a form that has direct physiologic significance and immediate applicability.

Monitoring of cardiopulmonary function in critically ill patients commonly entails continuous measurement of cardiac rate and rhythm and vascular pressures. Cardiac output and blood gas values are determined intermittently, usually at intervals of several hours. Therefore, accurate information regarding the key events of cardiopulmonary function – gas exchange in the lungs and gas exchange in the peripheral tissues – is available only sporadically.

The introduction of pulse oximetry has improved monitoring of pulmonary function considerably by allowing continuous measurement of arterial blood oxyhemoglobin saturation [1]. In a number of patients with mild to moderate pulmonary gas exchange defect, circulatory function can be assumed to be stable and largely unaffected by the pulmonary disease process and its treatment. When tissue oxygen balance is stable, alterations in arterial blood oxyhemoglobin saturation are effected primarily by the changes in the composition of alveolar gas and by the efficiency of pulmonary gas exchange. Pulse oximetry can be used in these patients to guide adjustment of respiratory therapy, without invasive monitoring.

In many critically ill patients, however, the underlying illness and therapeutic interventions may bring about rapid and unexpected changes in both pulmonary and cardiovascular function. Such patients cannot be managed appropriately without pulmonary artery catheterization and specific separate assessment of circulatory and respiratory function.

When arterial and mixed venous blood samples are available, the efficiency of pulmonary gas exchange can be assessed by calculating venous admixture, or physiologic right-to-left intrapulmonary shunting of blood (Q_{sp}/Q_t). Venous admixture is influenced by factors such as cardiac output, pulmonary blood flow distribution, and alveolar gas composition, that may not directly be related to the lung injury itself. However, Q_{sp}/Q_t still is the most accurate bedside method available to evaluate the extent of impairment in pulmonary gas exchange.

Sampling of arterial and mixed venous blood also enables assessment of peripheral oxygen use by allowing calculation of the oxygen utilization coefficient (O_2UC) [2, 3]. The oxygen utilization coefficient – the ratio between oxygen consumption and oxygen delivery – reflects the amount of oxygen carried in arterial blood, the systemic blood flow, and tissue oxygen demand. Therefore, it provides an estimate of the overall efficiency of the cardiopulmonary system in meeting tissue oxygen requirements.

Simultaneous consideration of Q_{sp}/Q_t and O_2UC permits integrated assessment of the two essential functions of the cardiorespiratory system, pulmonary gas exchange and tissue oxygen balance. Both Q_{sp}/Q_t and O_2UC are calculated from the oxygen contents of systemic and pulmonary arterial blood. Since the essential factor for determining oxygen content is oxyhemoglobin saturation, these variables can be estimated, given oxygen saturation values in pulmonary end-capillary, arterial, and mixed venous blood. Arterial blood oxyhemoglobin saturation (SaO_2) can be measured continuously using a pulse oximeter and mixed venous blood oxyhemoglobin saturation ($S\bar{v}O_2$) can be measured continuously using a pulmonary artery oximeter. Pulmonary end-capillary blood oxyhemoglobin saturation can be calculated. Therefore, continuous, real-time assessment of pulmonary gas exchange and tissue oxygen utilization is possible using integrated pulse and pulmonary artery oximetry – dual oximetry [4]. This is accomplished by calculating the ventilation perfusion index (VQI), an estimate of Q_{sp}/Q_t, and the oxygen extraction index (O_2EI), an estimate of O_2UC [5, 6].

Ventilation-Perfusion Index

The venvilation-perfusion index is calculated from a modified intrapulmonary shunt equation:

$$VQI = \frac{1.32 \cdot Hgb \cdot (1-SaO_2) + 0.0031 \cdot PAO_2}{1.32 \cdot Hgb \cdot (1-S\bar{v}O_2) + 0.0031 \cdot PAO_2}$$

where Hgb = blood hemoglobin concentration and PAO_2 = alveolar oxygen tension [5]. This calculation assumes that the amount of oxygen dissolved in arterial and mixed venous blood is negligible and, therefore can be discounted. It further assumes that pulmonary end-capillary blood is fully saturated with oxygen, and that alveolar carbon dioxide tension and the respiratory exchange ratio are normal and remain unchanged. Since oxygen dissolved in pulmonary end-capillary blood is included in the calculation, the VQI remains an accurate estimate of Q_{sp}/Q_t even with variable inspired oxygen concentration.

The VQI formula is applicable whenever SaO_2 is less than 100%. In the event that arterial blood oxyhemoglobin is fully saturated with oxygen, the difference between pulmonary end-capillary and arterial blood oxyhemoglobin saturations becomes zero. Since oxygen dissolved in the arterial blood is not included in the calculation, the numerator of the equation becomes a constant, and the relationship between VQI and Q_{sp}/Q_t becomes inaccurate. When VQI is used clinically, however, full saturation of arterial blood hemoglobin would indicate weaning from oxygen therapy, which would re-establish the accuracy of VQI, as SaO_2 decreases to a value less than 100%.

The pulse oximeter reads dysfunctional hemoglobins, such as carboxy- and methemoglobin, mainly as oxyhemoglobin, while the mixed venous oxygen saturation monitor reads them as deoxyhemoglobin. Since the assumption of 100% oxyhemoglobin saturation of pulmonary end-capillary blood ignores dyshemoglobins, the numerator of the VQI equation remains accurate even in the presence of dysfunctional hemoglobins. The error in the denominator results in slight, systemic underestimation of the absolute level of Q_{sp}/Q_t. Since the magnitude of this error is small and remains unchanged in most critically ill patients, it has little clinical significance.

The relationship between VQI and Q_{sp}/Q_t is linear, with a slope close to that of the identity line (Fig. 1) [5]. The accuracy of VQI is minimally influenced by changes in inspired oxygen concentration, when the calculation is appropriately updated for changes in PAO_2. Since $S\bar{v}O_2$ is included in the formula, the relationship between VQI and Q_{sp}/Q_t also is little affected by fluctuations in arteriovenous oxygen content difference during periods of circulatory instability. A correlation coefficient of 0.78 was calculated between Q_{sp}/Q_t and VQI in general surgical intensive care unit patients in a prospective clinical investigation [7]. Within individual patients, change in Q_{sp}/Q_t induced by alteration in contin-

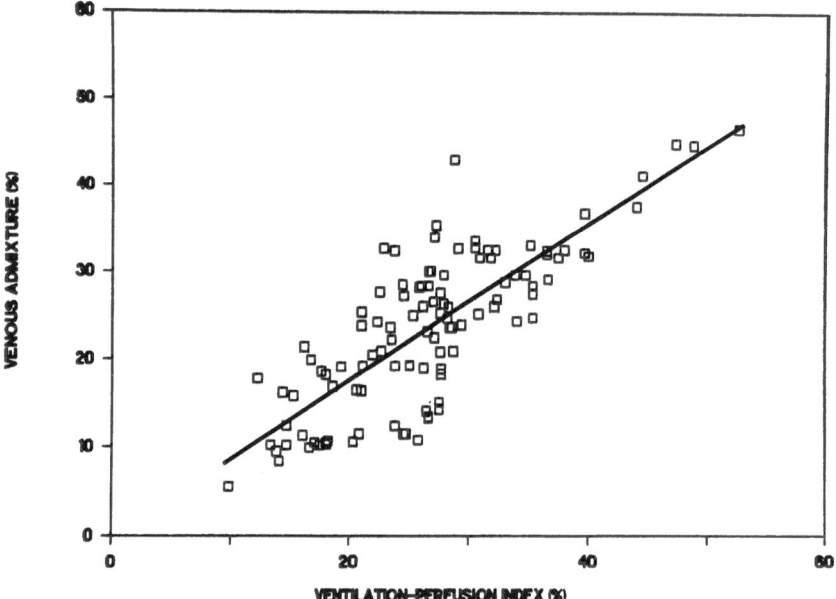

Fig. 1. Plot of ventilation-perfusion index and venous admixture at seven levels of continuous positive airway pressure in 17 patients with acute respiratory failure

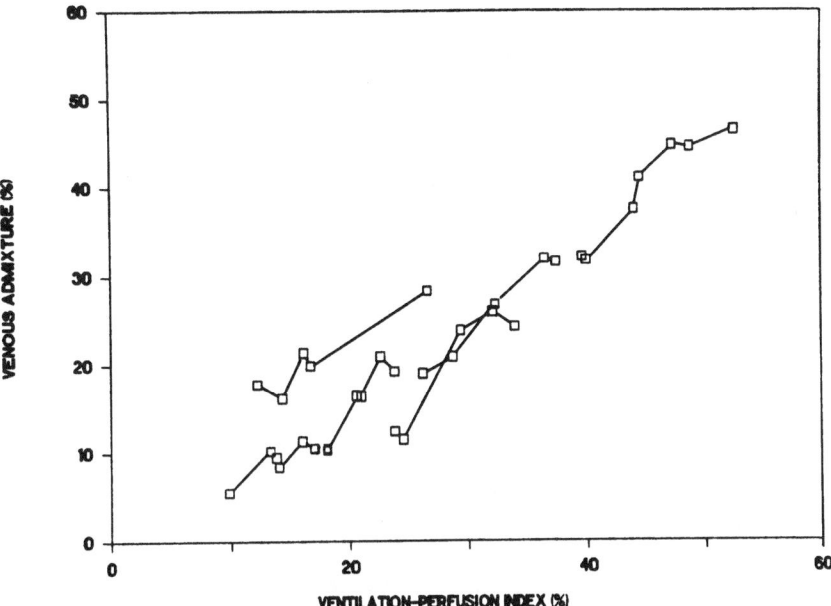

Fig. 2. Response of ventilation-perfusion index to alterations in venous admixture induced by changes in continuous positive airway pressure in six patients with acute respiratory failure

uous positive airway pressure was reflected accurately by VQI, with an average correlation coefficient of 0.94 ± 0.05 (Fig. 2).

Oxygen Extraction Index

The oxygen extraction index is derived from the oxygen utilization coefficient:

$$O_2UC = (CaO_2 - C\bar{v}O_2)/CaO_2$$

by discounting the contribution of dissolved oxygen in the oxygen content of arterial (CaO_2) and mixed venous ($C\bar{v}O_2$) blood.

$$O_2EI = (SaO_2 - S\bar{v}O_2)/SaO_2$$

The O_2EI has an excellent correlation with the O_2UC ($r = 0.96$) [6]. The slope of the relationship closely follows that of the line of identity, and the two variables have an identical physiological significance (Fig. 3).

Monitoring with Dual Oximetry

Monitoring with dual oximetry requires a pulse oximeter, a mixed venous oxygen saturation monitor and an interfacing device, such as a microcomputer. The computer performs the necessary calculations, allows updating of hemoglobin and inspired oxygen concentration, displays the variables and stores the data for

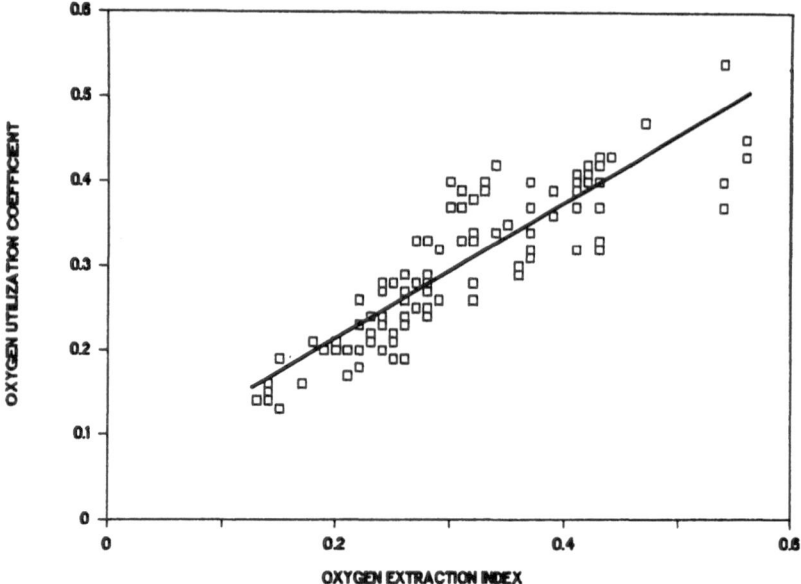

Fig. 3. Plot of oxygen extraction index and oxygen utilization coefficient at 7 different levels of continuous positive airway pressure in 17 patients with acute respiratory failure

later analysis. The dual-oximetry device requires calibration only on the part of the mixed venous oxygen saturation monitor. Drift in the accuracy of the measurements and calculations also depends primarily on the accuracy of the mixed venous oxygen saturation monitor. We have observed a drift of $1 \pm 3\%$ in VQI and 0.01 ± 0.03 in O_2EI during six hours of continuous monitoring, indicating that calibration of the device is necessary only once in 24 hours [8].

Clinical applicability of the information presented by a monitoring system depends on the ratio between clinically significant physiologic change in the patient and the random variability generated by the system. We have estimated that 95% of the random variability falls within a range of $\pm 5\%$ in VQI and within a range of ± 0.04 in O_2EI. These ranges also are suggested as guidelines for clinical interpretation of changes in VQI and O_2EI.

A prospective study revealed that when dual oximetry is used in routine monitoring of general intensive care unit patients, the device remains functional approximately 85% of the time, if no undue attention is focused on the equipment or on the training of the staff [8]. One half of the 15% failure time (8%) was due to 100% saturation of arterial blood oxyhemoglobin, which renders the VQI formula inaccurate. Other types of equipment failure included malfunctioning of the pulmonary artery catheter (5%), malpositioning of the pulse oximeter probe (3%), and inadvertent disconnection (2%). With proper attention directed to the equipment, training, and appropriate oxygen supplementation, the equipment failure time likely can be reduced to less than 5%.

Dual oximetry has been shown to provide a basis for accurate and effective titration of continuous positive airway pressure therapy in patients with acute lung injury, by allowing simultaneous assessment of the pulmonary and circulatory effects of elevated airway pressure [9]. Furthermore, this technique may significantly improve treatment of any critically ill patient with unstable cardiopulmonary function. The nearly instantaneous feedback provided by dual oximetry allows optimization of therapy without the time lag associated with conventional assessment of patient response.

Monitoring with dual oximetry produces no added risk to patients who require a pulmonary artery catheter. Blood loss for calibration of the equipment is minimal, and repeated patient assessments within the calibration period effect no increase in blood loss, cost, or danger of bacterial contamination. Since the physiological significance of VQI and O_2EI is well defined, the information provided by dual oximetry can be applied immediately in therapeutic decision-making without further processing by the observer. Therefore, cardiopulmonary support can be initiated, optimized, adjusted, and discontinued efficiently and safely using dual oximetry. Efficacious and timely therapy may decrease the frequency of complications, shorten the time of treatment, and thereby improve the general cost-effectiveness of critical care.

References

1. Yelderman M, New W (1983) Evaluation of pulse oximetry. Anesthesiology 39:349–352
2. Beach T, Millen E, Grenvik A (1973) Hemodynamic response to discontinuance of mechanical ventilation. Crit Care Med 1:85–90
3. Nelson L (1986) Continuous venous oximetry in surgical patients. Ann Surg 203:329–333
4. Downs JB, Räsänen J (1987) Dual oximetry in assessment of cardiopulmonary function. In: Vincent JL (ed) Update in Intensive Care and Emergency Medicine, vol 3. Springer, Berlin Heidelberg New York London Paris Tokyo, pp 342–348
5. Räsänen J, Downs JB, Malec D, Oates K (1987) Oxygen tensions and oxyhemoglobin saturations to assess pulmonary function during cardiopulmonary failure. Crit Care Med 15:1058–1061
6. Räsänen J, Downs JB, Malec DJ, Seidman P. Estimation of oxygen utilization by dual oximetry. Ann Surg (in press)
7. Räsänen J, Downs JB, Malec DJ, DeHaven B, Garner W. Real-time continuous estimation of gas exchange by dual oximetry. Int Care Med (in press)
8. Räsänen J, Downs JB, Hodges MR. Continuous monitoring of gas exchange and oxygen use with dual oximetry (Submitted for publication)
9. Räsänen J, Downs JB, DeHaven B. Titration of continuous positive airway pressure therapy by real-time dual oximetry. Chest (in press)

Cardiopulmonary Resuscitation

Automatic Detection of Cardiac Arrest Rhythms

G. W. N. Dalzell, S. R. Cunningham, and A. A. J. Adgey

The Need for Automatic Detection of Cardiac Arrest Rhythms

The majority of deaths from ischemic heart disease occur outside the hospital shortly after the onset of symptoms. When all age groups are considered 40% of the deaths occur within one hour of the onset of symptoms and among middle aged and younger male patients 63% of the deaths occur within 1 hour. Over 90% of these deaths are due to ventricular fibrillation which is both correctable and preventable.

It has been estimated in the UK that the expected incidence of acute myocardial ischemic attacks (including sudden death) is one or two cases per day per 100000 of the population. More than one-quarter of a million people in the UK have coronary attacks each year. The community mortality is of the order of 40% so that there are at least 100000 deaths from this cause annually. Among those aged less than 70 years there are some 55000 deaths from acute myocardial infarction in the UK annually. A conservative estimate indicates that there are some 20000 unnecessary deaths occurring among individuals under the age of 65 each year. Seventy percent of sudden cardiac deaths are witnessed and 50–60% of patients dying suddenly are free from symptoms at the time of or shortly ante-dating the event. It has also been recorded that 45% of cases of ventricular fibrillation occur in the patient's home, 12% at work and 43% in a public place.

Although coronary disease is the leading cause of death, the gap between what is therapeutically possible and what is accomplished remains wide. The problem therefore is getting effective therapy to the stricken individual quickly. Whilst cardiopulmonary resuscitation can maintain life for at least one hour if properly carried out the training involved in individuals only encountering 1–2 collapses per life span and maintaining the level of competence is very considerable. The definitive therapy for ventricular fibrillation is defibrillation and the shorter the time a patient is in ventricular fibrillation, i.e. the shorter the time to defibrillation the greater the patient's chance of immediate and long-term survival.

Mobile or out-of-hospital coronary care units have been very successful in the correction of ventricular fibrillation outside the hospital [1]. Nevertheless, in the USA only 1–3% of 300000 patients with out of hospital ventricular fibrillation are successfully resuscitated and discharged from hospital [2]. This is probably due to the time-lapse in getting trained personnel to a patient. In an average city this approximates to 10 minutes. In addition, the entire population cannot be covered by these out-of-hospital mobile coronary care units as some 40% of people live outside urban areas and the majority of sudden deaths take place at home. Therefore, in order to allow the spouse to carry out arrhythmia assessment and defibrillation in high risk patients, intelligent or smart defibrillators have been developed. Although it was intended at first that these smart or intelligent defibrillators should be given to the spouses of high risk patients they have also been used in the USA to train paramedic personnel. They are also being used by them in out-of-hospital cardiac arrests.

Automatic External Defibrillators

The first practical device "the heart aid" was used by Diack et al. (1979) at the University of Oregon Medical School [3]. This device employed a special airway placed over the tongue with a pregelled electrode applied over the epigastrium. These electrodes allowed monitoring of the electrocardiogram and detected respiratory movements. The device then automatically analyzed the input signals and made decisions on whether defibrillation was or was not appropriate.

Rozkovec et al. (1983) used electrocardiogram recordings from electrophysiological studies and cardiac surgery cases to test the accuracy of rhythm analysis [4]. The accuracy of the "Heart aid" left considerable room for improvement. In 50% of the recordings of ventricular tachycardia and supraventricular tachycardia the device made a decision to shock whereas in only 38 out of 82 recordings of ventricular fibrillation was the decision to shock. A major shortfall lay in the inability to detect fine (< 0.35 mV) ventricular fibrillation.

Cummins et al. [5] further tested the device in out-of-hospital cardiac arrests and reported 81% sensitivity (13 of 16 people with ventricular fibrillation received at least one countershock) and 100% specificity (all 21 non ventricular fibrillation rhythms) in out-of-hospital use by paramedics.

Jaggaroo et al. [6] used the device successfully in 11 patients and detected ventricular fibrillation in 5 out of 5 patients with ventricular fibrillation. The rhythm in the other 6 patients was identified as non ventricular fibrillation and no shock was administered. In 1983 the same group reported 6 cases of ventricular fibrillation inappropriately interpreted as asystole and in 2 cases inappropriate defibrillating shocks were delivered to patients in asystole [7]. In 1985 Cummins et al. reported a randomized controlled trial of automatic external devices versus manual defibrillators and noted no significant difference in survival to discharge from hospital between the 2 groups [8]. The automatic device did however reduce the time to first shock (p < 0.05). The number of patients in this study was small, 30 in one group, 37 in the other not sufficient to confidently state that the automatic external defibrillator was comparable to a manual device.

Stults et al. [9] in a large multicenter out-of-hospital cardiac arrest study compared 18 centers using either automatic external defibrillators with 18 centers using conventional defibrillators. Ambulance technicians using conventional defibrillators correctly diagnosed ventricular fibrillation more frequently than the AED's 98% vs 83%. Specificity was similar in the 2 groups: 100% for AED's vs 94% for technicians. Interestingly AED's delivered shocks more quickly 1.56 vs 2.77 min (p < 0.001). The ability of AED's to terminate ventricular fibrillation was 97% vs 70% for the control group. In 1 patient with medium amplitude ventricular fibrillation and 1 with coarse amplitude ventricular fibrillatition the AED delayed defibrillation for 6 and 7 minutes respectively. Neither patient survived. This is a worrying point and gives cause for concern.

In another randomized controlled trial of emergency medical technicians using automatic external defibrillators against EMT's with conventional defibrillators 321 cardiac arrest patients were treated: 116 with automatic external devices and 158 with standard defibrillators [10]. No significant difference in survival to hospital discharge was noted. The 2 groups did not differ significantly in the sensitivity for detecting VF or specificity. Time to first shock was marginally lower in the group with the automatic device. Despite initial optimism and the prediction of Friedberg 14 years ago that defibrillators would be made accessible to the community at large, the AED remains a device which is still developing. Promise for the future lies in the improved algorithms for ventricular fibrillation detection currently being produced.

Automatic Detection of Cardiac Arrest Rhythms

We first reported our results on the automatic detection of ventricular fibrillation in 1986 when Jack et al. recorded the efficacy of a microprocessor based algo-

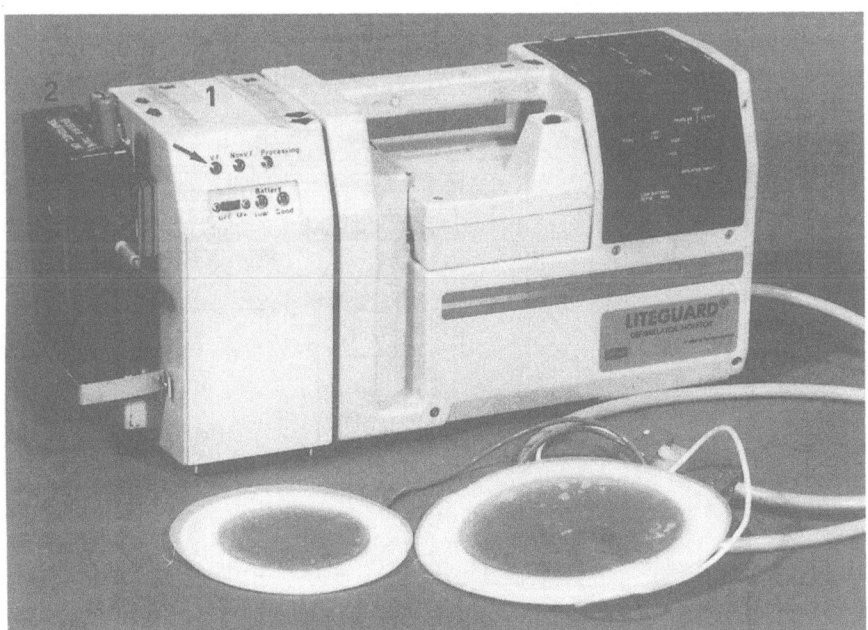

Fig. 1. Liteguard 6 with VF detection system (1) and self-adhesive ECG/defibrillator pads. Results of analysis are displayed visually on the unit (arrow), and recorded on tape (2) for later comparison

rithm which looked for the absence of an isoelectric segment, irregular energy density spectrum and irregular wave shape [11]. The electrocardiogram was analyzed every 8–18 seconds. Of the 223 analysis segments of ventricular fibrillation which occurred 165 were correctly determined by the system (sensitivity 74%). When the rhythm was non-ventricular fibrillation of 5002 episodes 4953 were correcty detected (specificity 99%). The results of testing an improved algorithm with an extended dynamic range have recently been reported by Dalzell et al. (1987) [12]. The sensitivity of the improved algorithm was 94.3% and specificity 97.5%.

We have now extended our investigations to 78 cardiac arrests in 74 patients (44 male, 30 female), aged 43–90 years (mean 67). Myocardial infarction was the cause of 29 arrests. The initial rhythm was ventricular fibrillation in 16 of the arrests and non-ventricular fibrillation in 62.

We use a microprocessor based system with ECG sensing during the cardiac arrest using disposable ECG/defibrillator pads (Fig. 1). The ECG is continuously analyzed every 4 seconds. The ECG and system's analysis are recorded on tape and later compared (Fig. 1). The algorithm for the detection of ventricular fibrillation uses 1) absence of isoelectric segment, 2) QRS width, variability

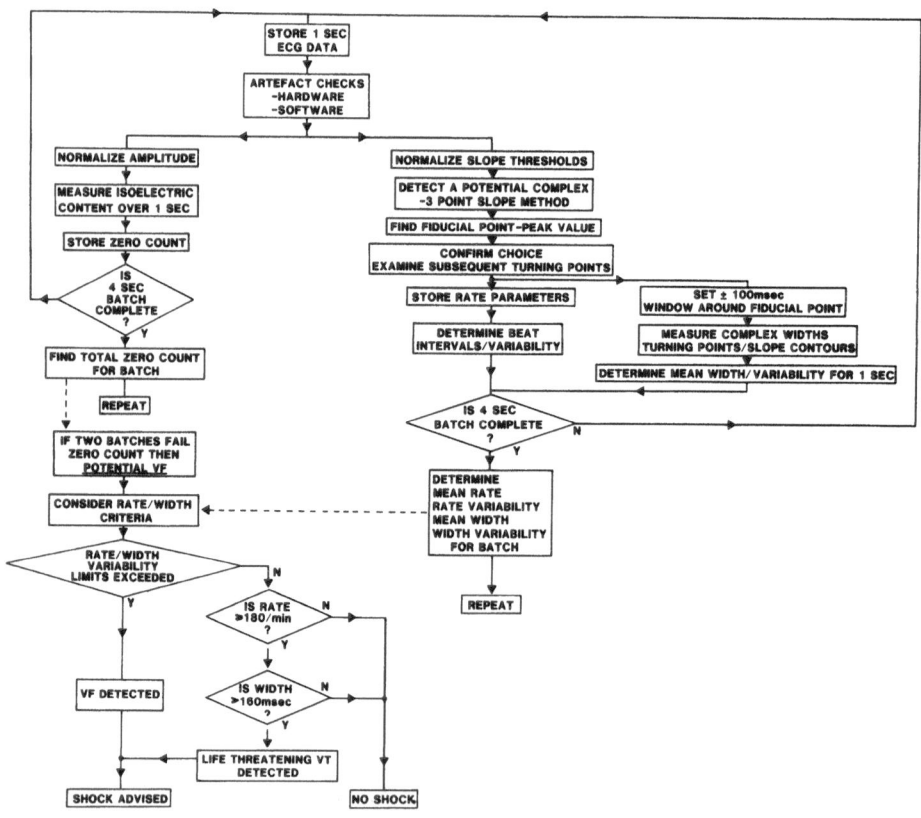

Fig. 2. VF detection algorithm

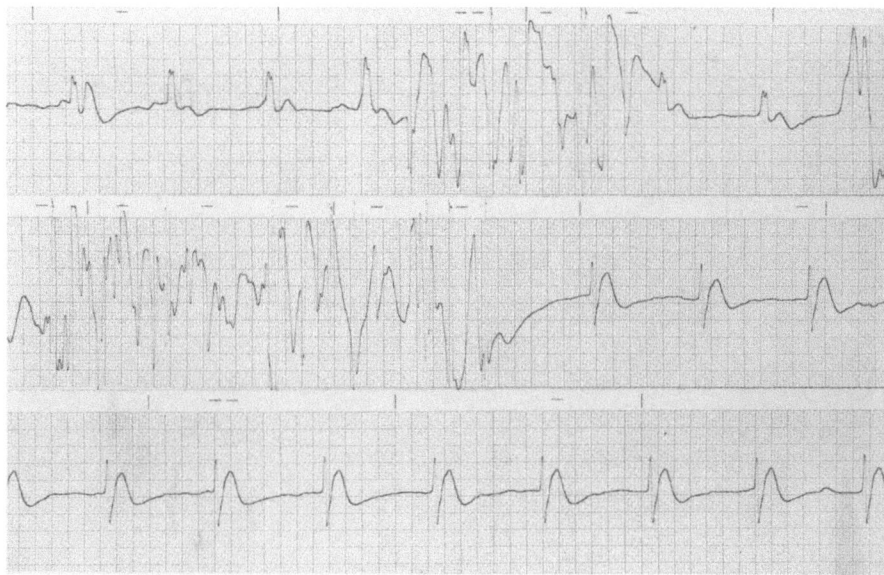

Fig. 3. Excessive CPR causes saturation of the amplifier, with resetting of the algorithm each second. In this continuous recording the cardiopulmonary resuscitation induced distortion is accompanied by single dash occurring each second. When CPR is stopped the underlying rhythm is correctly detected as non-ventricular fibrillation and 2 dashes are recorded

Table 1. Microprocessor vs physician interpretation in 10,994 episodes of cardiac arrest rhythms

	Correctly detected	Incorrectly detected	Total
VF	464	42	506
Non-VF	9791	697	10488

Sensitivity 91.7% (464/506)
Specificity 93.3% (9791/10488)

and regularity (Fig. 2). The zero content is optimized by input filtering. Excessive cardiopulmonary resuscitation induced artefact causes saturation with resetting of the system each second (Fig. 3). DC shock also causes saturation and resetting of the system (Fig. 4).

Of the 16 cardiac arrests where ventricular fibrillation was the initial rhythm, 14 were correctly identified by the system i.e. sensitivity of 87.5% (Fig. 5). For the 62 cardiac arrests where non-ventricular fibrillation was the initial rhythm, 59 were correctly identified by the system, i.e. specificity 95.2%. When the continuous 4 second ECG analysis was carried out (Table 1) sensitivity was 92% and specificity 93%. Of the 42 episodes of ventricular fibrillation where the system did not detect ventricular fibrillation, cardiopulmonary resuscitation was responsible in 24 episodes (Fig. 6), low amplitude ventricular fibrillation i.e. <0.35 mV

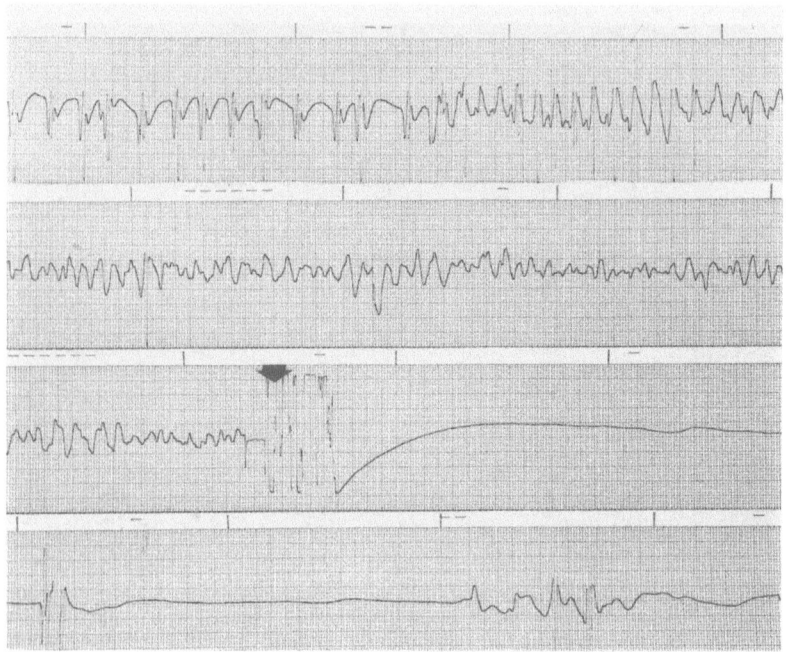

Fig. 4. Effect of DC shock (arrow). In this continuous recording ventricular fibrillation develops and is converted by countershock into an agonal rhythm, which is correctly detected as non-ventricular fibrillation. There has been resetting of the system between the DC shock and the detection of non-ventricular fibrillation

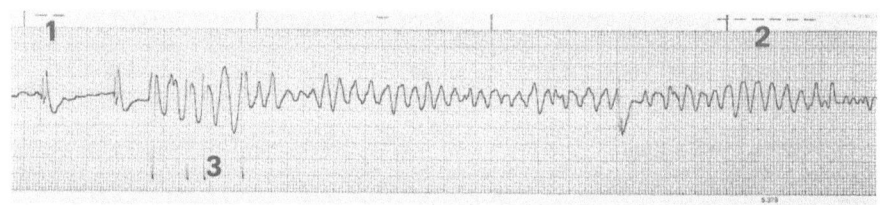

Fig. 5. Typical ECG recording showing a supraventricular rhythm deteriorating into ventricular fibrillation. The results of the analysis are displayed as horizontal dashes at the top of the recording. Non-ventricular fibrillation is indicated as 2 dashes (1) and ventricular fibrillation as 6 dashes (2). A single dash occurs every 4 seconds. The vertical deflections (3) are artefacts due to the recording process

in 13 (Fig. 7) and change of rhythm to ventricular fibrillation during analysis in 5 episodes (Fig. 8, Table 2). In the automatic/semi-automatic defibrillator envisaged cardiopulmonary resuscitation will not be ongoing during the analysis and if the rhythm changes during the 4 second analysis period the unit will continue to analyze and as the ventricular fibrillation persists ventricular fibrillation will

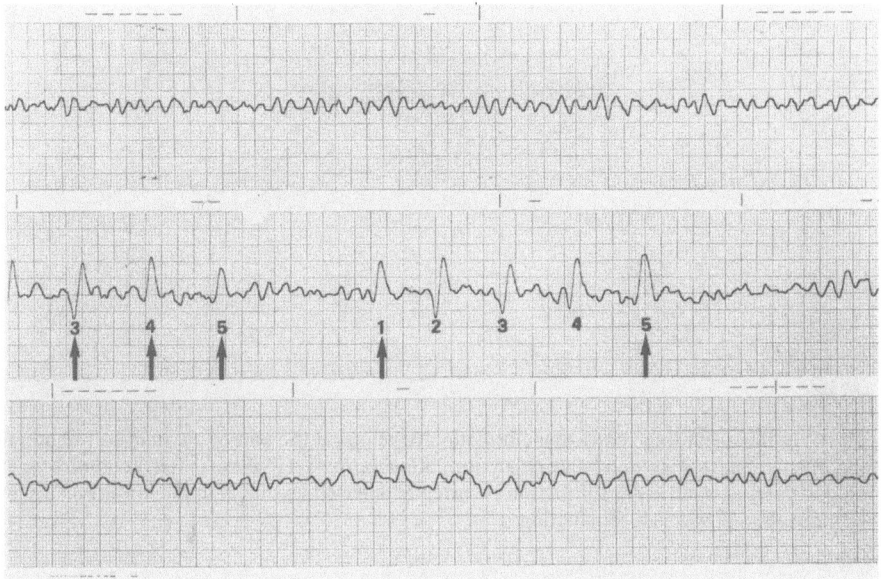

Fig. 6. In this continuous recording the rhythm is ventricular fibrillation, correctly detected by the system in the upper tracing. When CPR commences (middle tracing) the deflections on the ECG cause incorrect detection as non-ventricular fibrillation

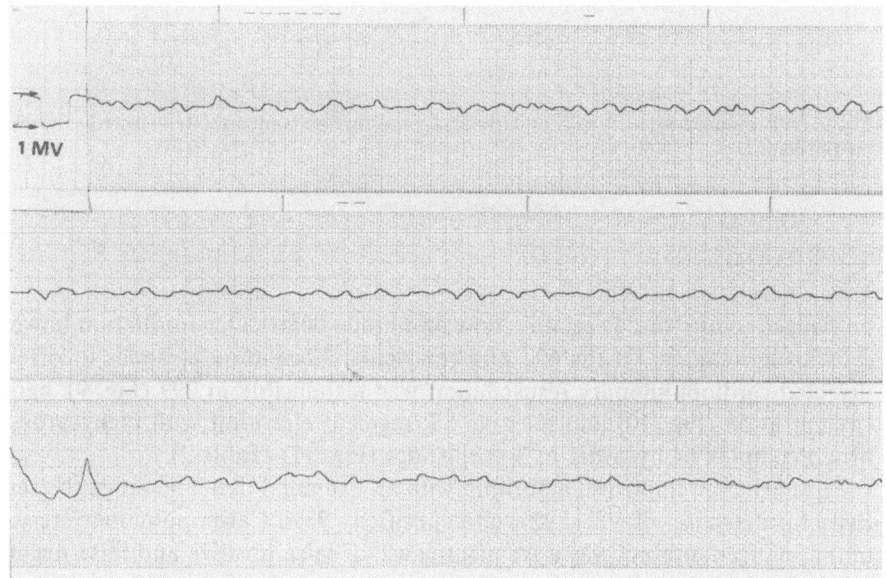

Fig. 7. This continuous recording is of low amplitude ventricular fibrillation initially correctly detected (upper trace). When the amplitude decreases further (middle trace) the rhythm is incorrectly detected as non-ventricular fibrillation

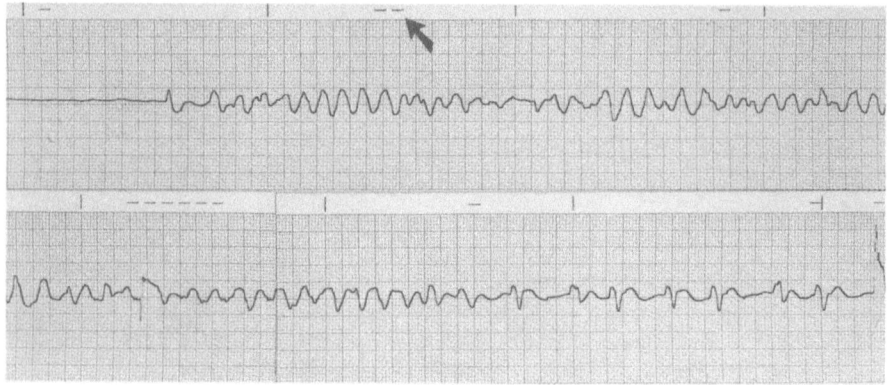

Fig. 8. In this recording ventricular fibrillation develops at the end of an analysis period and is incorrectly detected as non-ventricular fibrillation (arrow). However, after another 8 seconds analysis period, ventricular fibrillation is correctly detected as shown in the lower tracing. Interestingly, the VF was self-terminating

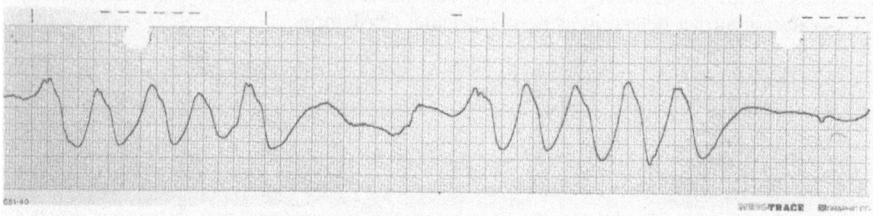

Fig. 9. CPR-induced artefact with underlying agonal rhythm is incorrectly detected as ventricular fibrillation

be flagged in another 4 seconds. Low amplitude ventricular fibrillation however remains an enigma. Of the 697 non-ventricular fibrillation episodes incorrectly detected cardiopulmonary resuscitation was responsible in 299 (Fig. 9), agonal rhythm in 58 (Fig. 10) and massive ST segment elevation with tachycardia or broad complex tachycardia in 340 episodes (Fig. 11) (Table 2).

Thus using an improved algorithm with an extended dynamic range the sensitivity for detection of VF is 92% and specificity 93%. Cardiopulmonary resuscitation induced artefact was a frequent cause of false positive and false negative results.

Weaver et al. [13] has also reported the results of improved automatic detection of VF. One hundred percent of patients with ventricular fibrillation were shocked at least once with the modified device.

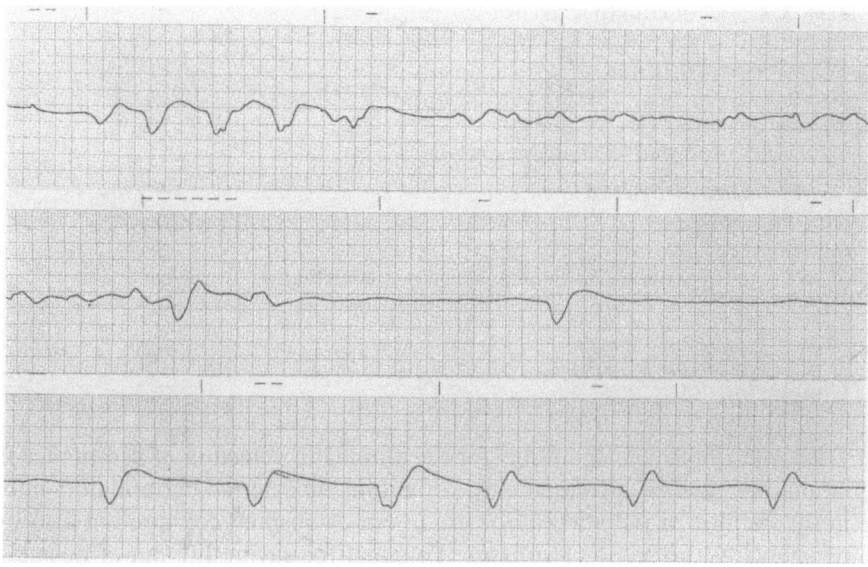

Fig. 10. Agonal rhythm, correctly detected in the upper tracing as non-ventricular fibrillation. However, in the middle tracing ventricular fibrillation has been falsely detected

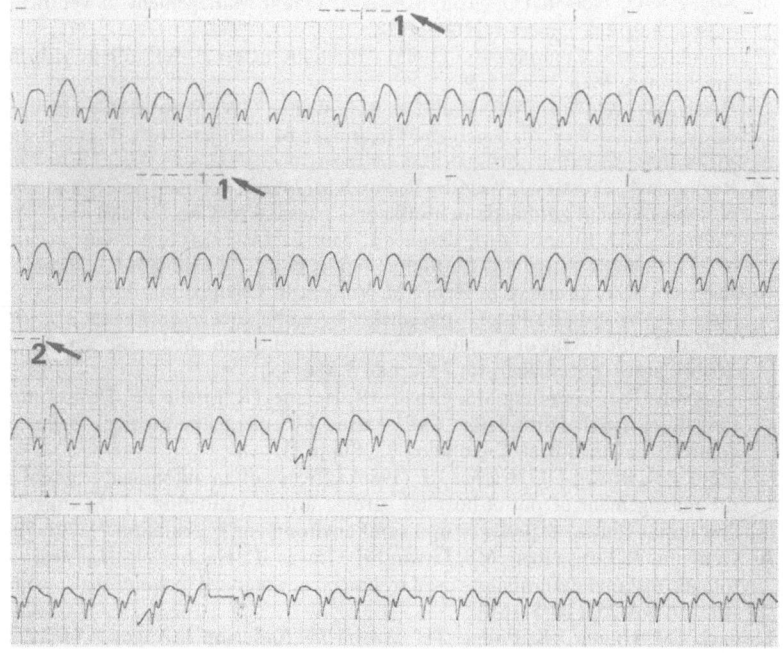

Fig. 11. Broad complex tachycardia, falsely detected as ventricular fibrillation in the upper 2 tracings (1). As the ORS complexes become more narrow in the lower tracings (2) the system correctly detects non-ventricular fibrillation

Table 2. Causes of erroneous results

VF Incorrectly Detected	*42/506*
(a) CPR	24
(b) Low amplitude VF (<0.35 mV)	13
(c) Change of rhythm to VF during analysis	5
Non-VF Incorrectly Detected	*697/10488*
(a) CPR	299
(b) Agonal rhythms	58
(c) ST segment abnormality (infarction, aberrant condition)	340

Conclusion

Thus with improved algorithms for the automatic detection of ventricular fibrillation there will be increased usage of automatic external defibrillators not only in the training of paramedics for use in out-of-hospital collapse but also by lay personnel at the scene of collapse. Potential for saving life out-of-hospital has increased significantly.

References

1. Adgey AAJ, Nelson PG, Scott ME, et al (1969) Management of ventricular fibrillation outside hospital. Lancet 1:1169–1171
2. Eisenberg MS, Cummins RO (1985) Automatic external defibrillation; bringing it home. Am J Emerg Med 3:568–569
3. Diack AW, Welborn WS, Rullman RG, Walter CW, Wayne MA (1979) An automatic cardiac resuscitator for emergency treatment of cardiac arrest. Medical Instrumentation 13:78–81
4. Rozkovec A, Crossley J, Walesby R, Fox KM, Maseri A (1983) Safety and effectiveness of a portable external automatic defibrillator – pacemaker. Clin Cardiol 6:527–533
5. Cummins RO, Eisenberg M, Bergner L, Murray JA (1984) Sensitivity, accuracy and safety of an automatic external defibrillator; report of a field evaluation. Lancet 2:318–320
6. Jaggarao NSV, Grainger R, Heber M, Vincent R, Chamberlain DA (1982) Use of an automated external defibrillator – pacemaker by ambulance staff. Lancet 2:73–75
7. Heber M (1983) Out of hospital resuscitation using the "heart aid" an automated external defibrillator – pacemaker. Int J Cardiol 3:456–458
8. Cummins RO, Eisenberg MS, Graves JR, Hearne TR, Litwin PE, Hallstrom AP (1985) Automatic external defibrillators (AED) used by emergency medical technicians (EMT): a controlled clinical trial. Circulation 72, Suppl III – 8
9. Stults KR, Brown DD, Kerber RE (1986) Efficacy of an automated external defibrillator in the management of out-of-hospital cardiac arrest: validation of the diagnostic algorithm and initial clinical experience in a rural environment. Circulation 73:701–709
10. Cummins RO, Eisenberg MS, Litwin PE, Graves JR, Hearne TR, Hallstrom AP (1987) Automatic external defibrillators used by emergency medical technicians – a controlled clinical trial. JAMA 257:1605–1610
11. Jack CM, Hunter EK, Pringle TH, Wilson JT, Anderson J, Adgey AAJ (1986) An external automatic device to detect ventricular fibrillation. Eur Heart J 7:404–411
12. Dalzell GWN, Beggs O, Bailey A, Anderson J, Adgey AAJ (1987) Accuracy in the automatic detection of ventricular fibrillation. JACC 9:206 A
13. Weaver WD, Hill D, Fahrenbruch C, et al (1986) Value of field experience in improving automatic external defibrillators. JACC 7:72 A

Teaching Citizen-CPR: A Belgian Experience

L. L. Bossaert

Introduction

More than 25 ears ago the modern techniques of CPR were first described by Kouwenhoven, Jude and Knickerbocker [1]. Since then the widespread knowledge and application of CPR by doctors, paramedics and the lay public has substantially changed the survival of sudden cardiac death.

The incidence of sudden cardiac death is estimated at about 1000 per day in the US, and about 55 per day in Belgium [2]. A number of reports have demonstrated the usefulness of CPR performed by the citizen: a survival rate as high as 43% was reported in selected subsets (witnessed, primary ventricular fibrillation) of sudden cardiac death victims when CPR was started within 3 minutes, and if Advanced Cardiac Life Support (ACLS) was continued within 8 minutes [3]. It was estimated that this best outcome could be obtained if about 20% of adult lay public is sufficiently trained in CPR [4].

The role of the American Heart Association (AHA) and the Red Cross Ligues was essential in the widespread teaching of citizen CPR according to internationally accepted standards and guidelines. The activities of the AHA are reflected by the CPR consensus meetings resulting in the publication of the standards and guidelines of CPR and Emergency Cardiac Care [5-10]. These reports are generally considered as essential for all CPR teaching programs throughout the world.

At the present time about 15000 Belgian citizens receive training in CPR each year in a number of local and regional training programs (e.g. Red Cross first aid courses, the action "ABC red mee", the "Instituut voor Medische Dringende Hulpverlening" ...). However, in order to reach the target of 20% of Belgian citizens trained in CPR, a large-scaled nationwide and institutionalized training program is required.

Teaching Citizen CPR in Belgium

In October 1986 a nationwide campaign for teaching citizen CPR was started in Belgium, entitled "three minutes for a life". The total duration of the campaign is 3 years, and the objective to train at least 100000 lay people in the techniques of basic CPR [11]. It was decided that five preconditions should be fulfilled:

- medical consensus;
- standardization;

- public awareness;
- professional planning, organization and implementation;
- scientific evaluation of the teaching program.

Medical Consensus

The worldwide medical consensus concerning the value of CPR is materialized in the CPR symposia of the WHO (1963), of the AHA (1973, '79, '85) and of the Ligue of the Red Cross associations (1981), where it has been agreed that CPR training of the lay public should be organized wherever feasible.

This consensus is also illustrated by the following statement of the AHA [9], and the words of P. Safar [12]:

"Since 60 to 70% of sudden cardiac deaths caused by cardiac arrest occur before hospitalization, it is clear that the community deserves to be recognized as the ultimate coronary care unit" and: "Now there is overwhelming scientific evidence about the usefulness, the feasibility and the safety of CPR teaching and CPR practice by the lay public".

The medical consensus concerning the Belgian nationwide CPR campaign is illustrated by:

- the structure of the steering committee of the campaign "3 minutes for a life", in charge of its direction and follow-up, consisting of representatives of the Belgian Heart Association, the Belgian Red Cross, and the Belgian Society for Intensive Care
- the approval and support of the campaign by representative Belgian CPR-experts.

Standardized Teaching Program

In the AHA conference on CPR (Dallas, July 1985) the following recommendations for CPR-educational programs have been formulated:

- CPR courses should be simple, uniform, compact,
- more attention should be paid to evaluation of the victim,
- a CPR course is a good opportunity for giving information about
  - prevention of cardiovascular disease by reduction of risk factors
  - recognition of warning signs preceding heart attack
  - activation of the Emergency Medical System (EMS)
- the teaching programs and their results should be scientifically evaluated.

The acutalized standards of this AHA conference for teaching CPR have been published in 1986 in a supplement issue of JAMA [10].

The educational package of the Belgian CPR-campaign "3 minutes for a life" has been elaborated according to these AHA recommendations and includes:

Motivation: the extent of the problem of sudden death and the possible role of CPR;

Knowledge: how to recognise warning symptoms preceding heart attack and how to activate the EMS system;

Prevention: how to reduce cardiovascular risk by risk factor reduction;

Skills: basic CPR by 1 rescuer is taught in a single 3-hour course;

Evaluation: a detailed evaluation program was started to study all aspects of the campaign.

Implementation

The educational package: The CPR instruction is limited to basic CPR by 1 rescuer of the adult cardiac arrest victim in a 2.5–3 hour course. Uniformity of the course is obtained by the development of a standard educational package used by every instructor, and consisting of

- a detailed instructors manual;
- a set of flip-charts;
- an action-plan-poster;
- a training manikin;
- a set of evaluation forms.

A limited number of 8–12 trainees is allowed per instructor.

Public awareness: A Gallup Study, performed in the US in 1977 has shown that 54% of the adult population was willing to be instructed in CPR [13]. A survey performed in 1981 by the American Red Cross has shown that 20% of the adult population had effectively followed a CPR-course. In Belgium, it is estimated that less than 10% of the adult population is trained in CPR.

To increase public awereness for the CPR campaign, a number of promotional methods have been used within a limited budget:

- involvement of media (press, television spot, radio);
- involvement of the organizing associations;
- involvement of a supermarket chain;
- a national CPR-telephone line.

Instructor recruitement and formation: To reach the target 100 000 trainees within 2 years, the existing number of competent first aid instructors was largely insufficient and not prepared for this task. Therefore, the additional help of 2 648 CPR-instructors/animators was obtained.

Instructor trainers: 50 experienced CPR instructors were extensively trained according to the guidelines outlined by the steering committee of the campaign, and became "instructor-trainers".

CPR instructors: all CPR- and first-aid instructors, participating in this campaign, were retrained for this purpose by the instructor-trainers in a one day course: 663 CPR-instructors have been trained.

CPR-animators: a number of motivated nurses, doctors and teachers, willing to participate in this campaign, equally received a one day training for this purpose by the instructor-trainers: 1985 CPR-animators have been trained.

The evaluation program: A detailed evaluation program was organized to answer the following questions:

- what is the attitude of the Belgian population towards CPR?
- what is the value of the promotional campaign?
- what is the profile of CPR-instructor and CPR-trainee?
- what is the initial knowledge, and attitude of the trainee concerning CPR?
- what level of theoretica knowledge and practical skills is finally reached?
- what is the degree of retention of knowledge and skills?
- what is the final impact on the quality and quantity of bystander-CPR?

To answer these questions, the evaluation program has been subdivided in four aspects:

1. *The promotional campaign:* By means of two telephone enquiries within one year, the perception of the promotional campaign and the basic knowledge and attitude concerning CPR is studied in a representative sample of the Belgian population.
2. *The instruction:* Basic knowledge and attitude, and the individual and socioeconomic profile of each individual CPR-trainee is studied. At the end of each course the final theoretical knowledge of each trainee is tested by a set of multiple choice questions, and the practical skills by a practical test. All individual evaluation forms are ready for computer analysis.
3. *Retention* of knowledge and skills: In a subset of trainees, the regression of skills and knowledge will be studied after 6 and 12 months, to identify factors influencing this retention [14].
4. *Impact* on quality and frequency of bystander CPR:
   Since 1983, the "Cerebral Resuscitation" study group of the Belgian Society for Intensive Care has compiled a data base describing more than 2000 incidents of out-of-hospital cardiac arrest. This registry includes data on timing, bystander CPR, subsequent treatment and outcome [15, 16]. The pre-campaign data (1983–86) will be compared with data collected in 1987–89.

Results After 1 Year

First Data on Attitude and Knowledge of the Belgian Population Concerning CPR, and on Penetration of the Promotional Campaign

In december 1986, two months after the beginning of the action "three minutes for a life", a first telephone enquiry was performed in a randomly selected, representative sample of the Belgian population. A total of 1231 adults (age ⩾ 18 years) have been questioned (Flanders FL = 638; Brussels BX = 208; Wallonie W = 385). This study sample was representative for the Belgian population in terms of age, sex, language, familial and, somewhat less, socio-economic characteristics.

At time of the study there was a significant difference in the overall perception of the campaign (Total = 30%; FL = 20%; BX = 33%; W = 45%). This difference between the 3 regions was even more striking if only spontaneous correct answers were taken into account (Total = 14%; FL = 6.5%; BX = 19%; W = 23%). However, there was an opposite trend in the intention to follow a CPR course (FL = 31%; BX = 11%; W = 22%). This confirms that it is not enough to have seen information about a campaign to take real action and subscribe for a course.

Also a large number of people gave no or a grossly incorrect interpretation for the slogan "3 minutes for a life" (FL = 23%; BX = 47%; W = 41%). It was equally important to note that the term "CPR" was poorly understood, especially in Flanders (not understood in 34% compared to BX = 1.5%; W = 10.5%).

The previous knowledge of CPR is also different in the 3 regions: 17% of the people in Flanders, only 4% in Wallonie and 10% in Brussels, had already followed a CPR-course. Within Flanders, marked local differences were found (e.g. Eastern Flanders 26%; Antwerp 8%). Two thirds of those who had followed a CPR-course were under 40 years of age, they were usually male (56%), with a higher educational level (82% at least high school).

A clearly different attitude concerning the accessibility of CPR by the lay public was observed: Flemish people seem to have a higher willingness for personal active involvement in case of a medical emergency, and more frequently estimate CPR as feasible. French-speaking people have more the tendency to call first for medical help, and they usually estimate CPR as rather difficult, requiring a high level of medical knowledge (Table 1).

Table 1. Attitude towards citizen CPR by the Belgian lay public

	Flemish	French
First reaction in presence of unconscious victim		
– personal active help	46%	26%
– call for medical help	19%	34%
Previous CPR training	17%	4%
Accessibility of CPR		
– difficult	42%	51%
– easy	57%	45%
Previous medical knowledge required	29%	42%
CPR restricted to professional people	18%	28%

First Quantitative and Qualitative Data on the CPR Instruction

So far 48949 individual evaluation forms have been received for analysis after 5,237 CPR courses (Table 2). There is an equal distribution of trainees and courses over the country, related to the total population of each region and province. The public consisted mainly of young people: (61% ≤ 36 years) with a majority of students (22%) and employees (33%). This finding demonstrates that a reorientation of the campaign towards older age groups and other socio-economic classes, such as working class (only 14%) and housewives (only 12%) is probably required. Since sudden cardiac arrest first concerns older male people, the main target group for teaching citizen CPR should not only be the youngster (not being at his parents home at the moment of the incident) or the person at risk himself! Indeed, if the aim of teaching citizen-CPR is to instruct the potential *bystander* of the cardiac arrest victim, all efforts should be directed towards this target group: the natural bystander of the person-at-risk. Therefore, this information is important for readjustment of the strategy of CPR campaigns.

Table 2. First quantitative data after 1 year of the CPR-campaign

CPR-Instructions

	Total	Flemish	French
CPR-course	5237	43%	57%
CPR-student	48949	48%	52%
CPR-instructor			
– doctor	4%	8%	1%
– nurse	28%	38%	20%
– teacher	22%	24%	19%
– other	46%	30%	60%

Profile of the CPR-student

Sex	Male	47%
	Female	53%
Age (year of birth)	Before 1920	1.5%
	1920–29	6.5%
	1930–39	12.5%
	1940–49	18.5%
	1950–59	22.5%
	After 1960	38.5%
Profession	Independent	4.7%
	Farmer	0.6%
	Working class	14.4%
	Employee	32.6%
	Executive	4.8%
	Housewife	12.1%
	Retired	5.2%
	Student	22.1%
	Unemployed	3.6%

Nationwide CPR-Actions in Europe

Sweden (8 million inhabitants): a nationwide CPR campaign was started early in 1985. Up to now 155000 people have been trained.

Norway (4 millions): the nationwide Norwegian CPR campaign was also started early in 1985. Sofar 25000 citizen have been trained.

Great Britain (52 millions): the British CPR campaign, with important involvement of BBC, has started in July 1986, and 122000 citizen have been trained.

Belgium (10 millions): in view of these European data the Belgian result (47800 people trained between October 1986 and October 1987) is encouraging. It is equally important to note that only the Belgian campaign will be able to provide detailed quantitative and qualitative data. Although an important additional effort is required for collection and analysis of these data, this information is of important value for the organization of similar actions and campaigns in public health education.

References

1. Kouwenhoven W, Jude R, Knickerbocker G (1960) Closed-chest cardiac massage. JAMA 173:1064–1067
2. Berghmans L, Heyerick P, De Backer G, et al (1985) Pilot projet for registering acute myocardial infarction in Belgium. Acta Cardiol 40:365–374
3. Cobb L, Baum R, Alvarez H, Schaffer W (1975) Resuscitation from out-of-hospital ventricular fibrillation: 4 years follow-up. Circulation 51/52 (suppl 3), III 223–235
4. Cummins R, Eisenberg M, Hallstrom A, Litwin P (1985) Survival of out-of-hospital cardiac arrest with early initiation of CPR. Am J Emerg Med 3:114–117
5. American Heart Association (1983) Textbook of Advanced Cardiac Life Support. American Heart Association, Dallas, USA
6. American Heart Association (1983) Manual for Basic Life Support for Physicians. Dallas, USA
7. American Heart Association (1985) Basic Life Support Instructors Manual. Dallas, USA
8. Standards for Cardiopulmonary Resuscitation and emergency cardiac care (1974) JAMA 227:834–868
9. Standards and Guidelines for Cardiopulmonary Resuscitation (CPR) and emergency cardiac care (ECC) (1980) JAMA 244:453–509
10. Standards and Guidelines for Cardiopulmonary Resuscitation (CPR) and emergency cardiac care (ECC) (1986) JAMA 255:2841–3044
11. Bossaert L, Van Rillaer L (1987) Drie minuten voor een leven. Nationale actie voor CPR onderwijs aan de bevolking. Tijdsch Geneesk 43:1115–1123
12. Safar P (1981) Cardiopulmonary Cerebral Resuscitation. WB Saunders-Laerdal. Philadelphia, Stavanger
13. Gallup G (1983) Campaign to educate Americans in CPR successful. Sunday Advocate (Baton Rouge), Nov 27
14. Van Kerschaver E, Moens G, Delooz H (1987) Effect van eenmalige en herhaalde cardiopulmonale reanimatietrainingen op de reanimatievaardigheid van de schoolpopulatie. Tijdsch Geneesk 43:753–765
15. Buylaert W, Mullie A, Corne L, et al (1986) Een multicentrische analyse van hartstilstand buiten het ziekenhuis behandeld door medische interventiegroepen. Tijdsch Geneesk 42:825–829
16. Studygroup "Cerebral Resuscitation" of the Belgian Society of Intensive Care Medicine (1984) A Multicenter registration project of CPR in Belgium. Acta Anesth Belg 35, S1:29

Pharmacology of Drugs in CPR

J. C. Mercier, J. F. Hartmann, and F. Beaufils

Introduction

Cardiac arrest results in cessation of organ perfusion. Circulatory standstill leads to immediate cellular ischemia, anoxia and finally death. The brain is the most rapidly damaged organ, already after 4 to 6 minutes of cardiac arrest in human beings [1], maybe longer in very special circumstances such as in the child, or after drowning in iced water [2]. The myocardium is the second most vulnerable organ, which may tolerate 15 minute anoxia and recover. However, at least in children, the longer the cardiac arrest the less the chances to recover a spontaneously beating heart [3].

Survival is first warranted by the immediate institution of cardiopulmonary resuscitation (CPR) which associates artificial ventilation [4] and closed-chest massage [5]. Its aim is to provide enough blood and oxygen to the vital organs. However, cardiac output provided by CPR is extremely low when compared to pre-arrest values [6]. CPR-induced blood flow is fortunately rather distributed to critical organs for survival, i.e. carotid and coronary blood flows [7]. This however, does not necessarily mean good cerebral or myocardial perfusion [8]. In recent years, an intensive experimental research has allowed a better understanding of the mechanisms of blood flow during CPR [9–11]. In fact, it appears

Table 1. Effectiveness of epinephrine administered by various routes in restoring circulation

Route of injection	No. of dogs	No. of dogs with restoration of circulation	Mean time from injection to restoration of circulation (s)
None	10	2	142
Intramuscular	10	4	50
Intralingual	10	2	292
Intravenous	10	10	127 ± 67
Intracardiac	10	9	139 ± 34
Intratracheal, not diluted	10	2	116
Intratracheal, diluted with saline	10	8	217 ± 142
Intratracheal, diluted with water	10	10	132 ± 44

Ten dogs with circulatory arrest for 5 minutes due to obstructive asphyxia received 1 mg of epinephrine by each route in addition to ventilation of the lungs with air, closed-chest massage, and electrical defibrillation when indicated. (After Redding et al. [14]).

that the best cerebral and myocardial blood flows were probably obtained in dogs with a combination of simultaneous chest compression and ventilation associated to epinephrine [12].

Nevertheless, the best circulatory blood flow is by far obtained by the spontaneously beating heart [13]. Thus, whereas CPR has been started as soon as possible, the main question is how to deliver drug therapy to its site of action to obtain the expected therapeutic effect? Redding et al. [14] have already addressed very practically this important problem many years ago. They systematically studied the effects of 1 mg of epinephrine administered by intralingual, intramuscular, intravenous, intracardiac, or intratracheal routes on survival of dogs. The results are listed in Table 1. Only intracardiac, intravenous, and intratracheal routes were effective either in terms of rapidity of action or in survival.

Intracardiac Route

In spite of the fact that the beneficial use of epinephrine in CPR is related to their effects on the peripheral vasculature, many physicians felt that intracardiac should be more effective than intravenous injection. However, a lot of good reasons plea for not using this route anymore. First, intracardiac injection is often accomplished after considerable delay, due to difficulty to introduce a needle in the ventricular cavity. Second, intracardiac injection has been occasionally followed by complications such as pneumothorax, hemopericardium, or even coronary artery injuries [15]. In addition, inadvertent intramyocardial injection of epinephrine has been mentioned as responsible of intractable ventricular fibrillation. Finally, closed-chest massage must be interrupted for an unacceptable period of time, when adequate blood flow must be obtained for efficient drug distribution. For all these reasons, intracardiac route is now definitely discourages [16], unless special conditions are present such as open-heart surgery.

Intravenous Route

Intravenous (IV) access is very difficult in CPR, for at least three reasons:

1. peripheral veins are often collapsed and hardly visible;
2. central venous catheterization is difficult, when the patient is shaken by external closed-massage;
3. external conditions are sometimes unfavorable (street, public location, general ward of a hospital ...) or stressful.

Furthermore, the most difficult venous access is in small children. Thus, Rossetti et al. [17] retrospectively reviewed the difficulties and the delay of vascular access in 66 pediatric arrests in a 3-year period. In 4 infants (6%), IV access was never achieved. An additional 24% (16/66) required 10 or more minutes. Cutdowns were placed at an average of 24 minutes into the code in 33% of the cases (22/66). Finally, successfully resuscitated patients had intravascular access established significantly sooner than did those not resuscitated (p < 0.05).

While several studies addressed the issue of endotracheal drug administration in the late 70s, it was not until 1981 that critical investigations of the relative efficacy of drug distribution from central venous and peripheral venous administration were undertaken. Kuhn et al. [18] compared the delivery of indocyanine green to a femoral artery sampling site when administered via a right antecubital or right subclavian vein in 6 patients undergoing closed-chest CPR who have failed resuscitation attempts. In their study, a large dye concentration was obtained at the femoral artery site within 30 seconds of central venous injection, and no dye was present from the peripheral injection for at least 90 seconds (Fig. 1). The dye concentration obtained with central venous injection was uniformly four times greater than the maximum dye concentration observed five minutes after peripheral administration. In view of these data, the authors advocated the routine establishment of central venous lines in patients requiring advanced cardiac life support.

In 1983, Hedges et al. [19] used a technetium–99m–labeled albumin to study drug delivery to the right and left ventricles via a peripheral forelimb vein versus the superior vena cava in dogs undergoing closed-chest CPR. Right ventricular half peak times averaged 5.7 seconds for the central venous group and 28.5 seconds for the peripheral venous group; left ventricular half peak times were 10.6 and 83.7 seconds. However, quantitative peak left ventricular activity for the groups was similar. The authors suggest that the 70-second advantage of the central venous over the peripheral venous route for drug delivery indicates that, when available, the central venous route should be preferred. Keats et al. [20] found also a significant delay in the onset of peak aortic diastolic pressure after epinephrine given either peripherally (114 ± 20 seconds) or centrally (82 ± 14 seconds) ($p < 0.02$) in dogs during cardiac arrest. However, the peripheral and cen-

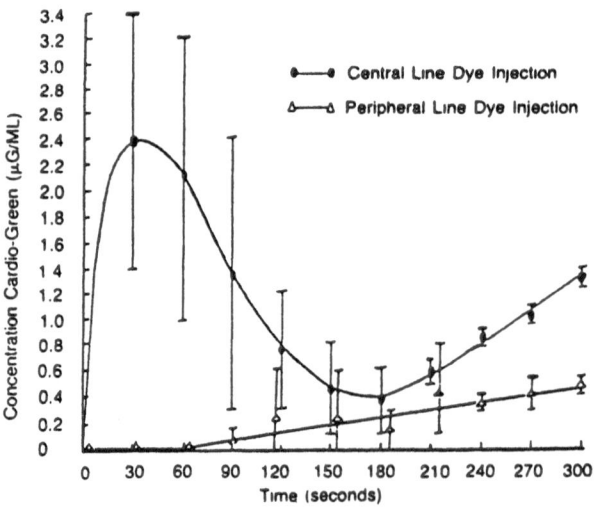

Fig. 1. Indocyanin green concentration at femoral artery following injection via right subclavian vein vs right basilic vein in 6 adults during CPR. ($p = 0.02$ at 30 sec.; $p < 0.005$ at 300 sec.). (From [18], with permission)

tral injection of epinephrine equally augmented aortic diastolic pressure. These three studies suggest, in fact, that during even properly performed CPR:

1. cardiac output is much lower than normal values;
2. blood flow is likely to be directed from a peripheral towards a central compartment which explains the delay in drug action when administered peripherally. The latter fact is in fully accordance with the concept of the heart as a passive conduit during CPR in which blood flow is the result of vascular beds compression in the lungs due to the increase in intrathoracic pressure [21].

In the same year Dalsey et al. [22], using a similar isotope technique, compared superior vena cava (SVC) and inferior vena cava (IVC) access during normal perfusion and closed-chest in dogs. The normal perfusion study demonstrated no significant difference between SVC and IVC delivery. During CPR, however, times to reach right and left ventricular half peaks were significantly shorter for the SVC group. Times to mean right ventricular half peak were 5.7 seconds and 20.2 seconds for the SVC and IVC groups, respectively; mean left ventricular half peak times were 10.6 and 27.8 seconds. Nevertheless, quantitative peak activity counts for the right and left ventricles were similar in the two groups. The authors concluded that their results support the preferential use of the SVC route over the IVC route during CPR. This conclusion is supported by the results obtained in dogs by Niemann et al., using either pressure-synchronized cineangiography [23] or cinefluoroscopic observations of bead flow-indicator catheters [24]. Their observations suggested that cardiac output obtained during CPR was essentially brachiocephalad at the expense of the subdiaphragmatic part of the body. In accordance to this, drug delivery through the subdiaphragmatic venous system may be substantially delayed due to the "to-and-fro" movement of the venous blood in the inferior vena cava.

Nevertheless, all these studies but the one by Kuhn's et al. [18] have been done in animals and their conclusions should be cautiously extended only to human beings. In the smaller pediatric patients, it is uncertain whether the site of injection is as important [16]. Practically, if immediately available, peripheral injection by any venous access is preferable. Whenever possible, however, central venous drug injection must be preferred to peripheral venous injection. Concerning the choice between supradiaphragmatic or subdiaphragmatic access, the more rapidly obtained central venous catheterization is the best: internal jugular vein, subclavian vein, or femoral vein. In infants, the most practical is catheterization of the superior saggital sinus through the anterior fontanel, whereas in neonates this is the umbilical vein catheterization [25].

Intraosseous Route

The concept of using the bone marrow for the administration of fluid and drugs is an old one, since its first description in 1922. In 1940, Tocantins [26] demonstrated the rapid absorption of substances injected into the bone marrow. Substances are thought to pass from the bone marrow cavity into sinusoids, large medullary venous channels, nutrient and emissary veins, and finally the systemic venous circulation. Tocantins et al. [27] established practical techniques and improved disposable IV needles. Intraosseous infusion fell into obscurity by the late 1950s. However, in 1984, this technique regained some favor when Ber [28] showed that catecholamines such as epinephrine could be administered in children that way when no vascular access could be found. The intraosseous access has been used also for bicarbonate infusion. In the largest single study of 1000 pediatric cases, Heinild et al. [29] reported 78 infusions of sodium bicarbonate without complications. He did not describe how the bicarbonate was infused (i.e., a slow infusion or rapid bolus) and did not address the reason for bicarbonate administration. Comparison of intraosseous, central and peripheral routes of sodium bicarbonate administration during CPR in pigs has been studied by Spivey et al. [30]. The intraosseous route was found to be as effective as the central venous route. An additional study concluded that $NaHCO_3$ does not have permanent adverse effects on the bone marrow in terms of roentgenographs, bone scans, and microscopic examination [31]. No data are available on the efficacy of epinephrine or bicarbonate during CPR in human beings but this route may be considered when venous cannulation is not readily available.

Endotracheal Route

During CPR, the endotracheal (ET) access is in fact the most important alternate route for drug administration. This route has several theorical and practical advantages. The enormous surface area and the fact that the lungs receive the entire cardiac output make them excellent candidates for drug absorption. If adequately dispersed sufficiently deep into the tracheobronchial tree, the drug would be directly delivered into the pulmonary capillaries, therefore just before the heart and the systemic arteries. This is very important for epinephrine which acts principally as a systemic peripheral vasoconstrictor [32]. In addition, the most effective step in CPR, at least when cardiac arrest is secondary to respiratory arrest, is to resume effective ventilation. Thus, endotracheal intubation should be performed as early as possible, and in most clinical settings, the ET route is practically available before a vascular access could have been established.

Pharmacokinetics of Endotracheal Drug Administration in Animals

The pharmacokinetic principles which govern drug administration via the ET route are similar to those of other routes of drug administration [33] and include the following:

1. nature and size of the particles;
2. drug delivery and absorption factors;
3. area of the respiratory tract;
4. distribution of the drug;
5. biotransformation; and
6. excretion and metabolism.

The application of these factors to the ET route of drug administration is crucial to be the effective and safe use of ET medication.

Nature and size of particles: The actual mechanism of drug absorption at the alveolar level is similar to absorption at other cell membranes. When considering lipid-insoluble drugs, absorption is almost exclusively based upon molecular size. The higher the molecular weight, the slower the rate of absorption. Any substance whose particle size approximates 0.1 to 6 µ or less is rapidly absorbed into the pulmonary capillaries. Conversely, large particles such as charcoal and silica are absorbed by the lymphatic system, and inorganic ions in a manner resembling the diffusion of gas molecules [34]. On the other hand, more highly lipid-soluble drugs are better absorbed.

Drug delivery and absorption factors: The diluent vehicle is of major importance for ET drug absorption. Since the passage of water across the alveolar capillary membrane is rapid, water seems to be the ideal diluent for ET drug absorption. However, Greenberg et al. [35] found in dogs that ET administered distilled water was more detrimental on arterial blood gases than normal saline solution. They hypothesized that distilled water may damage alveolar cells and surfactant. It is still unclear what recommendations should be given for human beings.

The status of the alveolar-capillary membrane also is a factor to consider. The integrity of the membrane may in fact be damaged in the earliest phases of sepsis or other shock events, and fluid tends to leak into the alveolar space. Whether this leak facilitates the uptake of medication into the blood is an unanswered question.

Diffusion probably plays the major role in the pulmonary absorption of drugs and involves molecular movement from an area of higher concentration (intra-alveolar space) to one of lower concentration (pulmonary capillary). This process is altered by any primary pulmonary pathology which affects the concentration gradient and hence the rate of lung absorption. Therefore, the clinical setting of pneumonia, atelectasis, obstructive pulmonary disease and hypoxia all may interfere to some degree with effective drug absorption, either by direct toxic effects or by inequalities in ventilation/perfusion ratios.

Area of absorption within the respiratory tract: Absorption occurs at all levels of the respiratory tract, from the trachea to the alveoli. By far the major area of absorption is the vast absorptive surface of the alveolar-capillary interface. Therefore, most efficient and rapid absorption is obtained if drugs are dispersed throughout the alveolar surface of the lung. However, it is necessary not to flood up the whole lung in order to keep enough lung for alveolar gas exchange. Thus, it appears that the best administration mode is to inject the diluted drug deep into the trachea followed by a few manual ventilations using bag [36].

Distribution of the drug: Distribution to sites of action is extremely rapid for all drugs studied via the ET route [14, 37, 38]. Although blood levels can be detected almost instantaneously, there also exists a depot-type prolonged release of medication from alveolar sites into the systemic circulation. When compared with IV injection, epinephrine and its metabolites remain at elevated levels for prolonged periods of time [38]. This sustained blood level is ascribed to a gradual continual absorption of drugs into the systemic circulation from the lungs. Nevertheless, there are some important differences in the kinetics of epinephrine following IV and ET administration. If circulation is intact, blood levels are approximately eight to ten times higher via the IV route when equal doses are studied, but the magnitude of changes in heart rate and blood pressure are only twofold to three-fold higher with the IV drug. Conversely, the effect of epinephrine is significantly prolonged following ET administration. Thus, five minutes after ET administration, 80% of the initial blood concentration is detected while only 20% of the original blood level is detected following IV injection.

The same results have been obtained in subhuman primates [39]. In that study, plasma catecholamine levels and hemodynamic responses to intratracheal epinephrine administration were assessed using a double-blind, randomized crossover design in 7 male baboons (Papio anubis) who received 5 ml of 1:10000 epinephrine on one day and 5 ml of 0.9% NaCl on another day. Intratracheal epinephrine significantly ($p < 0.05$) elevated heart rate to 120 ± 6 from 105 ± 6 beats/min, mean arterial pressure to 120 ± 4 from 112 ± 5 mmHg, and plasma epinephrine to 8882 ± 2143 from 928 ± 209 pg/ml within1 minute of administration, and these effects persisted for 30 minutes. Plasma norepinephrine levels did not change after intratracheal epinephrine administration. None of the four variables changed after intratracheal was given.

Biotransformation of the drug: The area of the biotransformation within the lungs remains to be fully investigated. It is well known that the lungs play a role in the metabolism of certain agents, such as prostaglandins and norepinephrine, but, to date, the local transformation of ET-instilled medication has not been extensively studied. Furthermore, significant pharmacological and physiological responses parallel those which would be expected in direct IV injection [37, 38]. These facts tend to speak against any significant local biotransformation for the drugs studied to date.

Excretion of the drug: The most critical phase of excretion in ET pharmacology is in fact in the preabsorptive phase. This involves the possible reflux of medication in a retrograde fashion out the ET tube for instance because of coughing. This potential problem may be minimized by the use of a long catheter-introducer to disperse the medication distally into the tracheobronchial tree as efficiently as possible. In addition, when a drug is absorbed into the circulation from the lung, it behaves as if given intravenously.

Experimental Validation of the Endotracheal Route During CPR

Ralston et al. [40] validated the value of the ET administration of epinephrine during CPR in dogs. In their study, blood flow to vital organs was measured at five-minute intervals during 20 minutes of CPR and ventricular fibrillation in

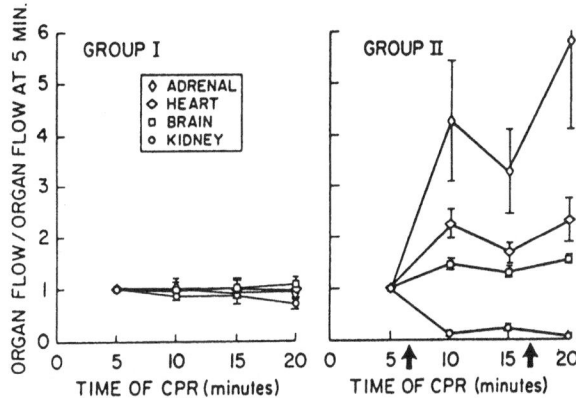

Fig. 2. Organ blood flows at 5-minute intervals during 20 minutes of CPR in Group I (control) and in group II (epinephrine-treated) dogs. Arrows indicate epinephrine intrapulmonary injection. (From [40], with permission)

two groups of anesthetized dogs (n = 15). In a preliminary study, a very important point was confirmed: it was clearly shown that epinephrine should be delivered deeply into the bronchial tree in order to obtain a significant raise in blood pressure in living dogs whereas the administration of epinephrine directly into the endotracheal tube had no effect. Intrapulmonary epinephrine significantly improved blood flow to the myocardium, the brain, and the adrenals in comparison to control dogs which received saline (Fig. 2). In addition, the relationship between organ blood flow and restoration of circulation after 20 minutes of ventricular fibrillation was assessed. A mean myocardial blood flow of less than 0.13 ml/min/g resulted in no survival, while a flow of greater than 0.16 ml/min/g consistently resulted in survival (Fig. 3). Thus, a critical level of myocardial blood flow is required to restore the ability of the heart to recover. When a drug has been delivered adequately to reach its systemic peripheral vascular receptors, that increase in myocardial blood flow improves resuscitation efforts.

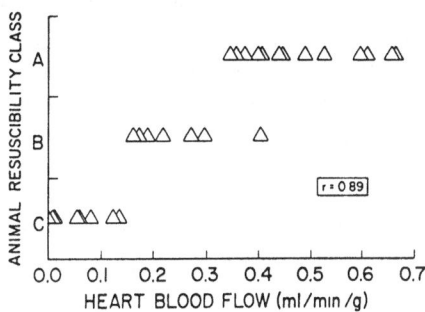

Fig. 3. Relationship between the animal's response to resuscitation and blood flow to the heart. Each data point represents the mean of four blood flow determinations in one animal. (From [40], with permission)

Clinical Use of the Endotracheal Route During CPR

The clinical use of epinephrine administration through the ET route has been reported for the first time by Roberts et al. [41] in a 57-year old woman who suffered asphyxial cardiac arrest during the course of an asthma attack. She was successfully resuscitated after having received 10 ml of 1:10000 epinephrine into the trachea. In the same report, was also mentioned the case of a 13-day old premature baby. This case was reported in more details elsewhere [42]. This baby was found apneic and pulseless at home. Proper CPR was administered en route to the hospital. No peripheral IV access was available. Saphenous, umbilical, and brachial cutdowns were unsuccessful. Epinephrine (0.01 mg) was administered via syringe directly into the endotracheal tube and a manual ventilation was supplied. With CPR continuing, the child quickly regained a pulse and spontaneous respiratory efforts. A coarctation of the aorta was discovered. However, there was a massive intraventricular cerebral hemorrhage and the child died from another cardiac arrest on the third hospital day. Following that report, Lindemann [43, 44] described successful ET administration of epinephrine in 7 newborns suffering birth asphyxia at birth and 3 babies with cardiac arrest from various causes.

The ET route may be used for administration of other drugs than epinephrine. Thus, ET lidocaine has been shown effective to treat arrhythmias in dogs [45] and in human beings [46]. Atropine was shown also to be effective after ET administration in a 74-year old patient suffering profound bradycardiac cardiovascular collapse [47].

The optimal drug dosages for the endotracheal route are currently unknown. According to the animal studies [37, 38] a larger dose (threefold?) than the intravenous dose should be used. It must be noticed, however, that in spite of the official recommendations of the American Heart Association [16] of 1 mg for adults and 10 µg/kg for children, no study has been specifically done to determine the optimal intravenous dosages in human beings. Thus, at least the same dose as used intravenously if not threefold dose may be given endotracheally. Quinton et al. [48] randomly allocated 12 patients with asystolic cardiac arrest to treatment with endotracheal epinephrine (5 patients) or peripheral intravenous epinephrine (7 patients). Femoral-artery blood samples were taken for assay of epinephrine and norepinephrine. After intravenous epinephrine there was a good clinical and biochemical response, but after endotracheal epinephrine there was no change in serum epinephrine and no measurable clinical response. On the basis of their data, the authors concluded that the endotracheal route of epinephrine administration is not a reliable in out-of-hospital cardiac arrest. However, Marchant [49] criticized that study by pointing out that the endotracheal dose should have been twofold the intravenous one, as the United Kingdom Resuscitation Council recommends. The debate is therefore still open, and more studies either experimental or clinical are needed.

Conclusions: Practical Recommendations

As soon as the diagnosis of cardiac arrest has been made, effective ventilation and closed-chest compression must be continuous. Effective ventilation, in fact, requires endotracheal intubation as soon as possible for at least three reasons:

1. it maintains the airway securely open;
2. it greatly facilitates CPR management, because it frees one rescuer who would have otherwise to maintain the "head tilt-chin-lift" position with one hand and to maintain the mask fitted on the mouth to the achievement of an airtight seal with the other hand;
3. it allows to use much higher insufflating pressure without the risks of deleterious hyperinflation of the stomach and the gastrointestinal tract.

Since the endotracheal tube is in place, it would be worthless not to use it for early drug administration. At least 1-mg for adults and 10-μg/kg for children (if not a threefold dose, i.e. 3-mg and 30-μg/kg) dose of *diluted* epinephrine (1:10000 i.e. 10 ml = 1 mg) must be administered as deep as possible into the tracheobronchial tree, followed by 5 deep manual ventilations using bagging to insure effective intrapulmonary absorption of the drug. An effective serum peak should be rapidly obtained, followed by a slow decrease due to depot-type release in the lung. Thus, epinephrine may rapidly reach its systemic peripheral receptors, provided an efficient and continuous artificial blood flow is insured by a well-done CPR. All of this would allow quite often return to spontaneous hemodynamic-efficient cardiac activity.

When this does not occur, epinephrine must be administered intravenously. A central venous access, if possible in the upper part of the body, must be found. The fastest i.e. the venous catheterization which the rescuer is the more confident in, must be attempt. The following venous catheterization may be advised: umbilical vein in newborns, saggital superior sinus in infants, (left) subclavian or (right) internal jugular veins in children or in adults. Nevertheless, as soon as the venous access is secured, a system including a short (small dead-space for the pediatric age) tubing and two stop-coks must be used in order to avoid epinephrine (pH 2.0–4.0) inactivation by sodium bicarbonate (pH 8.0–9.0) if the latter has to be employed.

In fact, a tremendous number of experimental studies has been done so far in understanding the pharmacology of drugs in CPR. However, numerous questions are to date unsolved. The optimal dosage of epinephrine is still unknown. It is uncertain whether it is appropriate to use the same dose through the endotracheal route as the intravenous one or higher doses (twofold, threefold?). To what extent is there a cephalad circulating central compartment and a non-circulating peripheral compartment during CPR in patients? Is it relevant enough to definitely exclude the peripheral drug injection, when a peripheral venous access was inserted prior to cardiac arrest occurrence? Is the adult model identical to the pediatric model? All these unanswered questions clearly justify to pursue experimental as well as clinical research.

References

1. Cole SL, Corday E (1956), Four-minute limit for cardiac resuscitation. JAMA 161:1454–1458
2. Southwick FS, Dalglish PH (1980) Recovery after prolonged asystolic cardiac arrest in profound hypothermia. A case report and literature review. JAMA 243:1250–1253
3. Ludwig S, Kettrick RG, Parker M (1984) Pediatric cardiopulmonary resuscitation. Clin Pediatr 23:71–75
4. Safar P, Scarraga LA, Elam JO (1958) A comparison of the mouth-to-mouth and mouth-to-airway methods of artificial respiration with the chest-pressure arm-lift methods. N Engl J Med 258:671–677
5. Kouwenhouven WB, Jude JR, Knickerbocker GG (1960) Closed-chest cardiac massage. JAMA 173:1064–1067
6. Voorhes WD, Babbs CF, Tacker WA (1980) Regional blood flow during cardiopulmonary circulation in dogs. Crit Care Med 8:134–136
7. Luce JM, Ross BK, O'Quin RJ, et al (1983) Regional blood flow during cardiopulmonary resuscitation in dogs using simultaneous and nonsimultaneous compression and ventilation. Circulation 67:258–265
8. Rodgers MC (1988) The physiology of cardiopulmonary resuscitation. Intensive Care Med (in press)
9. Criley JM, Blaufuss AH, Kissel GL (1976) Cough-induced cardiac compression. Self-administered form of cardiopulmonary circulation. JAMA 236:1246–1250
10. Rudikoff MT, Maughan WL, Effron M, et al (1980) Mechanisms of blood flow during cardiopulmonary resuscitation. Circulation 61:345–352
11. Maier GW, Tyson GS, Olsen CO, et al (1984) The physiology of external cardiac massage: High-impulse cardiopulmonary resuscitation. Circulation 70:86–101
12. Michel JR, Guerci AD, Koehler RC, et al (1984) Mechanisms by which epinephrine augments cerebral and myocardial perfusion during cardiopulmonary resuscitation in dogs. Circulation 69:822–835
13. Luce JM, Rizk NA, Niskanen RA (1984) Regional blood flow during cardiopulmonary resuscitation. Crit Care Med 12:874–878
14. Redding JS, Asuncion JS, Pearson JW (1967) Effective routes of drug administration during cardiac arrest. Anaesth Analg 46:253–258
15. Redding JS, Pearson JW (1962) Resuscitation from asphyxia. JAMA 182:283–286
16. American Heart Association (1986) Standards and guidelines for cardiopulmonary resuscitation (CPR) and emergency cardiac care (ECC). JAMA 255:2905–2992
17. Rossetti V, Thompson BM, Aprahamian C, et al (1984) Difficulty and delay in intravascular access in pediatric arrest. Ann Emerg Med 13:406 (abstract)
18. Kuhn GJ, White BC, Swetnam RE, et al (1981) Peripheral vs central circulation times during CPR: A pilot study. Ann Emerg Med 10:417–419
19. Hedges JR, Barsan WB, Doan LA, et al (1984) Central versus peripheral intravenous routes in cardiopulmonary resuscitation. Am J Emerg Med 2:385–390
20. Keats S, Jackson RE, Kosnik JW, et al (1985) Effect of peripheral versus central injection of epinephrine on changes in aortic diastolic pressure during closed-chest massage in dogs. Ann Emerg Med 14:495 (abstract)
21. Criley JM, Niemann JT, Rosborough JP, et al (1981) The heart is a conduit in CPR. Crit Care Med 9:373–374
22. Dalsey WC, Barsan WG, Joyce SM, et al (1984) Comparison of superior vena caval and inferior vena cava access using a radioisotope technique during normal perfusion and cardiopulmonary resuscitation. Ann Emerg Med 13:881–884
23. Nieman JT, Rosborough JP, Hausknecht M, et al (1981) Pressure-synchronized cineangiography during experimental cardiopulmonary resuscitation. Circulation 64:985–991
24. Nieman JT, Rosborough JP, Ung S, et al (1984) Hemodynamic effects of abdominal binding during cardiac arrest and resuscitation. Am J Cardiol 53:269–274
25. Mercier JC, Gaudelus J (1985) Voies d'abord vasculaires chez le nouveau-né et l'enfant. In: Perelman R, Pédiatrie pratique: Périnatologie. Maloine Paris, pp 1876–1897

26. Tocantins LM (1940) Rapid absorption of substances injected into the bone marrow. Proc Soc Exp Biol Med 45:292-296

27. Tocantins LM, O'Neill JF, Jones HW (1941) Infusions of blood and other fluids via the bone marrow: Applications in pediatrics. JAMA 117:1229-1234

28. Ber RA (1984) Emergency infusion of catecholamines into bone marrow. Am J Dis Child 138:810-811

29. Heinild S, Sondergaard T, Tudvad F (1947) Bone marrow infusions in childhood. Experiences from a thousand of infusions. J Pediatr 30:400-401

30. Spivey WH, Lathers CM, Malone DR, et al (1985) Comparison of intraosseous, central, and peripheral routes of sodium bicarbonate during CPR in pigs. Ann Emerg Med 14:1135-1140

31. Spivey WH, Unger HD, McNamara RM, et al (1987) The effect of intraosseous sodium bicarbonate on bone in swine. Ann Emerg Med 16:773-776

32. Otto CW, Yakaitis RW, Blitt CD (1981) Mechanisms of action of epinephrine in resuscitation from asphyxial arrest. Crit Care Med 9:321-324, 364-365

33. Greenblatt DJ, Koch-Weser J (1975) Clinical pharamcokinetics. N Engl J Med 293:702-705, 964-970

34. Dal Santo G (1977) Non-respiratory functions of the lungs and anesthesia. Little Brown Co Boston pp 61-90

35. Greenberg MI, Baskin SI, Kaplan AM, et al (1982) Effects of endotracheally administered distilled water and normal saline on the arterial blood gases of dogs. Ann Emerg Med 11:600-604

36. Greenberg MI, Roberts JR, Krusz JC, et al (1979) Endotracheal epinephrine in a canine anaphylactic shock model. JACEP 500-503

37. Roberts JR, Greenberg MI, Knaub M, et al (1978) Comparison of the pharmalogical effects of epinephrine administered by the intravenous and endotracheal routes. JACEP 7:260-264

38. Roberts JR, Greenberg MI, Knaub MA, et al (1979) Blood levels following intravenous and endotracheal epinephrine administration. JACEP 8:53-56

39. Chernow B, Holbrook P, D'Angona DS, et al (1984) Epinephrine absorption after intratracheal administration. Anesth Analg 63:829-832

40. Ralston SH, Voorhes WB, Babbs CF (1984) Intrapulmonary epinephrine during prolonged cardiopulmonary resuscitation: improved regional blood flow and resuscitation. Ann Emerg Med 13:79-86

41. Roberts JR, Greenberg MI, Baskin SI (1979) Endotracheal epinephrine in cardiopulmonary collapse. JACEP 8:515-519

42. Greenberg MI, Roberts JR, Baskin SI (1981) Use of endotracheally administered epinephrine in a pediatric patient. Am J Dis Child 135:767-768

43. Lindemann R (1982) Endotracheal administration of epinephrine during cardiopulmonary resuscitation. Am J Dis Child 136:753-754

44. Lindemann R (1984) Resuscitation of the newborn: Endotracheal administration of epinephrine. Acta Paediatr Scand 73:210-212

45. Elam J (1977) The intrapulmonary route for CPR drugs. In: Safar P (Ed) Advances in cardiopulmonary resuscitation. Springer Verlag Berlin Heidelberg New York, pp 132-140

46. Ward JT Jr (1983) Endotracheal drug therapy. Am J Emergy Med 1:71-82

47. Greenberg MI, Mayeda DV, Chrzanowski R, et al (1982) Endotracheal administration of atropine sulfate. Ann Emerg Med 11:546-548

48. Quinton DN, O'Byrne G, Aitkenhead AR (1985) Comparison of endotracheal and peripheral intravenous adrenaline in cardiac arrest: Is the endotracheal route reliable? Lancet 1:828-829

49. Marchant B (1987) Endotracheal adrenaline in cardiac arrest. Lancet 1:1098

Cerebral Resuscitation After Cardiac Arrest: The Role of Calcium Antagonists

R. O. Roine, M. Kaste, and P. Nikki

Introduction

The outcome of cardiac arrest victims is usually determined by the neurological state of the patient after restoration of spontaneous circulation. More than 50% of resuscitated patients die at hospital because of anoxic encephalopathy – a fact that usually cannot be discovered in mortality reports [1]. Of the surviving patients, at least 20% have unequivocal signs of anoxic brain injury, although the exact incidence of mental sequelae is not known because of the rarity of adequate neuro-psychological information on the cardiac arrest victims [2].

Cerebral resuscitation – or cardiopulmonary-cerebral resuscitation – is a relatively new concept, apparently first introduced by Safar in 1976, who raised the possibility to interfere with the developing cerebral injury after a global anoxic-ischemic injury [3]. Hossman et al. [4] had earlier demonstrated the ability of neurons under certain circumstances to recover their high energy metabolism, enzymatic functions and action potential generation even after 60 minutes of complete ischemia, suggesting that there is no "4-minute limit" of cerebral anoxia. In the broadest sense of the word, cerebral resuscitation can be understood to consist of all measures designed to limit the brain injury after ischemic, anoxic or traumatic insults of any kind. In case of pretreatment, it is more appropriate to use the term cerebral protection, which is sometimes used synonymously with cerebral resuscitation.

Pathophysiology of Global Cerebral Ischemia

New data of the pathophysiology of cerebral anoxia have conspicuously improved the theoretical possibilities of cerebral resuscitation. Firstly, a sufficiently long period of global ischemic anoxia of the brain is followed by initial hyperemia and by delayed hypoperfusion after restoration of the cerebral blood flow, reflecting a mismatch between metabolic rate and blood flow in the brain [5]. The cause and significance of this phenomenon are still incompletely understood [6, 7]. Loss of cerebrovascular autoregulation, arterial spasm, cellular swelling, platelet aggregation, intravascular coagulation and various metabolic factors, (e.g. acidosis) have been proposed to explain it [8]. Secondly, the ischemic-anoxic brain injury progresses during several hours of reperfusion – as does the accumulation of intracellular calcium, which has recently been documented in animal models (9–14).

The Calcium Hypothesis

The role of calcium in the pathogenesis of ischemic brain damage has been increasingly evident during the last decade. Calcium dependence of cellular injury was first revealed in the hepatocyte in 1979, when Schanne and coworkers suggested that calcium may be the final common pathway in cellular death in various toxic and hypoxic conditions [15]. The hypothesis of calcium-mediated ischemic neuronal injury was published two years later [14, 16, 17].

Calcium plays an essential role in the regulation of cellular homeostasis controlling the excitability of neuronal systems and neurochemical events at membrane and cytoplasmic levels. This requires the maintenance of a constant level of calcium in neurons. Intracellularly, the physiological effects of calcium are mediated via Ca^{++}-calmodulin complex. The calcium ion is actively maintained outside neurons with a concentration gradient of $1:10000$ by several ATP-dependent membrane mechanisms primarily Ca^{++}-ATPase. It is activated by the presence of calcium, which it then removes to the extracellular space.

Global ischemia induces depletion of high-energy phosphates and ATP in about 5 minutes, which seems to herald the ischemic cascade [18]. This is followed by potassium efflux, depolarization of the cell membrane and massive calcium influx resulting in intracellular calcium overload. The intracellular calcium accumulation is believed to cause cellular injury by the following mechanisms. The activation of phospholipases and proteases lead to destruction of cellular membranes, free fatty acid liberation and free radical formation. Arachidonic acid then activates the cyclo-oxygenase and lipo-oxygenase pathways leading to formation of thromboxane A_2 and leukotrienes, which in turn cause smooth muscle spasm and increased permeability in vascular walls. Intracellularly, calcium accumulates in mitochondria and uncouples the oxidative phosphorylation. Initially, calcium activates the calcium-dependent Ca^{++}-ATPase, the function of which rapidly ceases as the cellular ATP-stores are consumed, leading to further increase in intracellular calcium. Calcium influx also induces the liberation of excitatory neurotransmitters, such as glutamate, at synaptic terminals. As a result, wastage of ATP, membrane damage, increased permeability and smooth muscle spasm will ultimately lead to impaired blood flow and neuronal death [5, 11, 16].

Calcium Entry Blockers in Cerebral Resuscitation

No medical treatment has by now been shown to reduce neurological morbidity or mortality after cardiac arrest. Even the result of the thiopental study was negative [19]. Based on the above-mentioned calcium hypothesis, calcium entry blockers seem to be a rational choice. There are several possible mechanisms of beneficial action of calcium entry blockers in neuronal anoxia [5, 20, 21]. Calcium entry blockers may inhibit calcium influx into ischemic neurons [13, 14]. Another mechanism of action would be their ability to prevent the postischemic hypoperfusion state after global ischemia. This has been demonstrated in various in vitro and in vivo animal models [7, 22–25].

Nimodipine, a dihydropyridine derivative calcium entry blocking drug, has been shown to prevent this postischemic hypoperfusion phenomenon, and there is some evidence that it may also reduce the preceding hyperemia [7, 22–25]. Its effect on human cerebral blood flow after cardiac arrest is currently under study. Nimodipine seems to be the most promizing calcium entry blocking drug in cerebral resuscitation, partly because of its high selectivity for cerebral vessels and its high affinity for specific receptors in brain tissue. The dihydropyridine receptor has been shown to be identical with calcium channels [26, 27]. Nimodipine binding sites have been identified also in human cerebral cortex [28]. The uptake of nicardipine, another dihydropyridine derivative drug, has been shown to be enhanced in ischemic brain tissue [29]. A possible but unconfirmed beneficial effect of calcium entry blockers during ischemia and reperfusion could be the prevention of calcium influx into ischemic cells. On the other hand, there is substantial evidence that calcium entry blockers may inhibit the release of excitatory neurotransmitters. Nimodipine has been shown to inhibit noradrenaline release from human cerebral arteries and substance P and dopamine release in the rat [30, 32]. Experimentally, nimodipine has also an anticonvulsive effect against seizures produced by ischemia and reperfusion as well as certain convulsants although its therapeutic antiepileptic effect remains to be documented in humans [33]. Recent in vivo animal experiments indicate that calcium entry blockers may be useful in the treatment of cerebral ischemia [21, 34]. Steen et al. [34] have demonstrated that nimodipine improves neurological outcome in a primate global ischemia model, which is relevant clinically since the treatment was started 5 minutes after 17 minutes of complete cerebral ischemia. A nimodipine bolus dose of $10\mu g/kg$ body weight was given 5 minutes postischemia followed by an infusion of $1 \mu g/kg$ body weight/min for 10 hours, a dosage comparable to those used in clinical studies with nimodipine. Both the neurologic function and histopathologic findings in anoxic brain injury improved significantly in the nimodipine-treated animals compared to placebo-treated animals. The authors recommended controlled clinical trials in patients resuscitated after cardiac arrest.

Of other calcium entry blockers, positive results in experimental cerebral resuscitation have been published with lidoflazine and flunarizine [35, 36]. Many of the calcium entry blockers seem to have a cerebroprotective effect when given prior to global ischemia. Pretreatment is not relevant in cerebral resuscitation, but can be useful in cerebral protection, for instance during extracorporeal circulation and open-heart surgery or carotid endarterectomy, which can endanger the cerebral circulation. The beneficial effect on neurological recovery in animals has been documented for nimodipine and lidoflazine when administrated after global ischemia [24, 34, 35]. Nimodipine reduces reperfusion impairment after global ischemia in cats and dogs [22, 24, 25]. The ameliorating effect of flunarizine on the decrease in cerebral blood flow after complete cerebral ischemia has also been documented in dogs [36]. Lidoflazine, however, had no effect on cerebral blood flow following 12 minutes total cerebral ischemia [37]. Lidoflazine, in contrast to nimodipine, did not improve neurologic outcome in a primate model corresponding to that of Steen et al. [34, 38]. Nimodipine is one of the most potent and selective inhibitors of cerebrovascular spasm, and it is less likely to cause peripheral vasodilatation and hypotonia [22, 39, 40]. In consequence, it decreases blood pressure less than other calcium entry blockers, which is clearly an advantage after cardiac arrest. Nimodipine nearly doubles the coronary blood flow and is thus one of the most potent coronary vasodilatators; additionally, it markedly increases cardiac output, elevates PaO_2 and diminishes pulmonary vascular resistance without an effect on intrapulmonary shunting [41, 42]. Because of these cardiopulmonary effects, the hypothetical possibility of its size-limiting effect on myocardial infarction would also be tempting, but there is no clinical evidence to support it. Increase in intracranial pressure has been a feared complication of calcium antagonist therapy. Recently, nimodipine has been demonstrated to actually decrease the intracranial pressure (ICP) after carotid artery occlusion in baboons at all levels of ICP and PCO_2, and there is no evidence of a deleterious effect on intracranial pressure in other experimental models [43]. The potentially beneficial cardiovascular and cerebrovascular effects of nimodipine seem to increase its likelihood to improve the outcome of cardiac arrest victims.

Clinical Studies

A multicenter study of lidoflazine in out-of-hospital cardiac arrest is being carried out in the U.S.A. and Europe, but results have not been published so far.

There are no earlier human prospective studies of the effect of calcium blocking drugs in cerebral resuscitation. In an uncontrolled retrospective study of 29 patients, there was a trend toward improved neurological outcome, when verapamil and/or magnesium sulfate was used in 18 deeply comatose patients at some point after cardiac arrest. The patient material was not homogeneous and the treatment was not standardized, so that it is difficult to draw conclusions [44].

Our preliminary study of a calcium entry blocking drug in out-of-hospital ventricular fibrillation (VF) has been published in 1987 [45]. In this open pilot study, it was our aim to investigate the safety and efficacy of nimodipine in out-of-hospital cardiopulmonary and cerebral resuscitation. The study group consisted of 22 patients resuscitated from VF by the Mobile Intensive Care Unit (MICU) of Meilahti Hospital, Helsinki, from January to August, 1985. The control group consisted of matched historical controls resuscitated by the same team during the first half of 1984. The age and sex distribution, estimated cardiac arrest time, cardiopulmonary resuscitation time and duration of hypotonia did not differ significantly in the nimodipine and control group. The calculated total insult time of cerebral ischemia was 25 minutes in both groups (25.7 ± 15.7 min and 25.0 ± 11.7 min, respectively).

The intravenous dose of nimodipine was increased stepwise in the first 11 patients up to 0.5 μg/kg body weight/min as continuous infusion for 24 hours while the last 11 patients received a bolus dose of 10 μg/kg body weight followed by a 24 hour infusion of 0.5 μg/kg/min. The bolus dose was always given within 30 minutes after cardiac arrest by the physician of MICU. All patients received a standardized, brain-oriented treatment at the intensive care unit according to the principles described by Safar [46].

Why only patients with primary VF were chosen? During a three year period (1981–1983), the MICU of Helsinki attempted resuscitation of 1079 patients, 45.2% whom had primary VF. A total of 52.5% were admitted alive to the emergency department, and 18.2% were ultimately discharged alive from hospital – compared to $13.1 \pm 22.9\%$ and $1.3\% \pm 2.9\%$ of asystole and other pulseless rhythms, respectively. As a result, VF carries a better prognosis (about 10 times) compared to that of asystole and other pulseless rhythms. It is also the largest and apparently the most homogeneous one of all subgroups of resuscitated patients. Therefore, it is undoubtedly more appropriate for cerebral resuscitation studies than other rhythms. These figures mean also, that about two thirds (65%) of VF patients will die at hospital – most of them with an anoxic brain injury severe enough to preclude the recovery of consciousness. Only about 1% of all resuscitated patients will return back to their work whereas 1% will stay permanently at hospital.

Results of the Nimodipine Study

The results (Table 1) demonstrate that two thirds (14/22) of nimodipine-treated patients survived, compared to one third (7/22) of controls. The difference was significant ($p < 0.05$, Fisher's exact test). Twelve of 22 nimodipine-treated patients were discharged home from hospital, compared to 7 of 22 control patients.

Patients treated with a bolus dose plus continuous infusion of nimodipine seemed to have the best prognosis since 9 of 11 patients survived ($p < 0.05$) and were discharged home from hospital.

Three cases of primary pulseless rhythms were accidentally included in the nimodipine group and were also included in the analysis. The prognosis of these rhythms is known to be very bad – in fact less than 10% of the survival rates of patients with primary VF. We also analyzed the material without these three patients, who all died. The difference in survival was significant ($p < 0.01$) between the patients with VF and controls. The VF patients treated with nimodi-

Table 1. The 3 month outcome of cardiac arrest patients

	Survival		Discharge home	
	Nimodipine	Control	Nimodipine	Control
– All patients	14/22	7/22 $p < 0.05$	12/22	7/22 NS
– Patients after ventricular fibrillation	14/19	5/19 $p < 0.01$	12/19	5/19 $p < 0.05$
– id., treated with Nimodipine[a]	9/11	4/11 $p < 0.05$	7/11	3/11 NS

[a] Intravenous bolus of 10 µg/kg followed by a continuous infusion of 0.5 µ/kg/min for 24 h.

pine regained consciousness by the end of the first day and were even discharged home more often than controls (12 of 19 vs 5 of 19, p<0.05).

Nimodipine was well tolerated in this study. In some cases, a short drop of up to 40 mmHg in the mean arterial pressure was noted after the bolus dose of nimodipine. The blood pressure usually returned to normal spontaneously in 2 to 5 minutes. Volume loading or dopamine was used when necessary. No effect on the heart rate was observed.

Conclusion

The results of our pilot study, which provided the first human data on safety and efficacy of a calcium entry blocking drug in cerebral resuscitation, suggested that nimodipine can be safely used during out-of-hospital resuscitation, at least by a prehospital emergency care unit [45]. Nimodipine may also increase survival. A randomized placebo-controlled double-blind trial is needed to find out whether nimodipine therapy affects the survival, the extent and severity of the anoxic-ischemic brain injury and the outcome of patients resuscitated from VF outside hospital. We are now conducting such a study, which should be completed by the end of 1988.

Although the chances for some of the calcium entry blockers to be beneficial after cardiac arrest seem currently very promising, their clinical use still remains experimental. In the near future, clinical trials on cerebral resuscitation should apparently be based on the expanding background information of the mechanisms of neuronal injury in global ischemia – not merely the calcium hypothesis. In practice, this might implicate the combination of several methods, such as a glutamate receptor antagonist, inhibition of epileptic neuronal activity and reduction of cerebral metabolic rate for oxygen and glucose as well as regulation of cellular pH by controlled ventrilation and strict control of blood glucose, possibly in addition to a dihydropyridine calcium entry blocker. Presently, until results of controlled therapeutic studies are available, no drug can be recommended for routine clinical use in cerebral resuscitation.

References

1. Levy DE, Caronna JJ, Singer BH, Lapinski RH, Frydman H, Plum F (1985) Predicting outcome from hypoxic-ischemic coma. JAMA 253:1420–1426
2. Volpe BT, Hirst W (1983) The characterization of an amnesic syndrome following hypoxic ischemic injury. Arch Neurol 40:436–440
3. Safar P, Stezoski W, Nemoto EM (1976) Amelioration of brain damage after 12 minutes cardiac arrest in dogs. Arch Neurol 33:91–95
4. Hossmann K-A, Kleinhues P (1973) Reversibility of ischemic brain damage. Arch Neurol 29:375–384
5. Siesjö BK (1984) Cerebral circulation and metabolism. A review article. J Neurosurg 60:883–908
6. Jenkins LW, Powlishock JT, Lewelt W, Miller JD, Becker DP (1981) The role of postischemic recirculation in the development of ischemic neuronal injury following complete cerebral ischemia. Acta Neuropathol (Berlin) 55:205–220

7. White BC, Winegar CP, Henderson O, et al (1983) Prolonged hypoperfusion in the cerebral cortex following cardiac arrest and resuscitation in dogs. Ann Emerg Med 12:414–417
8. Safar P (1986) Resuscitation after brain ischemia. In: Grenvik A, Safar P (eds) Brain failure and resuscitation. Churchill Livingstone, New York, pp 155–184
9. Petito CK, Pulsinelli WA (1984) Delayed neuronal recovery and neuronal death in rat hippocampus following severe cerebral ischemia: Possible relationship to abnormalities in neuronal processes. J Cereb Blood Flow Metabol 4:194–205
10. Pulsinelli WA, Brierley JB, Plum F (1984) Temporal profile of neuronal damage in a model of transient forebrain ischemia. Ann Neurol 11:491–498
11. Raichle ME (1983) The pathophysiology of brain ischemia. Ann Neurol 13:2–10
12. Yanagihara T, McCall JT (1982) Ionic shift in cerebral ischemia. Life Sci 30:1921–1925
13. Hossmann K-A, Paschen W, Csiba L (1983) Relationship between calcium accumulation and recovery of cat brain after prolonged cerebral ischemia. J Cereb Blood Flow Metabol 3:346–353
14. Harris RJ, Symon L, Branston NM, et al (1981) Changes in extracellular calcium activity in cerebral ischemia. J Cereb Blood Flow Metabol 1:203–209
15. Schanne FAX, Kane AB, Young EE, Farber JL (1979) Calcium dependence of toxic cell death: A final common pathway. Science 206:700–703
16. Siesjö BK (1981) Cell damage in the brain: a speculative hypothesis. J Cereb Blood Flow Metabol 1:155–186
17. Hass WK (1981) Beyond cerebral blood flow, metabolism and ischemic thresholds: an examination of the role of calcium in the initiation of cerebral infarction. In: Meyer JS, Lechner H, Reivich M, et al (eds) Cerebral Vascular Disease. 3. Excerpta Medica, Amsterdam, pp 3–17.18
18. Hass WK (1983) The cerebral ischemic cascade. Neurol Clin 1:345
19. Brain Resuscitation Clinical Trial I Study Group (1986) Randomized clinical study of thiopental loading in comatose survivors of cardiac arrest. N Engl J Med 314:397–403
20. Godfraind T (1985) Calcium entry and calcium entry blockade. In: Godfraind T, Vanhoutte PM, Govoni S, Paoletti R (eds) Calcium Entry Blockers and Tissue Protection. Raven Press, New York, pp 1–20
21. White BC, Winegar CD, Wilson RF, Hoehner PJ, Trombley JH (1983) Possible role of calcium blockers in cerebral resuscitation: A review of the literature and synthesis for future studies. Crit Care Med 11:202–207
22. Kazda S, Hoffmeister F, Garthoff B, Towart R (1979) Prevention of the postischaemic impaired reperfusion of the brain by nimodipine (BAYe9736). Acta Neurol Scand 60 (Suppl 72):302–303
23. Harper AM, Craigen L, Kazda S (1981) Effect of the calcium antagonist, nimodipine, on cerebral blood flow and metabolism in the primate. J Cereb Blood Flow Metabol 1:349–356
24. Steen PA, Newberg LA, Milde JM, Michenfelder JD (1983) Nimodipine improves cerebral blood flow and neurologic recovery after complete cerebral ischemia in the dog. J Cereb Blood Flow Metabol 3:38–43
25. Steen PA, Newberg LA, Milde JH, Michenfelder JD (1984) Cerebral blood flow and neurologic outcome when nimodipine is given after complete cerebral ischemia in the dog. J Cereb Blood Flow Metabol 4:82–87
26. Bellemann P, Schade A, Towart R (1983) Dihydropyridine receptor in rat brain labeled with [3H]nimodipine. Proc Natl Acad Sci USA 80:2356–2360
27. Middlemiss DN, Spedding M (1985) A functional correlate for the dihydropyridine binding site in rat brain. Nature 314:94–96
28. Peroutka SJ, Allen GS (1983) Calcium channel antagonist binding sites labeled by [3H]nimodipine in human brain. J Neurosurg 59:933–937
29. Grotta JC, Pettigrew LC, Lockwood AH, Reich C (1987) Brain extraction of a calcium channel blocker. Ann Neurol 21:171–175
30. Porter ID, Gardiner IM, de Belleroche J (1985) Nimodipine has an inhibitory action on neurotransmitter release from human cerebral arteries. J Cereb Blood Flow Metabol 5:338–342

31. Woodward JJ, Leslie SW (1986) Bay K 8644 stimulation of calcium entry and endogenous dopamine release in rat striatal synaptosomes antagonized by nimodipine. Brain Res 370:397–400
32. Perney TM, Miller RJ (1987) Sensitivity of substance P release from cultured rat sensory neurons to nimodipine and other dihydropyridines. In: Proceedings of The International Symposium on Calcium Antagonists, New York, p 39 (abstract)
33. Meyer FB, Anderson RE, Sundt TM Jr, Sharbrough FW (1986) Selective central nervous system calcium channel blockers – a new class of anticonvulsant agents. Mayo Clin Proc 61:239–247
34. Steen PA, Gisvold SE, Milde JH, et al (1985) Nimodipine improves outcome when given after complete cerebral ischemia in primates. Anesthesiology 62:406–414
35. Vaagenes P, Cantadore R, Safar P, Alexander H (1984) The effect of lidoflazine and verapamil on neurological outcome after 10 minutes ventricular fibrillation cardiac arrest in dogs. Crit Care Med 12:228
36. White PC, Gadzinski DS, Hoehner PJ, et al (1982) Correction of canine cerebral cortical blood flow and vascular resistance after cardiac arrest using flunarizine, a calcium antagonist. Ann Emerg Med 11:118
37. Dean JM, Hoehner PJ, Rogers MC, Traystman RJ (1984) Effect of lidoflazine on cerebral blood flow following twelve minutes total cerebral ischemia. Stroke 15:531–535
38. Fleischer JE, Lanier WL, Milde JH, Michenfelder JD (1987) Lidoflazine does not improve neurologic outcome when administered after complete cerebral ischemia in primates. J Cereb Blood Flow Metabol 7:366–371
39. Mohamed AA, McCulloch J, Mendelow AD, Teasdale GM, Harper AM (1984) Effect of the calcium antagonist nimodipine on local cerebral blood flow: Relationship to arterial blood pressure. J Cereb Blood Flow Metabol 4:206–211
40. Peroutka SJ, Banghart SB, Allen GS (1984) Relative potency and selectivity of calcium antagonists used in the treatment of migraine. Headache 24:55–58
41. Satoh K, Kawada M, Wada Y, Taira N (1984) Cardiovascular actions of the dihydropyridine calcium antagonist nimodipine in the dog. Arzneim Forsch 34:563–568
42. Boldt J, Von Bormann D, Kling D, Ratthey K, Hempelmann G (1987) Influence of nimodipine and nifedipine on intrapulmonary shunting – a comparison to other vasoactive drugs. Intensive Care Med 13:52–56
43. Hadley MN, Spetzler RF, Fifield MS, Bichard WD, Hodak JA (1987) The effect of nimodipine on intracranial pressure. Volume-pressure studies in a primate model. J Neurosurg 66:387–393
44. Schwartz AC (1985) Neurological recovery after cardiac arrest: Clinical feasibility trial of calcium blockers. Am J Emerg Med 3:1–10
45. Roine RO, Kaste M, Nikki P, Kinnunen A (1987) Safety and efficacy of nimodipine in resuscitation of patients outside hospital. Br Med J 294:20
46. Safar P (1986) Cerebral resuscitation after cardiac arrest. A review. Circulation 74 (Suppl 4):138–153

Emergency and Trauma

Pre-hospital Trauma Care

C. E. Robertson and D. J. Steedman

Introduction

At a time when major re-organizations are occurring nationally and internationally in relation to ambulance services and emergency care facilities, it is appropriate to consider the most effective and rational use of pre-hospital and early hospital care given to such cases. This is particularly the case at times of financial restriction and at a time when all forms of medical care are under scrutiny for possible cost savings while maintaining service efficiency.

Although the concept of providing medical care at the scene of accidents was recognized by the Ancient Greeks and Romans, it was not until the time of the Napoleonic Wars that pre-hospital care was formed upon recognizable modern lines. Instrumental in the establishment of such a service was Dominique Jean Larrey whose teams of flying ambulances provided rapid evacuation and early medical care to injured soldiers. He was able to show dramatic effects on mortality and morbidity of the soldiers thus treated [1].

Subsequently, medical experience obtained during the First and Second World Wars, Korea, the Middle East and Vietnam, illustrated the benefits of providing immediate basic medical care and rapid evacuation [2]. The overwhelming message from such experience was that mortality was directly related to the time taken for the patient to reach definitive surgical care [3].

The European Experience

It would however be wrong to draw conclusions from combat situations and without careful review extrapolate them to a civilian milieu. In Western Europe, trauma is the principal cause of death in patients under 35 years of age. Approximately 25 000 people in Great Britain alone die annually as a consequence of trauma and a further 500 000 sustain major injury. But the forms of trauma that present to us are markedly different from both the combat and North American scenarios. In contrast to the situation of young fit, highly trained soldiers sustaining penetrating trauma on the battlefield, the situation that pertains in Western Europe involves a spectrum of age with clusters in the third decade and over 60's.

The US experience of 15–20% of major trauma cases due to penetrating injury from gunshot and knife wounds is fortunately uncommon here. In the United Kingdom few surgeons have ever seen a gunshot wound.

Our overwhelming problem is that of blunt trauma from road traffic accidents and falls from a height with a small mixed group of patients who have been assaulted or involved in industrial accidents [4].

Why Do Trauma Patients Die?

The trimodal distribution of trauma deaths in relation to time is well established [3]. Of those people who will die from trauma 50% die within 30 minutes. Death is due to such complex and severe injuries that for these patients survival is impossible within the constraints of our current technology. This must not be taken to imply that there is no role for pre-hospital care in these cases, but to direct such efforts towards prevention.

A further 30% of all trauma deaths occur within 4 hours of injury. These patients succumb due to a failure to provide and maintain an adequate airway, and to inadequate circulating blood volume. The contribution of these separate components in causing death varies, but between 5-40% of all patients who die do so as a consequence of airway obstruction [5, 6]. Yates' study indicated that for patients dying in hospital following trauma, those who had had airway obstruction died following less severe injury, than did those without such obstruction [8].

The contribution of hypovolemia to mortality is less well documented, but it is estimated that 7-25% of all trauma deaths are due to potentially treatable volume loss [7, 9]. In such cases the rate of blood loss is in excess of 100 ml/min and necessitates immediate operative surgical intervention.

The Contribution of Pre-hospital Care

From the above data, it would appear reasonable to provide advanced airway care and volume replacement in the expectation of improved survival and reduced morbidity for such cases. However, a considerable body of evidence is accumulating which indicates that this is not the case. Firstly, it is important to consider the operational constraints that exist. A recent major UK study has shown that in an urban and semi-urban environment, over 80% of emergency patients will have been transported to hospital within 30 minutes of the initial call [10].

Experience in the field demonstrates that to establish adequate intravenous access and give volume replacement exceeds site-to-hospital transit times and is merely delaying appropriate in-hospital surgical resuscitation [11–13]. The provision of advanced airway techniques is likely to be of most value in patients who are unconscious as a result of cerebral trauma. Those patients with head injuries accompanied by apnea are not salvageable. For the remainder achieving endotracheal intubation may be at the cost of further temporal delays and the possibility of causing or exacerbating a spinal injury. A recent study indicated that of over 26000 patients taken to hospital as an emergency, only 1 was likely to have derived long-term benefit from the use of advanced out-of-hospital trauma techniques [10]. Two assumptions were made in this study. Firstly, that ambulance personnel employing an advanced technique would always succeed in performing the procedure attempted and secondly, that maximum possible benefit would always occur. Since both are unlikely, the conclusion must be that to use advanced pre-hospital trauma techniques in urban/semi-urban areas is undesirable and unnecessary.

The above comments should however not be taken to imply that there is no role for any pre-hospital care. The importance of basic airway clearance and maintenance techniques together with appropriate splintage and pressure techniques is emphasized [10]. Previous attempts to assess the benefits of extended ambulance training have failed to consider the ability of ambulance staff to achieve successful outcomes using existing basic training.

Furthermore, in certain clinical settings, the operational techniques may require modification. In situations involving entrapment with delays in extrication, mass casualty situations, or in environmental or geographical locations where unavoidable delays will occur before reaching hospital, then advanced pre-hospital techniques will be required. Helicopter transportation both to and from the scene is currently the most rapid and safe system in these special cases.

In the UK, hospital-based mobile accident flying squads have partially fulfilled this role [14]. Until recently, objective evidence of the value of these squads has been limited, but evidence is accruing to suggest that for a few such patients lives can be saved by medical staff using advanced techniques [15–17]. While arguments can be put forward for advanced trained ambulance personnel to provide this role, such a mechanism is wasteful of resources and training, while the number of cases managed with each year by any individual would be insufficient for expertise to be gained and maintained in these trauma cases.

Trauma Service Regionalisation

Finally, given all of the above constraints, it is erroneous to imagine that trauma patients should necessarily be taken to the nearest hospital. For this situation the North American and West German experiences are invaluable [3]. A series of studies have shown that when major trauma cases are primarily directed to a designated regional trauma centre, that preventable deaths can be cut by 5 fold [3, 18, 19]. The view that for such a centre to function optimally, approximately 400 major trauma cases should be seen annually [20], may not be practicable in Western Europe, but it does focus our attention on the direction and need to concentrate such human and technical resources appropriately. If we continue to triage such cases to small, inadequately staffed and equipped hospitals, then preventable deaths will still occur.

References

1. Richardson R (1974) Larrey: Surgeon to Napoleon's Imperial Guard. Murray
2. Eisman B (1967) Combat Casualty Management in Vietnam. J Trauma 7:53–63
3. Trunkey DD (1983) Trauma. Scientific American 249:20–27
4. O'Byrne GA, Bodiwala GG (1987) Use of the resuscitation room for trauma. Arch Emerg Med 4:83–90
5. Ruffnell-Smith (1970) Time to die from injuries received in road traffic accidents. Injury 1:2
6. Lauppi E (1954) Die aspiration bei Opfern des Straßenverkehrs. Schweiz Med Wschr 84:335
7. Hoffman E (1981) On-site resuscitation. In: Wilson DH, Marsden AK (eds) Proc. of V International Congress of Emergency Surgery. John Wiley & Sons, Chichester, pp 77–80
8. Yates DW (1977) Airway patency in fatal accidents. Br Med J II:1249–1251
9. Adams R (1981) Evidence "for" immediate care. John Wiley & Sons, Chichester, pp 65–72
10. Anderson IWR, Black R, Ledingham IMcA, Little K, Robertson CE (1987) Early Emergency Care Study: the potential and benefits of advanced pre-hospital care. Br Med J 294:228–231
11. Bodai BI, Walton CB, Smith JP (1987) Mistakes in treatment of accident cases before reaching hospital. Injury 18:18–20
12. Smith JP, Bodai BI, Hill AS, Frey CF (1985) Prehospital stabilisation of Critically Injured Patients: A failed concept. J Trauma 25:65–69
13. Border JR (1983) Prehospital trauma care – stabilise or scoop and run. J Trauma 23:708–711
14. Robertson CE, Steedman DJ (1985) Are Accident Flying Squads really cleared for take-off? Lancet 2:434–436
15. Little K (1976) The Hospital based Accident Flying Squad. M. D. thesis. University of Edinburgh
16. Steedman DJ, Robertson CE (1985) Accident Flying Squads: an objective evaluation of their role in trauma. J Roy Coll Surg Ed 31:80–84
17. Gorman DF, Coals J (1983) Evaluation of a hospital-based flying squad using an injury scoring system. Injury 14:513–518
18. West JG, Trunkey DD, Lim RC (1979) Systems of trauma care: A Study of Two Counties. Arch Surg 114:455–460
19. Shackford SR, Hollingworth-Fridlund P, Cooper GF, Eastman AB (1986) The effect of regionalisation upon the quality of trauma care. J Trauma: 26:812–820
20. Tuefel W, Trunkey DD (1977) Trauma Centres: a pragmatic approach to need, cost and staffing patterns. J. A.C.E.P. 6:546–551

Emergency Medical System in Tokyo

Y. Yamamoto, Y. Ohtomo, and T. Otsuka

Introduction

It is well known that special and highly sophisticated medical treatment in university hospitals or other comprehensive general hospitals is essential for severely ill emergency patients. It is in practice, however, impossible to give adequate and satisfactory medical treatment for a number of reasons in Japan. The Ministry of Health and Welfare and other local authorities as well as the Japan Medical Association and Local Medical Associations are making every effort to establish critical care medical (CCM) centers in each community. Each functions as a central organization for emergency medical care in its community and gives adequate treatment to those patients with severe injury or life-threatening conditions.

In the present Japanese medical education curriculum, however, there has been little or no systematic training in critical care medicine nor in emergency medicine during the undergraduate or postgraduate courses. For this reason, it is quite likely that physicians who are actually working in the emergency medical care services in the local CCM centers or emergency medical care facilities may encounter difficulties due to inadequate training or experience.

Authors' CCM Center of Nippon Medical School was established, in cooperation with the Japan Fire Defence Agency, in April 1975. During the past 12 years since its foundation, the Center has been highly regarded by various parties with respect to its practice in this field.

Condition of Patients

In the CCM Center of Nippon Medical School, there is no outpatient department for the third level emergency patients. First to third level emergency patients and their related medical facilities are considered as follows:

First level emergency patient:
   Outpatients only (hospitalization unnecessary)
Second level emergency patient:
   Necessary for Hospitalization
   Operation performed, if necessary
Third level emergency patient:
   Necessary for cardio-pulmonary support, severe head trauma, extensive burns

There are 513 emergency facilities in Tokyo and our CCM Center is the one of the largest and oldest facilities in Japan (Fig. 1). Our Center has 35 beds includ-

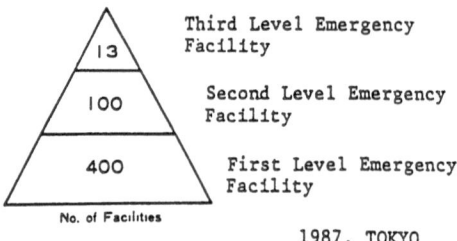

Third Level Emergency
Facility

Second Level Emergency
Facility

First Level Emergency
Facility

No. of Facilities

1987. TOKYO

population: about 12 million

Fig. 1. Number of emergency medical facilities in Tokyo

ing 4 beds of the burns unit, and only extremely severe patients can be admitted. During the 11 years from April 1, 1975 to March 31, 1987, 7409 patients were admitted to the Center: 5322 males and 2087 females. Of these 2054 died, the mortality being 27.7%. The mortality, excluding DOA (dead on arrival) cases, was 27.7%, and the average hospital stay were 9.4 days. When the patients were judged to be out of danger, they were transferred to the relevant department of the university hospital, the affiliated hospitals, or to the original medical institutions from where they had been admitted.

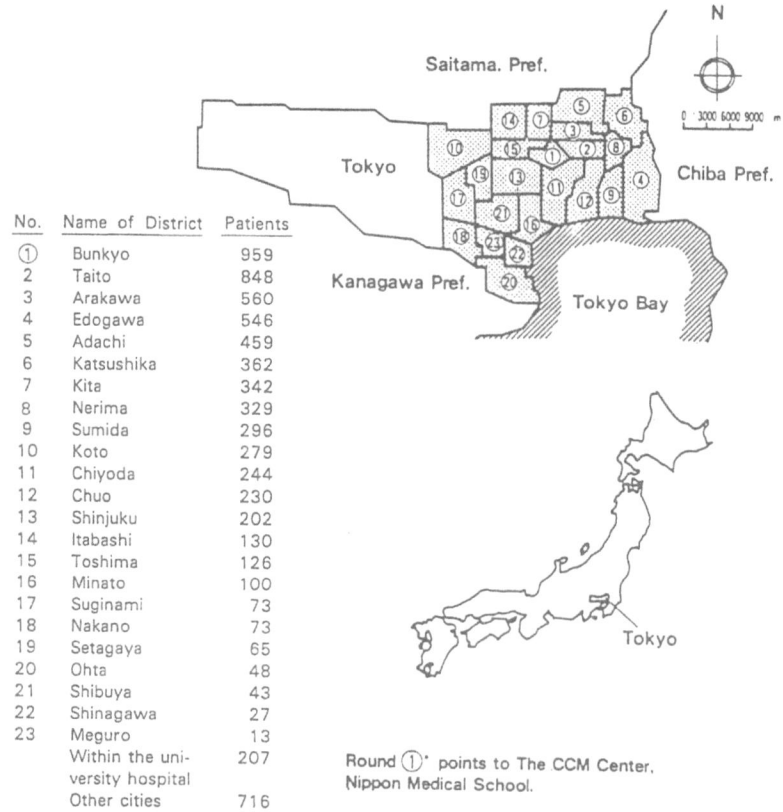

No.	Name of District	Patients
1	Bunkyo	959
2	Taito	848
3	Arakawa	560
4	Edogawa	546
5	Adachi	459
6	Katsushika	362
7	Kita	342
8	Nerima	329
9	Sumida	296
10	Koto	279
11	Chiyoda	244
12	Chuo	230
13	Shinjuku	202
14	Itabashi	130
15	Toshima	126
16	Minato	100
17	Suginami	73
18	Nakano	73
19	Setagaya	65
20	Ohta	48
21	Shibuya	43
22	Shinagawa	27
23	Meguro	13
	Within the university hospital	207
	Other cities	716

Round ① points to The CCM Center,
Nippon Medical School.

Fig. 2. Geographical source of patients (April 1975 – March 1987)

Geographical Source of Patients (Fig. 2)

The patients were admitted from all parts of Tokyo, but because of the locality of the Center, patients from the Jotoh Area (east part of Tokyo) accounted for a high percentage. In addition, patients were also received from the satellite towns in the surroundings of Tokyo or nearby prefectures. This indicates that the establishment of CCM centers in urgently needed in these areas.

When critically ill patients need to be admitted from the Izu Islands or the Pacific Ocean, they are transported by helicopters or rescue airplanes with the help of the Tokyo Fire Department or Japan Self Defence Force.

Classification by Diseases (Table 1)

Patients with various types of diseases were admitted. The breakdown shows that there were 3353 injuries including traffic accidents, industrial accidents, falls

Table 1. Classification of diseases and mortality (Dept. of Emergency and CCM, Nippon Medical School). (April 1975 to March 1987)

Disease	No. of Cases	%	No. of Deaths	%
Trauma	3353	45.3	743	22.2
Cerebro-vascular disorder	786	10.6	377	48.0
Burns	623	8.4	149	23.9
Acute abdomen (GI perforation, ileus, etc)	502	6.8	54	10.8
Acute poisoning	327	4.4	48	14.7
Death on arrival (Unknown cause)	283	3.8	255	90.1
Digestive tract bleeding	280	3.8	54	19.3
Acute respiratory failure	251	3.4	45	17.9
Acute circulatory failure	157	2.1	48	30.6
Asphyxia	95	1.3	39	41.1
Acute myocardial infarction	91	1.2	62	68.1
Severe infection (Meningitis, encephalitis, UTI, etc)	83	1.1	25	30.1
Mental disease	66	0.9	4	6.1
Vascular disease (Aneurysm, arterial occlusion)	56	0.8	28	50.0
Acute hepatic failure	47	0.6	20	42.6
Terminal stage of malignant disease	46	0.6	23	50.0
Renal failure (Acute or chronic)	41	0.6	18	43.9
Foreign body in the airway or digestive tract	39	0.5	3	7.7
Tetanus/gas gangrene	34	0.5	5	14.7
Near drowning	31	0.4	13	41.9
Diabetic coma	28	0.4	4	14.3
Gynecological disease	25	0.3	6	24.0
Heat stroke	11	0.1	2	18.1
Congenital anomaly	10	0.1	6	60.0
Caisson disease	7	0.1	0	0
Others	137	1.8	23	16.8
Total	7409	100.0	2054	27.7

or self inflicted injuries in intended suicide. These accounted for 45.3% followed by cerebrovascular diseases, extensive burns over 20% body surface area, acute abdomen, and acute poisoning. There were only 95 cases of acute myocardial infarction admitted to the general section of the CCM Center.

There is, however, a CCU within the CCM Center, which admits directly about 170 patients with acute myocardial infarction in a year.

Surgical Operation Rate (Table 2)

Of the total of 7409 patients, 2571 patients were subjected to some kind of operations or surgical procedure; the rate performance of operations was 34.7%, in which simultaneous multiple operations and repeated operations were included. The operative mortality was as high as 23.8%. It is a special characteristic of third level emergency centers that high risk patients need to undergo operations. Various types of operative procedures are necessary throughout the whole body from head to toe by CCM doctors ourselves.

Emergency Patient Delivery System

There are two methods of delivery of emergency patients: indirect delivery and direct delivery. The indirect delivery is that patients are referred through "First to second level emergency medical facilities" and the direct delivery is that patients are delivered directly to the Center by the Ambulance Emergency Technicial (AEMT). During the 11 years 3209 patients were sent by indirect delivery and 4200 patients were by direct delivery.

Table 2. Analysis of operations performed between April 1975 and March 1987

	No. of cases	(%)
Total No. of admissions	7409	
Operative procedures		
Neurosurgical	710	27.6
Thoracic	315	12.3
Abdominal	979	38.1
Orthopedic	440	17.1
Others	401	15.6
Total	2845	
Surgical operations	2571	34.7
Operative deaths	613	23.8

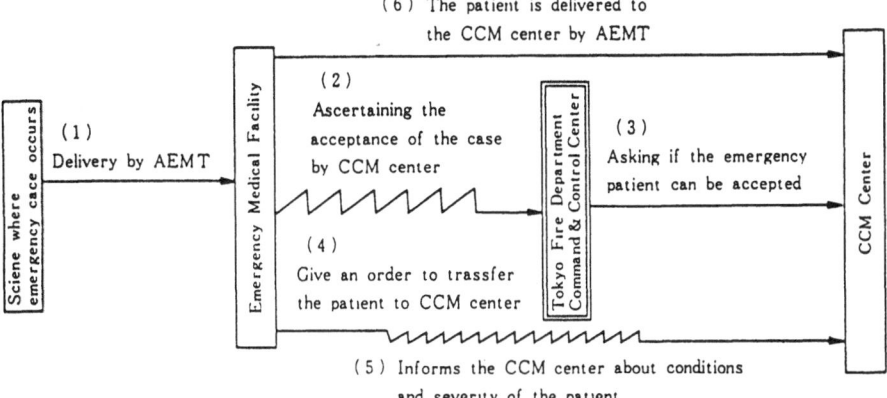

Fig. 3. Indirect delivery way: 3209 cases

Indirect Delivery System (Fig. 3)

1. AEMT of Tokyo Fire: Department sends the patient from the initial location to the nearest "emergency medical facility" where the patient is given the necessary primary medical treatment;
2. If the emergency physician thinks it necessary to send him/her to the CCM Center, the attending doctor contacts the Command and Control Center of Tokyo Fire Department while the primary treatment is being given;
3. The Command and Control Center immediately contacts the CCM Center to ascertain whether a patient can be accepted;
4. After confirming that the CCM Center is ready to accept the patient, the Command and control Center gives an order to the AEMT to transfer the patient to the CCM Center;
5. At the same time, the physician responsible for the primary treatment reports to the CCM Center concerning the condition or severity of the patient to be sent to the Center;
6. The patient is transferred to a CCM Center designated by the Command and Control Center.

Direct Delivery System (Fig. 4)

1. Upon arrival, the AEMT judges that the patient should be immediately delivered to the CCM Center, and
2. requests the CCM Center to accept the patient through the Command and Control Center;
3. The Command and Control Center informs AEMT of the result;
4. AEMT then delivers the patient directly to the CCM Center designated by the Command and Control Center.

494   Y. Yamamoto et al.

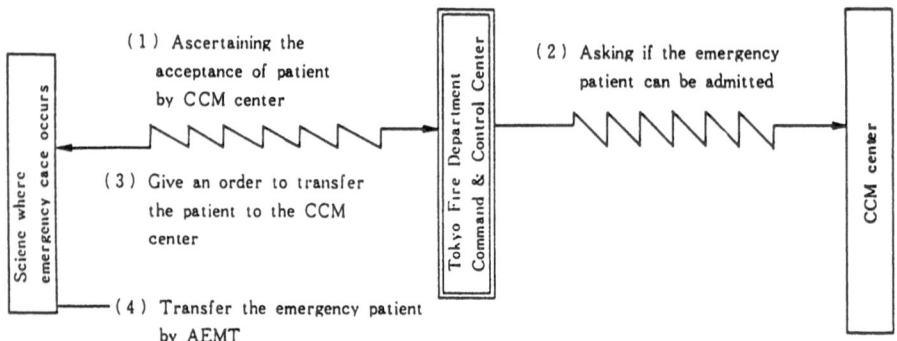

Fig. 4. Direct delivery way: 4200 cases

As shown above, patients are to be delivered to the CCM Center either by Method (1) or (2), so that a comprehensive communication net work is indispensable.

Urban Bomb Blast: Mechanisms of Injury and Principles of Management

C. J. van der Merwe

Introduction

A disaster is an emergency of such magnitude as to require extraordinary mobilization of emergency services [1]. As a sign of the times, the frequency of such disasters will inevitably increase [2–4]. The number of terrorist incident has steadily increased worldwide. From the beginning of 1976 up to 30 September 1986 there were 581 incidents in the Republic of South Africa (RSA) of which 492 (84.7%) involved explosive devices of some kind. There were 25 landmine incidents, 146 hand grenade attacks, 140 limpet mine blasts, 8 demolition mine explosions and 173 incidents caused by self-assembled explosion devices. Altogether 133 people died in these attacks [40]. The most devastating incident in the RSA was a bomb blast that occurred in Pretoria during 1983.

A bomb blast initiates one of the most fulminating of epidemics known to man with a point prevalence rate escalating from zero to maximum within a matter of seconds. It is imperative for clinicians and paramedical personnel involved in emergency care to have a sound knowledge of the mechanisms responsible for injuries and thus of the type of injuries that can be expected when a bomb blast occurs. This will ensure early recognition and management of the great variety of possible injuries, including the "not-so-obvious" serious injuries (Table 1).

Blast Dynamics

Several forces which have adverse effects on the human body come into effect when a charge of high explosives is detonated. Detonation of an explosive charge results in a high speed chemical decomposition of a solid or liquid explosive into a gas and the space previously occupied by the explosive is filled with gas under high pressure and with a high temperature [5–7].

High explosives such as trinitrotoluene (TNT) detonate rapidly and release large amounts of energy which generates enormous amounts of expanding gas. One gram of TNT releases 1120 calories of blast energy and, at the moment of detonation, generates pressures of approximately 10 psi within the initial gas [7]. The energy is released so rapidly and the pressures generated rise so quickly that objects in close proximity can be shattered by the force of the explosion. This shattering power is referred to as the "brisance effect" (Fig. 1). Brisance is the difference between high explosives and low (ordinary) explosives, like gunpowder, which releases its energy slowly and therefore does not possess brisance.

Table 1. Injuries possible in a bomb explosion

I. **Primary injuries**

Ear injuries:
Tympanic membrane rupture [18]
Dislocation of the ossicles
Inner ear injuries
Tinnitus
Sensorineural hearing loss (all frequencies)

Lung injuries:
a) Alveolar capillary membrane damage:
  Pulmonary edema (shock lung) [2]
  Intra alveolar hemorrhage [1]
b) Lung lacerations:
  Alveolar rupture (pulmonary hematoma and contusion) [7]
  Tearing of the visceral pleura [3]
  (pneumohemothorax and pneumomediastinum)
  Alveolar venous fistulae with air emboli (neurological abnormalities)

Intestinal injuries:
Serosal hemorrhages
Bowel perforations [2]

Central nervous system injuries:
Concussion [16]
Intracranial hemorrhage (seldom survive) [1]

Cardiovascular injuries:
Myocardial ischemia due to air emboli

II. **Secondary injuries**

Lacerations caused by glass, shrapnel etc.:
Penetrating wounds of the abdomen, thorax [3]
Foreign bodies embedded [16]
Large vessel injuries [1]

III. **Tertiary injuries**

Crush injuries:
Myocardial contusion [1]

Fractures of:
Skull, cervical vertebrae [4]
Extremities (closed, compound or amputations) [24]
Diaphragmatic rupture [1]
Abdominal injuries [3]
Thoracoabdominal injuries [3]

Acceleration-deceleration injuries:
Rupture of the thoracic aorta [1]

Primary Force (Shock Wave)

A very high pressure within the gas produced by detonation is the primary force
in a blast incident and forms the basis for the development of the shock wave
(primary force). The high pressure is transmitted to the surrounding medium e.g.

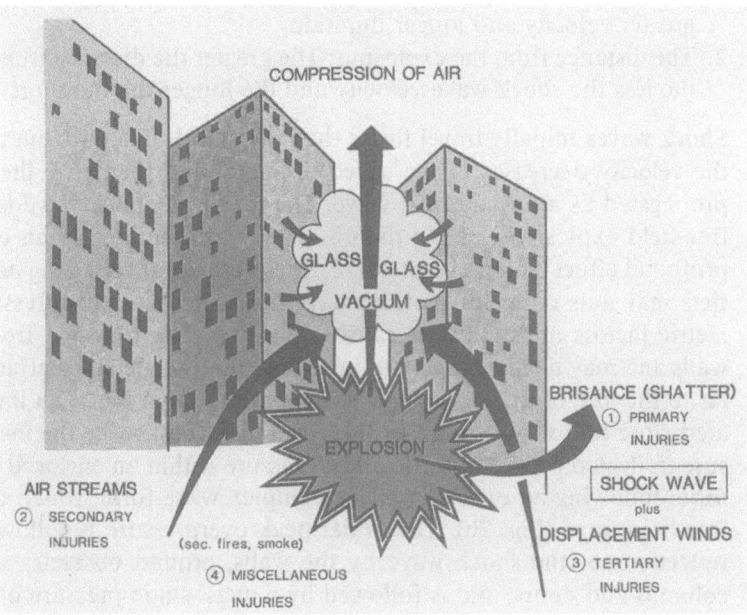

Fig. 1. Dynamics and mechanisms of injury caused by a bomb blast

air or water. The velocity and duration of the shock wave depends on the size of the explosive charge and the surrounding media, be it air or water. The lethal radius around an explosion in water is about three times what it would be in the air [8]. If the explosion occurs in free-field conditions, it is transmitted in the form of a layer of compressed air, which is propagated as a positive pressure wave or shock wave (primary force) that travels out radially at a very high intensity from the explosion [7]. The intensity of the positive pressure wave produced is measured in tens of thousands of atmospheres released within a thousandth of a second. Air is a medium of low density and high velocity, therefore the shock wave of an explosion in air expands faster than the speed of sound and its intensity decreases by a power of three of the distance from the center of the explosion [9].

Water, on the other hand, is of high density and explosions in water produce shock waves of greater peak pressure and longer duration [5, 10]. The shock wave travels at the corresponding speed of sound, which in water is 4 to 5 times faster than in air. Because of the higher peak pressures, the distance at which effects can occur is much greater than those for an explosion in the air. The idealized shock wave that is produced by overpressure in air under free-field conditions is a steep-fronted pulse that rises instantaneously to a maximum peak overpressure and then decays over a longer period (positive phase overpressure) to a minimum of less than the previous ambient (atmospheric) pressure. Thereafter, the environmental pressure returns to the normal baseline pressure (Fig. 2a). The velocity of the shock wave and the duration of the positive overpressure component is determined by two factors:

1. The size of the explosive charge: Bigger explosions produce shock waves of greater velocity and longer duration.
2. The distance from the explosion: The greater the distance from the explosion, the less the shock wave velocity and the longer the duration.

Shock waves initially travel faster than the speed of sound, but as they expand, the velocity decreases to the speed of sound and thereafter the shock wave is propagated as an accoustical wave. The idealized shock wave is found only in free-field explosions, as the nature of the surroundings of an explosion has a profound effect on the overpressure. The presence of reflecting or absorbing barriers may thus radically alter the wave form and peak overpressure. These geometric factors are critical, because a blast wave is reflected from surfaces e.g. walls and may be magnified two- to three-fold by reflecting surfaces perpendicular to the line of travel. It can thus be expected that when an individual is situated close to a wall he may be subjected to at least twice the incident overpressure (reflected pressure) [6]. The overpressure within an enclosed space such as a room following an explosion has a complex wave form, which differs from the free-field form (Fig. 2b). The initial peak overpressure is followed by multiple reflections of the shock wave by the walls, around obstacles such as people, columns and doors, and is followed by a quasi-static pressure of long duration,

a

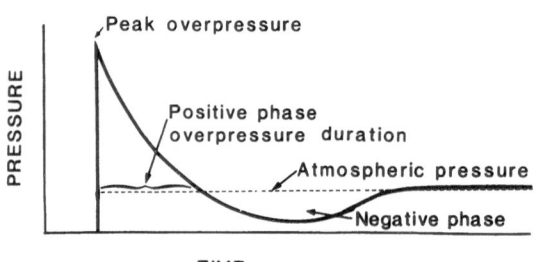

b

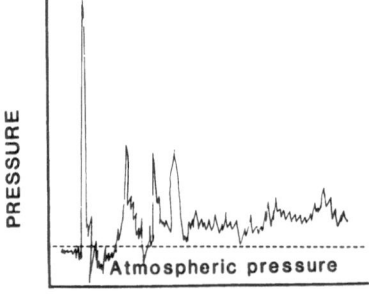

Fig. 2a, b. Blast overpressure in air. a An idealized shock front resulting from the detonation of an explosive under free-field conditions. b A pressure/time profile following an explosion in an enclosed space the intensity and duration of which are dependent upon the size of the room and the degree of venting through doors and windows. These factors create not only a complex wave form, but also cause variations in the peak overpressure and durations to which people are subjected at various positions in the room. The effect of the reflection depends on the strength of the incoming wave and how the surface is orientated to the direction of travel of the shock wave [11]. A blast wave that will cause only modest primary injury in the open can be lethal if the victim stands near a reflecting surface, such as a wall [12].

Secondary Force (Displacement Wave)

Air is compressed during the positive pressure phase of the shock wave, which results in the creation of a vacuum (negative pressure) with a suction effect behind the shock wave. The displacement wave is the result of the pressure variations and the vacuum that is produced by the shock wave [13] (Fig. 1). High velocity displacement air streams (waves or winds) can be produced by even small changes in pressure due to the low density of air. A peak pressure of 0,25 psi corresponds to a wind velocity of 125 mph (200 km/hour). Although loose objects can be accelerated by the shock wave itself, the ultimate velocity is determined by the corresponding displacement wave velocity. The high velocity of the displacement wave results in the rapid acceleration of light objects or debris over short distances, and they can reach a high speed even at low peak pressures [14]. Because water is denser than air, the displacement wave in water has a very low velocity and rarely produces significant damage.

Mechanisms of Blast Injuries

The mechanisms of blast injuries have been discussed by many researchers [5, 15–17), and they are related to the effects of the shock wave (causing primary and tertiary injuries), the effects of the displacement waves (causing secondary injuries) and various miscellaneous effects, e.g. smoke and gas inhalation and burns by secondary fires (causing miscellaneous injuries).

Effects of the Shock Wave (Fig. 3)

A shock wave can damage living tissue by four mechanisms, spalling, implosion, pressure differentials (all of which are responsible for primary injuries) (Fig. 3) and acceleration-deceleration, which is responsible for tertiary injuries [5].

Spalling: Spalling occurs when a shock wave reaches an interface between media of different densities e.g. blood and air in the lung. At the interface of the different non-homogeneous density media of the body tissues, it causes reflec-

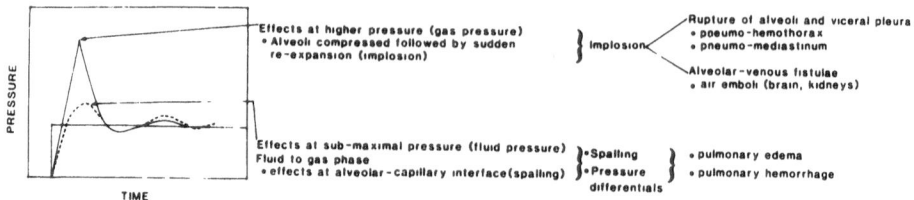

Fig. 3. Pulmonary effects of a shock wave

tion which creates turbulence. As a result of turbulence, the surface between the media is disrupted, and particles of fluid are thrown from the more dense medium (vascular) into the less dense medium (air) (fluid-to-gas phase). This is similar to the phenomenon witnessed when a depth charge explodes under water and the surface erupts into a shower of drops. As the shock wave travels through tissue containing both liquid and gas, particles are spalled into the gaseous compartment, causing e.g. pulmonary edema.

Implosion: As the shock travels through a gas-containing organ such as the lung, each gas pocket can be compressed. The gas is compressed to an extremely small volume by the pressure effect of the surrounding fluid, thereby absorbing a substantial amount of energy. As soon as the shock wave has passed, the energy is released and a rebound expansion of each gas pocket takes place, causing minute secondary internal explosions which may result in lung lacerations, lung hematomas, pneumo- or hemothorax, pneumomediastinum and air emboli (gas-to-fluid phase).

Pressure differentials: At the moment of impact of a shock wave upon a victim, a difference in pressure may evolve between the outer body surface and the internal organs. The pressure on the exterior and within the fluid-containing tissues and vascular system remains equal. However, the alveolar gas is easily compressible and at the moment of impact of a shock wave, a pressure differential may exist between the vascular system and the alveoli, and blood is forced from the pulmonary edema and hemorrhage seen in primary injuries.

Acceleration-deceleration: Acceleration-deceleration injuries occur as the victim is either accelerated away from an explosion or impacted against a stationary solid object. Organs with different densities, masses or attachments may be accelerated at different rates, causing tears at the pedicles (e.g. liver and spleen) or at the attachments of structures (e.g. thoracic aorta) due to a shearing motion. This mechanism is significant in causing tertiary blast injuries. The instantaneous acceleration of large objects is less, but may be significant if it is close to an explosion. For a typical adult of 75 kg, a peak pressure of 15 psi from an explosion can produce an instantaneous acceleration of 137 m/sec (approximately 14 gravities). For common terrorist bombs the acceleration would last only a few milliseconds and the victim would reach only a low ultimate velocity. This differs from explosions from nuclear devices, where the very long period of the positive pressure component of the shock wave means that a significant time exists in which to accelerate the victim [18]. The instantaneous acceleration itself is usually tolerable for the victim, but when the victim impacts a hard stationary object, damage is done by the force of the sudden deceleration.

Extrapolation of animal experiments to a 75 kg man predicts a 50% mortality from a vertical impact against a flat, concrete surface at a velocity of 30 km/hour [14]. Impacts of 3.4 to 4.9 m/sec) onto hard surfaces with the knees locked can produce fractures of the lower extremities [18]. Impacts of 4.6 to 7 m/sec can cause skull fractures [20].

Effects of the Displacement Wave

Rapid acceleration of debris and small fragments by displacement waves is a major factor in secondary blast injuries. Small fragments of debris are commonly accelerated to velocities of several hundred feet per second and are thus converted into high velocity missiles that are responsible for secondary injuries. The skin is easily lacerated by small missiles with velocities of 1.24 m/s, and with velocities of 121 m/s, serious wounds, including penetration of body cavities, are seen [18]. The abovementioned velocities are commonly produced by terrorist bombs. Most of the morbidity from terrorist explosions is caused by secondary injuries as a result of flying glass, shrapnel and debris.

Classification of Blast Injuries

Around any explosion there are concentric zones of injury [16] (Fig. 4). Although many factors, as have been discussed, are important in determining the type of injury, the major determinant is the position of the victim in relation to the explosion. Injuries caused by explosions are commonly classified into four catego-

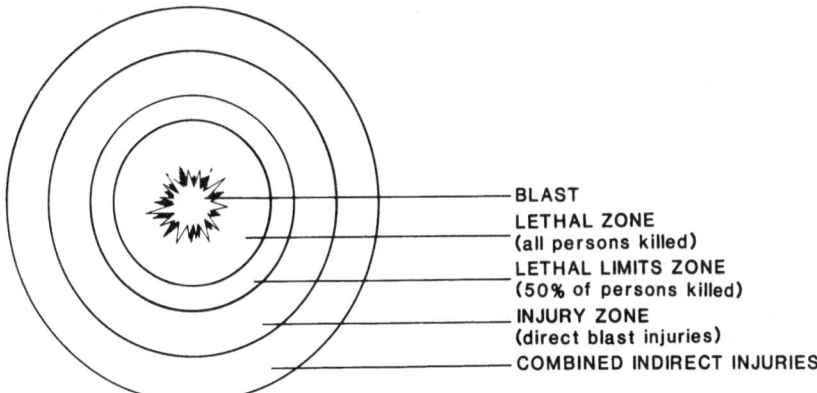

Fig. 4. Concentric zones of injury around any explosion

ries: viz. primary, secondary, tertiary and miscellaneous injuries. A great variety of injuries are possible (Table 1).

Primary Blast Injuries

This category includes all injuries inflicted by the sudden changes in environmental pressure due to the shock wave. Direct exposure to the blast of air is a requirement for these types of injuries. Most organs are, however, virtually incompressible and therefore little or no internal changes or displacements take place. The organs most commonly affected by primary blast injuries are the ears, lungs, bowel, central nervous system and cardiovascular system [21].

Ear injuries: Primary blast injury to the ear results in rupture of the tympanic membrane at 5 psi. The shape of the perforations are either "punched-out" or "slit-like" [22–24]. Eardrum ruptures are extremely common due to the low pressure that is required to inflict this injury [25]. In one study 18% of bomb blast victims had perforations and 36.9% presented with ear complaints [22]. In the Pretoria bomb blast incident we found that 18 of 27 seriously injured victims (66%) had perforated tympanic membranes [40]. The frequency of ear injuries and the possibility that they might go undetected, make it imperative for all injured victims to be examined by an ear specialist at the earliest opportunity. Although the most common effect on the ear is rupture of the tympanic membrane, dislocation of the ossicles is also occasionally found [24]. Fortunately, most ruptured tympanic membranes heal spontaneously. The inner ear can be damaged at pressures that are insufficient to rupture the tympanic membrane. The initial sensorial deafness caused by the damage recovers spontaneously quite rapidly and sufficiently for normal speech frequencies. Tinnitus usually presents in most of the victims experiencing deafness and it generally disappears at the recovery of hearing [24].

Pulmonary injuries: Lung damage is the result of pressure differentials which cause inward displacement of the chest wall towards the spinal column, similar to displacement due to impact of a non-penetrating missile. The lungs become compressed, not only by the chest wall moving towards the vertebral column, but also by the upward thrust of the diaphragm due to compression of the abdominal wall [26]. This mechanism leads to a high transient overpressure within the thoracic cavity, causing the tearing of alveolar septae [27] and creating alveolar-venous fistulae [28]. Zuckerman's theory proposes that positive pressure is transmitted directly down through the tracheo-bronchial tree into the lungs, causing rupture of the alveoli and capillaries [29].

Whatever the mechanism, primary blast injuries to the lungs occur at 15 psi and produce damage to alveolar parenchyma (edema) and hemorrhage into the interstitial and intra-alveolar spaces [9, 26, 39–34]. The results of this pulmonary hermorrhage and alveolar wall destruction can be summarized as follows: bleeding into the airways [25], contusion with infiltration and edema formation [45] and pulmonary edema due to imbalance in the fluxes of fluid across the damaged alveolar-capillary gas exchange membrane [27] (Fig. 3). Lacerations can occur at any site in the lung tissue. Rupture of the alveolar wall and tearing the visceral pleura can result in pneumothorax, pneumomediastinum, hemothorax and intrapulmonary hematomas [30].

The clinical picture of a victim with a blast injury is remarkably consistent for 24–48 hours, but it eventually results in respiratory distress and hypoxia. During the initial period the patient shows few signs of respiratory distress and the blood gas analysis may be normal [26]. After an initial period, signs and symptoms such as dyspnea, coughing, rhonchi, crepitations in both lung fields, hemoptysis, chest pain and varying degrees of cyanosis may set in [30]. Tachypnea is usually present [31].

Respiratory failure that develops a few days after exposure to a blast may also be due to factors other than blast effects. These may include fat embolism syndrome, fluid overload, aspiration pneumonia, or a combination of these factors [29]. It is important to note that although the clinical picture of bomb victims with primary lung injuries may initially not reveal pulmonary injury, radiological evidence of pulmonary contusion and edema can be detected as early as 2 to 4 hours and reveals marked changes 8 to 11 hours after the blast in spite of a relatively benign clinical presentation. The initial X-rays are thus more impressive than the initial clinical picture. It is therefore important that all victims who have been in the injury zone, even though they may appear clinically satisfactory, should be admitted to hospital for control X-rays and observation [32].

Bowel injuries: The bowel is gas-containing, with pockets of gas especially present in the colon. For this reason the bowel can be injured by the same mechanisms as described for blast lung and may present with serosal hemorrhages and tears [30]. However, air blast injury is less likely to produce gastrointestinal injury. In most fatal cases reported, pulmonary injury occurs, leaving the probably gastro-intestinal injuries undetected. Most reported cases of blast injury to the gastrointestinal tract have occurred in underwater blast incidents [36, 37]. It must however be noted that secondary and tertiary forces can cause bowel perforations (Table 1).

Central nervous system involvement: Brain injury can occur due to the effects of a shock wave causing hemorrhages in the meninges, brain substance and nerve roots [38]. Unconsciousness may be caused by brain contusion and neurological manifestations due to air emboli [32, 35]. The admission of unconscious victims with brain damage despite normal X-rays has been reported [25]. The precise mechanism of head injuries is often difficult to determine because either secondary forces (e.g. fallen masonry) or tertiary forces (the victim impacts a hard stationary object) may be responsible. Victims with intracerebral hematomas rarely survive.

Cardiovascular system involvement: Air embolism in the coronary artery (and cerebral vessels) has been reported [30].

Secondary Blast Injuries

The majority of victims of a bomb blast present with secondary injuries which include lacerations by glass, shrapnel lacerations and other missiles, penetrating wounds by the abovementioned missiles, embedded foreign bodies, fractures and amputations of extremities. Fortunately the majority of the victims usually sustain only trivial injuries. Out of 1532 victims reported in one study only 250 (16%) required admission. (Nine of those that were admitted died and there were approximately 50 deaths before admission) [39].

Tertiary Blast Injuries

These injuries are caused by acceleration-deceleration. The victims are situated in the lethal and lethal limit zones (Fig. 4). If the victim is impacted against a stationary solid object it may result in various crush injuries e.g. fractures of the ribs, pelvis, extremities, skull and cervical spine or injury to thoracic and abdominal organs. In addition, serious damage may result from the deceleration e.g. rupture of the thoracic aorta and shearing of the pedicles of solid abdominal organs with resultant hemorrhage.

Miscellaneous Blast Injuries

These include flash burns caused by the explosion and burns of various degrees due to secondary fires. Exposure to dust and smoke inhalation occur frequently. The inhalation of the smoke of incinerating synthetic material is especially damaging to the lungs. Burns of the upper respiratory tract must be considered a possibility in large explosions.

Injury Profile of the Pretoria Incident

Comparative Results

The Pretoria explosion of 1983 killed 17 people outright and injured a further 204, one of whom died of exsanguination from a severed femoral artery and other injuries shortly after admission. A second victim succumbed on the 5th day from multiple severe injuries, bringing the death rate to 8.6%. The death rate in patients reaching the hospital alive in this series was 1.0% (N = 204) [41] as compared with 0.6% in Belfast [39] and 2.5% in Birmingham incidents [40].

The 202 survivors (treated in 3 different hospitals) suffered 453 injuries, documented according to the Injury Coding Manual (ICM), 1980 [42].

Skin lacerations comprised 214 (47.2%) of all the documented injuries, with exposed areas of the body being particularly at risk. Apart from lacerations, the only other specific injuries reaching a frequency exceeding one per cent were perforation of the tympanic membrane (18; 4.0%), physiological stress (15; 3.3%)

and compound fractures of the lower leg (1.3%). There were 13 (2.9%) eye injuries recorded which included 4 lacerations, 5 perforations and 2 ruptures of the eyeball. In Birmingham, the proportion of ruptured tympanic membranes was 18.0% (n = 111) [22]. Abdominal injuries comprised 6 (1.3%).

The ISS classification [43] of 203 injured were as follows: 0–24 (194; 95.6%), 25–49 (7; 3.4%) and 50–74 (2; 1.0%).

The patients in the last group, of whom one died and one survived, both scored 66. At the Emergency Department, 6 (3.0%) patients were intubated and ventilated mechanically, 8 (4.0%) required central venous monitoring and 3 (1.5%) required intercostal drainage. Blood was administered to 21 (10.4%) patients.

In an Israeli report, only 3.6% of patients needed a blood transfusion [44]. Ninety seven patients (48%), including all the seriously injured, were admitted to the H F Verwoerd Hospital in Pretoria. Laparotomy was performed in 8 (4.0%) patients for the following injuries: ruptured spleen (1), ruptured livers (2), ruptured diaphragm (1) and perforations of the bowel (3). In one patient the laparotomy was negative. Isolated nerve injuries necessitating exploration and repair occurred in 2 (1.0%) patients and vascular injury (excluding amputations) in 5 (2.5%). There were 42 fractures amongst 24 (11.9%) patients, of which 26 (61.9%) were compound, hence a mean of 1.75 fractures per patient. This is comparable to a mean of 1.2 and 1.5 fractures per patient in Bologna [45] and Belfast [46], respectively. In the Belfast series 4.6% of patients suffered fractures [39]. If the distribution of permanent disability following the bomb blast in Pretoria [40] and Belfast [35] is compared, it is noted that in Pretoria the proportion of permanently disabled (10.8%) was significantly greater (p < 0.001) than in Belfast (4.0%). The individual disabilities, with the exception of permanent limp, are, however, remarkably similar, although the numbers are too small for meaningful statistical comparison. In the Pretoria bomb blast incident, the causes and approximate percentages of fatalities were [40]: brain damage 30%, multiple injuries 55%, blood loss 10%, burns 5%.

The most common factors observed in bomb blast fatalities in Northern Ireland (8/1969–8/1977) were [27]: brain damage (66%), skull fractures (51%), diffuse contusion (47%), eardrum rupture (45%), liver lacerations (34%).

Discussion of Injury Profiles and Course

Bomb blasts kill mainly through brain injury (with or without skull fracture), lung contusion, or lacerations of the liver [25, 27] and up to 25% of the dead and severely wounded will sustain some kind of traumatic amputation [47]. Only a very small proportion of deaths will occur after admission [39, 41] and the large majority of these will be unavoidable. Admission rate vary greatly [39, 41, 44, 45], but 15% to 25% seems to be a fair figure [27, 39, 41], with the most common causes for admission being fractures, burns and concussion. In other series [40, 48] burn injuries were rare. The incidence of flash burns, fractures and soft tissue damage will be higher if an explosion occurs in a confined space [27, 49]. One third of all patients will have head injuries and a further third will also sustain injuries to the legs [48]. Although only 10% of injuries will be to the trunk, of which only 10% will be penetrating [48], these constitute a large proportion of the fatal injuries [25].

Primary "blast lung" in surviving patients is rare [29, 39, 47]. A very high frequency of tinnitus, temporary (and sometimes permanent) deafness and perforation of the tympanic membrane occurs [22, 27]. Most perforations involving less than 80% of the tympanic membrane surface will heal spontaneously while the remaining will need intervention, usually after 6 months [24]. Permanent hearing loss over the speech frequency range will occur in 5% of patients with initial sensorineural impairment [24].

When fractures occur they are often multiple, and of 107 cases, 58% of trunk and limb fractures and 28% of skull fractures were compound [39]. Up to 70% of fractures may develop wound infection [46].

The most common injuries remain skin lacerations and contusions, with the legs and head suffering the most [39]. Tetanus following injury due to civil war violence is rare [50]. Psychological effects of civil violence have been described by Lyons [51] and Sims et al. [52].

In all bomb blast incidents that occurred in the United Kingdom from 1951 to 1971, 50 or more cases were admitted on only 5 occasions and on only 21 occasions were more than 15 but fewer than 50 patients admitted [1]. In 78 explosions, only 13 (16.8%) resulted in more than 20 patients being brought to hospital or more than two patients being admitted [53]. A large regional hospital should be able to deal comfortably with 15 acute admissions without activating a disaster plan.

Principles of Management

Management at the Site of the Incident

Sorting is one of the most important functions of the pre-hospital care provider and it is the responsibility of the most senior and most experienced of the team (Table 2). Sorting entails determining by necessity which patients require immediate resuscitation (life-threatening injuries) (Priority I), which patients are urgent but can wait if necessary (Priority II) and those who must wait if necessary (Priority III). In a multiple casualty incident, e.g. the Pretoria bomb blast with 204 injured [40], it was impractical for the pre-hospital care team to assess patients precisely according to an injury severity index, because the transportation time to the main receiving hospital was only 6 minutes. However, it is of paramount importance for Priority I patients to be recognized and stabilized immediately so that they can be transported to the hospital first. Even when a pre-hospital care provider has been trained in advanced life support, the time spent at the scene should be limited to the minimum required to provide the patient with an adequate airway, ventilation, circulation (e.g. M.A.S.T. application) and immobilization of fractures prior to transportation. The immobilization of major fractures is essential for several reasons. It reduces pain and thus shock, reduces

Table 2. Principles of determining priorities in a catastrophe ("Sorting" or categorizing of victims)

Priority I (Emergencies)
A. Require immediate resuscitation and immediate surgical intervention e.g. major vascular injuries.
B. Require immediate resuscitation, but surgical intervention can be somewhat delayed, e.g. splenic rupture, respiratory insufficiency with other reparable injuries, shock and maxillary injuries.

Priority II (Semi-emergencies)
Serious injuries that are not immediately life-threatening e.g. long bone fractures.

Priority III
Relatively minor injuries that require hospitalization.

Priority IV
Minor injuries that can be treated.

Priority V
Patients with massive injuries that have been classified as unsalvageable e.g. 80% burns and extensive open brain injuries.

---

blood loss and thus shock, lowers the incidence of post-traumatic fat embolism and prevents further local tissue damage.

The management will be influenced by the number of injured persons, the number of pre-hospital care providers and the distance to an appropriate facility (transportation time). If the distance to the receiving hospital is short, all that will probably be necessary will be sorting, ensuring an open airway, instituting ventilation if indicated and rapid transportation to the receiving facility where intravenous therapy can be instituted under more ideal conditions. In severely shocked victims, stabilization of the circulatory status must, however, be achieved prior to transportation.

Patients with a clear airway can be adequately ventilated by positive mask ventilation. A well-fitting mask and bag and ventilation with 100% oxygen provide excellent oxygenation of the blood. If any doubt exists as to the adequacy of ventilation, an endotracheal airway should be inserted and ventilation administered using a bag-valve device. A direct airway (cricothyrotomy) may rarely be necessary. Patients with head injuries should be hyperventilated initially and during transportation, in an attempt to decrease intracranial pressure by decreasing the $PaCO_2$ [66].

Where patient can be rapidly evacuated, formal triage, documentation or treatment (other than life saving procedures) should not be performed on the site [1, 54–60]. Metropolitan areas with sophisticated facilities may send doctors to the site as a routine [56, 61–63]. Triage stations near the site are necessary only if the disaster is of catastrophic proportions or if a long delay in evacuation is inevitable [60]. The area must be cordoned off immediately, by the police or military; crowds must be controlled and law and order maintained [63, 64].

The only documentation needed at the site is that of drugs administered. These can be written on the triage tag or on the patient's forehead [3]. Triage at the site should be done according to vital signs [3] to determine the priority of victims. If no doctor is present, the senior ambulance officer at the site can decide on the priority and destination of the evacuees [2, 55, 63]. A standardized [65] colour tag may be employed [2, 63]. Health care workers at a disaster site should also be easily recognizable [2, 63]. An emergency vehicle assembly area should be established near the site, from which all vehicles can be controlled. The critically injured should be transported in specialized ambulances, which should include those of the private sector [64]; the seriously injured should be transported in standard ambulances, and patients with minor injuries can be transported in minibuses or by private vehicles. The three systems can operate independently and simultaneously. Medical rescue teams are usually only needed if victims are trapped [55]. Traffic police must ensure an open lane for ambulances [63, 66] and must seal off the feeder road to the Hospital at its nearest junctions. Attempts to control traffic at the hospital entrance gate will only result in chaos. The police or military will immediately sweep the area for additional explosive devices, as it has become fashionable to arrange for a second and even bigger explosion to coincide with the maximum expected crowd gathering.

Management in the Emergency Department

Sorting and stabilization constitute the first steps in the management of emergencies [66] (Table 2). All patients should be directed to one of the following areas [59, 60, 66, 67]: Ambulant patients treatment areas, admission area, intensive care area, resuscitation area, operating room or the mortuary. The initial management should be carried out by way of the Emergency Department [1] and the normal routine should be followed where possible [59].

The most common causes of death associated with bomb blast injuries are inadequate airway or breathing, organ injuries and inadequate circulation as a result of massive blood loss. In patients with multiple injuries, treatment of these aspects is top priority and the initial management in the Emergency Department rests on five principles:

1. Re-sorting (categorization) (Table 2). Priority I patients should be divided into two groups: those requiring immediate surgical intervention and those where surgical intervention can be delayed after evaluation and stabilization if necessary. Other categories are shown in Table. 2.
2. Resuscitation: Evaluation and stabilization of the vital signs.
3. Evaluation of the injuries: Details of the injuries are necessary for resuscitation and the immediate management of life-threatening problems.
4. Planning for definitive management.
5. Continued life support and surveillance until the patient has reached the operating room or the intensive care unit.

Priorities in resuscitation are: ensuring adequate ventilation, ensuring adequate micro-circulation, management of life-threatening injuries, correction of acid-base disturbances, treatment of pain and restlessness, prevention of hypothermia and prevention and treatment of coagulation abnormalities. The essential steps in the initial care of the severely injured victims are outlined in Table 3.

Controversy exists as to the method of ventilation of patients with blast injuries to the lung and as to the need for prophylactic bilateral pleural drainage when the patient is mechanically ventilated. However, the intra-alveolar edema and hemorrhage plus alveolar atelectasis (from plugging of the bronchioles with blood clot) with blast injuries to the lungs probably result in a decrease in functional residual capacity (FRC), a lowering of the ventilation/perfusion ratio (V/Q) and an increase in right-to-left shunting (non-ventilated alveoli). This may be severe enough to result in acute respiratory failure. The objective of treatment is to restore arterial blood gases to near normal until the lungs have recovered. This may require positive pressure ventilation (PPV) with variable oxygen concentrations. The dangers of this procedure are the possibility of introducing air into the pulmonary veins thru alveolar-venous fistulae [32] and that patients are liable to develop a pneumothorax. However, it must be noted that a substantial part of the pressure required during PPV to inflate the lungs is dissipated in overcoming the concomitant increased resistance in the bronchial tree, and also that pressure changes in the alveoli are reduced and it is even less in those alveoli which are damaged because they are filled with blood. For these reasons, some authors are of the opinion that it is unlikely that PPV will increase the risk of air embolism in the management of blast injuries to the lung, but that regular examination for sequelae of air emboli is indicated e.g.: focal neurological signs, ECG evidence of transient myocardial ischemia, or opthalmoscopy, which may reveal air bubbles in the retinal arteries [35]. Continuous positive pressure venti-

Table 3. Initial care of severely injured victims

1. Secure airway
   Oxygen by mask; endotracheal intubation; mechanical ventilation as indicated
2. Peripheral venous lines (2 or more)
   Crystalloid/colloid solutions; blood; drugs
3. Central venous line
   Serial CVP measurements
4. Chest X-ray
   Routine; 100 cm for assessment of mediastinum (preferably sitting up)
5. Chest drains if indicated
6. Blood gas analyses
   Arterial line
7. Bladder catheter inserted
   Consider urethrogram prior to catheterization
   Measure urine output; test for blood
8. Naso-gastric tube
9. Other X-rays as indicated:
   Skull and cervical spine
   Urogram
   Extremities
   Angiography

lation (CPPV) has been advocated, but it carries the same dangers of air embolism and pneumothorax. The question also arises as to whether the advantages of PEEP (improvement in arterial oxygenation with lower oxygen concentration by clearing fluid-filled alveoli or opening up collapsed alveoli) outweigh the disadvantages (hemodynamic deterioration). CPPV is advocated by several authors [26, 31] and a case has been made for prophylactic pleural drainage [31] but others and ourselves suggest careful monitoring as this procedure is not without complications [35].

There is no other specific treatment for blast injuries to the lung. Removal of blood and secretions from the tracheo-bronchial tree is important. Administration of steroids has been advocated [26] and methylprednisolone was given to some patients by Caseby and Porter [35]. It is standard practice in our unit to administer methylprednisolone sodium succinate (Solu-Medrol) to all severely injured patients as prophylaxis against possible adult respiratory distress syndrome (ARDS) [68, 69]. In blast victims with multiple secondary injuries, tertiary injuries and burns, infections are a major hazard [35]. Septic shock is a contraindication for steroid administration and it should probably not be administered to blast victims because they have a high risk of secondary infections.

Hypovolemia due to blood or plasma loss as a result of other injuries should be monitored and corrected, as hypovolemia may result in a fall in cardiac output and a decrease in the systemic venous saturation, which will aggravate any existing hypoxia due to lung damage [33]. If the heart function is normal, the circulatory blood volume should be assessed by monitoring the CVP response to the administration of 200 ml fluid over 10 minutes (fluid challenge) if hypovolemia is suspected.

Conclusion

Several important conclusions can be drawn:

1. In a bomb blast various mechanisms may cause injury and each mechanism can be responsible for specific injuries. It is imperative that the clinician remains acutely suspicious of all the possible entities in blast casualties.
2. The number of victims will depend on several factors, viz.
   a) Size of the TNT charge.
   b) Locality and surrounding environment (open field, enclosed area and possible reflecting surfaces).
   c) The number of persons in the area.
   d) Distance of victims from the explosion.
   e) Clothing worn in the event of "flash" and other burns.
3. The majority of victims usually only require treatment for superficial soft-tissue damage, but victims in the injury zone are usually seriously injured.
4. Every victim should undergo a careful, painstaking examination to evaluate for all the possible injuries that can be associated with a bomb blast incident. All the victims who were situated in the balst affected area should be admit-

ted for a 24–48 hour observation period to recognize the delayed development of e.g. a "blast lung" in victims.

The presence of blunt abdominal injury may not be evident initially and monitoring and repeated re-examination of the abdomen is usually necessary to come to a diagnosis.

5. Flash burns, fractures, serious soft-tissue damage and tympanic membrane ruptures are the predominant injuries in victims close to the blast.

6. "Blast lung" is uncommon in explosions of small magnitude but it may be significant in explosions from larger explosive charges, especially if they occur is an enclosed space.

7. Brain injury is the most common injury seen in the fatally wounded.

8. Sorting and, if indicated, stabilization at the site of the incident and after admission to the Emergency Department are important aspects of the management of blast victims.

References

1. Rutherford WH (1973) Experience in the Accident and Emergency Department of the Royal Victoria Hospital with patients from civil disturbances in Belfast 1969–1972, with a review of disasters in the United Kingdom 1951–1971. Injury 4:189–199

2. Baker FJ (1980) Hospital physician's role in disaster planning and in management of the disaster site: the City of Chicago disaster plan. In: Frey R, Safar P (eds) Types and event of disasters organization in various disaster situations. Springer, Berlin Heidelberg New York, pp 247–253

3. MacMahon AG (1985) Sorting out triage in urban disasters. S Afr Med J 67:555–556

4. Cowley RA, Myers RAM, Gretes AJ (1984) EMS response to mass casualties. Emerg Med Clin North Am 2:687–693

5. Schardin H (1950) The physical priniciples of the effects of detonation. In: German Aviation Medicine, World War II; 2: Washington DC, US Government Printing Office, pp 1207–1224

6. Cook MA (1958) Shock waves in gaseous and condensed media. In: The Sciences of High Explosives. Reinhold Publishing Corp New York, chap. 13, pp 322–352

7. Kinney GA (1962) Explosive Shocks in Air. New York, The MacMillan Co.

8. Benzinger T (1950) Physiological effects of blast in air and water. German Aviation Medicine, World War II; 2: Washington, DC, US Government Printing Office

9. Hirsch M, Bazini J (1969) Blast injury of the chest. Clin Radiol 20:362–370

10. Rawlins JSP (1978) Physical and pathophysiological effects of blast. Injury 9:313–320

11. Swisdak MM (1975) Explosion effects and properties, Part I – Explosion effects in air. NSWC/WOL/TR 75-116, White Oak Laboratory, Naval Surface Weapons Center, White Oak, Silver Spring, Maryland pp 1–139

12. White CS, Jones RK, Damon EG, et al (1971) The biodynamics of airblast. Report DNA. Washington, DC, US Government Printing Office, 2738T, p 1–124

13. White, CS (1959) Biological blast effects. US Atomic Energy Commission Technical Report TID-5564. Albuquerque, Lovelace Foundation for Medical Education and Research

14. Stapczynski JS (1982) Blast injuries. Ann Emerg Med 11:687–694

15. De Candole LA (1967) Blast injury. Can Med Assoc J 96:207

16. Hamit HF (1973) Primary blast injuries. Ind Med 42:14

17. White CS, Richmond DR (1959) Blast biology, Washington DC, US Atomic Energy Commission Report, Tid-5764

18. White CS (1961) Biological effects of blast. Defense Atomic Support Agency Report DASA-1271. Albuquerque, Lovelace Foundation for Medical Education and Research

19. Richmond DR, Bowen IG, White CS (1961) Tertiary blast effects: Effects of impact on mice, rats, guinea pigs, and rabbits. Aerospace Med 32:789–805

20. Gurdjian ES (1975) Deformation studies of the skull: Mechanisms of skull fracture, in Impact Head Injury. Springfield Charles C Thomas pp 113–138

21. Chiffelle TL (1966) Pathophysiology of direct air-blast injury. Defense Atomic Support Agency Report DASA-1778. Albuquerque, Lovelace Foundation for Medical Education and Research

22. Pahor AL (1981) The ENT problems following the Birmingham bombings. J Laryngol Otol 95:399–406

23. Pahor AL (1979) Blast injuries to the ear: An historical and literary review. J Laryngol Otol 93:225–251

24. Kerr AG (1980) Trauma and the temporal bone. The effects of blast on the ear. J Laryngol Otol 94:107–110

25. Hill JF (1979) Blast injury with particular reference to recent terrorist bombing incidents. Ann Royal Coll Surg Engl 61:4–11

26. Gray RC, Coppel DL (1975) Intensive care of patients with bomb blast and gunshot injuries. Br Med J 1:502–504

27. Cooper GJ, Maynard RL, et al (1983) Casualties from Terrorist Bombings. J Trauma 23:955–967

28. Freund U, Kopolovic J, Durst AL (1978) Compressed air emboli of the aorta and renal artery in blast injury. Injury 12:37–38

29. Coppel DL (1976) Blast injuries of the lungs. Br J Surg 63:735–737

30. Huller T, Bazini Y (1970) Blast injuries of the chest and abdomen. Arch Surg 100:24–30

31. McCaughey W, Coppel DL, Dundee JW (1973) Blast injuries to the lungs. A report of two cases. Anaesthesia 28:2–9

32. Weiler-Ravell D, Adatto R, Borman JB (1975) Blast injury of the chest. A review of the problem and its treatment. Israeli J Med Sci 11:268–274

33. Pontoppidan H, Laver MB, Geffin B (1970) Acute respiratory failure in the surgical patient. In: Welch C (ed) Advances in Surgery 4: Chicago, Year Book, 163

34. Coppel DL (1976) Blast injuries of the lungs. Br J Surg 63:735–737

35. Caseby NG, Porter MF (1976) Blast injuries of the lungs, clinical presentation, management and course. Injury 8:1–12

36. Goligher JC, King DP, Simmons HJ (1949) Injuries produced by blast in water. Lancet 2:119–123

37. Greaves FC, Draeyer RH, Brines DA, et al (1943) An experimental study of underwater concussion. US Navy Med Bull 41:339–363

38. Murthy JMK, Chopra JG, Gulati DR (1979) Subdural hematoma in an adult following a blast injury. J Neurosurg 50:260–261

39. Hadden WA, Rutherford WH, Merrett JD (1978) The injuries of terrorist bombing: a study of 1532 consecutive patients. Br J Surg 65:525–531

40. Coetzer PWW, Smith FCA, van der Merwe CJ, et al (1987) The epidemiology of terrorism. J Acc Emerg Med 4:15–21

41. Waterworth TA, Carr MJT (1975) Report on injuries sustained by patients treated at the Birmingham General Hospital following the recent bomb explosions. Br Med J 2:25–27

42. Petrucelli E, States JD, Huelke DF, Hames LN (1980) Injury Coding Manual 1980. Washington DC: US Department of Transportation

43. Committee on Injury Scaling (1980) The Abbreviated Injury Scale: 1980 Revision. Morton Grove: American Association of Automotive Medicine

44. Adler J, Golan E, Golan J, Yitzhaki M, Ben-Hur M (1983) Terrorist bombing experience during 1975–79: Casualties admitted to the Shaare Zedek Medical Center. Israeli J Med Sci 19:189–193

45. Brismar B, Bergenwald L (1982) The terrorist bomb explosion in Bologna, Italy, 1980: an analysis of the effects and injuries sustained. J Trauma 22:216–220

46. Calderwood JW (1975) Analysis of fractures treated in the Royal Victoria Hospital, Belfast, in 1972, with special reference to gunshot wounds and bomb blast injuries. Injury 6:206–305

47. Owen-Smith M (1979) Bomb blast injuries; in an explosive situation. Nurs Mirror 149:35–39
48. Kennedy TL, Johnston GW (1975) Civilian bomb injuries. Br Med J 1:382–383
49. Waterworth TA, Carr MJT (1975) An Analysis of the post-mortem findings in the 21 victims of the Birmingham pub bombings. Injury 7:89–95
50. Johnston GW, Kennedy TL (1976) Limb and abdominal injuries: principles of treatment. Br J Surg 63:738–741
51. Lyons HA (1979) Civil violence: the psychological aspects. J Psychosom Res 23:373–393
52. Sims ACP, White AC, Murphy T (1979) Aftermath Neurosis: psychological sequelae of the Birmingham bombings in victims not seriously injured. Med Sci Law 19:78–81
53. Central Statistical Services (1985) South African Life Tables: 1979–81; Pretoria Government Printer
54. Crockhard HA, Coppel DL, Morrow WFK (1973) Evaluation of hyperventilation in treatment of head injuries. Br Med J 4:634–640
55. Rutherford WH (1980) Triage and urban terrorism. In: MacMahon AG, Jooste M (eds) Disaster Medicine: report of proceedings of the International Conference on Disaster Medicine, Cape Town, August 1979. Balkema, Cape Town, pp 94–96
56. MacMahon AG (1980) Regional medical disaster control and communications. In: MacMahon AG, Jooste M (eds) Disaster Medicine Balkema Cape Town, pp 90–93
57. Irving M (1976) Major disasters: hospital admission procedures. Br J Surg 63:731–734
58. Tucker K, Lettin A (1975) The Tower of London bomb explosion. Br Med J 3:287–290
59. Gann DS, Nagel EL, Stafford JD, Walker F (1979) Mass casualty management. In: Zuidema GD, Rutherford RB, Bellinger WF (eds) The management of trauma. 3rd ed, Saunders Philadelphia, pp 780–793
60. Rutherford WH (1975) Disaster procedures. Br Med J 1:443–445
61. Scheidler K (1980) Immediate reaction of the health service in a disaster. In: Frey R, Safar P (eds) Types and events of disasters: organization in various disaster situations. Springer, Berlin Heidelberg New York, pp 163–165
62. Holloway RM (1980) Organizational response to multiple casualty incidents: experience in New York City. In: Frey R, Safar P (eds) Types and events of disasters: organization in various disaster situations. Springer, Berlin Heidelberg New York, pp 125–127
63. Coetzee MM (1980) The advantages of a regional ambulance service. In: MacMahon AG, Jooste M (eds) Disaster Medicine Balkema Cape Town, pp 179–184
64. Mesnick PS (1980) Value of disaster critiques as demonstrated by the management of two "L" crashes in the City of Chicago. In: Frey T, Safar P (eds) Types and events of disasters; organization in various disaster situations. Springer, Berlin Heidelberg New York, pp 133–139
65. Broekman RJ (1985) The hospital's role in managing civil disasters. S Afr Hosp Supplies (Des):17–23
66. Savage PEA (1980) Hospital disaster planning. In: MacMahon AG, Jooste M (eds) Disaster Medicine Balkema, Cape Town, pp 20–24
67. White MES, Gann DS (1979) Emergency department organization. In: Zuidema GD, Rutherford RB, Ballinger WF (eds) The Management of trauma. 3rd ed. Saunders, Philadelphia, pp 767–779
68. van der Merwe CJ, Louw AF, Welthagen D, Schoeman HS (1985) Adult respiratory distress syndrome in cases of severe trauma – the prophylactic value of methylprednisolone sodium succinate. S Afr Med J 67:279–283
69. Lindeque BGP, Schoeman HS, Dommisse GF, et al (1987) Fat embolism and the fat embolism syndrome. A double-blind therapeutic study. J Bone Joint Surg 69:128–131

Difficult Intubation

R. Scherer

Introduction

Tracheal intubation is a common routine procedure for anesthesiologists and intensive care physicians. It is anesthesiologists a simple procedure, but if the attempt proves unexpectedly difficult the patient may be seriously at risk. Unfortunately, intubation is often done poorly and taught improperly, so that easy intubations often become difficult or even impossible. The plan for this review includes causes of difficult intubation, approaches and strategies to difficult intubation, intubation assist devices and possible complications of attempted intubation.

Causes of Difficult Intubation

The most frequent causes of difficult intubation are shown in Table 1. The variations of the normal head and neck anatomy are the most frequent causes of unexpected difficulties of intubation. However, there is also a long list of diseases and syndromes primarily affecting other parts of the body which may contribute [1].

Table 1. Causes of difficult intubation

---

1. *Variations of the normal head and neck anatomy*
   (short muscular neck, high larynx, large and protruding teeth, large tongue, long high-arched palate, small mouth, receding mandibule

2. *Reduced temporo-mandibular joint mobility*
   (rheumatoid arthritis, spondylarthritis)

3. *Reduced neck movement*
   (cervical trauma, luxation, spondylarthritis, Klippel-Feil syndrome)

4. *Facial anomalies*
   (Pierre-Robin syndrome, Treacher-Collins syndrome, Apert syndrome, M. Crouzon, Acromegaly, Cockayne's syndrome, Cleft palate, Le Fort II and III fractures, facial burns, radical head-neck surgery)

5. *Space-occupying lesions in the upper respiratory tract*
   (mandibular fracture, tumors, hemangioma, thyroid carcinoma)

Approach to Difficult Intubation

Examination of the Patient

Careful clinical examination of the patient usually reveals some signs of a potentially difficult intubation. The systemic steps for patient examination are:

- Examine the patient from the lateral position, look for micrognatia and maxillary overgrowth;
- extend and bend the neck maximally to disclose restricted neck mobility;
- examine and palpate the neck anteriorly;
- look for a narrow submental angle, a reduced suprahyoid notch to chin distance (<6 cm) suggesting that direct laryngoscopy will be impossible [2];
- examine mouth opening (normaly 35–40 mm in adults), teeth and oral cavity. If the fauces of a seated patient protruding his tongue could not be visualized adequately direct laryngoscopy may be difficult [3];
- determine the patency of the nostrils.

X-ray examination has been advocated to analyze anatomical features for identification of factors predicative of difficult intubation. However, no single anatomical factor determines the ease of intubation [4], so that the X-ray examination is not a useful predictor of difficult intubation.

Positioning of the Patient

Successful direct laryngoscopy requires alining the oral, pharyngeal and laryngeal axes such that the passageway from the incisor teeth to glottis is nearly a straight line. This can be achieved by extension of the head at the atlanto-occipital joint, while the neck is bended at the cervical spine [5]. This posture is described as the "sniffing position" and is easily achieved by elevating the head about 10 cm with pads under the occiput. Raising the head is not required for intubation in infants and children because of the relatively large size of their head. Vigorous attempts to improve visualization by extending the cervical spine can bow it forward, and lift the larynx of some patients too anteriorly [6].

Intubation Assist Devices

The laryngoscope: Traditionally, the laryngoscope is the most frequently used device to visualize the larynx directly for endotracheal intubation. The choice of laryngoscope blade is often based on personal preference and experience. The two basic types of blades are the curved blade (MacIntosh) and the straight blade with a curved tip (Miller). The curved blade has the advantage of reducing trauma to the teeth and the epiglottis and offering more room for passage of the tracheal tube through the oropharynx. Because of anatomic differences, a straight blade is preferred for exposure of the infant's larynx. Opening of the glottis is greater permitting observation of the tube as it passes through the glottis.

Whatever blade is used, a change of blade may make a difficult intubation possible. The blade should be selected on the basis of its length, degree and character of curvature, the need to compress tongue and soft tissues into the mandibular space, the need to avoid prominent upper teeth and the need to improve blade maneuvrability in a small mouth.

In order to reduce teeth damage in patients with reduced mouth opening a modified MacIntosh blade has been proposed [7]. The depth of the proximal part of the blade was carved 0.5–2 cm shallower and the corresponding part of the blade was made smaller in the horizontal plane. In addition, the distal end of the blade was bent slighly at the tip. In order to further improve visualization of the larynx by increasing the blade's pressure on the base of the tongue the author proposed a modified MacIntosh blade with carved proximal end and an adjustable tip (Fig. 1) [8]. The 5 cm tip of the blade was made adjustable in its angle by means of a joint controlled by a screw-lock fixation via a small wire parallel to the blade. Another modified MacIntosh blade is characterized by a reduced overall curvature combined with a distinctly curved tip [9]. Other devices to improve visualization of the larynx include mirrors and prisms attached to the blade. By improving the angle of refraction, a prism brings the larynx and the tip of the tube into view without the need of excessive traction on the laryngoscope handle.

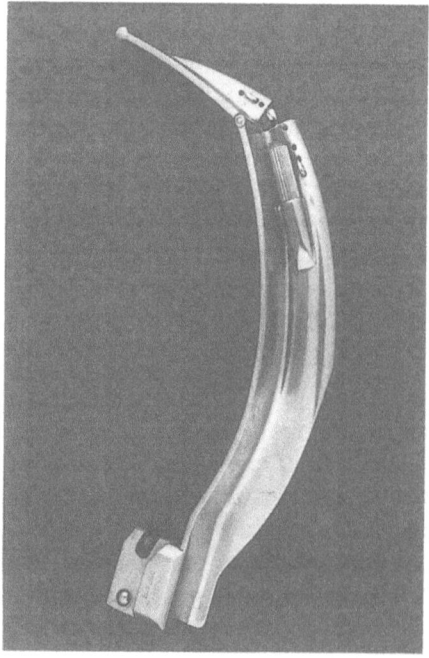

Fig. 1. Modified MacIntosh-blade with carved proximal part and adjustable tip

Stylets: MacIntosh popularized the concept of threading the Oxford non-kinkable tube over lubricated gum-elastic stylets. With the aid of a laryngoscope the stylet is introduced into the larynx, even without adequate exposure. After withdrawal of the laryngoscope, the tube is threaded over the introducer [10]. The Salem-Resce intubation guide (Flexiguide) is a flexible plastic introducer with a distal tip, that can be mechanically tilted anteriorly or posteriorly as well as sideways be means of a proximal handle [11, 12]. A well lubricated introducer is placed inside the tube and direct laryngoscopy is performed. Even if the larynx is not visualized, the tip of the introducer can be passed into the trachea utilizing important landmarks, i.e. esophageal surface of the larynx, arytenoids, or the epiglottis.

Maleable stylets incorporating a light (Tube-Stat) have been used successfully for oral and nasotracheal intubation [13, 14]. Under dimmed operating-room light the lighted stylet and tube are inserted into the oropharynx, and the transillumination is shown in the neck. When the trachea is entered a bright area of illumination appears in the midline just below the cricoid cartilage and the endotracheal tube is slid off the stylet and into the trachea. The manufacturer has encased the bulb and wire in a firm plastic coating, thus preventing disconnection of the bulb from the stylet [15].

Forceps: The Magill forceps is the most widely used device to direct the tip of the tube between the vocal cords. Other devices such as the Bearman wire hook [16] or the tracheal tube retractor [17, 18] may be used to guide the endotracheal tube particularly during nasotracheal intubation. Furthermore, tongue forceps and malleable tongue retractors may be used to increase the size of the oral cavity [13].

Oro-, nasopharyngeal airways and special endotracheal tubes: Special oropharyngeal airways not only facilitate ventilation by face-mask, but also accommodate blind intubation by directing the endotracheal tube into larynx [19, 20], and channel the fiberscope during orotracheal brochoscopic intubation. Nasopharyngeal airways (Wendl-tubes) 28 to 34 French lubricated with lidocaine (2%) jelly have been successfully used for sequential dilatation of the nose reducing blood loss from nasotracheal intubation [21]. Finally, endotracheal tubes that incorporate a tip moving device are very helpful in patients with an "anterior" larynx and should be available together with various other types of endotracheal tubes [22].

All intubation assist devices should be contained in a special tray available for difficult intubation [23]. This protects all concerned from the frustration caused by an uninformed person gathering unfamiliar things from unfamiliar places.

Intubation Strategies

The unexpected difficult intubation: If the anesthesiologist is unfortunate enough to render a patient apneic and fail to intubate a plan of action is suggested in Table 2.

Table 2. Plan of action in unexpectedly difficult intubation

First attempt failure
1. Keep calm
2. Assure adequate ventilation by face mask
3. Improve position of the head
4. Maintain cricoid pressure
5. Deepen the anesthesia (relaxation?)
6. Choose appropriate material

Second attempt failure
1. Keep calm
2. Establish "surgical" anesthesia with spontaneous ventilation
3. Fiberoptic intubation if available
4. Blind intubation if unavailable

Third attempt failure
1. Consider inhalational anesthesia by face mask (for surgery)
2. Consider tracheostomy

If direct laryngoscopy using the various intubation assist devices fails, fiberoptic intubation should be considered early. The fiberoptic bronchoscope to visualize the laryngeal inlet in difficult cases is well accepted and has revolutionized procedures in patients with known intubation difficulties [3]. Although this method sounds attractive in cases of unexpected difficult intubation, it has shortcomings, which include difficulty to identify the structures, secretions or condensations of water obscuring the field. Numerous attempted intubations using conventional laryngoscope invariably result in pharyngeal trauma and once bleeding starts fiberoptic bronchoscopy becomes difficult. Furthermore, during emergency situations, time required to set up a fiberoptic bronchoscope, the required expertise of the physician and finally the cost of the fiberoptic bronchoscope may limit its use. In the authors' opinion fiberoptic intubation is a first attempt procedure for expected difficult intubations rather than a "rescue" maneuver.

Blind intubation, however, is a frequently helpful "rescue" manoeuver in unexpected difficult intubation. Basic requirements are a well lubricated tube and topical anesthesia of the larynx in awake patients or in anesthetized spontaneously breathing patients. With the bevel facing the nasal septum, the tube is introduced along the floor of the nose to the hypopharynx and is then advanced into the trachea while listening to exhaled air passing from the tube. In the presence of excessive extension or flexion of the head the tube may be deviated into the anterior commissure or to the esophagus, respectively.

Retrograde intubation is another "rescue" procedure. This term implies threading the tube over a catheter or J-wire introduced through puncture of the cricothyroid membrane and passed via the larynx to the mouth or nose [24, 26]. Dislodgment of the tube when the translaryngeal wire is removed or partial obstruction of the tube are distressing complications of this method. However, the retrograde technique is rarely necessary, but is useful in the presence of very severe and complex anatomical difficulties.

The expected difficult intubation: Unfortunately difficult intubations cannot always be recognized before intubation. In cases of expected difficulties however, prophylactical measures are of outmost importance [23]. The most important measures which can prevent risks are listed in Table 3. Examination and positioning of the patient and the choice of the necessary equipment and drugs have been discussed previously. Prevention of aspiration includes fasting, administration of histamine-2-blockers, e.g. ranitidine 150 mg orally both the night before and early the day of surgery [27] or 100 mg intravenously 1 to 2 hours prior to induction of anesthesia [28]. In addition, 30 ml of 0.3 M sodium citrate have proved effective to elevate gastric pH within 15 minutes [29]. Before intubation is attempted a nasogastric tube should be inserted to evacuate as much gastric contents as possible. Cricoid pressure properly applied is the simplest and most effective measure for minimizing the risk of aspiration.

The safest intubation strategy to manage patients with known or suspected difficult airways is to perform it when they are awake [30]. Intubation using a fiberoptic bronchoscope is becoming the method of choice in airway management prior to induction of anesthesia [3]. Initially the nose was used as a logical guide to the larynx for fiberoptic bronchoscopic intubation. Recently, a variety of oral airway obturators or guides have been described to enable easier and safer use of the fiberoptic bronchoscope through the mouth [19, 31]. Local anesthesia of the upper respiratory tract can easily be achieved by inhalation of nebulized lidocaine 4% before fiberoptic-assisted awake intubation [32]. Other maneuvers include bilateral block of the superior laryngeal nerve at the apex of the greater cornu of the hyoid bone, which blocks the vagal distribution to the larynx and trachea. Injections of local anesthetic through the cricothyroid membrane into the trachea produces anesthesia below the vocal cord.

Complications

Acute respiratory obstruction may occur during attempts to intubate a patient. Percutaneous cricothyroidotomy employing various devices is an effective method to relieve obstruction permitting adequate short-term to-and-fro ventilation [33]. Percutanous transtracheal or transcricothyroid membrane ventilation via a large bore canula (14 gauge) is possible but frequently leads to CO_2 retention. It also has an increased risk of barotrauma to the lungs. In every case of expected difficult intubation a surgeon must be available to perform emergency tracheostomy.

Table 3. Preventive measures prior to an expected difficult intubation

1. Examination of the patient
2. Optimal positioning of the patient
3. Aspiration prophylaxis
4. Choice and preparation of intubations assist devices and drugs
5. Provide adequate oxygenation and ventilation before any attempt

Unrecognized esophageal intubation is another major risk factor for patients difficult to intubate. End-tidal CO_2 measurement is at present the most reliable means to determine proper airway position [34, 35]. All other conventional methods to insure proper tube placement like bilateral breath sounds, bilateral hemithorax elevation, epigastric auscultation, reservoir bag compliance, presence of exhaled tidal volumes, endotracheal cuff palpation in the neck and condensation of water vapor in the tube lumen have been documented to fail under certain circumstances.

Trauma of oral or nasal mucosa with bleeding is a frequent and almost inevitable consequence of difficult intubation. Nasotracheal intubation may be associated with penetration and dissection of mucosa and formation of a retropharyngeal abscess in the postoperative period. Other intubation-related lesions include trauma to lips and tongue, dental damage, temporo-mandibular joint dysfunction and trauma to the cervical spine.

Conclusion

By paying meticulous attention to the patients' history and physical examination, the anesthesiologist will develop a high degree of suspicion that intubation may be difficult. Provided the necessary intubation assist devices are readily available the anesthesiologist following the intubation strategies for expected and unexpected difficulties will be able to minimize the risk for his patient. Finally, the more difficult is an intubation the more careful should be the extubation.

References

1. Jones AEP, Pelton DA (1976) An index of syndromes and their anaesthetic implications. Can Anaesth Soc 23:207-226
2. Mallampati SR, Gatt SP, Gugino LD, et al (1985) A clinical sign to predict difficult tracheal intubation. Can Anaesth Soc J 32:429-434
3. Patil VU, Stehling LC, Zauder HL (1983) Fiberoptic endoscopy in anaesthesia. Year Book Medical Publishers Inc
4. Van der Linde JC, Roelofse JA, Steenkamp EC (1983) Anatomical factors relating to difficult intubation. S Afr Med J 63:976-977
5. Gordon RA (1972) Anesthetic management of patients with airway problem. Int Anesthesiol Clin 10:37-59
6. Nichol HC, Zuck D (1983) Difficult laryngoscopy - the "anterior" larynx and the atlanto-occipital gap. Br J Anaesth 55:141-143
7. Ibler M (1983) Modification of MacIntosh laryngoscope blade. Anesthesiology 58:200
8. Scherer R, Habel G (1987) Ein modifizierter MacIntosh-Spatel mit abwinkelbarer Spitze für schwierige Intubationen. Anaesthesist (Suppl) 36:254
9. Wiemers K (1972) Modifizierter Laryngoskopspatel (Freiburger Modell). Anaesthesist 21:147
10. Alsop AF (1955) Non-kinking endotracheal tubes. Anaesthesia 10:401-403
11. Salem MA, Mathrubhutham, Bennett EJ (1976) Difficult intubation. N Engl J Med 295:879-881
12. Rao TLK, Mathru M, Gorski DW, Salem MR (1982) Experience with a new intubation guide for difficult tracheal intubation. Crit care med 10:882-883
13. Ducrow M (1978) Throwing light on blind intubation. Anaesthesia 33:827-829

14. Ellis DG, Jakymec A, Kaplan RM, et al (1986) Guided orotracheal intubation in the operating room using a lighted stylet: a comparison with direct laryngoscope technique. Anesthesiology 64:823–826
15. Stone DJ, Stirt JA, Kaplan MJ, McLean WC (1984) A complication of lightwand-guided nasotracheal intubation. Anesthesiology 61:780–781
16. Bearman AJ (1962) Current comments: device for nasotracheal intubation. Anesthesiology 23:130–131
17. Chester MH (1979) A new endotracheal tube retractor. Anesthesiology 51:274
18. Chester MH (1984) Trachealtube guide to facilitate nasotracheal intubation. Anesthesiology 60:522–523
19. Berman RA (1977) A method for blind oral intubation of the trachea or esophagus. Anesth Analg 56:866–867
20. Williams RT, Harrison RE (1981) Prone tracheal intubation simplified using an airway intubator. Can Anaesth Soc J 28:288–289
21. Kay J, Bryan R, Hart HB, Minkel DT, Munshi C (1985) Sequential dilatation: a useful adjunct in reducing blood loss from nasotracheal intubation. Anesthesiology 63:A 259
22. Fry ENS (1985) Difficult tracheal intubation. Anaesthesia 40:206
23. Bonfils P (1983) Prophylaktische Maßnahmen vor einer schwierigen Intubation. Anaesth Intensivther Notfallmed 18:17–20
24. McLellan J, Mac Leod GF (1981) Use of an epidural cannula for a difficult intubation. Anesthesia 36:231–232
25. Borland LM, Swan DM, Leff S (1981) Difficult pediatric endotracheal intubation: a new approach to the retrograde technique. Anesthesiology 55:577–578
26. King HK (1985) Translaryngeal guided intubation using a sheath stylet. Anesthesiology 63:567
27. Francis RN, Kwik RSH (1982) Oral ranitidine for prophylaxis against Mendelson's syndrome. Anesth Analg 61:130–135
28. Maile CJD, Francis RN (1983) Pre-operative ranitidine: effect of a single intravenous dose on pH and volume of gastric aspirate. Anaesthesia 38:324–329
29. Gibbs CP, Banner TC (1984) Effectiveness of Bicitra as a preoperative antacid. Anesthesiology 61:97–99
30. Duncan JAT (1977) Intubation of the trachea in the conscious patient. Br J Anaesth 49:619–623
31. Rogers SN, Bennmof JL (1983) New and easy techniques for fiberoptic endoscopy aided tracheal intubation. Anesthesiology 59:569–572
32. Sutherland AD, Williams RT (1986) Cardiovascular responses and lidocaine absorption in fiberoptic-assisted awake intubation. Anesth Analg 65:389–391
33. Fisher JA (1979) A "last ditch" airway. Can Anaesth Soc J 26:225–230
34. Linko K, Paloheimo M, Tannisto T (1983) Capnography for detection of accidental oesophageal intubation. Acta Anaesthesiol Scand 27:199–202
35. Birmingham PK, Cheney FW, Ward RJ (1986) Esophageal intubation a review of detection techniques. Anesth Analg 65:886–891

Severe Birth Asphyxia

M. I. Levene

Introduction

Birth asphyxia is one of the two most important conditions which predispose to serious brain injury in the neonatal period. Asphyxia refers to a basic patho-physiological insult comprising simultaneous hypoxia and hypoperfusion at a cellular level which results in an accumulation of acidic products of anaerobic metabolism. A clinical definition of asphyxia is much more difficult and depends on a number or factors including the gestational age and the duration of the asphyxial insult. The effects of birth asphyxia involves the whole body although the brain, myocardium and kidneys are most vulnerable to injury. Effective management is directed towards the early prenatal diagnosis of this condition, rapid delivery and effective early resuscitation, followed by neuro-intensive care in those infants in whom this is necessary. Unfortunately there is little evidence that intensive management after the initial period of resuscitation is likely to make a considerable impact in limiting the extent of eventual pathology. More recently new methods have become available to predict the final extent of brain injury as well as possible means of treating the early effects of injury [1].

Timing of the Asphyxial Insult

Over 90 precent of infants who sustain asphyxial insult do so during passage through the birth canal and the rest are affected following birth. This latter group represents those infants found collapsed due to infection, intra-operative complication or the victims of "near-miss sudden infant death syndrome". The fetus is entirely dependent on the placenta for gas exchange and any compromise of utero-placental function may cause the fetus to be asphyxiated. This is usually due to placental dysfunction, but in approximately 10 percent of cases direct obstruction of the umbilical cord may occur. This is usually due to cord prolapse and less commonly is associated with the cord around the infants neck or a knot in the umbilical cord.

Some fetuses are more likely to suffer intrapartum asphyxia as they have been compromised prior to the onset of labor. Intra-uterine growth retardation may be the result of longstanding placental dysfunction and fetuses affected by this condition are less able to withstand the rigors of labor and are consequently more liable to develop metabolic compromise with metabolic acidosis. In one study 25% of asphyxiated full-term infants had evidence of intra-uterine growth retardation [2].

Detection of Intrapartum Asphyxia

Meconium staining of the amniotic fluid has long been considered feature of intrapartum asphyxia but this is probably a relatively late and imprecise sign of fetal compromise. Cardiotocography is widely used to monitor the fetus during labor. A variety of abnormal patterns are recognized including loss of beat-to-beat variability, late decelerations and persistent fetal tachycardia. Unfortunately cardiotocography does not appear to be a very sensitive test for detecting intrapartum asphyxia. An estimate of pH from the fetal scalp is a useful test in the presence of an abnormal cardiotocography and a value below 7.25 is considered indicative of fetal asphyxia with acidosis and rapid delivery is recommended.

Asphyxia and Gestational Age

It is most important to consider the effect of gestational age on the clinical and pathological abnormalities found in infants who have suffered intrapartum asphyxia. The full-term infant in general shows a quite different spectrum of pathological as well as clinical features following asphyxia than those seen in premature infants. Macroscopic examination of the brain of a full-term infant who has suffered severe birth asphyxia is often unremarkable unlike that of the premature infant. Periventricular hemorrhage and periventricular leukomalacia both commonly occur in brain of premature infants and the underlying abnormality is often associated with an intrapartum event. Some infants show established periventricular leukomalacia at birth indicating that they had received a severe asphyxial or hypotensive event well before the onset of labor.

The full-term infant, unlike the premature, shows a consistent pattern of clinical signs following asphyxia and can be graded on the basis of the clinical ab-

Table 1. A classification system for post-asphyxial encephalopathy. (From [1])

Grade I (Mild)	Grade II (Moderate)	Grade III (Severe)
Irritability, "Hyperalert ness"	Lethargy	Coma
Mild differential tone	Marked differential tone with hypertonus	Severe hypotonia
Poor sucking	Requirement for tube feeding	Failure to maintain spontaneous respiration
No seizures	Seizures	Prolonged or frequent seizures

normality as mild, moderate or severe encephalopathy [2, 3,] and this is shown in Table 1. Infants with mild post-asphyxial encephalopathy (PAE) usually recover by 48 hours after birth, and those with moderate PAE show signs of recovery by one week from birth. Death is only likely to occur in infants with severe encephalopathy.

What Is Asphyxia?

Birth asphyxia has been defined in a variety of ways but the three most commonly reported are depression of Apgar score, delay in establishing spontaneous respiration and postasphyxial encephalopathy. Depression of Apgar score is widely used as the method for diagnosing perinatal asphyxia but may be considerably influenced by non-asphyxial factors including maternal drugs, prematurity and rarely neuromuscular disorders. Donald in 1959 [4] defined "asphyxia neonatorum" as failure to establish spontaneous ventilation at birth, but like depression of the Apgar score there may be many causes for this. Unlike other methods, behavioral abnormalities in the newborn infant is a more sensitive indicator of significant preceding asphyxia. Even if the infant is born with a depressed Apgar score be is most unlikely to have sustained significant cerebral insult if he subsequently shows no abnormality in behavior. I believe that evidence of post-asphyxial encephalopathy is the best diagnostic criterion with which to diagnose intrapartum asphyxia.

General Management

The asphyxiated infant must be carefully assessed in order to detect and treat non-cerebral complications. Table 2 lists the common systemic complications

Table 2. Systemic complications of birth asphyxia

Renal:	Acute tubular necrosis
	Oliguria
Cardiovascular:	Myocardial failure
	Myocardial infarction
	Hypotension
Pulmonary:	Meconium aspiration
	Pulmonary hypertension
Metabolic:	Inappropriate ADH secretion
	Hypoglycemia
	Hypocalcemia
	Metabolic acidosis
	Hyperglycemia
	Hyperammonemia
Hematological:	Disseminated intravascular coagulation
Gastrointestinal:	Stress ulceration
	Necrotizing enterocolitis

associated with asphyxia. Regular blood gas estimates should be performed in order to detect respiratory compromise due either to associated lung disease (meconium aspiration) or central respiratory depression. We would electively ventilate an infant if the $PaCO_2$ exceeded 6 KPa and ensure that the infant is adequately oxygenated. Careful attention must be paid to maintaining the infant in the appropriate environmental temperature and to avoid heat or cold stress. Hypoglycemia must be anticipated and regular assessment of blood sugar should be made. A high index of suspicion should be maintained for infection and broad spectrum antibiotics used if this is likely.

Brain Orientated Care

The principals of management of severe birth asphyxia are to maintain an adequate systemic blood pressure, control of neonatal seizures and treatment of intracranial hypertension.

Hypotension: Systemic hypotension occurs commonly in severely asphyxiated infants. The blood pressure is often extremely labile and intermittent or indirect assessment may be misleading. Continuous monitoring of direct arterial pressure is recommended, and treatment should be started when systolic pressure falls below 35 mmHg in a very premature infant and 50 mmHg in a full-term infant. Plasma infusion (10 ml/kg) followed by the administration of an inotropic agent (dopamine 5–10 μg/kg/h) is most effective.

Seizures: These occur in all infants who have sustained significant birth asphyxia. They may be clinically obvious in the form of tonic or clonic convulsions but may often be subtle in nature [5]. Continuous monitoring of EEG activity is the most sensitive method for detecting cortical seizure activity, but it is known that infants may show clinical signs of seizures with no abnormal features on the EEG [6]. These "seizures" may be extremely resistent to treatment. First line anticonvulsant medication is phenobarbitone (20 mg/kg loading dose, and 3 mg/kg maintenance given 12 hourly). In my unit I use clonazepam as the second line drug [1]. This is reserved for full-term infants and is given as a loading dose of 0.25 mg intravenously with a maintenance of 0.05 mg, 12 hourly. It may also be given by continuous infusion in infants with severe and prolonged fits.

Intracranial Hypertension: This does not occur in all infants with severe birth asphyxia. A sustained rise in intracranial pressure (ICP) of 10 mmHg or more lasting an hour or more occurred in 14 of 23 infants in whom ICP was continuously measured [7]. Furthermore there was little evidence that treatment using dexamethasone or mannitol made a significant improvement in outcome. The indication for direct measurement of ICP is discussed below.

Monitoring the Severely Asphyxiated Infant

Infants with moderate or severe post-asphyxial encephalopathy require careful observation and monitoring in an intensive care unit in which neurological function can be closely observed. It is clear that ICP monitoring is of only limited value and it is therefore necessary to know which babies are likely to benefit from this form of management.

Doppler ultrasound assessment of cerebral blood flow velocity (CBFV) has been used to assess the cerebral circulation in asphyxiated full-term infants [8]. An index of flow pattern was used to quantify abnormalities and is referred to as Pourcelot's Resistance Index (PI). A low PI (0.55 or below) has been shown to correlate with adverse outcome in a group of 43 asphyxiated infants. A low PI predicted adverse outcome (severe handicap or death) in 86% of cases and had a sensitivity of 100%. This is considerably better than assessment of outcome based on severity of PAE. The PI becomes abnormal shortly after birth, and in the majority of cases within 24 h, and presumably reflects abnormal hemodynamics due to asphyxial injury of the brain.

We recommend that ICP monitoring be reserved for infants who have normal PI values at 24 h. Intracranial hypertension occurs as the result of asphyxial injury and develops in the second 24 h of life. We believe that the brain swelling is a secondary phenomenon in the process of brain injury and its treatment is unlikely to reduce cerebral injury if the brain has already sustained a major ischemic insult. Doppler assessment prior to direct ICP monitoring will avoid unnecessary invasive procedures and effective treatment of intracranial hypertension will be directed only at those infants with a relatively good prognosis.

Conclusion

Birth asphyxia is a common condition and in full-term infants can only be reliably diagnosed in the presence of a well recognized pattern of clinical signs. In the premature infant specific hemorrhagic and ischemic lesions may be recognized on ultrasound scanning but they rarely show obvious clinical signs of encephalopathy. Management is directed towards effective treatment of hypotension, seizures and monitoring of ICP in those with normal Doppler assessment of cerebral hemodynamics. In the future more effective methods for the early protection of neuronal tissue may become available, but at the present time this has not been evaluated in the newborn infant.

References

1. Levene MI (1987) Current Reviews in Paediatrics. Neonatal Neurology. Churchill Livingstone, Edinburgh
2. Levene MI, Kornberg J, Williams THC (1985) The incidence and severity of post-asphyxial encephalopathy in full-term infants. Early Hum Develop 11:21–26

3. Sarnat HB, Sarnat MS (1976) Neonatal encephalopathy following fetal distress. A clinical and electroencephalographic study. Arch Neurol 33:696–705
4. Donald I (1959) Adaptation from intrauterine to extrauterine life. In: Holland E, Bourne A (eds) British Obstetric Practice. Heinnemann, London
5. Volpe JJ (1986) Neurology of the Newborn. 2nd ed. Saunders Co, Philadelphia
6. Connell J, Oozeer R (1988) Neonatal electroencephalography. In: Levene MI, Bennet M, Punt J (eds) Fetal and Neonatal Neurology and Neurosurgery. Churchill Livingstone, Edinburgh. (In press)
7. Levene MI, Evans DH, Forde A, Archer LNJ (1987) Value of intracranial pressure monitoring of asphyxiated newborn infants. Develop Med Child Neurol 29:311–319
8. Archer LNJ, Levene MI, Evans DH (1986) Cerebral artery Doppler ultrasonography for prediction of outcome after perinatal asphyxia. Lancet ii:1116–1118

Clinical Use of Benzodiazepine Antagonists

P. Lheureux and R. Askenasi

Introduction

The benzodiazepins were introduced in the early sixties. Their various pharmacological properties and their high toxic/therapeutic ratio explain the wide development of their clinical use (and abuse?). Their mechanism of action on the central nervous system (CNS) was only elucidated in 1977 when high affinity binding sites, closely related to GABA-ergic synapses, were discovered in the mammalian cerebral cortex and related to the pharmacologic action of benzodiazepines [1, 2]. A specific antagonist of benzodiazepine-receptors (Ro 15-1788 – flumazenil), able to inhibit all the effects of classical benzodiazepines without inducing any own action, was discovered by Hunkeleer et al. in 1981 [3].

Benzodiazepine Receptors

Two types of benzodiazepine-receptors are now recognized:

Central Receptors

Although widespread in the CNS, they are present in larger amounts in the cerebral and cerebellar cortex. They are closely related to the GABA receptors and the chloride channels [4]. The GABA-dependent opening of the Cl channel is modulated (gabamodulin) by the benzodiazepine-receptor activation. In the presence of benzodiazepine, GABA receptor shifts from low to high affinity state and the frequency of Cl channel opening is increased. This results in an hyperpolarization of the cellular membrane, responsible for the inhibition induced by the GABA-ergic neurotransmission. Reciprocally, binding of an agonist ligand (GABA, muscimol) to the GABA receptor enhances ("GABA-shift") the affinity of benzodiazepine-receptors for their agonist ligands. The picrotoxine – barbiturate binding site modulates also the function of the GABA receptor – Cl channel complex. Functional supramolecular stucture with multiple binding sites (GABA, benzodiazepine, barbiturate) has been proposed [5].

Peripheral Receptors

Another type of benzodiazepine binding sites (independent of the – GABA-receptor related) has been discribed in several tissues such as heart, lung, kidney, liver, uterus, adrenal cortex and blood cells. They were called "peripheral receptors", although they are also present in the CNS. They were initially considered as simple acceptors rather than as true receptors [6], but this concept was recently challenged by the possible implication of peripheral benzodiazepine-receptors in pathologic conditions, in the antiarrhythmic properties of diazepam, or in the electophysiologic effects of Ro 5-4864 [7], a selective peripheral ligand. This pharmacological actions could be mediated through a benzodiazepine-receptor/Ca channel coupling [8].

Subclasses of Receptors

Several studies have suggested the existence of subclasses of receptors in both groups. Their signification remains controversial.

Ligands of the Benzodiazepine-Receptors   (see Table 1)

The spectra of affinity of both binding sites are not identical:

Benzodiazepine Derivatives

Both types bind diazepam and flunitrazepam, but clonazepam and flumazenil only bind to the central receptor. Ro 5-4864 seems to be a selective agonist of the peripheral type [6]. A close relationship between receptor affinity and pharmacologic potency has been demontrated for both types of receptors.

Non-benzodiazepine Derivatives

Several non-benzodiazepine compounds present a specific affinity for the benzodiazepine-receptors: triazolopyridazine (agonists), pyrazolo-quinolinones (agonists and antagonists) and β-carboline-3-carboxylate derivatives (partial

Table 1. Affinity of some benzodiazepine and isoquinoline-carboxamide derivatives for central and peripheral benzodiazepine-receptors

Central receptors	Both sites	Peripheral receptors
Ro 15-1788 (Flumazenil)	Diazepam	Ro 5-4864 (?)
Clonazepam	Flunitrazepam	PK 11212, PK 11195

agonists, antagonists and (partial) inverses agonists) are ligands of central benzodiazepine-receptors. PK 11195, an isoquinoline carboxamide compound is a specific antagonist of peripheral binding sites [9].

Antagonization of Benzodiazepine Pharmacological Properties

A classification of the coumpounds able to antagonize the pharmacological effects of benzodiazepines on their central receptors, after the mechanism of action, is reported in Table 2.

Clinical Use of Benzodiazepine Antagonists

Clinical Toxicology

Benzodiazepines are implicated in a lot of suicidal attempts by drug overdose, alone or associated to other drugs with CNS depressant effect. Wide use of these compounds is also responsible for accidental poisonings in high risks groups such as elderly, children, patients with chronic obstructive respiratory disease or liver failure. Previous attempts to reverse the CNS depression and to shorten the duration of coma induced by benzodiazepine abuse (methylxanthines, physostigmine, naloxone) had been disappointing.

Pure benzodiazepine overdose: Several studies [10–12] clearly demonstrated the diagnostic and therapeutic values of flumazenil for benzodiazepine overdosed patients. A dose of 3.5 ± 1.5 mg is able to produce a quick arousal and to keep the patient awake during 3–5 h in pure benzodiazepine abuse, despite the short plasmatic half-life (1.3 ± 0.6 h) of the drug [13]. Relapse of profound drowsiness is observed mainly with flunitrazepam but also with other low liposoluble compounds (triazolam, alprazolam, clobazam). In a recent double-blind randomized study, we have observed that lower doses (1.1 ± 0.5 mg) seem sufficient to wake up the patient, but readministrations (after 2 or 3 hours) are more often required. A definite way of antidote administration remains thus to be determined in long-acting benzodiazepine overdose. An initial bolus of 1–2 mg, slowly (1 mg/ 5 min) administered through an intravenous line, seems usually adequate to wake up the patient. Continuous infusion of flumazenil as been proposed to prevent relapses of coma, but the infusion rate and duration must be determined in each case. It will depend on the relative affinity of both agonist and antagonist for the central benzodiazepine-receptor, the drug (and metabolites) pharmacokinetics and plasma level, and the possible acquired tolerance of the patient. As an exemple, in midazolam or diazepam induced coma, 25 μg/min flumazenil (after a bolus of 2.5 mg) appears sufficient to maintain arousal [14]. Repeated bolus administration seems easier and perhaps more efficient for competition antagonism at the receptor level.

Table 2. Classification and site of action of benzodiazepine antagonists

Site and mechanism of effect		Type	Antagonists
Central receptors			
GABA ergic neuron	*GABA Synthesis*	NS	isoniazide
		NS	thiosemicarbazide
	GABA Release	NS	tetanus toxin
Primary target cell			
GABA receptor		NS	bicuculline
Barbiturate-picrotoxin receptor		NS	picrotoxin
Benzodiazepine-receptor	*Antagonists*	S	imidazobenzodiazepines: Ro 15-1788, Ro 15-3505
		S	other: B-CCPr, ZK 43426, CGS 8216
	Inverse agonists	S	phenylpyrazoloquinolinones: CGS 9896
		S	B-carboline derivatives: B-CCE, B-CCM, DMCM, FG 7142
Secondary (or further) target cells		NS	physostigmine
		NS	methylxantines: caffeine, aminophylline, …
		NS	naloxone
Peripheral receptors		S	isoquinoline carboxamide derivatives PK 11195, PK 11212.

S = specific antagonism, NS = non-specific antagonism   B-CC: ester de beta-carboline-3-carboxylate   Pr = propyl   E = ethyl   M = methyl

Mixed (including benzodiazepines) drug poisoning and non-benzodiazepine poisoning: In multiple drugs poisoning including benzodiazepines, a transient improvement of the consciousness is generally observed. The unresponsiveness of the non-benzodiazepine poisoned patient highly suggests that the antidotal effect is quite specific. However, observations of durable improvement in benzodiazepine-ethanol or pure ethanol intoxication [11, 15] have been reported and are currently controlled in a double-blinded randomized study. The doses required to wake up the patient seem higher (3–5 mg) than for benzodiazepine overdose.

Tolerance of the treatment and side effects: The local and general tolerance of flumazenil is remarkable. The lack of significant cardiovascular effect observed in poisoned patient is in agrement with the observations made during flumazenil-induced recovery of benzodiazepine anesthetized patients [16]. However, withdrawal syndrome may occur after rapid administration to chronic benzodiazepine "addicts" [17]. It is usually mild and short, but seizures have been reported. Occurrence of seizures should also suggest concomitant ingestion of other drugs with convulsant properties. This situation could be a relative contraindication to the use of flumazenil, as is profound hypothermia and aspiration pneumonia requiring assisted ventilation. Other mild side effects rarely reported are anxious awakening, vomiting and shivering.

Usefulness of partial inverse agonist of the benzodiazepine-receptor in poisoning due to other CNS depressants [18] (such as barbiturate or meprobamate) is still to be investigated. The role of peripheral receptors as site of the antidotal effect of diazepam in cloroquine overdose remains hypothetical. Experimental studies with specific ligands of the peripheral benzodiazepine-binding (PK 11195, Ro 5-4864) should help to explain this mechanism.

Anesthesiology

Many studies [16, 19–21] have disclosed flumazenil as efficient and safe to reverse benzodiazepine-induced sedation in anesthesiology. The only side effect reported is a mild increase in the occurrence of postoperative nausea. The incidence of anxious reaction is controversial. No changes in hemodynamic parameters are recorded. Flumazenil was also of value in paradoxical benzodiazepine reactions which are sometimes observed.

An intravenous dose of less than 1 mg is often sufficient to reverse midazolam induced sedation, without relapse of coma. Flumazenil should mainly be useful for benzodiazepine-induced short sedation during endoscopy or for neurologic evaluation of benzodiazepine-sedated patients in intensive care units.

Hepatic Encephalopathy

During the last years, the role of GABA in the pathophysiology of hepatic encephalopathy has been emphasized. Hypersensitivity to benzodiazepines in this condition is not only related to decreased hepatic clearance or increased blood/

brain barrier permeability, but also to increase number and affinity of benzodiazepine central receptors [22]. Animal [23] and isolated human [24, 25] observations suggest that benzodiazepine antagonists (or partial inverse agonist) could be useful in encephalopathy related to liver failure. However, randomized studies are still required.

Conclusions

Specific benzodiazepine-receptor antagonists have widely contributed to the knowledge of the pharmacological properties of benzodiazepines and other ligands in the CNS. The discovery of peripheral binding sites and specific ligands will probably explain some other effects of benzodiazepine, especially on the heart.

Flumazenil undoubtedly represents an important step in the diagnosis and treatment of common drug poisoning and should belong to the limited category of antidotes lacking of own toxic effects. The development of "one day" clinics, requiring rapid recovery of neurological function after anesthesia, will probably increase its use in this field.

The evaluation of benzodiazepines antagonists or inverse agonists is still experimental in ethanol intoxication or hepatic encephalopathy, but first results are promising.

References

1. Squires RF, Braestrup C (1977) Benzodiazepine receptors in rat brain. Nature 266:732–734
2. Molher H, Okada T (1977) Benzodiazepine receptor: demonstration in the central nervous system. Science 198:849–851
3. Hunkeleer W, Mohler H, Pieri L, et al (1981) Selective antagonists of benzodiazepines. Nature 290:514–516
4. Mohler H, Richards JG, Wu JY (1981) Autoradiographic localisation of benzodiazepine receptors in immunocytochemically identified GABA ergic synapses. Proc Natl Acad Sci 78:1935–1938
5. Polc P, Bonetti EP, Schaffner R, Haefely W (1982) A three-state model of the benzodiazepine receptor explains the interaction between the benzodiazepine antagonist Ro 15-1788, BZD tranquilizers, B-carbolines, and phenobarbitone. Naunyn-Schmiedelberg's Arch Pharmacol 321:260–264
6. Richards JG, Mohler H, Haefely W (1982) Benzodiazepine binding sites: receptors or acceptors? TIPS 3:233–235
7. Mestre M, Carriot T, Belin C, et al (1984) Electrophysiological and pharmacological characterization of peripheral benzodiazepine receptors in guinea pig heart preparation. Life Sci 35:953–962
8. Mestre M, Carriot T, Belin C, et al (1985) Electrophysiological and pharmacological evidence that peripheral-type benzodiazepine receptors are coupled to calcium channels in the heart. Life Sci 36:391–400
9. Le Fur G, Vaucher N, Perrier ML, et al (1983) Differentiation between two ligands for peripheral benzodiazepine binding sites, (3H) Ro 5-4864 and (3H) PK 11195 by thermodynamic studies. Life Sci 33:449–457

10. Hofer P, Scollo Lavizzari G (1985) Benzodiazepine antagonist RO 15-1788 in self-poisoning: diagnostic and therapeutic use. Arch Intern Med 145:663-664

11. Lheureux P, Askenasi R (1987) Specific treatment of benzodiazepine overdose. Human Toxicology (in press)

12. O'Sullivan GF, Wade DN (1987) Flumazenil in the management of acute drug overdosage with benzodiazepines and other agents. Clin Pharmacol Ther 42:254-259

13. Klotz U, Ziegler G, Reimann IW (1984) Pharmacokinetics of the selective benzodiazepine antagonist RO-15-1788 in man. Eur Clin Pharmacol 27:115-117

14. Klotz U, Ziegler G, Ludwig L, Reimann IW (1985) Pharmacodynamic interaction between midazolam an a specific benzodiazepine antagonist in humans. J Clin Pharmacol 25:400-406

15. Lheureux P, Askenasi R (1986) Benzodiazepine antagonist RO 15-1788 in acute alcohol intoxication. Toxicology Letters 31(s):155 (abstract)

16. Louis M, Forster A, Suter PM, Gemperle M (1984) Clinical and hemodynamic effects of a specific benzodiazepine antagonist (Ro 15-1788) after open heart surgery. Anaesthesiology 61:A61

17. Lheureux P, Askenasi R (1986) Treatment of benzodiazepine overdose with RO 15-1788. Arch Intern Med 146:1241 (letter)

18. Havoudjian H, Reed GF, Paul SM, Skolnick P (1987) Protection against the lethal effects of pentobarbital in mice by a benzodiazepine inverse agonist, 6,7-dimethoxy-4-ethyl-3-carbomethoxy-B-carboline. J Clin Invest 79:473-477

19. Sage, JD, Close A, Boas RA (1987) Reversal of midazolam sedation with anexate. Br J Anaesth 59:459-464

20. Ricou B, Forster A, Bruckner A, Chastonay P, Gemperle M (1986) Clinical evaluation of a specific benzodiazepine antagonist (Ro 15-1788). Studies in elderly patients after regional anaesthesia under benzodiazepine sedation. Br J Anaesth 58:1005-1011

21. Wolff J, Carl P, Clausen TG, Mikkelsen BO (1986) Ro 15-1788 for post operative recovery. A randomized clinical trial in patients undergoing minor surgical procedures under midazolam anesthesia. Anaesthesia 41:1001-1006

22. Samson Y, Bernuau J, Pappata S, Chavoix C, Baron JC, Maziere MA (1987) Cerebral uptake of benzodiazepine measured by positron emission tomography in hepatic encephalopathy. N Engl J Med 316:414-415

23. Baraldi M, Zeneroli ML, Ventura E, et al (1984) Supersensitivity of benzodiazepine receptors in hepatic encephalopathy due to fulminant hepatic failure in the rat: reversal by a benzodiazepine antagonist. Clin Sci 67:167-175

24. Scollo-Lavizzari G, Steinmann E (1985) Reversal of hepatic coma by benzodiazepine antagonist (Ro 15-1788) (letter). Lancet 1:1324

25. Bansky G, Meier PJ, Ziegler WH, Walser H, Schmid M, Huber M (1985) Reversal of hepatic coma by benzodiazepine antagonist (Ro 15-1788). Lancet 1:1324-1325 (letter)

Outcome After Trauma

Factors Influencing Outcome
After Severe Head Trauma

M. Hemmer

Introduction

There are three essential reasons for identifying the prognostic factors and measuring the outcome from brain injury: definition of subpopulations with a similar
potential for recovery, evaluation of prophylactic and therapeutic modalities and
demonstration that head injury is a major public problem with important psychological, sociological and financial consequences. Multiple numerical assessment
scales of the neurological status based on selected parameters have been devised
to describe the severity of injury and to predict prognosis. The generalized use of
Glasgow Coma Scale (GCS) with its subdivision into severe, moderate and mild
head injury together with the classification based on Cerebral Computed Tomography (CT) findings permits an uniformed description of the brain-injured patients [1, 2]. More complex categorization, based on the order of disappearance
of brain stem reflexes due to the rostro-caudal spread of the injury is sometimes
employed [3]. The creation of International Data Bank and the US National
Traumatic Coma Data Bank has stimulated most of neurosurgical centers to
prospectively collect data concerning patients' characteristics, circumstances of
accidents, type of injury, evolution of cerebral and general disorders and use of
therapeutic modalities [4, 5]. Statistical analysis of data obtained from well comparable groups of patients permits to identify both the single factors and the
groups of factors indicating prognosis.

The generally adopted assessment of outcome in individual patient is the
Glasgow Outcome Scale (GOS) proposed by Jennett and Bond in 1975 [6]. This
five point scale is based rather on functional than on neurological aspects of
recovery (good outcome, moderate disability, severe disability, permanent vegetative state and death). In the majority of studies on factors influencing prognosis, a binary assessment of outcome (survival/death) or a three point assessment
("good outcome" corresponding to both good outcome and moderate disability
of Jenett and Bond, "bad outcome" corresponding to severe disability and permanently vegetative state and "death") are used for statistical comparisons [6, 7].

When outcome is assessed, the time from the injury to the measurement has to
be defined because the recovery from head trauma is a dynamic condition. The
first evaluation usually takes place at least six months after trauma with repetitive measurements up to two years after injury [7].

Neuropsychological outcome of the survivors of brain injury who are, in majority, in the categories of good outcome and moderate disability of Jennett and
Bond Scale may also be assessed by a battery of standard neuropsychological

tests which examine higher cognitive functioning, new problem solving skills, focused attention, concentration and memory.

Prognosis After Head Injury

Several studies have shown that the severity of initial injury is the major determinant for prognosis of head trauma. The severity of initial injury may be assessed by the use of standard scales, by CT classification of injury patterns and by the presence of abnormalities in multimodal evoked potentials [8].

The poor outcome is also associated with the secondary ischemic hypoxic brain damage which may be due to several intracranial and extracranial factors, namely the quality of pre-hospital care, presence of associated lesions leading to hypotension, hypoxia and anemia and secondary alterations in cerebral hemodynamics [9, 10].

Recently, an assessment based on biochemical evaluation of the severity of trauma has been proposed in addition to clinical, radiological and electrophysiological data [11]. Biochemical markers of the injury indicate the magnitude of stress response, the impairment of cellular metabolism and the extent of cellular destruction and are considered as good indicators of both the initial injury and the secondary brain damage.

The age of the head trauma patient and the clinical course of the disease (duration of coma and of posttraumatic amnesia PTA) are also important in the prediction of prognosis [12, 13].

Finally the effect of all prophylactic and therapeutic regimens which include initial resuscitation, surgical treatment, mechanical ventilation, treatment of intracranial hypertension, cerebral metabolic protection and nutritional support have to be regularly evaluated [14–19].

The Predictive Value of Standard Assessment Scales

The Glasgow Coma Scale and, in particular, its motor response score, shows a good inverse correlation with outcome. A confident prediction of prognosis may be obtained in about 60% of patients [1, 20]. However, the confidence of prediction is much better for low (3 or 4) and high (8 to 15) scores than for the intermediate (5 to 7) scores [20]. Some studies have shown that the combination of abnormal motor response with impaired or absent pupil light reflexes and eye movements indicating brain stem involvement is a better indicator of outcome than the GCS alone. Therefore, the Glasgow-Liège Coma Scale which includes a score based on brain – stem reflex activity seems to have a better predictive value than the GCS, especially for the patients with the GCS = 5 [3].

CT Injury Patterns

The type of injury defined by the first CT at admission indicates the severity of the initial lesion. However, the first multicenter study, which proposed the categorization of the CT type of injury according to its influence on outcome has demonstrated that both the GCS and the CT type of lesion must be considered together to predict the prognosis [20]. Other authors have shown that the midline shift is associated with poor outcome [10]. A more recent study by Lobato et al. classified the CT findings into eight distrinctive patterns related to outcome [2]. Three of these patterns, namely extracerebral hematoma with acute hemispheric swelling (pattern 2), multiple unilateral brain contusions with or without subdural hematoma (pattern 4) and diffuse axonal injury (pattern 7) were related in a very significant way to poor outcome. Multiple bilateral brain contusions and normal CT patterns have yielded both good and bad outcome scores and the highest incidence of good outcome has been observed in patients with pure extracerebral hematoma (pattern 1), general brain swelling without focal injury (pattern 6) and single contusion (pattern 3).

The initial CT patterns alone are indicative of the severity of brain injury but do not allow an absolute prognosis. Serial CT scanning together with the neurological assessment and ICP monitoring may enhance the prediction of outcome.

The Influence of Age on the Outcome from Brain Injury

Several studies have shown that the outcome in head injury is better in children than in adults. This difference may be explained by the relatively low incidence of mass lesion and the higher incidence of general brain swelling in younger age groups [10, 21]. Moreover, the threshold for neurophysiological dysfunction and the potential for neurophysiological recovery may be different in children. A very high incidence of bad outcome scores has been shown in brain injured patients over seventy years of age [10].

Assessment for the Outcome by Multimodality Evoked Potentials

Multimodality Evoked Potentials (MEP's) are good indicators of outcome in brain injury [8, 15]. It has been shown that mild abnormalities (grade I and II MEP's) recorded early after injury are indicative of a favorable outcome, while severe deficits (grade III and IV MEP's) are rarely compatible with survival or recovery of consciousness with the exception of a focal abnormality.

The Influence of Altered Cerebral Hemodynamics on the Outcome from Brain Injury

Intracranial Pressure (ICP) and Cerebral Perfusion Pressure (CPP)

There is overhelming evidence that increased ICP is associated with poor prognosis in head injury. Several studies have also shown a good correlation between the ICP and outcome [10, 15, 22]. ICP above 20 torr is related to the increase in morbidity and ICP above 50–60 torr is almost uniformely fatal, irrespective of the other features of the head injury.

Two types of patients who present with intracranial hypertension can be distinguished. In some cases the brain swelling and the elevated ICP are the principal pathology responsible for the patients' neurological status and the outcome may improve with effective treatment. In the second group of patients the intracranial hypertension is just a secondary manifestation and a marker of irreversible brain swelling due to an unknown progressive biochemical lesion of the neurons and the endothelial cells by either the initial traumatic insult or the secondary ischemic/hypoxia brain damage. In these cases ICP is often uncontrollable and its temporary decrease with a very aggressive treatment does not improve the outcome. In these patients, other indicators, in particular the biochemical markers, may better reflect the severity of neurological insult [11].

Moreover, ICP alone is not a sufficient indicator of prognosis in head trauma patients because its variations are influenced by changes in mean arterial systemic pressure (MAP). Arterial hypotension increases the frequency of elevated ICP and decreases the cerebral perfusion pressure (CPP) [22]. An intimate relation between these three variables exists (CCP = MAP − ICP) so that change in any of them may influence the degree of secondary brain damage [22, 23]. Average CPP seems to have a better predictive value than ICP or MAP alone, its normal value is superior to 80 mmg Hg and the "critical" level of CPP, lower than 40 torr is very important in the development of secondary brain damage [22, 23].

Cerebral Blood Flow (CBF) and Cerebral Metabolic Rate (CMRO₂)

Several studies of CBF in acute head injury have shown that posttraumatic coma is associated with CBF levels ranging from extremely low values to pronounced hyperemia. Different CBF patterns are observed in patients with different types of injury. Abnormally elevated CBF, clearly in excess of metabolic need, is significantly related to brain swelling and intracranial hypertension and may be considered as a "luxury" perfusion. Lowest levels of CBF are observed in patients with severe focal injuries. Because of these large variations of early posttraumatic measurements the initial CBF values are not predictive of outcome, at least in terms of Glasgow Outcome Scale [24].

$CMRO_2$ values are uniformly low in acutely comatose patients and are better predictors of outcome than CBF [24]. However, when serial measurements are performed, CBF declines to very low levels in patients who die, while in patients who survive a coupling of CBF and $CMRO_2$ with increases in both values accompanies the neurological improvement [24].

The presence of early hyperemia especially when related to intracranial hypertension has been shown to influence the neuropsychological outcome in conscious survivors of severe head injury tested one year after trauma [25].

Early hyperemia has been shown to correlate with overall intellectual and memory impairment, and intracranial hypertension has been associated with both general and specific memory deficits.

Biochemical Markers of Head Injury

Biochemical markers of severe head injury directly result from neurological lesions, and their concentration in CSF reflects the extent of structural brain damage. The principal markers are glycolytic and mitochondrial enzymes such as creatinine kinase (CK), lactate dehydrogenase (LDH) and neuron-specific enolase (NSE), released from the membranes of destructed cells. CSF CK – BB seems the most promising of these markers and provides the best correlation with the impairment of consciousness assessed by Glasgow – Liège Coma Scale [26]. Early posttraumatic elevation of CK-BB activity has a high predictive value of outcome and reflects the severity of initial lesion. Delayed CK – BB elevations, also associated with poor outcome, may reflect secondary cerebral damage.

Metabolic Markers of Head Injury

Traumatic brain injury activates the sympathetic nervous system, induces a massive catecholamine release and initiates a cascade of deleterious events resulting in severe metabolic and systemic disorders. Elevated plasma catecholamine levels (norepinephrine, epinephrine, dopamine) have been shown to reflect the severity of neurological insult, to enhance the reliability of GCS in assessing the gravity of injury and to be independent predictors of outcome in both the acute and chronic phases of traumatic brain injury [27].

Brain tissue acidosis inferred by CSF lactic acidosis can play an important role in the clinical course of severe head injury. To is probably due to cellular hypoxia or impaired metabolism. High ventricular CSF lactate concentration is observed early after trauma and its resolution in the following 48 hours is a reliable sign of improvement. Ventricular CSF lactate levels that remain elevated or that increase over time indicate the patient's deterioration. Serial CSF lactate measurements via a ventricular catheter is useful in the evaluation of prognosis [28].

The Influence of Pre-hospital Care and the Impact of Associated Lesions on the Mortality in Severe Head Injury

Improved pre-hospital care and rapid transport has been shown to decrease mortality rate in head injury [29]. It has been demonstrated that surgical decompression within four hours improves the prognosis of acute subdural hematoma which usually carries the highest mortality rate of all traumatic lesions [30].

High quality pre-hospital medical care is important for patients with acute respiratory disturbances and systemic hypotension following the brain injury. A recent study demonstrated that 40% of brain injured patients with treatable injuries, assessed by the Abbreviated Injury Scale (AIS) and the Injury Severity Score (ISS) died at the scene of the accident and that the associated organ lesions were the dominant cause of death in patients with high ISS. In patients who survived over 24 h, 52% of deaths were due to the brain injury itself and 48% to associated systemic causes (respiratory failure 31%, pulmonary infection

12%, sepsis, peritonitis and cardiac disorders 5% [31]. The importance of respiratory disorders and infectious complications in head injury patients has been stressed by several authors. [32].

The Outcome with Aggressive Treatment

Several reports have claimed that a standardized management regimen which includes early detection and removal of an intracranial hematoma, routine mechanical ventilation and routine application of medication to lower the ICP and to provide cerebral protection improve outcome in patients with severe brain injury [10, 14]. However, some recent studies demonstrated that such an aggresive "multimodal" management does not improve outcome. Moreover, the routine administration of neuroprotective medication (corticosteroids, barbiturates, other anesthetic substances) has not been shown to improve outcome in large randomized clinical trials [15–17, 33]. The apparent failure of these therapies in randomized trials in spite of frequently encountered good results in individual patients is due to the complex dynamic pathology of brain injury. New means of investigation of the cerebral metabolic impairment (magnetic resonance spectroscopy, PET scanning) will allow to define more specific subpopulations of brain-injured patients and to better determine the choice and the timing of therapeutic regimens.

Neuropsychological Outcome and Residual Complaints of Severe Head Trauma Patients

Neuropsychological outcome and residual complaints of conscious survivors of head trauma are significantly related to the severity of brain injury and the pre-injury IQ of the patient [34]. The majority (80%) of brain-injury victims have some residual neuropsychological deficit [35]. Slowness, impaired memory, anticipatory behavior deficit, dizziness, fatigue, depressive moods, restlessness and inability to relax are the most frequently encountered complaints. [34–36]. This permanent neuropsychological deficit is observed even in the "good outcome" patients of Jennett and Bond's classification [34, 35]. Therefore not only the permanently vegetative and severely disabled but also the patients in good outcome categories need continuity of care, prolonged rehabilitation programs and psychosocial counseling for both the family and the patient.

Severe brain injury carries the mortality rate of 30 to 50% in spite of early and aggressive treatment. Head trauma remains the single most common cause of death under the age of fourty in industrialized countries. Of brain injury victims 10 to 20% become severely disabled or permanently vegetative and even the remaining 40 to 50% who are classified in good outcome categories wave persistent neuropsychological deficits. For these reasons not only a better pre-hospital care and new therapeutic modalities but also large preventive programs which may lower the incidence of brain injury should be developed.

References

1. Teasdale G, Jennett B (1974) Assessment of coma and impaired consciousness: A practical scale. Lancet 2:81-84
2. Lobato RD, Cordobes F, Rivas JJ, et al (1983) Outcome from severe head injury related to the type of intracranial lesion. J Neurosurg 59:762-774
3. Born JD, Hans P, Dexters G, et al (1982) Evaluation pratique du dysfonctionnement encé-phalique chez le traumatisé crânien. Neuro-chirurgie 28:1-7
4. Jennett B, Teasdale G, Galbraith S, et al (1977) Severe head injury in three countries. J Neurol Neurosurg Psychiatry 40:291-298
5. Marshall LF, Becker DP, Sharon A, et al (1983) The National Traumatic Coma Data Bank. J Neurosurg 59:276-284
6. Jennett B, Bond M (1975) Assessment of outcome after severe brain damage: A practical scale. Lancet 1:480-484
7. Langfitt TW (1978) Measuring the outcome from head injuries. J Neurosurg 48:673-678
8. Greenberg RP, Newlon PG, Hyatt MS, et al (1981) Prognostic implications of early multi-modality evoked potentials in severely head injured patients. J Neurosurg 55:227-236
9. Langfitt TW, Genarelli T (1982) Can the outcome from head injury be improved? J Neurosurg 56:19-25
10. Miller JD, Butterworth JF, Gudeman SK, et al (1981) Further experience in the management of severe head injury. J Neurosurg 54:289-299
11. Bakay RAE, Ward AA (1983) Enzymatic changes in serum and cerebrospinal fluid in neurological injury. J Neurosurg 58:27-37
12. Berger MS, Pitts LH, Lovely M, et al (1985) Outcome from severe head injury in children and adolescents. J Neurosurg 62:194-199
13. Lyle DM, Pierce JP, Freeman EA, et al (1986) Clinical course and outcome of severe head injury in Australia. J Neurosurg 65:15-18
14. Marshall LF, Smith RW, Shapiro HM (1979) The outcome with aggressive treatment in severe head injuries, part I and II. J Neurosurg 50:20-25 and 26-30
15. Ward JD, Becker DP, Miller DJ, et al (1985) Failure of prophylactic barbiturate come in the treatment of severe head injury. J Neurosurg 62:383-388
16. Dearden NM, Mc Dowall DG (1985) Comparison of Etomidate and Althesin in the reduction of increased ICP after head injury. Br J Anaesth 57:361-368
17. Dearden NM, Gibson JS, Mc Dowall GD, et al (1986) Effect of high dose dexamethasone on outcome from severe head injury. J Neurosurg 64:81-88
18. Hemmer M (1985) Ventilatory support for pulmonary failure of the head trauma patient. Bull Eur Physiopat Respir 21:287-293
19. Rapp, R, Young B, Twyman D, et al (1983) The favorable effects of early parenteral feeding on survival in head - injured patients. J Neurosurg 58:906-912
20. Genarelli TA, Spielmann GM, Langfitt TW, et al (1982) Influence of the type of intracranial lesion on outcome from severe head injury. J Neurosurg 56:26-32
21. Bruce DA, Raphaely RC, Goldberg AL, et al (1978) Patophysiology, treatment and outcome following severe head injuries in children. J Neurosurg 48:679-688
22. Changaris DG, Mc Graw PC, Richardson JD, et al (1987) Correlation of CPP and GCS to outcome. J Trauma 27:1007-1013
23. Tsutsumi H, Ide K, Mizutani I, et al (1985) The relationship between ICP, CCP and outcome in head injured patients; the critical level of CPP. Intracranial Pressure VI. Springer, Berlin Heidelberg New York Tokyo, pp 661-666
24. Obrist WD, Genarelli TA, Segawa H, et al (1979) Relation of cerebral blood flow to neurological status and outcome in head injured patients. J Neurosurg 51:292-300
25. Uzell BP, Obrist WD, Dolinskas CA, Langfitt T (1986) Relationship of acute CBF and ICP findings to neuropsychologic outcome in severe head injury. J Neurosurg 65:630-635
26. Hans P, Born JD, Chapelle JP, Milbauw G (1983) Creatin kinase isoenzymes in severe head injury. J Neurosurg 58:689-692
27. Woolf PP, Hamill RW, Lee LA, et al (1987) The predictive value of catecholamines in assessing outcome in traumatic brain injury. J Neurosurg 66:875-882

28. De Salles AAF, Kontos HA, Becker DP, et al (1986) Prognostic significance of ventricular CSF lactic acidosis in severe head injury. J Neurosurg 65:615–624
29. Klauber MR, Marshall LF, Toole BM, et al (1985) Cause of decline in head injury mortality rate in San Diego Country, California. J Neurosurg 62:528–531
30. Seelig JM, Becker DB, Miller JD, et al (1981) Traumatic acute subdural hematoma. Major mortality reduction in comatose patients treated within 4 hours. N Engl. J Med 304:1511–1518
31. Kraus J, Conroy C, Cox P, et al (1985) Survival times and case fatality rates of brain – injured persons. J Neurosurg 63:537–543
32. Frost EAM (1977) Respiratory problems associated with head trauma. Neurosurgery 1:300–305
33. Gelpke GJ, Braakman R, Dik J, et al (1983) Comparison of outcome in two series of patients with severe head injuries. J Neurosurg 59:745–750
34. Williams JM, Gomes F, Drudge OW, Kessler M (1984) Predicting outcome from closed head injury by early assessment of trauma severity. J Neurosurg 61:581–585
35. Van Zomeren AH, van den Burg W (1985) Residual complaints of patients two years after severe head injury. J Neurol Neurosurg Psychiatry 48:21–28
36. Freedman PE, Bleiberg J, Freedland K (1987) Anticipatory behaviour deficits in closed head injury. J Neurol Neurosurg Psychiatry 50:398–341

Prognosis of Head Injured Patients

D. Scheidegger

Head trauma is internationally recognized as a major cause of death and disability, with an estimated incidence of 200 victims per 100000 population per year [1]. Reports of mortality rates from severe head injury range from 30 to 50% among those patients who had an initial significant neurologic deficit. Sevitt [2] reported that 50% of deaths related to head injury occurred within the first two hours, 60% within 24 hours and 75% within 48 hours. About 50% of the mortality from head injury occurs therefore in patients who never reached a hospital.

It is not only the high mortality that is a matter of major concern for the patient, his family, and the whole society but also the quality of survival after a severe head trauma. However, it remains very difficult to assess outcome in head traumatized patients for different reasons. First, the patient himself may lack insight so that the full degree of disability would only become clear through the relative's view. The purely physical sequelae of severe head injury are easy to recognize and well documented, but it is becoming increasingly evident that the most serious long term morbidity after head injury is psychological; involving cognitive, behavioral, and social and family disturbance [3, 4]. Second, it is very important to realize that every description of outcome after head injury is observer dependent. If the one was involved in the therapy of the patient his view may be too optimistic.

To be able to compare outcomes of head injured patients from different institutions it is mandatory that the assessment was made at the same time interval after injury. Division into deaths and survivors can reasonably be made at the time of discharge from the Intensive Care Unit. To get a more accurate idea of late sequellae after head injury the status of the patient has to be evaluated after one year. In the Data Bank study, 90% of all patients had reached their final outcome by six months already [1]. Most studies looking for late outcome of head traumatized patients, however, have used the 12 month interval [5-8].

As we and others have previously reported about 25% of the head injured patients admitted to an Neurointensive Care Unit will die. In the past, concerns have often been expressed that the intensive treatment of head injury may result in some reduction of mortality, but causes patients to survive with severe morbidity, resulting in more patients requiring chronic long term institutional care. All of our patients received a full aggressive intensive treatment program. However only 3% of all patients were in that situation after one year. This and the finding that almost 50% of the patients returned to work at one year lead to the conclusion that while head injury may cause significant disability, it appears to leave a lesser long term social burden than many authors have predicted.

There are many studies on the outcome of head injured patients [9, 10]. What the clinician would be interested in is a possibility to predict outcome of a patient at the time of admission to the ICU. We know from the Data Bank study that age, depth and duration of coma are factors with predictive power [11]. All other factors have only little relation to outcome.

For the physician who cares for an individual patient it would be important to know the outcome for that patient by combining the favorable and adverse factors. This can be done by a computer-assisted method described by Teasdale an coworkers [12], who conducted a pilot survey of neurosurgeons to discover their opinions about making predictions, about the influence of prognosis on management and about the potential of a formal computer-based predictive system. A total of 89% of the physicians stated that they tried to estimate prognosis preoperatively, and 74% estimated prognosis at 24 h. Of them, 60% considered that their preoperative estimate greatly influenced their decision to operate and 42% allowed their 24 h estimate to affect management decisions. To judge how a neurosurgeon's concept of prognosis might affect management they asked the doctors: "At what percentage prospect of a dead or severely disabled outcome for a patient would you not advise operation for a traumatic intracranial hematoma?" To this question, 39% replied 99–100%, 21% said 95–98%, 30% said less than 95%. When they were asked to put themselves in the position of the patient, over 50% replied that they would not like to be operated on unless they had better chances of a reasonable outcome than they had required for a patient.

Only 33% of the neurosurgeons thought that the computerized data bank would be more accurate than an experienced clinician, 40% thought they were as good and 19% thought those predictions were less reliable. To evaluate how accurate predictions from an experienced clinician are we performed a prospective study asking the same neurosurgeon an outcome score (1. dead or vegetative, 2. severely disabled, and 3. good recovery) for each patient after 12 h. All patients were then reexamined 2 years after the accident. Only 50% of the patients predicted to have an outcome 1 died, and 40% of that group had a good recovery. In the group predicted to remain severely disabled, 71% made a good recovery. Only 83% of the group predicted to have a good outcome had actually a good recovery.

These results show again, that even for an experienced clinician it is impossible to predict the outcome for an individual head traumatized patient.

References

1. Jennett B, Teasdale G (1981) Management of Head Injuries. FA Davis Company
2. Sevitt S (1973) Fatal road accidents in Birmingham: times to death and their cause. Injury 4:281–293
3. Levin HS, High WM, Goethe KE, et al (1987) The neurobehavioural rating scale: assessment of the behavioural sequelae of head injury by the clinician. J Neurol Neurosurg Psychiatry 50:183–193
4. Brooks, N. Campsie L, Symington C, Beattie A, McKinlay W (1986) The five year outcome of severe blunt head injury: a relative's view. J Neurol Neurosurg Psychiatry 49:764–770

5. Alberico AM, Ward JD, Choi SC, Marmarou A, Young HF (1987) Outcome after severe head injury. J Neurosurg 67:648–656
6. Williams JM, Gomes F, Drudge OW, Kessler M (1984) Predicting outcome from closed head injury by early assessment of trauma severity. J Neurosurg 61:581–585
7. Vapalahti M, Luukkonen M, Puranen M, Hernesniemi J, Tapaninaho A (1986) Early clinical signs and prognosis in children with brain injuries. Ann Clin Res 18:37–42
8. Lyle DM, Pierce JP, Freeman EA, Bartrop R, et al (1986) Clinical course and outcome of severe head injury in Australia. J Neurosurg 65:15–18
9. Jane JA, Rimel RW, Pobereskin LH, Tyson GW, Steward O, Gennarelli TA (1982) Outcome and Pathology of Head Injury. Head Injury: Basic and Clinical Aspects. Raven Press, New York
10. Thienprasit P, Fisher SV, Alcorn MH (1985) Longterm Outcome of Closed Head Injury. Minnesota Medicine 68:559–561
11. Teasdale G, Skene A, Spiegelhalter D, Murray L (1982) Age, Severity, and Outcome of Head Injury. Head Injury: Basic and Clinical Aspects. Raven Press, New York
12. Barlow Ph, Teasdale G (1986) Prediction of Outcome and the Management of Severe Head Injuries: The Attitudes of Neurosurgeons. Neurosurgery 19:989–991

Posttraumatic Stress Disorders

K. Kuch and R. P. Swinson

Introduction

Freud assumed in the early stages of his career that neuroses could be explained by childhood trauma. Later he considered it a phantasy. Recent statistics on child-abuse suggest that Freud's early theories had a realistic basis.

The history of posttraumatic stress disorder (PTSD) includes descriptions of railway spine, shell shock, combat fatigue and accident neurosis. Kardiner (1941) considered it a "physioneurosis" [1] and described several of the current diagnostic criteria. PTSD gained prominence during the Viet Nam war, the Stockholm hostage crisis and the Coconut Grove fire. It gained recognition by West German authorities as a compensable consequence of concentration camps. But it is still seen as a condition limited to wars, violence and disasters.

Minor traffic and industrial accidents seem less credible as a source of disability than disasters but are also followed by anxiety, pain and drastic changes in life-style. Only 25% of the patients on disability for chronic low back pain had demonstrable anatomical abnormality according to one study [2]. Pain is common in patients with PTSD. Diagnostic screening for nightmares, panic and posttraumatic phobias should help to reduce enigmatic disability after assault, industrial and traffic accidents.

Definitions

The Diagnostic and Statistical Manual (DSM III-R) defines PTSD as following events that are outside the range of usual experience and would be distressing to almost anyone [3]. The traumatic event is reexperienced by distressing recollections that intrude against the patient's will, by nightmares, flashbacks and sudden feelings of recurrence. Exposure to reminders of the trauma triggers intense distress and is avoided. General responsiveness is numbed. Persistent symptoms of increased arousal develop with insomnia, outbursts of anger and poor concentration. PTSD may re-emerge after a latency period of months or years [3].

An intense preoccupation with injury, loss and helplessness sets PTSD apart from the other anxiety disorders. The victim's perception of daily life are altered. Situations that seem safe to others remind him of his experience and are perceived as threatening. This understandable loss of trust grows into a disorder when it interferes with the tasks of daily living.

PTSD shares some behavioral abnormalities with phobic disorder. Phobias are thought to be atavistic fears that had survival value at an earlier evolutionary stage and are characterized by persistent, excessive and maladaptive fear of a harmless situation. Exposure to it is avoided or endured with dread. Typical posttraumatic phobias replicate the conditions experienced during the trauma.

DSM III-R does not define what a pathogenic stressor is beyond describing it as seriously distressing to almost anyone. Stress can be "without distress" according to Selye. Distress is caused by events that are neither desirable nor controllable [4]. A study of Viet Nam veterans confirms that PTSD symptoms depended on the degree of combat exposure [5]. A similar "dose-response relationship" was found in the Mount St. Helens eruption [6]. An experience "outside the range of usual experience" does not have to be uncommon. Serious distress accompanies serious illness. Myocardial infarction can be as traumatic as assault. PTSD is comparatively rare as a primary diagnosis. But its symptoms contaminate other disease entities and complicate their course.

Epidemiology

The Ontario statistics for 1986 include 187 286 road traffic accidents with 102 fatalities and 73 703 personal injuries (informal report). Statistics Canada reports 65 887 assaults. Sexual and child-abuse are included but likely underreported. The Workers Compensation Board informally reported 186 662 claims including 108 fatalities. Ontario's population was 9 181 900. A rough calculation suggests, that the chances of being assaulted, or injured on the road and at work were 35 per 1000.

We found few statistics on postaccidental psychopathology. An inter-ministerial task force of the Province of Ontario surveyed 1525 survivors of traffic accidends by questionnaire 4 years after the event. Only survivors who had been taken to hospital were included in the survey and 34.4% returned a completed questionnaire. Legal action had been taken by 26.6% of the respondents. 26.1% had required admission. About one-third reported emotional after-effects. Most common were a fear of driving (19%), nervousness (15%), insomnia (11%) and depression (10%), anxiety and other fears (6%). No correlation between these complaints and the severity of injury was found by the task force [7].

Theory

Classical Conditioning

Pavlov's dogs salivated in response to the ringing of a bell after the unconditioned stimulus of food and the conditioned stimulus of the ringing bell had been presented together repeatedly. Watson and Rayner conditioned an emotional reaction in "little Albert", who was taught to fear a white rat. The rat was presented repeatedly together with a frightening bang and little Albert became very frightened of rats [8]. Mary Cover Jones helped "little Peter" over a fear of a rabbit by bringing it closer gradually while he was enjoying some favorite food [9]. Jones [10] noted that it was unclear how Peter might have acquired his fear and later studies found, that fear-acquisition could not be reproduced at will. The development of a phobia likely requires a preparedness for it [10].

Classical conditioning theory offers a testable hypothesis within these limitations. Sofar we have only observed patients with concussion who developed generalized fearfulness, not specific post-accidental driving phobias. A combination of concussion and specific posttraumatic phobia would disprove the role of classical conditioning as pathogen.

Many studies of *experimental neuroses in animals* used severe aversive stimuli as a pathogen and should be considered models for posttraumatic neurosis. Differences in stimulation produced different results. Baum conditioned rats to become fearful of electrically chargeable floors and deconditioned their fear through re-exposure in a procedure that has become a cornerstone of exposure therapy [10]. Seligman trained 150 dogs to jump from one compartment of a cage into another to escape from a painful electrical foot-shock. A barrier was then erected that prevented escape. Two-thirds of the dogs developed "learned helplessness" after exposure to inescapable shock. They would no longer attempt to escape from the pain even after the barrier was lowered again. Seligman then dragged the passive animals across the lowered barrier in an attempt to teach escaping once more. He was successful only with some animals. The others remained passive [1, 10].

Neurophysiology

Opiates suppress the conditioning of fear. A dose of morphine that would be too low to interfere with general behavior also abolishes the distress-calls of separated animals. Separation-distress is re-instated by the opiate antagonist naloxone [1].

Endorphines are the body's own analgesics and are released by stress. Thyer exposed a woman with a severe fear of snakes to a large snake and monitored concomitant plasma endorphin levels. He observed a substantial elevation which returned to normal at the cessation of fear [11]. Beta-endorphin may mediate declining foot-shock avoidance by raising the pain-threshold. Pain-inhibition following stress is also observed on the battlefield and during athletic performance. Endorphin effects were reduced, when painful shock was continued for 11 days, suggesting that levels of endogenous opioids vary with the duration of stress and that tolerance may develop [1].

These are isolated observations but they invite speculation about neuroendocrine mediation of conditioning and learned helplessness in PTSD. Kolb [12] hypothesizes that prolonged sensitizing stimulation leads to impaired habituation. Accordingly, PTSD-patients may fail to down-regulate their excessive neuronal exitation [12]. One might add that exposure therapy is effective as long as it elicits a homeostatic endorphinergic response leading to down-regulation.

More evidence demonstrating a relationship between stress and *immunomodulation* is accumulating. Foot shock can reduce the resistence to tumor challenge in rats, an effect apparently mediated by opioid peptides [13].

Operant Learning and Illness-Behavior

Skinner [14] demonstrated that external circumstances influence behavior through reward and punishment and that behavior is driven less by "inner states" than commonly assumed. *Behavioral assessment* is a clinical technique that applies Skinner's observations. It investigates sequences of stimulus-response-effect in order to identify the rewards and punishments that influence pathological behavior and has spawned an impressive literature.

Fordyce [15] adapted Skinner's principles to the clinical treatment of pain by monitoring the effects of the environment on illness-behavior. His basic presumption is that illness behavior like excessive pill-taking can persist beyond recovery from the original disease and that it is shaped according to the laws of reinforcement. Attention is a potent reward. Overprotective care may perpetuate illness behavior by rewarding inactivity and ignoring "well-behaviors". Physicians ask more about complaints than enjoyment. Overprotective families take over tasks the patient could perform. Some lawyers advise against vigorous outdoor activities when claimants risk being followed by private investigators. Illness behavior expands to fill the time available as predicted by Parkinson's law. Fordyce's treatment approach uses selective reinforcement of "well behaviors" and tapering analgesics disguised in syrup to reduce cues for pilltaking.

Clinical Observations

Characteristics of the Stressor

Allodi [16] reports *previous accidents* in 38% of his 50 compensation cases referred by law firms and the Workers Compensation Board of Ontario. One-third of the previous accidents had also resulted in work stoppage and compensation. 20% had a family history of accidents. Accident repeaters are in our experience more avoidant and more difficult to rehabilitate. For some patients the worst comes after the accident. Some experience a virtual domino effect, when impairment means giving up valued activities, losing friends and status.

One of us investigated 78 *concentration camp survivors*. The majority had suffered overwhelming stress, had been imprisoned for at least 1 year, had suffered from near starvation and had lost several close family members. The survivors also had to adapt to a foreign culture. Their complaints were dominated by depression and chronic pain. They were more globally impaired and more depressed than the phobic accident litigants described below.

Host Factors

The patient's ability to cope with impairment depends on his *vocational, social and leisure-time skills*. In Allodi's study [16], 68% of patients spoke little English. Workoholic individuals cope poorly with retirement and inactivity. Good social and verbal skills enable an insurance claimant to deal better with the medico-legal process. Social skills may have played a role in an observation on Viet Nam veterans. Veterans suffering from PTSD were 1½ years younger on average than Viet Nam veterans without it and more likely to come from broken homes [17].

A past history of anxiety disorder was a strong predictor of posttraumatic phobias in our recent sample of 44 motor vehicle accidents. Their injuries were minor: 16 reported preexisting phobias not related to traffic and 2 had suffered from generalized anxiety disorder. Almost all were litigating and should have been inclined to underreport any pre-traumatic pathology. The majority were women as expected for a phobic population.

Posttraumatic Phobias

Specific travel phobias were observed in 17 out of the 44 cases. An additional 4 had illness fears as well and 10 more experienced generalized insecurity fears and panic symptoms. 7 also met DSM III criteria for agoraphobia. The posttraumatic phobias interfered seriously with rehabilitation. Their strong representation in this sample reflects the diagnostic acumen of our referral sources. Parker's 296 accident litigants may have been less pre-selected. He still diagnosed an astonishing 35% of the motor accidents and 6% of the industrial accidents as phobic [18].

PTSD and Pain

Benedikt and Kolb [19] found PTSD in 10% of 225 referrals to a Veterans Administration pain clinic. Hodge [20] described a "whiplash neurosis" in patients with sprained necks he had expected to recover in 4 to 8 weeks. Instead he found anxiety, insomnia, recurrent dreams of accidents, fear of road travel, hostility, a preoccupation with symptoms and a prolonged period of convalescence.

Of the 44 road accident victims described above, 21 also complained of spinal pain. The pain did remit in some cases rapidly in tandem with the associated anxiety disorder. In others no such link existed but patients who recovered from their psychiatric condition coped much better. Similar findings were reported earlier [21]. Sofar we have not been able to predict which patients would experience a remission of pain. The hypothesis of anxiety causing increased muscle tone that irritates a neck sprain is somewhat overused but may have limited application here.

Assessment and Treatment

Compensation

The difficulty inherent in the assessment of compensation claims has led to a sizable literature that can only be mentioned briefly. Kelly [22] rejects four common assumptions about litigating patients: that no-one recovers and returns to work before litigation is settled, that PTSD does not occur in situations for which there is no compensation, that it never follows severe head injuries and is in inverse proportion to the severity of the injury and that it never occurs in the managerial and professional classes. Tarsh and Royston [23] followed 35 claimants with accident neurosis without demonstrable organic pathology. Recovery appeared unrelated to the time of compensation. This agrees with our own experience: phobic patients recovered during exposure therapy well before their case came to trial. We have observed PTSD when there was no hope for compensation and have treated posttraumatic phobias in professionals.

We do not suggest, that malingering and aggravation never occur. Nor is every patient who returns to work fully recovered. Some take lower paying jobs and continue to suffer from anxiety and pain. A return of leisure activities to premorbid levels can be a more sensitive indicator of improvement than work attendance.

Behavioral Assessment

A *distress diary* offers a simple method of assessing the reactivity of symptoms. Distress is rated by the patient on a 0 to 8 (minimum to maximum) scale. When an event rates 4 or more it is recorded in terms of when, where and what activity was involved. A month of monitoring will demonstrate any consistent pattern.

Exposure tests require of the patient that he enters a potentially phobic situation. A trained observer notes signs of excessive arousal like a change in heart rate, respiration and perspiration and any signs of phobic avoidance. Exposure tests are useful as preparation for exposure therapy and for medico-legal purposes. A test drive also helps to identify other problems. Some patients turn into anxious "back-seat drivers" and arguments between spouses add to the distress of driving.

An adequate replication of the traumatic situation can be as challenging as solving a crime. A patient who had been caught in a conveyor belt dreaded escalators and any moving machinery. A cab-driver who almost had his throat cut by a midnight passenger would not go out alone in the dark and became very anxious when anyone stood behind him. A woman who had remained conscious because of anesthetic failure combined with subconvulsive electrochoc therapy would not recline, was unable to cooperate with an EEG and was even uncomfortable with wearing head-phones. A stockbroker who had a myocardial infarction treated successfully with bypass surgery developed panic disorder and experienced recurrent attacks on the highway where he had experienced severe angina. None of these patients seemed fully aware of the cues that triggered their discomfort. The connection was made by diaries and behavioral tests.

Exposure Therapy

There is no treatment exclusively designed for PTSD. Freud's and Breuers early techniques for treating hysteria encouraged an abreaction of childhood trauma. Abreaction under sodium amytal or pentothal was used in the management of war neuroses. Sodium pentothal is still a valuable adjunct in the exploration of enigmatic pain.

Little has been published on the results of exposure in postaccidental phobias [21] but the remedial effects of exposure therapy on phobias have been established beyond reasonable doubt. Exposure therapy requires that the patient attend the feared situation until the urge to leave fades [10]. This may take between 20 minutes to three hours and approximately 12 hours total should be allowed for a series of closely spaced sessions.

Psychotherapy

It is often difficult to convince a patient to expose himself again to risks that have been so drastically demonstrated by the trauma. He may benefit from a review of the effect the trauma had on his outlook. His way of discriminating between safe und unsafe situations should be discussed. Horowitz [1] defined successful resolution as the capacity to recall the trauma at will but without intrusive recollections that would interfere with one's capability to turn one's mind to other matters.

Pharmacotherapy

Anxiolytics serve as an adjunct to exposure therapy but are not essential. In declining dose desensitisation a phobic patient receives declining doses of an anxiolytic before each of a series of exposure tasks until he can master them drug-free [24]. Posttraumatic panic disorder may be treated with alprazolam, clonazepam. phenelzine and imipramine. Nightmares may be suppressed by amitriptyline [1]. The pharmacotherapy of panic disorder is discussed in another chapter in this volume.

Screening and Advising Patients

The symptoms of PTSD overlap with the symptoms of phobic and panic disorder. Checklists based on DSM III-R criteria (see above and under "acute anxiety disorder") combined with questions about a change in life style will identify the more chronic patients. Acute trauma patients should be examined for signs of psychogenic amnesia and a history of panic during the accident. Patients may benefit from visiting the scene of the accident and from discussing the experience soon after. They should be advised to return if anxiety, nightmares and phobic avoidance persist beyond six months or surface at a later date.

References

1. van der Kolk BA (1987) Psychological trauma. American Psychiatric Press, Washington DC
2. Loeser JD (1980) Low back pain. In: Bonica JJ (ed) Pain. Raven Press, New York
3. The diagnostic and statistical manual III-R (1987) American Psychiatric Assn, Washington DC
4. McFarlane AH, Norman GR, Streiner DL, Roy RG (1983) The process of social stress: Stable, reciprocal and mediating relationships. J Health & Social Behavior 24:160–173
5. Atkinson RM, Sparr LF, et al (1984) Diagnosis of posttraumatic stress disorder in Viet Nam veterans: Preliminary findings. Am J Psychiatry 141:5, 694–696
6. Shore JH, Tatum EL, Vollmer WM (1986) Psychiatric reactions to disaster: The Mount St. Helens experience. Am J Psychiatry 143:590–595
7. Slocum R & Interministerial task force report (1981) Injury: An Ontario survey of the societal and personal costs of hospitalized motor vehicle accident victims. Government Press
8. Watson JB, Rayner R (1960) Conditioned emotional reactions. In: Eysenck HJ (ed) Behavior therapy and the neuroses. Pergamon
9. Jones MC (1960) A laboratory study of fear: The case of Peter. In: Eysenck HJ (ed) Behavior therapy and the neuroses
10. Marks IM (1987) Fears phobias and rituals. Oxford University Press, Oxford New York
11. Thyer BA, Mathews J (1986) The effects of phobic anxiety on plasma beta-endorphin: a single subject experiment. Behav Res Ther 24; 2:237–241
12. Kolb LC (1987) A neuropsychological hypothesis explaining posttraumatic stress disorder. Am J Psychiatry 144:8, 989–995
13. Shavit Y, Terman GW, Martin FC, et al (1985) Stress, opioid peptides, the immune system and cancer. J Immunology 135(2):834–837
14. Skinner BF (1974) About behaviorism. Vintage Books, New York
15. Fordyce WE (1976) Behavioral concepts in chronic pain and illness. In: Davidson PE (ed) The behavioral management of anxiety depression and pain. Brunner Mazel, New York
16. Allodi FA (1974) Accident neurosis – Whatever happened to male hysteria? Can J Psychiatry 19:291–295
17. Figley CR (1987) Trauma and it's wake. Brunner Mazel Psychosocial stress series, New York
18. Parker N (1977) Accident litgants with neurotic symptoms. Aust Med J 2:318–322
19. Benedikt RA, Kolb L (1986) Preliminary findings on chronic pain and posttraumatic stress disorder. Am J Psychiatry 143:908–910
20. Hodge JR (1971) The whiplash neurosis. Psychosomatics 12:4, 245–249
21. Kuch K, Swinson RP, Kirby M (1985) Posttraumatic stress disorder after car accidents. Can J Psychiatry 30:426–427
22. Kelly R (1975) The posttraumatic syndrome: a iatrogenic disease. Forensic Science 6:17–24
23. Tarsh MJ, Royston C (1985) A follow-up study of accident neurosis. Br J Psychiatry 146:18–25
24. McCormick WP (1973) Declining dose desensitisation for phobias. Can J Psychiatry 18:9–12

Cerebral Crisis – Psychological Support

Management of Acute Cerebral Edema

M. Zimpfer and A. Aloy

Introduction

Edema formation is a basic response of many organs or tissues to injury. However, *cerebral edema* with increased intracranial pressure, transtentorial herniation and consequent brain stem compression, edema or hemorrhage is a very serious complication of any underlying neurological disease. The insults causing edema formation can be focal or diffuse, brief or prolonged, single or multiple, mild or severe. The present chapter delineates the pathophysiology and classification of cerebral edema formation and reviews the current therapeutic principles.

Pathophysiology

Cerebral edema is not a single pathological entity. Although it may be classified according to the type of injury that produces it, it is most often classified in terms of the pathological mechanism [1]. The latter classification distinguishes mainly between "vasogenic" and "cytotoxic" forms of cerebral edema. The former involves injury to the blood-brain barrier that permits a plasma filtrate to extravasate into the cerebral extracellular space. A wide variety of physical, chemical, infectious, allergic, and neoplasic insults may increase the ability of the bloodbrain barrier to produce *vasogenic edema*. After head injury, vasogenic edema commonly occurs in the vicinity of cerebral hemorrhages or contusions but may also occur diffusely with minimal gross evidence of structural brain damage [2] (Fig. 1). In addition, this form of edema may be exacerbated by hypoxemia, hypercapnia, and epileptic seizures, all of which may occur after head injury. The vasogenic origin is now generally accepted to be based on a breakdown of the tight junctions within the central nervous system, capillary bed as well as alterations in glial membrane structure. On the other hand, *cytotoxic edema* involves an increase in intracellular water due to defective osmoregulation. This results from a disturbance in cellular metabolism and/or maintenance of normal transmembrane ionic gradients. This form of edema is produced, at least initially, by cerebral ischemia, which is also a common complication of clinical head injury. It is however important to know that these two types of cerebral edema are not exclusive. They may develop simultaneously or in succession after various insults and may be produced by the same injury agent, e.g. ischemia. Furthermore, there is evidence that either type of edema can itself induce development of the other [3].

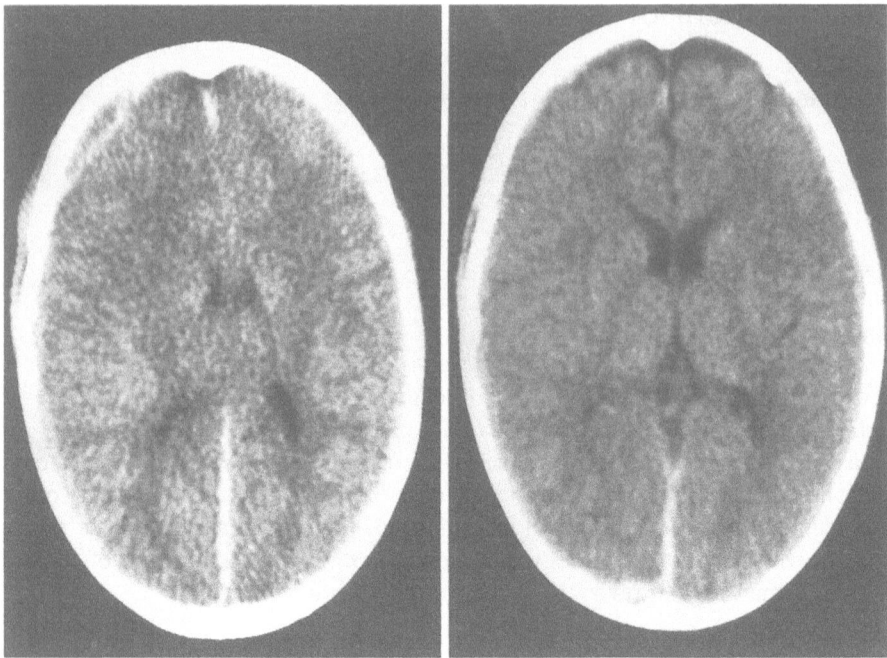

Fig. 1. Computed tomographic scan of a three-year-old boy who hit the ground after falling out of the window from approximately 6 meters. On admission (left), both cerebral hemispheres are diffusely swollen and of decreased density. The ventricles are mostly obliterated. Three weeks after injury (right), the follow up examination shows a marked decrease of the cerebral edema with a reexpansion of the ventricular system. After two weeks of volume-cycled controlled ventilation, concurrent unspecific treatment of the raised intracranial pressure and consecutive weaning the child was discharged with no residual neurological deficit

Treatment

Structural and Physiologic Causes of Elevated Intracranial Pressure

When intracranial pressure reaches a level of 20–25 mm Hg and, therefore, a decision is made to treat, three approaches have to be taken in a systemic fashion.

1. It is verified whether the measured increase in intracranial pressure is true, i.e., the wave form of the intracranial pressure tracing is assessed, the offset determined and the gain of the equipment calibrated.
2. It is determined what the causes are for this increase and
3. concurrently the treatment of the elevated intracranial pressure itself is adapted to the cause if possible.

There are both structural and physiologic causes for elevated intracranial pressure. *Structural causes* such as delayed intraventricular hemorrhage, postoperative hematomas, hydrocephalus and cerebral edema can be excluded by a CT-scan. Any patient who develops elevated intracranial pressure, from an initially normal range, should have repeated CT-scans to evaluate the presence of these causes. However, particularly cerebral edema cannot be treated immediately as, in the case of vasogenic edema, the repair of the blood-brain barrier begins within 15 to 24 h after injury [4] and the clearance of edema takes several days [5]. Before unspecific treatment is begun, physiologic causes such as elevated $PaCO_2$, hyponatremia, hyperthermia, poor ventilation, agitation, and seizures are checked and ruled out by the appropriate tests. Consequently, arterial blood gases are checked to see if the $PaCO_2$ is being adequately controlled. Serum electrolyte concentrations are drawn to be sure that there is no serum hypo-osmolarity that would cause a shift of water to the brain tissue. Temperature is assessed since increased temperature will increase the need of the brain for oxygen and, therefore, increase cerebral blood flow. The patient's activity is observed to be sure that he is not out of phase with the respirator causing increased intrathoracic pressure and impaired venous return from the head [6, 7].

Unspecific Treatment

Patient positioning (Fig. 2): The patient is positioned with an about 30 degree head-up tilt to facilitate venous drainage from the brain. Care is taken not to rotate the head to any side, i.e., the patient should "look straight".

Hyperventilation: The patient is carefully adapted to the respirator. Arterial $PaCO_2$ is lowered to between 25 and 30 mm Hg. This can be particularly useful if cerebral edema is secondary to a hyperemic response to brain injury [8]. Hypocarbia generally reduces blood flow [9]. During moderate hypocarbia blood may be shunted from normal tissue to ischemic zones [10]. With continued hyperventilation cerebral blood flow and intracranial pressure gradually presume nearly normal levels as cerebral spinal fluid, hydrogen, ion and bicarbonate concentrations reequilibrate.

Superimposed high frequency ventilation (Fig. 3): High frequency ventilation (8–12 Hz), superimposed to the conventional volume-cycled ventilation, can decrease intracranial pressure by enhanced venous return, due to the decreased intrathoracic pressure.

Ventricular drainage (Fig. 4): If a ventricular catheter is in place, the patient's ventricles are decompressed and drained down to approximately 15 mm Hg. However, in cases of severe cerebral edema it is almost impossible to insert ventricular catheters as the ventricular cavities are shrinked down.

Hypertonic solutions (Fig. 3): Hypertonic solutions such as mannitol, sorbitol and glycerol reduce brain water content by creating an osmotic gradient between the vascular compartment and the brain parenchyma across an intact blood-brain barrier [11]. However, the duration of intracranial pressure reduction following these agents has been controversial and all agents in this category have been alleged to potentially induce a rebound phenomenon by which the post-

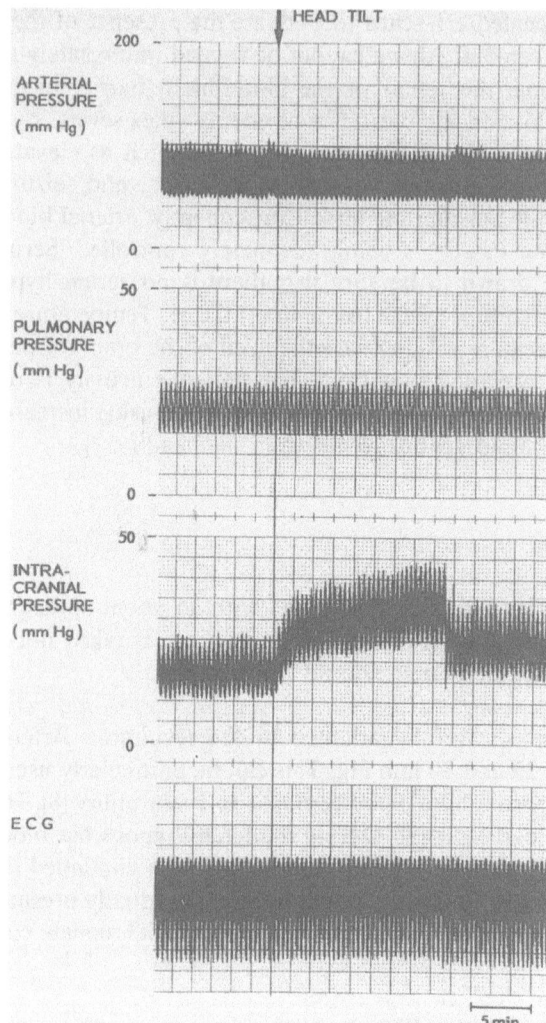

Fig. 2. Measurements of ECG, intracranial pressure and arterial pressure in a patient positioned with a 30 degree head-up tilt "looking straight forward" to facilitate venous drainage. Accidental tilting and rotating the head away from the upright "straight forward looking" position caused a distinct increase in intracranial pressure which partly returned towards control levels after repositioning of the patient

treatment intracranial pressure is higher than the baseline value. The mechanism is felt to be exceeding the threshold of the blood-brain barrier for these agents ultimately causing movement of water from the intravascular compartment of the brain parenchyma. The main toxic effects of glycerol, which can be avoided by careful slow administration, are hemolysis, hemoglobinuria and renal failure [12]. Also oxalic acid poisoning has been reported following the intravenous administration [13]. Furosemide can also be added to potentiate the effect of mannitol.

Steroids: While steroids are clearly effective in the treatment of edema associated with brain tumors [14], clear evidence of their beneficial effects in traumatic edema is lacking, despite widespread use.

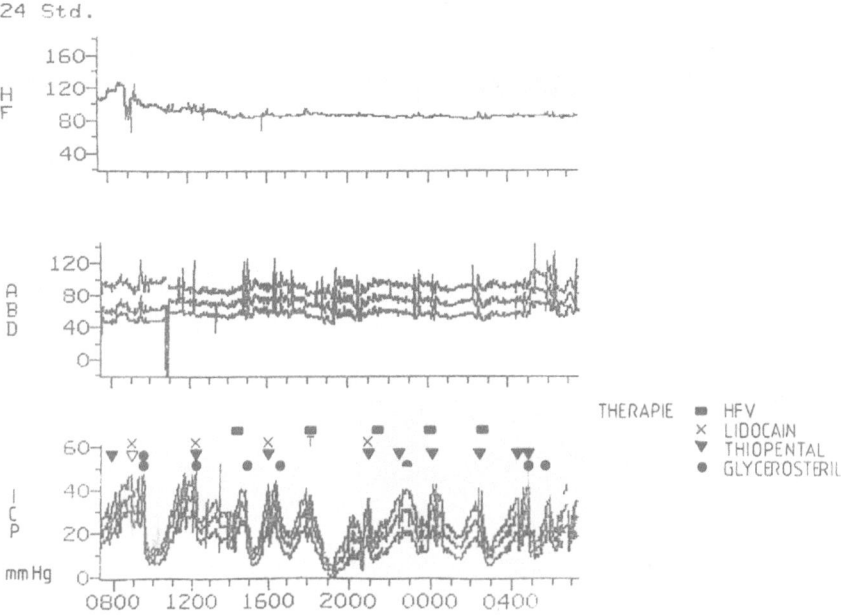

Fig. 3. Twenty-four-hour trend recording of heart rate (HF), systolic, diastolic and mean arterial pressure (ABD) and systolic, diastolic and mean intracranial pressure (ICP) in a patient with brain edema and volume-cycled controlled ventilation. Various pharmacologic interventions and to the regular respiratory cycle superimposed high frequency ventilation (HFV) are successfully employed to control the raised intracranial pressure

Barbiturates (Fig. 3): Barbiturates have been subject of considerable interest because of evidence of efficacy in providing protection from generalized and focal cerebral ischemia. Reduction of intracranial pressure has also been reported [15]. Barbiturate protection, at least partly, results from depressed metabolic demand for oxygen. Barbiturates also cause vasoconstriction in normal tissue and secondary shunting of blood to ischemic tissue [16, 17]. Other properties of barbiturates that may play a role in their protective effect include stabilisation of lysosomal membranes, suppression of the rate of edema formation, attenuation of fatty acid liberation, quenching of free radical reactions, reduction of intracellular calcium in ischemic tissue, reduced release of neurotransmitters during ischemia, and the inherent anesthetic property of barbiturates (see [18] for review).

Lidocaine (Fig. 3, Fig. 5): Lidocaine, which has been recommended just prior to suctioning [19], suppresses synaptic transmission and inhibits metabolism in normal tissue. It reduces membrane leak of sodium and potassium in ischemic brain by lowering membrane permeability, primarily for sodium. Because ion leaks are reduced, ion pumps are partially relieved of their load and the energy demand is decreased [16].

Acid-base buffering: The rational for cerebral protection from ischemia and hypoxia by administration of the buffer THAM (tris-hydroxymethyl-amino-me-

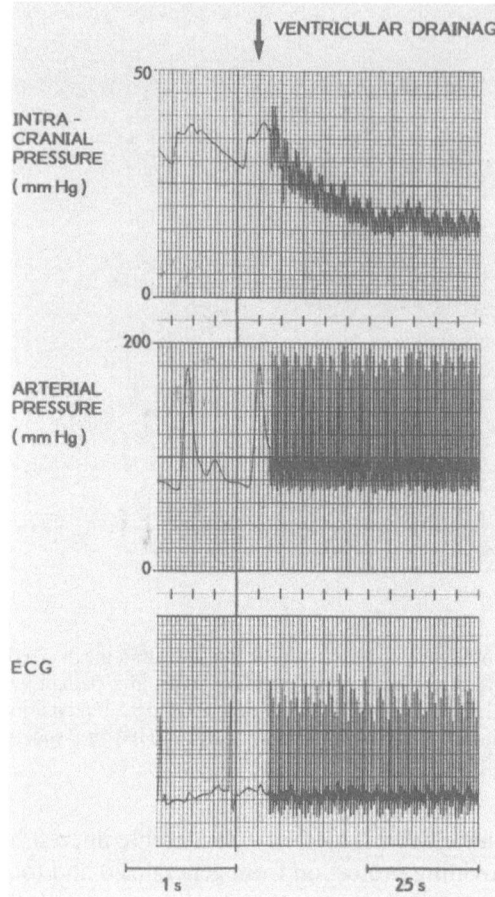

Fig. 4. Original tracings of intracranial pressure, arterial pressure and ECG in a patient with elevated intracranial pressure. Opening the ventriculostomy (ventricular drainage) lowers the intracranial pressure substantially. However, in the case of severe cerebral edema the insertion of a ventricular catheter may be impossible due to obliteration of the ventricular cavity

thane: tromethamine) is based upon its intracellular alkalinizing properties, its blood-brain barrier permeability, and its potential to reverse the harmful effects of tissue acidosis that follow an ischemic/hypoxic insult [20]. Its alkalinizing effect on tissues is similar to that of hypocarbia, but without reducing regional cerebral blood flow, jeopardizing aerobic glycolysis, and increasing tissue lactic acid, the by-product of anaerobic metabolism. However, our own experience has failed to demonstrate clear and reliable beneficial effects of THAM.

Substrate manipulation: While glucose is the primary fuel of brain metabolism, excessive amounts are harmful to ischemic and hypoxic brain tissue because the anaerobic metabolic end-product, lactic acid, may increase tissue acidosis sufficiently to interrupt cell function. For example, hypoglycemia caused by glucocorticoids aggravates ischemic brain damage [21]. Brain injury may also occur if the blood glucose level is too low, a situation commonly seen in patients comatose from insulin overdose.

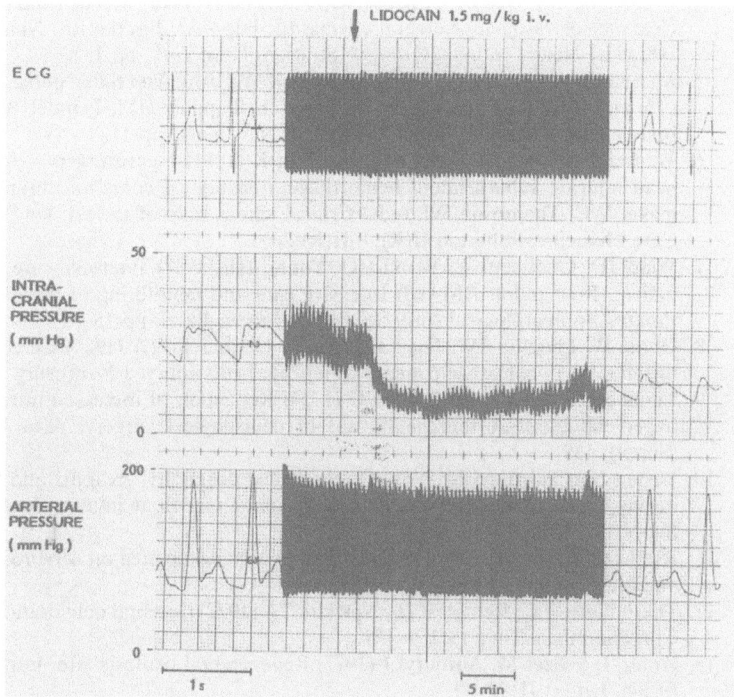

Fig. 5. Effects of lidocaine in a patient with increased intracranial pressure due to cerebral edema. Cerebral perfusion pressure rose substantially as intracranial pressure fell markedly while mean arterial pressure remained essentially unchanged

Conclusions

In summary, protection of the brain from cerebral edema and thus the harmful effects of ischemia and hypoxia is a multifactorial, complicated problem and will not be solved by the discovery of pharmacological panacea. At the same time, it is acknowledged that the injury by ischemia or hypoxia can be altered favorably in certain circumstances by various approaches and a variety of drugs with many different modes of action.

References

1. Klatzo I (1967) Neuropathological aspects of brain edema. J Neuropathol Exp Neurol 26:1
2. Tyson GW, Jane JA (1982) Pathophysiology of head injury. In: Cowley RA, Trump BF (eds) Pathophysiology of shock, anoxia, and ischemia. Williams & Wilkins, Baltimore London, pp 570–600
3. Fujimoto T, Walker JT Jr, Spatz M, Klatzo I (1976) Pathophysiologic aspects of ischemic edema. In: Pappius HM, Feindel W (eds) Dynamics of brain edema. Springer, Berlin Heidelberg New York, pp 171

4. Bruce DA, Ter Weeme C, Kaiser G, Ghostine S (1976) Mechanisms and time course for clearance of vasogenic cerebral edema. In: Popp AJ, Bourke RS, Nelson LR, Kimbelberg HK (eds) Neural trauma. Grune & Stratton, New York, pp 155
5. Marmarou A, Shulman K, Shapiro K, Poll W (1976) The time course of brain tissue pressure and local CBF in vasogenic edema. In: Pappius HM, Feindel W (eds) Dynamics of brain edema. Springer, Berlin Heidelberg New York, pp 112
6. Ward JD, Becker DP, Mickell J, Keenan R (1981) Neurosurgery - intracranial pressure, head injuries, subarachnoid hemorrhage, nonsurgical coma and brain tumors. In: Shoemaker WC, Thompson WL (eds) Critical care - state of the art, vol 2. Society of Critical Care Medicine, Fullerton II(R):1–II(R):26
7. Ward JD, Gadisseux P, Wood CO, Young HF (1987) Intensive care of the head-injured patient. In: Landolt AM (ed) Intensive care and monitoring of the neurosurgical patient. Progress in neurological surgery, vol 12. Karger, Basel, pp 15–52
8. Obrist W, Langfitt TW, Jaggi JL, Cruz J, Gennarelli TA (1984) Cerebral blood flow and metabolism in comatose patients with acute head injury. J Neurosurg 61:241–253
9. Lundberg N, Kjällquist A, Bien C (1959) Reduction of increased intracranial pressure by hyperventilation. A therapeutic aid in neurological surgery. Acta Psychiatr Scand 34 (Suppl): 139
10. Lassen NA, Palvölgyi R (1968) Cerebral steal during hypercapnia and the inverse reaction during hypercapnia observed by the 133 Xenon technique in man. Scand J Clin Lab Invest Suppl 102:XIII D
11. Reed DJ, Woodbury DM (1962) Effects of hypertonic area on cerebrospinal fluid pressure and brain volume. J Physiol 164:252–264
12. Tourtellotte WW, Reinglass JL, Newkirk TA (1972) Cerebral dehydration action of glycerol. Clin Pharmacol Ther 13:159–171
13. Krauz T, Sellzer M, Abrouryl I (1977) Renocerebral oxalosis after intravenous glycerol infusion. Lancet II:89–90
14. Galicich JH, French LA (1961) The use of dexamethasone in the treatment of cerebral edema resulting from brain tumors and brain surgery. Am Pract 12:169–174
15. Piatt JH Jr, Schiff SF (1984) High dose barbiturate therapy in neurosurgery and intensive care Neurosurgery 15:427–444
16. Astrup J, Sorensen PM, Sorensen HR (1981) Inhibition of cerebral oxygen and glucose consumption in the dog by hypothermia, pentobarbital, and lidocaine. Anesthesiology 55:263–268
17. Feustel PJ, Ingvar MC, Severinghaus JW (1981) Cerebral oxygen availability and blood flow during middle cerebral artery occlusion: effects of pentobarbital. Stroke 12:858–863
18. Hoff JT (1986) Cerebral protection. J Neurosurg 65:579–591
19. Bedford RF, Persing JA, Pobereskin L, et al (1980) Lidocaine or thipental for rapid control of intracranial hypertension. Anesth Analg 49:435
20. Rosner MJ, Becker DP (1984) Experimental brain injury: successful therapy with the weak base, tromethamine, with an overview of CNS acidosis. J Neurosurg 60:961–971
21. Koide T, Wieloch J, Siesjö BK (1986) Chronic dexamethasone pretreatment aggravates ischemic brain damage by inducing hyperglycemia. J Cereb Blood Flow Metab 5 (Suppl 1):S251–S252

Recent Advances in the Management of Subarachnoid Hemorrhage

B. Ljunggren, L. Brandt, and H. Säveland

Introduction

Four hundred years ago the French philosopher Michel de Montaigne (1533–1592), regarding the usual attitude of the scientific world towards new ideas and achievements, noticed:

– *Whenever a new discovery is reported to the scientific world, they say first: It's probably not true.* (Stage 1).

Thereafter, when the truth of the proposition has been demonstrated beyond question, they say: Yes, it may be true, but is it important? (Stage 2).

Finally, when sufficient time has elapsed to fully evidence its importance, they say: Yes, surely it is important, but it is no longer new. (Stage 3).

Background

At the Meeting of the Harvey Cushing Society in 1951, Arthur Ecker from Syracuse, New York presented a study published later the same year in *Journal of Neurosurgery* with Paul Riemenschneider. This publication dealt with arteriographic demonstration of spasm of the intracranial arteries with special reference to saccular arterial aneurysms [1]. As the talk began, Ecker noticed negative head shaking by some of the senior members in the rear of the auditorium. However, another man in the front seemed to smile approval. Ecker addressed the rest of his remarks to him. In the subsequent discussion some of the older men denied the existence of cerebral arterial spasm. Some younger neurosurgeons responded that, not only had they seen spasm at operation, but they had also deliberately produced it by touching the vessel. When the session was over, Ecker went to the unknown smiling man in front to thank him for his encouragement. He answered, still smiling, "I don't speak English" [2].

For several years cerebral vasospasm was met with reluctance. However, only six years after Ecker and Riemenschneider's original contribution, at the Society Meeting of British Neurological Surgeons a group of far-seeing Manchester neurosurgeons suggested that subarachnoid blood clot could maintain narrowing of cerebral arteries and cause serious ischemia and that this might be an indication for early surgery in an attempt to free the main vessels quite apart from treatment of the aneurysm itself [3].

Such attempts at an early surgical intervention had been reported in 1953 by Norlén and Olivecrona, but the mortality exceeded 50% and could at this time not be recommended [4]. In 1970 Drake reported on renewed attempts to perform early surgery but of 5 patients in good condition prior to operation, 4 became hemiplegic or demented, or both, and the 5th patient died [5]. 32 years earlier Wilder Penfield have said: "Brain surgery is a terrible profession, if I did not feel it will become different in my life time, I should hate it". Fortunately the results of early aneurysm surgery have been improved in the lifetime of today's neurosurgeons.

Up to the late 1970s ruptured intracranial aneurysms could obviously not be approached in the acute phase without disastrous surgical results. Consequently the case for delayed aneurysm surgery was at this time strongly stated and advocated by the neurosurgical expertise. Apart from rebleeds in patients awaiting surgery after a recovery phase of 12–14 days cerebral vasospasm or ischemic deterioration took a further heavy toll from the victims who has survived the first ictus. At this time there was no medical management available to combat such delayed ischemic dysfunction (DID). As late as in 1986 Wilkins stated that "numerous approaches to the prevention and treatment of intracranial arterial spasm have been made during the past three decades ... there has been some progress toward the satisfactory management of this detrimental condition, but much remains to be done" [6].

With the introduction of microneurosurgery a new era took place in the 1970s and renewed attempts to operate in the acute stage were made. At the Harvey Cushing Society in 1981 we presented a consecutive series of 81 patients subjected to operation in the acute stage [7]. The aim of early surgical intervention was not only to prevent rebleeds but also to reduce delayed ischemic deterioration by intraoperative removal of blood-contaminated cerebrospinal fluid (CSF) an clots from the basal cisterns. Not many of the audience smiled approval and negative head shaking could be observed from several neurosurgeons. Today, 7 years later, it is apparent that experienced aneurysm surgeons operating upon good risk patients in the acute stage can obtain similar morbidity and mortality rates as with delayed surgery just a decade ago.

Concerning the management of patients with a subarachnoid hemorrhage (SAH) controversial opinions, however, still exist. How are deleterious aneurysm rebleeds best prevented? Which management protocol offers the best protection against further cerebral damage after the initial bleed? How should delayed cerebral ischemia, elicited by the extravasation of blood to the subarachnoid spaces be prevented? What is the overall outcome with different treatment regimes? Has antifibrinolytic treatment any therapeutical place? What is the cognitive status and quality of life following aneurysmal SAH? Is there a difference in cognitive outcome in patients subjected to early versus late surgery? Do patients with SAH of unknown origin, who usually recover without any discernible neurological dysfunction, also show a complete cognitive recovery?

Prevention of Rebleeds

Kassell et al. recently emphasized that rebleeding is the most irreversible and disastrous complication of aneurysmal SAH and presented data indicating a high rate of rebleeding on the first 2 days following the initial bleed [8]. Using data from the Cooperative Aneurysm Study [9], Flamm suggested that the peak of early rebleeds occurs within the first 24 h and that there is no delayed peak [10]. He concluded that "since it is unlikely that most major centers will be also able to operate on all patients with aneurysmal SAH within the first 24 h, we may have to reconsider the idea that early surgery will significantly impact on eliminating rebleeding as a cause of death and disability" [10]. This statement is certainly highly controversial and merits a further evaluation. It appears that the data from the Cooperative Aneurysm Study, suggesting that the rate of rebleeding is highest on the first 2 days and then decreased rapidly [8], may be viewed with some precaution. This study involved 115 hospitals in 15 countries with 43% of the cases arriving at the centers after a delay of at least 3 days.

Vermeulen et al. performed a study on causes of acute deterioration in 150 patients with aneurysmal SAH and found a maximum incidence of rebleeds at the end of the 1st week, and in addition another peak seemed to emerge during the 3rd week [11]. In a similar study of 110 consecutive SAH-patients, confirmed rebleeding showed a flat distribution curve during the first 3 weeks after the presenting hemorrhage [12]. Episodes of non-hemorrhagic deterioration peaked between days 4 to 12. In yet another study of 150 consecutive patients admitted within 6 h of the initial bleed, 33 patients reblend, 23 of them within 6 h (15%) [13]. These authors found that the rebleeding rate was higher the more severe the initial SAH had been. Similar findings were reported from the prospective Danish Aneurysm Study Group reporting significantly fewer rebleeds in patients with good clinical grades as compared to those in a poor clinical condition [14]. This latter study revealed only a 0.8% rebleed rate during the first 24 h with a maximum risk of rebleeding between Day 4 and Day 9 [14]. In a study of 480 patients who were alive upon admission following an aneurysmal SAH in Sweden 21 initially good to fair risk patients (4% of the total SAH population) rebled fatally before surgery and within 48 h despite an early referral system and a policy to operate such patients as soon as possible [15]. In a recent British study [16] from 2 centers with a policy to operate good grade patients as soon as logistically possible 14% of good grade (Hunt & Hesse Grades I–II) [17] patients rebled, fatally in ⅓. Of the Hunt & Hess Grades III–V patients 13% rebled, fatally in over 50%. Since less than 50% of the patients in this British population were referred within four days after ictus, the authors concluded that their figure for early rebleeds probably represented an underestimation.

It may be concluded that rebleeds can only be prevented with a good and efficient referral system. This must be organized so that patients with a subarachnoid hemorrhage are admitted immediately to neurosurgical centers with a policy to operate as soon as possible.

Prevention of Delayed Ischemic Dysfunction (Vasospasm)

In patients who have survived their first aneurysmal SAH delayed neurological deterioration is now well recognized as a major determinant of outcome. The underlying pathophysiology of this syndrome and the significance of the various mechanisms possibly involved in the phenomenon are controversial [6]. With the introduction of computerized tomography (CT) it has been possible to demonstrate that there is a direct relationship between the amount and distribution of CT-visualized subarachnoid blood and later development of cerebral vasospasm or ischemic dysfunction. Fisher and coworkers thus found that when subarachnoid blood was not detected or was diffusely distributed on CT, severe vasospasm was almost never encountered. In the presence of subarachnoid blood clots or layers of blood in fissures and vertical cisterns, severe spasm followed almost invariably and there was a close correlation between the site of the major subarachnoid clots and the location of severe vasospasm [18].

A wide variety of different vasoconstrictive substances occurring in post-hemorrhagic CSF from patients with ruptured aneurysms have been suggested to account for the pathogenesis of delayed cerebral hypoperfusion and the list has grown as new vasoactive substances have been discovered. However, none has been shown to be more important than the others, and no antagonist of a single mediator candidate has been demonstrated to be therapeutically effective.

In 1979, we showed that perivascular application of nifedipine in cats invariably induced a marked dilatatory response of pial arterioles. Importantly this dilatation also occurred when vessels were constricted by the presence of subarachnoid blood [19]. This effect made us conclude that calcium channel blockers might be of potential use in the treatment of cerebral vasospasm and ischemia. Other investigators the same year were able to dilate cerebral blood vessels in dogs given oral nifedipine [20].

Further experimental studies on calcium channel blockers of the dihydropyridine family were summarized in a doctoral thesis from Lund in 1981 [21]. It was documented that the calcium channel blocker nimodipine dilates pial arterioles *in situ* and the response increased with decreases arteriolar size. The dilatatory response occurred also in the presence of perivascular human hemorrhagic CSF from patients with aneurysmal SAH and cerebral vasospasm. Such CSF in itself constricts cerebral arterioles. Pial arterioles brought to constriction by middle cerebral artery (MCA) occlusion were also dilated by nimodipine. In very small arterioles which stasis was present following occlusion of the MCA, there was a return of flow.

With these laboratory works the way was paved for further clinical trials. In 1983 Allen et al. reported a benefit of oral administration with the calcium channel antagonist nimodipine [22]. This multicenter trial was conducted in good grade patients and revealed a significant reduction in the number of patients having an unfavorable outcome ascribed to vasospasm alone. The following year 2 clinical trials [23, 24] with intravenous nimodipine were published with almost identical results. In these studies early clipping using microsurgical techniques with evacuation of post-hemorrhage CSF and clots combined with i.v. nimodipine therapy resulted in an incidence of DID with permanent deficit in less than 3% in a total of 125 patients. The appearance and severity of late angiographic vasospasm did not seem to be affected by nimodipine [23]. Since these studies were neither randomized nor placebo controlled, the results were mostly met with scepticism. Although most experienced aneurysm surgeons now confess themselves to an early surgical approach in good risk patients [25], some neuro-surgeons are still sceptic towards the benefit of an early surgical intervention [26]. Concerning the possible antiischemic effects of nimodipine the opinions are even more controversial.

In 1987 Weir and coworkers announced the results of a 17-center, random-ized, placebo-controlled, double-blind trial of oral nimodipine in 154 poor grade aneurysm patients [27]. Repeat angiography after day 4 in 124 patients showed no difference in the incidence of moderate or severe diffuse spasm. Nimodipine treatment was nevertheless associated with a significantly better outcome and a reduction in the number of patients suffering delayed neurological deterioration. The authors concluded that this effect must occur by a mechanism other than prevention of large vessel spasm as visualized on angiography.

A statistically significant beneficial antiischemic effect of i.v. nimodipine has also been reported in a placebo controlled, double-blind trial of patients ran-domly subjected to operation at different time intervals following SAH [28].

Antifibrinolytic Treatment?

In the 1960s great expectations were put on the use of antifibrinolytics [29–32]. There has, however, accumulated an abundance of evidence against the use of such drugs [33–41]. As early as in 1972, Kågström and Palma drew attention to the fact that antifibrinolytic treatment might be associated with an increase of delayed cerebral ischemic dysfunction [33]. Referring to a controlled study from the University of Western Ontario in 1973 [31], Girvin concluded that "the con-troversy regarding the use of antifibrinolytic therapy in the preoperative treat-ment of ruptured aneurysms has been resolved – the therapy has no benefit" [35] and Maurice-Williams made the same observations [36].

A randomized controlled clinical trial from Umeå University (1980) showed a reduced incidence of rebleeds using tranexamic acid in patients with recently ruptured aneurysms [37]. The total mortality from cerebral ischemia *and* re-bleeding was, however, higher in the group treated with antifibrinolytics as compared to the control group during the 6 weeks observation time [38]. In a review from the same center on the use of antifibrinolytics in SAH in 1982, it was summarized that antifibrinolytics evidently reduce or postpone the inci-dence of rebleeding but at the same time vasospasm and cerebral ischemic de-ficits appear more frequently in patients treated with tranexamic acid [39]. Kas-sell et al. 2 years later also reached the same conclusion, that patients receiving antifibrinolytic therapy (aminocaproic acid and/or tranexamic acid) had a sig-nificantly lower rebleeding rate, but higher rates of ischemic deficits and hydro-cephalus so that the net results was no difference in mortality in the first month following the initial SAH [40]. Finally, the anxiously awaited Rotterdam-Am-sterdam-Glasgow-London randomized, controlled, double-blind study revealed in 1984 that tranexamic acid is of no benefit in patients with subarachnoid he-morrhage [41].

Overall Outcome Following Different Regimes

The difference in total outcome in two populations subjected to early versus late management is depicted in Figure 1, which shows the results from 40% of the Swedish population during a 3-year period and the results from the Kingdom of Denmark during 1975–1983 [42].

Cognitive Status and Quality of Life Following SAH

Does early aneurysm operation, while lowering the overall management mortality, result in an unacceptable morbidity in terms of increased cognitive disturbances and psychosocial maladjustment? This important matter was dealt with in a recent study [43] showing that the pattern and distribution of cognitive and psychosocial sequelae after late aneurysm operation did not differ substantially from those in patients subjected to early operation. These results offer strong support to the concept that remaining disturbances in cognition are mainly related to their impact of the initial hemorrhage per se. The late surgery group of this study represented a selected subpopulation of patients who had not deteriorated as a consequence of further bleeds or delayed ischemic dysfunction, whereas the early surgery group included the individuals at risk of both rebleeding and developing secondary ischemic brain damage. The lack of clear-cut differences in cognitive outcome between the 2 groups offers a further strong argument for early clipping of ruptured intracranial aneurysms.

It is well documented that SAH of unknown origin represents a less severe stroke as compared to SAH of aneurysmal origin. Nevertheless, a recent study revealed that the extravasation of blood, also in patients where this was not visualized on CT, in most instances had demonstrable negative effects on higher brain function(s) [44].

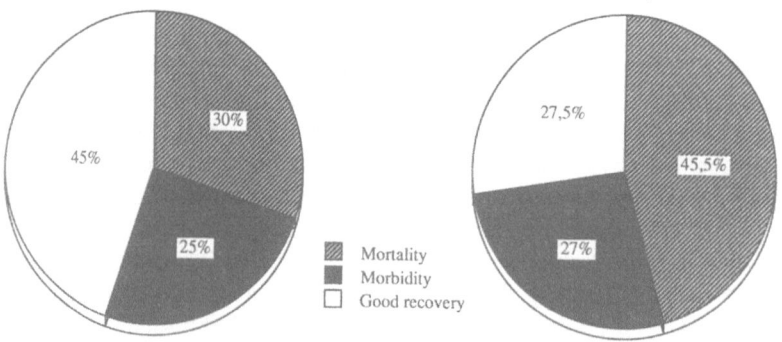

Fig. 1. Overall outcome in 480 patients who were alive upon admission to three neurosurgical centers in Sweden (covering 40% of the total population) with a policy of early operation *(left)*. Overall outcome in 1076 patients who were alive upon admission to all neurosurgical centers in the Kingdom of Denmark with a policy of delayed operation *(right)*

Conclusions

When looking back on the achievements in the last decade with regard to improvement in the management of patients with ruptured intracranial aneurysms Montaigne's three phases may be recognized:

Early timing of aneurysm operation in good condition patients has in the last decade passed Montaigne's phases and now appears to have reached stage 3. Thus, it is now generally agreed upon that surgery should no longer be delayed but performed as soon as possible in the acute stage in patients who have survived their first bleed in an acceptable condition. By this management deleterious rebleeds are eliminated. Early surgery furthermore permits a partial evacuation of blood clots and blood-contaminated cerebrospinal fluid (CSF) from the cisterns and subarachnoid spaces most probably resulting in a reduction of delayed hemorrhage-induced cerebral ischemia.

Concerning cerebral ischemic dysfunction following aneurysmal subarachnoid hemorrhage (SAH) the effects of additional preventive measures, by using a calcium channel blocker such as nimodipine, are called in question. Some are sceptic and mean that it is probably not true that such pharmacological treatment is beneficial while others waver and think that it may be true but still has to be proven in double-blind, placebo-controlled large trials. A few enthusiasts believe that the scientific proof has already been delivered and claim that additional nimodipine treatment of patients with aneurysmal SAH is important, but that it is no longer new.

References

1. Ecker AD, Riemenschneider PA (1951) Arteriographic demonstration of spasm of the intracranial arteries: With special reference to saccular arterial aneurisms. J Neurosurg 8:660–667
2. Ecker A (1982) The discovery of human cerebral arterial spasm in angiograms: an autobiographical note. Neurosurgery 10:90
3. Johnson RJ, Potter JM, Reid RG (1958) Arterial spasm in subarachnoid hemorrhage: mechanical considerations. J Neurol Neurosurg Psychiat 21:68
4. Norlén G, Olivecrona H (1953) The treatment of aneurysms of the circle of Willis. J Neurosurg 10:404–415
5. Drake CG (1971) Discussion of Symon L: Vasospasm in aneurysm. In: Moossy J, Janeway R (eds) Cerebral Vascular Diseases. Seventh Princeton Conference. Grune and Stratton, New York, pp 241–244
6. Wilkins RH (1986) Attempts at prevention or treatment of intracranial arterial spasm: an update. Neurosurgery 18:808–825
7. Ljunggren B, Brandt L, Kågström E, Sundbärg G (1981) Results of early operation for ruptured aneurysms. J Neurosurg 54:473–479
8. Kassell NF, Haley EC, Torner JC (1986) Antifibrinolytic therapy in the treatment of aneurysmal subarachnoid haemorrhage. Clin Neurosurg 33:137–45
9. Kassell NF, Torner JC (1983) Aneurysmal rebleeding A preliminary report from the cooperative aneurysm study. Neurosurgery 13:479–81
10. Flamm ES (1983) The timing of aneurysmal rebleeding A preliminary report from the cooperative aneurysm study. Neurosurgery 13:479–81

11. Vermeulen M, van Gijn J, Hijdra A, van Crevel H (1984) Causes of acute deterioration in patients with a ruptured intracranial aneurysm. A prospective study with serial CT scanning. J Neurosurg 60:935–939

12. Maurice-Williams RS (1982) Ruptured intracranial aneurysms: has the incidence of early rebleeding been over-estimated? J Neurosurg Psychiatry 45:774–779

13. Inagawa T, Kamiya K, Ogasawara H, Yano T (1987) Rebleeding of ruptured intracranial aneurysms in the acute stage. Surg Neurol 28:93–99

14. Rosenörn J, Eskesen V, Schmidt K, Rönde F (1987) The risk of rebleeding from ruptured intracranial aneurysms. J Neurosurg 67:329–332

15. Ljunggren B, Fodstad H, von Essen C, Säveland H, Brandt L, Hillman J, Romner B, Algers G (1988) Aneurysmal subarachnoid haemorrhage: Overall outcome and incidence of early recurrent haemorrhage despite a policy of acute stage operation. Br J Neurosurg (submitted)

16. O'Neill P, West CR, Chadwick DW, Conway M, Foy PM, Maloney P, Pickard JD, Spillane JA, Shaw MDM (1988) Recurrent aneurysmal subarachnoid haemorrhage: incidence, timing and effects. A reappraisal in a surgical series. Br J Neurosurg (in press)

17. Hunt WE, Hess RM (1968) Surgical risk as related to time of intervention in the repair of intracranial aneurysms. J Neurosurg 28:14–19

18. Fisher CM, Kistler JP, Davis JM (1980) Relation of cerebral vasospasm to subarachnoid hemorrhage visualized by computerized tomographic scanning. Neurosurgery 6:1–9

19. Brandt L, Andersson KE, Bengtsson B, Edvinsson L, Ljunggren B, MacKenzie ET (1979) Effects of nifedipine on pial arteriolar calibre: an in vivo study. Surg Neurol 12:349–352

20. Allen GS, Bahr AL (1979) Cerebral arterial spasm 10. Reversal of acute and chronic spasm in dogs with orally administered nifedipine. Neurosurgery 4:43–47

21. Brandt L (1981) Aspects on cerebral vasospasm; a clinical and experimental study. Lund University; Doctoral Thesis

22. Allen GS, Ahn HS, Preziosi TJ, et al (1983) Cerebral arterial spasm – a controlled trial of nimodipine in patients with subarachnoid hemorrhage. N Engl J Med 308:619–624

23. Ljunggren B, Brandt L, Säveland H, et al (1984) Outcome in 60 consecutive patients treated with early aneurysm operation and intravenous nimodipine. J Neurosurg 61:864–873

24. Auer LM (1984) Acute operation and preventive nimodipine improve outcome in patients with ruptured cerebral aneurysms. Neurosurgery 15:57–66

25. Adams CBT (1987) Effect of early aneurysm surgery and nimodipine administration. J Neurosurg 66:482–483

26. Kikuchi H, Fukushima T, Watanabe E (eds) (1986) Intracranial aneurysms. Surgical timing and techniques. Proceedings of the First International Workshop on Intracranial Aneurysms (IWIA). Japan: Nishimura; 1–376

27. Weir B, Disney L, Grace M (1987) Prospective randomized placebo control study of the calcium antagonist nimodipine in the prevention of vasospasm and ischemic neurologic deficit. Presented at the 8th European Congress of Neurosurgery (Abstract volume page 269)

28. Öman J, Heiskanen O (1987) Results of intravenous nimodipine treatment in patients randomly selected for surgery at three different time intervals following aneurysmal subarachnoid hemorrhage. Proceedings of 2nd World Congress of Neuroscience (IBRO). Budapest; Pergamon Press Suppl 22 (abstract)

29. Gibbs JR, O'Gorman P (1967) Fibrinolysis in subarachnoid haemorrhage. Postgrad Med J 43:779–784

30. Mullan S, Dawley J (1968) Antifibrinolytic therapy for intracranial aneurysms. J Neurosurg 28:21–23

31. Norlén G, Thulin CA (1967) Experiences with epsilon-amino-caproic acid in neurosurgery. Neurochirurgia 10:81–86

32. Norlén G, Thulin CA (1969) The use of antifibrinolytic substances in ruptured intracranial aneurysm. Neurochirurgia 12:100–102

33. Kågström E, Palma L (1972) Influence of antifibrinolytic treatment on the morbidity in patients with subarachnoid hemorrhage. Acta Neurol Scand 48:257

34. Girvin JP (1973) The use of antifibrinolytic agents in the preoperative treatment of ruptured intracranial aneurysms. Trans Amer Neurol Assoc 98:150–152

35. Girvin JP (1976) The failure of antifibrinolytic agents to improve the operative treatment of ruptured intracranial aneurysms. In: Morley TP (ed) Current controversies in neurosurgery Saunders Company, pp 279–281

36. Maurice-Williams RS (1978) Prolonged antifibrinolysis: an effective non-surgical treatment for ruptured intracranial aneurysms? Br Med J 1:945–947

37. Fodstad H (1980) Tranexamic acid as therapeutic agent in aneurysmal subarachnoid haemorrhage: Clinical, laboratory and experimental studies. Umeå University Medical Dissertation New Series No 60, pp 1–74

38. Fodstad H, Forssel Å, Liliequist B, Schannong M (1981) Antifibrolysis with tranexamic acid in aneurysmal subarachnoid hemorrhage; a consecutive controlled clinical trial. Neurosurgery 8:158–165

39. Fodstad H (1982) Antifibrinolytic treatment in subarachnoid haemorrhage: present state. Acta Neurochir 63:233–244

40. Kassell NF, Torner JC, Adams Jr HP (1984) Antifibrinolytic therapy in the acute period following aneurysmal subarachnoid haemorrhage. J Neurosurg 61:225–230

41. Vermeulen M, Lindsay KW, Murray GD, Cheah F, Hijdra A, Muizelaar JP, Schannong M, Teasdale GM, van Crevel H, van Gijn J (1984) Antifibrinolytic treatment in subarachnoid hemorrhage. New Engl J Med 311:432–437

42. Rösenörn J, Eskesen V, Schmidt K, et al (1987) Clinical features and outcome in 1076 patients with ruptured intracranial saccular aneurysms: a prospective consecutive study. Brit J Neurosurg 1:33–45

43. Sonesson B, Ljunggren B, Säveland H, Brandt L (1987) Cognition and adjustment after late and early operation for ruptured aneurysm. Neurosurgery 21:279–287

44. Sonesson B, Säveland H, Ljunggren B, Brandt L (1987) Cognition and adjustment after subarachnoid hemorrhage of unknown versus aneurysmal origin. J Neurol Neurosurg & Psychiatry (submitted)

Possible Role of Calcium Antagonists in Acute Ischemic Stroke

O. Busse

Introduction

Due to a rapid onset of morphological changes of the brain tissue after ischemic stroke all drug treatments have so far been insufficient. There are three different mechanisms of improving the chances of survival of the nerve cells:

1. improvement of ischemic tolerance of the brain tissue
2. improvement of the microcirculation.
3. prevention of secondary damage during the reperfusion phase due to the formation of additional harmful substances.

The barbiturate therapy and hypothermia for improvement of ischemic tolerance of the brain tissue have not been as successful as hoped for and cannot be used in clinical practice. The hyper- or isovolemic hemodilution is well accepted, even if the success of the hemorheological treatment has not proven [1, 2]. So far a well accepted therapy regimen does also not exist for the prevention of secondary damage. However the calcium channel blockers seem to prevent the development of damages after focal cerebral ischemia.

The Ischemic and Calcium Cascade

As seen in Figure 1 there is a loss of functions of the neurons after a decrease of cerebral blood flow (CBF) below a level of 20 ml/min/100 g. If the regional CBF falls to a level below 10 mg/min/100 g, the oxygen supply to the brain tissue is reduced, the energy reserves are depleted and lactic acidosis develops.

A membrane damage of the nerve cells causes an efflux of potassium and an influx of calcium and sodium with development of cell necrosis. Predominantly in the initial phase after an ischemic stroke there are cells without any functions which are still viable. In this area the r-CBF is between 10–20 ml/min/100 g. It is called the ischemic penumbra [3, 4].

The increased influx of calcium into the nerve cells due to ischemia triggers off a cascade of dangerous reactions. The development of additional harmful substances is favored due to oxygen supply during reperfusion. A loss of ATP caused by ischemia results in a reduced transport of calcium to the extracellular space. This results in an overload of calcium in the cytosol, the endoplasmic reticulum, and in the mitochondria which leads to an interruption of oxidative

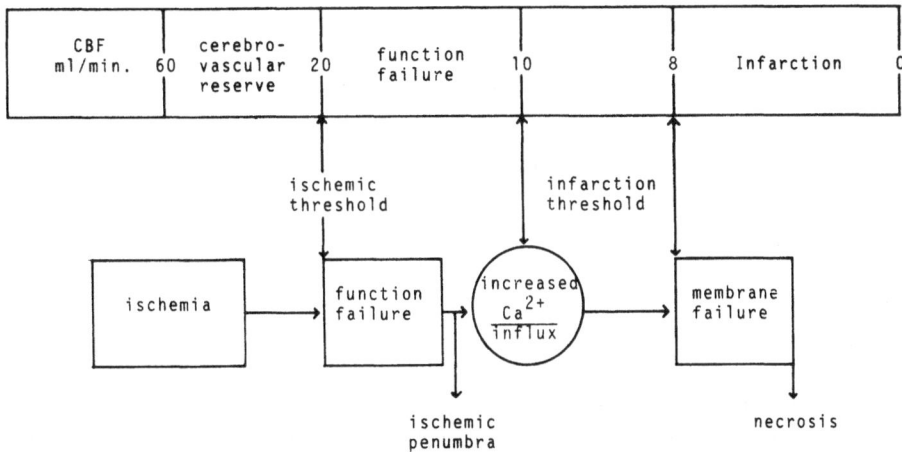

Fig. 1. The ischemic cascade

phosphorylation. The intracellular accumulation of calcium ions activates phospholipase A2 in the cell membranes and free fatty acids and in particular arachidonic acid is released. Vasoconstrictive prostaglandins, leukotrienes and free radicals are formed during reperfusion and oxygen supply. These substances now cause further membrane lesions (Fig. 2).

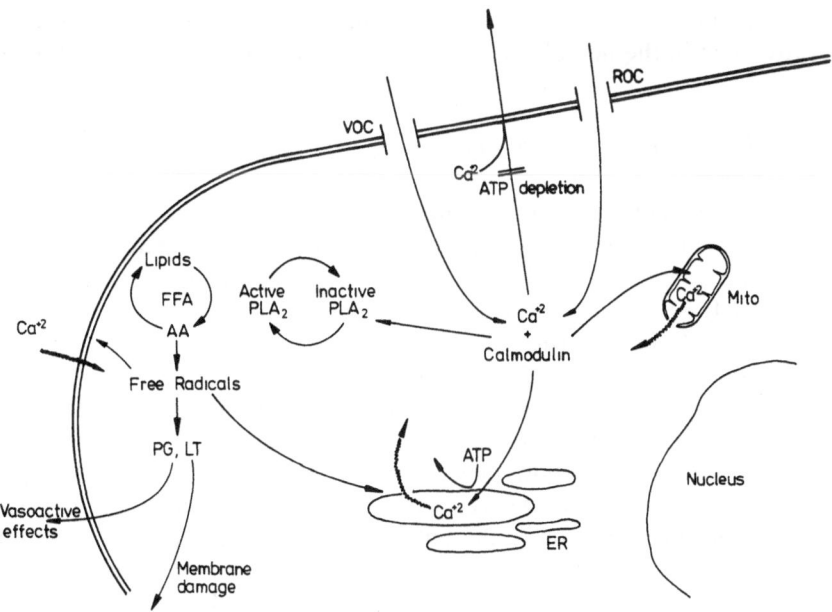

Fig. 2. The calcium cascade

Mode of Action of the Calcium Channel Blockers

Two modes of action are attributed to calcium channel blockers:

1. A cytoprotective effect with prevention of calcium overload in the neurons.
2. Increase of r-CBF due to the antivasoconstrictive effects: the calcium channel blockers act directly on the smooth muscle cells and secondarily via the production of vasoconstrictive substances.

A third mode of action could be the influence on red blood cell shape changes.

The efficacy of the calcium channel blockers is well documented for flunarizine and the dihydropyrine (DHP)-derivates nimodipine and nicardipine. Although the DHP's act on the potential operated channels (POC) and have a more marked effect on the cerebral vessels than on the brain tissue, nimodipine penetrates the blood brain barrier (BBB) and reacts with receptor operated channels too. Flunarizine should selectively prevent the calcium influx in the cell due to ischemia [6].

Pretreatment with flunarizine showed a dose-dependent reduction of the structure damages in different animal models of global ischemia; in addition an overload of calcium in the nerve cells could be proven histochemically [7]. Hossmann et al. [8] did not find any effect with flunarizine on the calcium concentration of the brain tissue in models of global ischemia given after the damage. Grotta et al. [9] demonstrated an improvement in neuronatal function by SSEP in rats after subcutaneous infusion of nicardipine before and after global ischemia. After a seven minute lasting interruption of the cerebral circulation in cats the "no-reflow phenomenon" could be prevented in comparison to control animals after pretreatment with 10 mg/kg nimodipine orally [10]. After a seventeen minute lasting global ischemia in monkeys Steen et al. [11] showed an improvement in the neurological outcome after treatment with nimodipine.

Experiments on Focal Cerebral Ischemia

The effects of the calcium channel blockers on focal cerebral ischemia is best documented for the DHP's. Sauer and Rodin [12] investigated the effect of the DHP-derivate PN 200–110 on the infarct size with the magnetic resonance imaging (MRI) 24, 48 and 72 hours after unilateral occlusion of the middle cerebral artery (MCA) in rats. The infarct size as well as the neurological outcome could be favorable influenced (Fig. 3). The best results were achieved if the calcium channel blocker was given before the occlusion. In the same trial the result with nimodipine given after the occlusion was not favorably. However Germano et al. [13] were able to show that pre- and posttreatment with nimodipine in a model of focal ischemia (MCA-occlusion) showed a reduction of the size of the infarction in comparison to the untreated animals and the placebo group (Fig. 4). Barnett et al. [14] could not demonstrate a reduction of the infarct size in cats after a four hour lasting MCA-occlusion when nimodipine was given before or during occlusion.

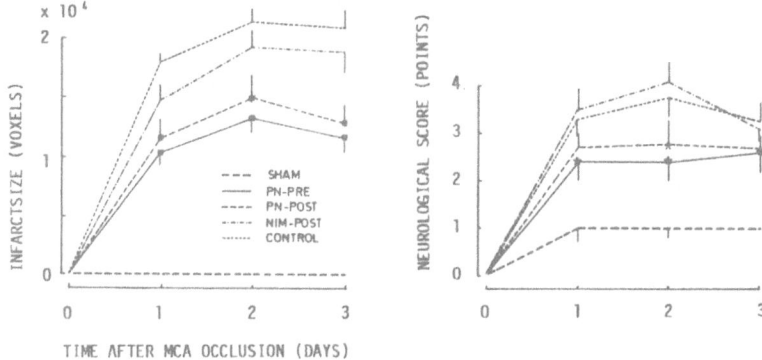

Fig. 3. Time course of infarct size and neurological score after MCA occlusion. *SHAM:* sham operated rats; *PN-PRE:* PN pretreated rats; *PN-POST:* PN posttreated rat; *NIM-POST:* Nimodipine posttreated rats; *CONTROL:* Vehicle treated rats. (From [12])

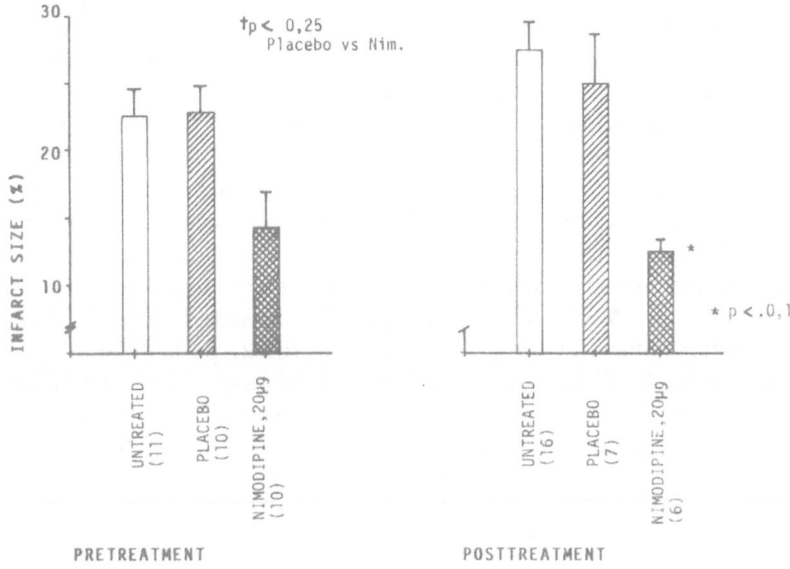

Fig. 4. Infarct size 24 h after MCA occlusion of the rat in MRI pre- and posttreatment Nimodipine 20 μg/kg. (From [13])

Clinical Studies

So far there are four completed studies with nimodipine in patients with acute ischemic stroke. In a first open pilot study [15] 29 patients received nimodipine in addition to a standard therapy (10% dextran for 5 days) while 31 patients received only dextran. Mortality and neurological outcome looks promising for nimodipine. Thereafter some double-blind placebo controlled studies were performed. In a multicenter, double-blinded study [15] 164 patients with acute is-

Table 1. Outcome of patients treated with nimodipine 120 mg daily for 3 or 4 weeks

Treatment	Placebo	Nimodipine	
Complete recovery	7,7%	9,6%	
Improvement	49,3%	65,3%	
			p-value <0.01
Unchanged or worse	27,2%	18,4%	
Death	15,8%	6,7%	
N	221	239	

chemic stroke (diagnoses proven by clinical signs and CT-scan) were included, 85 being treated with nimodipine (4 × 30 mg/day) and 79 with placebo. All patients were older than 45 years and were treated during the first 48 hours after the ictus. All patients received 10% dextran for 5 days and the same physiotherapy. Neurological outcome was measured with the Mathew-scale.

The four-weeks mortality was 21.2% in the placebo group and only 7.6% in the nimodipine group which was significantly and better in favor of nimodipine. Also the neurological outcome was much better in the nimodipine group than in the placebo group. Nimodipine was well tolerated.

In the meantime several double-blind placebo controlled studies in Europe and USA have been carried out or are finished up to now but are not yet reported. A meta-analysis of the four finished studies and the interim analysis of one running study showed a significant good result in favor of nimodipine looking for the clinical outcome at the end of the therapy (p<0.01). Of 239 patients treated with nimodipine, 6.7% of these are judged as complete recovered, 63.5% as improved, 18.4% as unchanged or impaired and 6.7% died. The corresponding values for the placebo group with 221 patients are: 7.7% completely recovered, 49.3% improved, 27.2% were unchanged, 15.8% died (Table 1).

The results of the studies and the meta-analysis showed that there will be a great hope in the near future for a new drug for these patients.

References

1. Grotta JC (1987) Current status of hemodilution in acute cerebral ischemia. Stroke 18:689–690
2. Scandinavian Stroke Study Group (1987) Multicenter trial of hemodilution in acute ischemic stroke. Stroke 18:691–699
3. Gelmers HJ (1985) Calcium-Channel Blockers: Effects on cerebral blood flow and potential use for acute stroke. Am J Cardiol 55:144B–148B
4. Astrup J, Siesjö BK, Symon L (1981) Thresholds in cerebral ischemia – the ischemic penumbra. Stroke 12:723–725
5. Welch KMA, Barkley GL (1986) Biochemistry and pharmacology of cerebral ischemia. In: Barnett HKM, Mohr JP, Stein BM, Yatsu FM (eds) Stroke. Churchill Livingstone, pp 75–90
6. Borgers M (1985) Morphological assessment of tissue protection. In: Godfraind T et al (eds) Calcium entry blockers and tissue protection. pp 173–181

7. Van Reempts J, Borgers M, Van Dael L, Van Eyndhoven J, Van de Ven M (1983) Morphological assessment of tissue protection. Arch Int Pharmacodyn Ther 262:76–88
8. Hossmann KA, Paschen W, Csiba L (1983) Relationship between calcium accumulation and recovery of cat brain after prolonged cerebral ischemia. J Cereb Blood Flow Metabol 3:346
9. Grotta J, Spydell J, Pettigrew C, Ostrow P, Hunter D (1986) The effect of nicardipine on neuronal function following ischemia. Stroke 2:213–219
10. Kazda S, Garthoff B, Krause WP, et al (1982) Cerebrovascular effects of the calcium antagonistic dihydropyridine derivative nimodipine in animal experiments. Arzneimittelforsch 32:331–338
11. Steen PA, Gisvold SE, Milde JH, Newberg LA, Scheithauer BW, Lanier WI (1985) Nimodipine improves outcome when given after complete cerebral ischemia in primates. Anaesthesiology 62:406–414
12. Sauter A, Rudin M (1986) Calcium antagonists reduce the extent of infarction in middle cerebral artery occlusion model as determined quantitative magnetic resonance imaging. Stroke 6:1228–1234
13. Germano I, Bartkowski H, Nishimura M, Cassel B, Pitts L (1986) The effects of nimodipine in acute experimentel cerebral ischemia in the rat. 11th International joint conference on stroke and cerebral circulation, San Francisco
14. Barnett GH, Bose B, Little JR, Jones SJ, Friel HT (1986) Effects of nimodipine on acute focal cerebral ischemia. Stroke 5:884–890
15. Gelmers HJ (1987) Nimodipine in ischemic stroke. Clin Neuropharm 5:pp 412–422

The Child's Central Nervous System: Assaults, Monitoring, and Therapy

P. R. Holbrook

Introduction

There has been an explosion of interest in child's brain in the last decade. Summarized in the following are some of the assaults, monitoring modalities, and therapy currently playing roles in the pediatric ICU.

Assaults

Head Trauma

The importance of the problem of pediatric head trauma cannot be overstated. Several new studies cast light on the magnitude of the problem. Kraus et al. [1, 2] note that 185 of every 100000 children will experience head trauma of sufficient degree to be brought to the hospital each year. 6 of 100 brain injured children will die, many before they receive medical attention. Of those who are admitted to the hospital, 12% will have a serious injury (Glasgow coma scale of 12 or less, at least 48 h in hospital, and brain surgery or an abnormal computed tomographic (CT) scan). Ward and Alberico [3] reviewed the care of 100 children with head trauma and Glasgow coma scale of 8 or less. 24% had surgical mass lesions. 94% had intracranial pressure (ICP) monitoring. Outcome was evaluated at 3 and 12 months after injury (Table 1). One quarter of the patients were dead at 12 months. Of significance is the relatively low incidence of chronic severe disability after 1 year.

Observing the problem from a different perspective, it is well established that trauma is the most common cause of death in the patient over 1 year of age. 80% of traumatized patients have sustained neurologic injury and in 60% the injury is the most severe. All patients who died in 1 series had some head injury [4].

Table 1. Outcome after pediatric head trauma. (From [3])

Outcome	3 months	1 year
Good	34	55
Moderately disabled	26	14
Severely disabled	11	5
Vegetative	8	2
Dead	21	24

Anoxic Ischemic Encephalopathy

There is a paucity of information which relates to the effects of hypoxic ischemic encephalopathy on the child's brain despite the fact that this condition is a major cause of death in the pediatric population. Further understanding of the pathophysiology of this problem will have await more fundamental discoveries. Therapy for this frustating problem has not advanced recently.

Brain Death

As a defined clinical entity, brain death in children has lagged behind its counterpart in adults. Many facets of the original adult clinical diagnosis of brain death were not applicable to the child. A multi-organizational task force has recently published their findings regarding brain death in small children (Table 2) [5].

In addition to the operational definition of brain death in children, there has been the issue of the legality of the definition. Many major organizations in the United States have endorsed the following statement.

> An individual who has sustained either (1) - irreversible cessation of circulatory and respiratory functions or (2) - irreversible cessation of all functions of the entire brain, including the brainstem, is dead. A determination of death must be made in accordance with accepted medical standards.

Current practice in determining brain death is governed by local institution policies and the jurisdiction in question. Since the above mentioned guidelines represent the work of a special task force and the work has been endorsed by the represented organizations, the practitioner is utilizing accepted medical standards if the above guidelines are followed.

Table 2. Guidelines for brain death in children. (From [5])

History: Determine proximate cause of coma

Physical examination:
1. Coexisting coma and apnea
2. Absent brainstem function
3. Normothermic and normotensive for age
4. Tone - flaccid, no movements spontaneous or induced (except spinal cord events)
5. Persisting results throughout observation period

Observation period:
    Birth - seven days: Criteria not applicable
    Seven days - two months: two exams, two EEG's 48 hours apart
    Two months - 12 months: two exams, two EEG's 24 hours apart; second exam obviated by
        absence of flow through cerebral arteries
    Older than one year: two exams, 12-24 hours apart; lab testing not required

Laboratory tests:
  EEG endorsed
  Cerebral radionuclide angiography endorsed
  Other tests being investigated

Reye Syndrome

Because Reye syndrome played such an important role in the development of pediatric critical care it deserves mention as an important assault on the central nervous system. The syndrome, first described by the late RDK Reye [6], is an acute syndrome of pernicious vomiting, altered mentation progressing to coma with increased intracranial pressure (ICP) in the more severe cases, and hepatic function abnormalities. The cause in unknown. In the United States an association between aspirin (acetylsalicylic acid) ingestion and the occurence of the syndrome has been noted. However, this association has not been noted in other areas [7]. The syndrome is diminishing in frequency, especially as an ICU entity. Reye syndrome, in its full form, is a dramatic condition which lead to the development of aggressive measures of ICP control in an attempt to support the patient while the disease ran its course. As such it was a major stimulus to the development of the techniques of pediatric critical care.

Monitoring Techniques

Computerized Tomography (CT) Scanning

Computerized tomography (CT) scanning of the brain has become common as an adjunct for modern neurointensive care. Unfortunately, the CT scanner has never been applicable as an ICU monitoring technique in its current form. Patients necessarily have to be transported to a CT scanner and the critically ill patient may be unable to tolerate such transportation. Furthermore, although CT scans are good for the definition of anatomical changes, these frequently lag behind the metabolic, electrophysiologic, or brain cellular functions important to the clinican as he attempts to assess the damaged and/or healing brain. Thus, while it is mandatory to have a CT scan available to any intensive care unit delivering sophisticated neurointensive care, even repeated CT scanning does not provide sufficient information to understand brain function.

Intracranial Pressure (ICP)

Intracranial pressure (ICP) can be monitored with a variety of different techniques. The intraventricular catheter was the original technique used to monitor intracranial pressure and became the gold standard [8]. Subsequently, investigators have monitored the intracranial pressure in the subdural space, and in the epidural space. In infants the pressure across the anterior fontanel has been measured, but meaninful numbers are difficult to obtain. Intraventricular catheters have become the primary method because other modes of intracranial pressure monitoring are either plagued with technical problems or are excessively expensive. Additionally, only intraventricular catheters permit drainage of cerebrospinal fluid which can be an important therapeutic intervention.

With experience in monitoring ICP, theoretical and practical problems have emerged. Intracranial pressure may not always be transmitted equally in all directions; thus, the ICP at a monitored site may not reflect ICP throughout the brain. Weaver et al. [9] recorded differential ICP in patients with unilateral mass lesions. In their experience, 50% of patients with mass lesions had different ICP on ipsilateral and contralateral subarachnoid spaces. Thus, pressure is not the same at all places inside the skull, and the significance of a given measured pressure is not clear.

A second consideration regards the absolute values of the ICP which require therapy. Normal daily activities produce transient increases in ICP to levels which would be considered pathological it they were discovered in the intensive care unit. Furthermore, some patients with pseudotumor cerebri have markedly elevated ICP without apparent pathologic findings. In the actually ill patient levels of greater than 20 mm Hg are considered abnormal in our ICU, but not always treated.

Practical problems in the monitoring of ICP pressure also occur. When a dampened pressure wave form appears on the monitoring screen, an immediate analysis of the dampened trace is mandatory. Dampened traces can be caused by clotting of the monitoring device, obstruction of the monitoring device, air bubbles in the system or dislodgement of the catheter from the space in which it was thought to rest. Furthermore, collapsed ventricles in the case of intraventricular monitoring can cause a dampened trace. Interpretation of a dampened trace is nearly impossible and the presence of a dampened trace calls for immediate manipulation of the pressure device until reasonable tracing are achieved. Otherwise, critical increase in ICP may be missed.

Electrophysiologic Events

Electrophysiologic events may be monitored in the intensive care setting. These events reflect neural discharge and, thus, measure a function of the brain cell itself. The utility of measurement of electrophysiologic events is limited by technical problems such as the presence of numerous electrical artifacts inherent in an intensive care unit.

The electroencephalogram (EEG) is monitored in the intensive care environment in the author's hospital for the patient receiving therapy (e.g. a paralyzing agent) which prevents neurologic assessment of the patient, for the patient receiving anesthetic doses of barbiturates for intracranial pressure or seizure control, or for the patient who may be having subclinical seizures. The EEG machine is positioned at the bedside and turned off and on by the ICU physicians as necessary.

The use of evoked response techniques which are derived from auditory, visual or somatosensory stimulation, has also been extensive over the last 5–15 years. These techniques, in general, fall to identify patients who will have meaningful recovery from those who will not. Further research may yet lead to clinical utility for the techniques. It should be recognized, however, that intact brainstem evoked responses are related to relatively primitive functions and life with only brain stem evoked responses intact would indeed be primitive.

Measurement of Cerebral Blood Flow

Techniques which allow the measurement of cerebral blood flow are now being used in some intensive care units [10]. A number of techniques have evolved and each involves different fundament principles. That there are numerous techniques to measure cerebral blood flow is indicative that no technique is demonstrably superior to others. It is not yet clear whether measurement of global cerebral blood flow is appropriate or whether it provides too crude an estimate to be meaningful. Regional blood flow, on the other hand, may be too sensitive a measure. Most techniques assume some degree of consistency between pathologic and normal tissues. These assumptions are probably not warranted. In addition, simple cerebral blood flow studies do not correlate with cerebral metabolic rates for the affected tissues. Finally, those studies of cerebral blood flow which have been published to date are not showing compelling clinical relevance. Much work needs to be done in this exciting area.

Brain Metabolism of Various Chemicals

The study of brain metabolism of various chemicals (oxygen, glucose, etc.) has been studied for some time. Under normal conditions metabolism is coupled to blood flow. In various pathologic conditions this coupling is disrupted. Thus, study of the metabolic rates may yield insights into pathophysiology and therapy [11]. The methodologies utilized to study these metabolic rates are quite varied. Use of the Fick principle is often made, but inherent in these measurements are problems of contamination with extracranial blood flow, sampling techniques and global vs regional information. Again, much work needs to be done in these areas.

Examination of Cellular Function

Several new technologies permit examination of cellular function of the brain. These technologies offer an opportunity to look literally inside the cell. Magnetic resonance spectroscopy is becoming increasingly widespread. This technique utilizes the spin characteristics of the nucleus of certain atoms. By subjecting these nuclei to perturbation by a radio wave impulse while they are maintained in a magnetic field and then measuring the spin characteristics while the nuclei return to their original alignment, a signal can be obtained which corresponds to the concentration of a given atom. Utilizing applied computer technology, the intracellular concentration of specific ions can be established. Magnetic resonance spectroscopy, therefore, provides a beginning look at function of the cells themselves. Other techniques, such as positron emission tomography (PET) scanning, utilize different methodologies but again reach toward the goal of establishing individual cellular function.

An additional technique, near infrared spectroscopy, is showing some promise. This technique utilizes the principle that biologic tissues are relatively permeable to light in the near-infrared spectrum. Jobsis [12] pointed out that hemoglobin, both oxygenated and deoxygenated, and cytochrome aa3 have absorption spectra between 700 and 1300 nanometers (near infrared). Thus, when infrared light is transmitted through biologic tissues these absorption spectra can be utilized to determine the state of oxygenation and deoxygenation of hemoglobin and the state of oxidation/reduction of cytochrome aa3, the enzyme responsible for the final redox reaction in the respiratory chain. Adding oxygenated and deoxygenated hemoglobin concentrations as measured by the quantity of light absorbed allows for calculation of blood volume as well. In addition, measurement of cerebral blood flow can be achieved if arterial injection of infrared absorbing dyes or administration of other infrared absorbing materials is utilized. It should be pointed out that the technique is noninvasive except for the infrared light and any injected substances. This technique has been applied to premature infants [13] in an attempt to monitor cerebral oxygen sufficiency as well as blood volume and oxygenation/deoxygenation status of the hemoglobin. Further work [14, 15] is showing the utility of this technique as a research tool and a significant improvement in our understanding of brain oxygenation may be forthcoming.

Therapy

Treatment of Increased Intracranial Pressure

ICP monitoring and subsequent treatment played a major role in the growth and development of pediatric intensive care as a separate discipline. The application of knowledge gained in the 1960s and the 1970s on ICP monitoring and treatment was invaluable when applied to certain patients, especially those with Reye syndrome.

The value of ICP monitoring has been established in Reye syndrome [16]. As the brain swells in this condition ICP may increase. The volume of blood, interstitial fluid and/or cerebrospinal fluid can be reduced by a number of well-established techniques. Thus, pressure can often be kept below critical levels while the disease process runs its course. It is now reasonably clear that ICP is elevated as a by product of the primary defect, and if the primary disease process is sufficiently severe, the brain may be destroyed even if ICP is controlled. Conversely, permitting uncontrolled elevation of ICP will add to the brain injury. Therefore, most centers monitor ICP when the patient reaches Stage 3 [17]. As noted above the decreased incidence of Reye syndrome in the U.S. has limited recent experience.

The ICP monitoring in patients who have sustained head trauma is widely practiced, but its utility is not firmly established. Elevated ICP in head trauma patients is a reflection either of the primary injury or of secondary reperfusion and/or ischemic injuries. Pressure, again, is a byproduct of other pathologic processes. It is clear that those patients who have increased ICP following trauma have a poorer outcome than those with normal pressure. Aggressive control of ICP has resulted in (apparent) improved survival in a limited number of flawed studies [18, 19]. In children, ICP is generally monitored when a Glasgow coma scale of 8 or less is achieved. It is not yet convincingly established that such monitoring is ultimately beneficial.

The ICP monitoring after anoxic and/or ischemic injuries is even more controversial. While it is true that ICP is elevated in some postanoxic ischemic patients, the benefit of monitoring and treating abnormalities in ICP is not established. It is now recognized that patients who have elevated ICP after anoxic/ ischemic injuries do poorly and aggressive attempts to control ICP in these patients have not been shown to alter outcome. Thus, it is currently commonplace not to monitor ICP on patients who have sustained anoxic/ischemic injuries, because the outcome of those who develop increased ICP is so poor.

Barbiturate Therapy

One of the most widely discussion if not widely used therapies in neurointensive care has been the use of various derivatives of barbiturate acid. Barbiturates have been used for anesthesia, sedation, seizure control, increased ICP, and protection against the effects of anoxic ischemic injuries. All but the last are still indicated. Because there has been so much discussion of these drugs, albeit with less frequency and passion in the pediatric world, a brief review is indicated.

Barbiturates affect the central nervous system in a variety of possibly unrelated ways. Barbiturates stabilize neuronal cell membranes, reduce cerebral blood flow, reduce cerebral oxygen consumption, possibly consume free radicals, and have numerous metabolic effects on the intracellular reactions [20]. These processes alone or in combination could theoretically explain each of the putative benefits of barbiturates in the above mentioned conditions.

On the negative side, barbiturates depress myocardial function, may alter the body's compensatory response to shock, inhibit some immune functions, depress respirations, and alter neurologic responsiveness, any of which may be a significant in the clinical situation.

At the present time barbiturates are indicated for seizure control, treatment of increased ICP, sedation, and anesthesia in selected situations. They are not indicated for protection of the brain from the effects of anoxia ischmia after perinatal asphyxia [21] or in the adult following cardiac arrest [22]. There is no reason to suspect they will benefit children not studied in either of these studies. Similarly, they are not indicated for the prophylactic treatment of patients following severe head trauma [23].

Supportive Therapy

With the recognition that the utility of barbiturates is limited to its traditional functions (seizure control, sedation, and ICP control) some investigators have turned their attention to the pursuit of other "magic bullets" (medications which, by themselves, will yield major improvements in outcome from brain injury). Among these are lidoflazine and other calcium channel blockers, oxygen radical scavengers, and inhibitors of xanthine oxidase. Such approaches seem fruitless for dealing with the enormously complicated processes involved with acute brain injury. A much more fruitful path is the systematic investigation of the pathophysiology of the diseases with stepwise application of appropriate findings.

Until such time as there has evolved a more sophisticated approach to the problem of acute brain assault, supportive care will continue to be the mainstay of therapy. The importance of preservation of good respiratory and circulatory function, the avoidance or early detection and treatment of infection, the provision of appropriate nutrition and metabolic support, and the provision of appropriate supportive and rehabilitative services cannot be overemphasized.

References

1. Kraus JF, Fife D, Conroy C (1987) Pediatric brain injuries: The nature, clinical course, and early outcome in a defined United States' population. Pediatrics 79:501–507
2. Kraus JF, Fife D, Cox P, Ramstein K, Conroy C (1986) Incidence, severity, and external cause of pediatric brain injury. Am J Dis Child 140:687–693
3. Ward JD, Alberico AM (1987) Paeditric head injuries. Brain injury 1:21–25
4. Mayer T, Walker ML, Johnson DG, et al (1981) Causes of morbidity and mortality in severe pediatric trauma. JAMA 245:719–721
5. Task Force Report (1987) Guidelines for the determination of brain death in children. Pediatrics 80:298–302
6. Reye RDK, Morgan G, Baral J (1963) Encephalopathy and fatty degeneration of the viscera: A disease entity in childhood. Lancet 2:749–752
7. Orlowski JP (1987) A catch in the Reye. Pediatrics 80:638–642
8. Lundberg N (1980) Continuous recording and control of ventricular fluid pressure in neurosurgical practice. Acta Psychiatr Neurol Scand 36 (Suppl) 149–53
9. Weaver DD, Winn HR, Jane JA (1980) Differential intracranial pressure in patients with unilateral mass lesions. J Neurosurg 56:660–665
10. Kirsch JR, Traystman RJ, Rogers MC (1985) Cerebral blood flow measurement techniques in infants and children. Pediatrics 75:887–895
11. Obrist WD, Langfitt TW, Jaggi JL, et al (1984) Cerebral blood flow and metabolism in comatose with acute head injury. Relationship to intracranial hypertension. J Neurosurg 61:241–245
12. Jobsis FF (1977) Noninvasive infrared monitoring of cerebral and myocardial oxygen sufficiency and circulatory parameters. Science 198:1264–1266
13. Brazy JE, Lewis DV, et al (1985) Noninvasive monitoring of cerebral oxygenation in preterm infants: Preliminary observations. Pediatrics 75:217–225
14. Cairns CB, Fillipo D, Proctor HJ (1985) A noninvasive method for monitoring the effects of increased intracranial pressure with near infrared spectrophotometry. Surg Gynecol Obstet 161:145–148
15. Piantadosi CA, Hemstreet TM, Jobsis-Vandervliet FF (1986) Near-infrared spectrophotometric monitoring of oxygen distribution to intact brain and skeletal muscle tissues. Crit Care Med 14:698–705
16. Shaywitz BA, Rothstein P, Venes JL (1980) Monitoring and management of increased intracranial pressure in Reye syndrome: Results in 29 children. Pediatrics 66:198
17. Lovejoy FH, Smith AL, Resnan MD, et al (1974) Clinical staging in Reye syndrome. Am J Dis Child 128:36
18. Miller JD, Butterworth JF, Gudeman SK, et al (1981) Further experience in the management of severe head injury. J Neurosurg 54:289–299
19. Bowers SA, Marshall LF (1980) Outcome in 200 consecutive cases of severe head injury treated in San Diego country: A prospective analysis. Neurosurgery 6:237
20. Trauner DA (1986) Barbiturate therapy in acute brain injury. J Pediatr 109:742–746

21. Goldberg RN, Moscoso P, Bauer CR, et al (1986) Use of barbiturate therapy in severe perinatal asphyxia: A randomized controlled trial. J Pediatr 109:851–856
22. Brain Resuscitation Clinical Trial I Study Group (1986) Randomized clinical study of thiopental loading in comatose survivors of cardiac arrest. N Engl J Med 314:398–402
23. Ward JD, Becker DP, Miller D (1985) Failure of prophylactic barbiturate coma in the treatment of severe head injury. J Neurosurg 62:383–388

Acute Anxiety Disorders

K. Kuch and R. P. Swinson

Introduction

Anxiety has a psychological, behavioral and physiological dimension. It is experienced as fear, a sense of forboding and anxious expectation. It may be without an apparent object, as in Westphal's description of panic [1] and strike out of the seemingly clear blue sky.

Anxiety behaviors include scanning for, avoiding and escaping from situations perceived as dangerous. Phobics go to great lengths to avoid situations that they fear, gather advance intelligence before venturing into unfamiliar territory and may not confront their fear for decades.

The physiological dimension of anxiety has come under intense scrutiny. We view it no longer as a homogeneous continuum stretching from mild to moderate to severe, but instead distinguish between panic and anticipatory anxiety. Panic is treated as a distinctive medical event, characterized by rapid intensification and a subjective sense of incapacitation.

The anxiety disorders have been reclassified according to the roles played by anticipatory anxiety, avoidance and panic. Treatment effects are assessed along the same three dimensions. Anticipatory anxiety, avoidance and panic may not change simultaneously. – This review is limited to anxiety disorders characterized by panic because of their importance to primary care.

Classification

The Diagnostic and Statistical Manual of Mental Disorders (DSM III-R) defines *panic* as discrete periods of intense fear and discomfort characterized by rapid intensification leading within minutes to a sense of impending incapacitation and loss of control [2]. Panic attacks usually last minutes and rarely hours. At least four associated symptoms occur during an attack.

They include shortness of breath, dizziness, palpitations, tachycardia, trembling, shaking, sweating, choking, nausea, abdominal distress, depersonalisation, derealisation, numbness, paresthesias, hot flashes, chills, chest pain, a fear of dying, of going crazy or of doing something uncontrolled. *Limited symptom attacks* involve fewer than four symptoms but meet the other criteria.

Panic disorder is diagnosed when four attacks have occurred within a 4-week period and if no organic factor initiated or maintained the disturbance. Recently the criteria were loosened to include cases where sporadic panic was followed by a persistent fear of attacks lasting at least one month.

Unexpected panic occurs without preceding anticipatory anxiety and patients may awaken at night experiencing it. *Situational panic* follows anxious anticipation and occurs in phobic situations.

DSM III-R defines *phobia* as a persistent fear of a circumscribed and harmless situation that is avoided or endured with dread. Fear and avoidance interfere significantly with the person's normal routine and he recognizes his fear as excessive and unreasonable.

Simple phobias involve a dread of heights, animals and enclosed spaces like elevators or airplanes. *Social phobics* dread being scrutinized during activities like public speaking, eating, drinking or writing and may feel deeply humiliated if they tremble or blush. On the whole they are more disabled than simple phobics because their fears impede a greater range of activities. *Agoraphobics* are the most restricted. They dread being in places from which escape might be difficult or where help in the case of panic might be unavailable. This includes many situations like tunnels, bridges, highways and traveling alone beyond "safe" territory. Agoraphobia is commonly associated with panic disorder and understood as it's behavioral manifestation.

Posttraumatic stress disorder may be associated with panic disorder and panic disorder may start after trauma. Panic occurs in *major affective disorder* and *drug-induced states*. Delirious patients are frightened but disoriented. Dementing patients get anxious about loosing their way in unfamiliar surroundings. DSM III-R is organized hierarchically, from the *organic mental disorders* downwards to the psychoses, major affective disorder and at last anxiety disorder. Anxiety disorder is only diagnosed after higher ranking conditions have been ruled out and only if anxiety is persistent, excessive and maladaptive.

Relevance to Emergency and Intensive Care

Anxiety disorder is distressing and potentially disabling. Careers change to accomodate public speaking phobias. Promotions are lost because of a fear of flying, a condition now recognized by airlines. Many agoraphobics are too anxious to attend meetings and job interviews. They see their social lives dwindle because of restricted mobility.

Anxiety disorder is also common. The New Haven Study found a current rate for all anxiety disorders of 4.3/100. Panic disorder accounted for 0.4/100, phobic disorder for 1.4/100 and generalized anxiety disorder for 2.5/100 [3]. Ulenhuth found 1.2/100 as the 1 year prevalence of agoraphobia with panic attacks and the 1 year prevalence of all other phobias as 2.3/100. The male to female ratio for agoraphobia with panic was approximately 1:3.5 [4].

Patients with anxiety disorder are amongst the highest users of outpatient facilities and may not volunteer any insight into their condition when they come to the emergency room to have heart attacks and other illness ruled out. Noyes et al. [5] assessed 60 patients with panic for hypochondriasis with an illness behavior questionnaire. Before treament their scores were comparable to those of a group of hypochondriacal psychiatric patients. The panic disorder patients who improved with treatment showed significant reductions in somatic preoccupation, disease phobia and disease conviction. Early diagnosis and treatment can prevent wasteful use of medical resources [5].

Masked psychiatric diagnosis are a major public health problem particularly in socio-economically depressed areas. Von Korff et al. [6] identified over one-half of all persons seen in a primary medical care clinic as suffering from anxiety or depressive disorder with anxiety disorder ranking first. Most patients with a potentiality treatable mental disorder did not receive treatment for it [6]. The differential diagnosis of panic disorder includes cardiovascular illness and serious psychiatric complications. It should not be removed from a primary care setting. Coryell et al. [7] found excess mortality due to suicide and cardiovascular disease in 155 former outpatients with panic disorder over a 12-year period, confirming an earlier observation with former inpatients [7].

Clinical Presentation

Simple phobias rately present in medical settings with some notable exceptions. Over the years we have observed 3 patients who injured themselves during a panicked escape and several others that only luck had saved from injury. If nothing else these cases demonstrate the intensity that panic may reach. Phobias occasionally become management problems. *Needle phobics* may experience bradycardia and faint. They should recline before venipuncture. *Illness phobics* can be irritating with their persistent requests for reassurance. A *claustrophobic* may be forced unwittingly into a confined space for a radiographic procedure or worse be immobilized in a cast. He may suddenly sign out on some pretense.

Exercise avoidance is found in patients, who fear heart attacks. Pathological fear may impede rehabilitation after myocardial infarction. An extension of this phenomenon is found when patients refuse to leave the security of an intensive care unit or get unduely upset when their oxygen-supplement is disconnected.

A decision to seek help depends not only on symptoms. Swinson investigated agoraphobics who considered themselve cured. A large percentage was still sufficiently impaired to meet the diagnostic criteria for agoraphobia with panic attacks (unpublished data). When patients seek help it often is in times of crisis. Roy-Byrne et al. [8] compared 44 patients with panic disorder with 44 matched healthy controls regarding the number, type and effect of life-events that had occurred during the year that preceded the onset of panic. The patients had a significantly greater number of also more distressing negative live events than the controls [8].

Panic is often relieved by arrival in the safety of an emergency room. The patient will then appear physically healthy and in no acute distress. *Screening questions* about sudden unexplained fearfulness and restricted mobility may lead to the diagnosis. The SCL-90 is a checklist to be completed by the patient and may serve as a functional enquiry of psychological symptoms. It allows diagnostic subscoring [9].

Below are some common complaints: Male patients are particularly prone to develope persistent fears of heart disease that are fuelled by *palpitations* and intercostal pains. Panic is more than a subjectively distressed state. Taylor had patients wear an ambulatory solid state *heart-rate* monitor. 58% of the panic episodes reported occurred at heart rates that were disproportionate to activity levels and contrasted from surrounding heart rates [10]. Freedman et al. [11] monitored heart rate and finger temperature changes in 12 panic disorder patients and 11 controls. Seven of 8 self-reported panic attacks were accompanied by heart rate increases up to 130 beats/min. Finger temperature increased prior to panic [11].

Dizziness is triggered in some phobic patients by heights, open spaces and shiny floors. Otoneurological tests were negative in our sample.

Swinson (unpublished data) investigated 28 *hyperventilators* that visited a general hospital emergency room. Of them, 39% did not fully meet any psychiatric diagnostic criteria, 35.6% were diagnosed as uncomplicated panic disorder, 7% suffered from agoraphobia with panic attacks, 7% from simple and social phobias and 7% from depression. Three fourths were female. Of the total, 14.5% had been injured in car accidents, 32% were bereaved and 18% found themselves in financial difficulties.

Transient bowel disturbances are common after emotional upheavals. Nausea and diarrhea occur during or after panic. Panic may also complicate an irritable colon. Lydiard et al. [12] described 5 patients with panic disorder and irritable bowel syndrome. In 2 the onset of gastrointestinal symptoms had occurred prior to panic. Both panic disorder and bowel syndrome responded rapidly to psychopharmacological treatment. Four cases improved with alprazolam and one with phenelzine [12].

Unremitting pain may be associated with phobic disorder. We have observed concurrent "fibromyalgia" and spinal pain in travel phobics that had experienced acceleration/deceleration injuries. The pain may improve dramatically with successful treatment of phobic disorder or remain unaffected.

Panic may lead to *alcohol dependence* in vulnerable personalities. Self-medicating patients use spirits as a tranquillizer before going out. Some avoid intoxication studiously and carry a flask more for reassurance than for actual use. Weiss and Rosenberg [14] found that 22.6% of 84 subjects hospitalized with a diagnosis of alcoholism met criteria for anxiety disorder [13]. Thyrer et al. [14] screened 156 patients meeting DSM III criteria for panic disorder and phobic disorder. Of these, 17% scored in the alcoholic range. The strongest associated with alcoholism was found in depressed agoraphobics.

Few anxiety disorder patients are without *benzodiazepines*. In our sample of several hundred consultations actual addiction was rare. Most cases presented, when discontinuation was attempted without tapering, when benzodiazepine doses were inappropriately timed or too low to suppress panic and when symptoms re-emerged after benzodiazepines had been tapered.

Aspects of Differential Diagnosis

Routine screening for mitral valve prolapse (MVP), thyroid disease, hypoglycemia, pheochromocytoma, and temporal lobe seizures is not recommended [15]. Some studies estimate the prevalence of MVP is estimated between 4 and 17%. Mazza et al. [16] screened 48 patients with MVP and 49 controls for anxiety disorder. Neither group contained any cases of phobia or panic disorder, a finding that does not support a theory of MVP causing panic [16].

Fishman et al. [17] examined 82 patients with panic attacks for evidence of *thyroid disease*. None had an abnormal T_3 or T_4 resin uptake, while 22% had an undetectable TSH level, an incidence that is higher than expected but unexplained. Several of our patients gave a past history of hyperthyroidism but had normal laboratory values. Panic disorder had emerged during the course of hyperthyroidism and then ran an independent course.

Laboratory-induced *hypoglycemia* is not associated with panic. As a screening test it should be limited to patients with postprandial attacks and attacks associated with hunger [15].

Anxiety is common in *pheochromocytoma*, but none of the patients reviewed met DSM III criteria for panic disorder. Phobic avoidance was not observed. The literature reports cases of *temporal lobe lesions* associated with panic disorder but this association is rare [15].

Phobias and their symptoms have a unique *territorial quality* that is revealed by monitoring the timing and geographical occurrence of symptoms. Such a diary is easy to keep. Only an intensity rating and a brief description of the situation are required.

Neurophysiological Studies

The learning of fear has evolutionary aspects. Fear may be learned more easily in response to some situations than to others. The first panic in a patient's history typically occurs in crowds or on trips, not in the safety of his home. A preparedness for agoraphobic fears may have atavistic survivor value [18].

A vulnerability to panic may be genetically transmitted. Torgersen [19] compared 32 MZ twins with 53 DZ twins for concordance of anxiety disorder with panic: It was five times more frequent in the MZ twins.

A number of studies support the theory of a neurophysiological mechanism of panic linked to catecholamine metabolism. Panic is provoked by a variety of agents including CO_2, sodium lactate but also anxious expectation. A critical review would go beyond the scope of this chapter and the following studies are cited as examples.

Lactate blood levels were of interest ever since Cohen found in 1947, that patients with neurocirculatory asthenia experienced nervousness after vigorous exercise. Pitts and McClure broke new ground when they managed to provoke panic attacks by administering 10 ml/kg of a 0.5 molar solution intravenously over 20 min. Liebowitz et al. [20] tested 43 patients with panic and 20 normal controls. 31 of the 43 patients responded with panic and none of controls did. Panic disorder patients treated successfully with MAOI lost their vulnerability [20]. Reiman et al. [21] used positron emission tomography to study 8 patients with panic disorder who were vulnerable to lactate, 8 patients with panic disorder who were not vulnerable to lactate and 25 normal controls with positron emission tomography. The lactate-vulnerable patients had a number of abnormalities in the resting non-panic state: an abnormal hemispheric asymmetry of parahippocampal blood flow, oxygen metabolism, abnormally high whole brain metabolism and an abnormal susceptibility to episodic hyperventilation [21].

Outcome Studies

The effectiveness of exposure therapy in simple *phobias* has been demonstrated beyond reasonable doubt. Social phobias also respond to behavioral management but are more complex. They often represent a blend of performance anxiety and social skills deficits. Agoraphobia improves with programmed exposure to feared situations [18].

Panic disorder responds to appropriate drug therapy. In a crossnational double-blind placebo-controlled trial of 500 patients alprazolam was shown to be efficacious in reducing the frequency and intensity of panic attacks within a dosage range of 2–10 mg/day (Ballenger, in print). Earlier investigations, including the original work by Sargeant and by Klein, demonstrated the effect of phenelzine and imipramine in panic and Max investigated the efficacy of clonazepam.

There is disagreement regarding drug-effects in agoraphobia [22]. Much of the current debate deals with three questions: Does drug therapy alone reduce phobic avoidance? Does behavior therapy reduce panic? Does improvement last beyond treatment and what are the long-term results? Mavissakalian and Michelson [23] followed 62 agoraphobic patients for 2 years after treatment. They had suffered from panic attacks but had been free of concomitant affective disorder. The patients had completed a controlled study comparing therapist-assisted flooding, imipramine and programmed self-exposure practice. Imipramine and flooding had an initial advantage over programmed practice which disappeared over 2 years of follow-up. Lasting improvement of agoraphobia was observed in 25 patients and 22 required no further help. Compliance to long term follow-up was poor with 28% of patients no longer attending the clinic after 6 months [23]. The results highlight the difficulties faced by investigators in obtaining controlled outcome data, and also caution against automatic prescribing since there is a subgroup of patients that do well without medication.

Management

The three dimensions of anxiety, anxious anticipation, avoidance and panic, should be assessed before, during and after treatment. *Alprazolam* should be given with small amounts of food and in 4 to 5 divided doses to prevent interdose withdrawal. Drug response is best titrated by gradually raising the dosage. Suppression of panic is the criterion for improvement. Treatment with benzodiazepines may lead to dependence [24]. Alprazolam should be discontinued only by slow tapering. Rapid withdrawal may lead to a rebound of symptoms (Pecknold, Swinson, Kuch et al. in press). Klein et al. [25] reported three cases of successful treatment of withdrawal from alprazolam with carbamazepine, an anticonvulsant without abuse potential. Doses were between 600 and 900 mg/day.

Patients with major depressive disorder, with depression preceding panic disorder and with alcoholism complicating panic disorder may do well with *imipramine*. Effective doses range widely from 25–250 mg/day. Patients may complain of caffeine-type side-effects. An adequate trial on this medication requires at least 4 weeks. *Phenelzine* in daily doses from 30–90 mgs may be useful to patients who suffer from intense feelings of depersonalisation and dysphoria and who are intolerant of imipramine. Phenelzine requires a diet low in tyramine and special precautions against adverse drug interactions.

Patients with agoraphobia may improve with *exposure therapy* alone or with medication as an adjunct. Target behaviors are monitored to assess change. They are chosen from everyday activities that represent a life-style that would be normal for the patient. Programmed practice may be prescribed as a self-help technique ("Living with Fear" by I. M. Marks, McGraw-Hill 1978).

References

1. Westphal C (1871–2) Die Agoraphobie: Eine neuropathische Erscheinung. Arch Psychiatrie Nervenkr 3:138–171, 219–221
2. Diagnostic and statistical manual of mental disorders, ed III–R (1987) American Psychiatric Association, Washington DC
3. Weissmann MM, Myers JK, Harding PS (1978) Psychiatric disorders in a US urban community. Am J Psychiatry 135:459–463
4. Ulenhuth EH, Balter MB, Mellinger GD, et al (1983) Symptom checklist syndromes in the general population. Arch Gen Psychiatry 40:1167–1173
5. Noyes R, Reich J, Clancy J, O'Gorman TW (1986) Reduction of hypochondriasis with treatment of panic disorder. Br J Psychiatry 149:631–633
6. Von Korff M, Shapiro S, Burke JD, et al (1987) Anxiety and depression in a primary care clinic. Arch Gen Psychiatry 44:152–156
7. Coryell W. Noyes R, House JD (1986) Mortality among outpatients with anxiety disorder. Am J Psychiatry 143:508–510
8. Roy-Byrne PP, Geraci MG, Uhde TW (1986) Life events and the onset of panic disorder. Am J Psychiatry 143:1424–1427
9. Derogatis LR, Rickles K, Rock AF (1976) The SCL-90 and the MMPI. Br J Psychiatry 128:280–289
10. Taylor BC, Sheikh J, Agras WS, et al (1986) Ambulatory heart rate changes in patients with panic attacks. Am J Psychiatry 143:478–482
11. Freedman RR, Ianni P, Ettedgui E, Puthezhath N (1985) Ambulatory monitoring of panic disorder. Arch Gen Psychiatry 42:244–248
12. Lydiard KB, Laraia MT, et al (1986) Can panic disorder present as irritable bowel syndrome? J Clin Psychiatry 47:470–473
13. Weiss KJ, Rosenberg DJ (1985) Prevalence of alcoholism among alcoholics. J Clin Psychiatry 46:3–5

14. Thyrer BA, Parrish, Hilme J, et al (1986) Alcohol abuse among clinically anxious patients. Behav Res Ther 24:357–359
15. Raj A, Sheehan DV (1987) Medical evaluation of panic attacks. J Clin Psychiatry 48:309–313
16. Mazza DL, Martin D, Spacavento L, et al (1986) Prevalence of anxiety disorder in patients with mitral valve prolapse. Am J Psychiatry 143:349–352
17. Fishman SM, Sheehan DV, Carr DB (1985) Thyroid indices in panic disorder. J Clin Psychiatry 46:432–433
18. Marks IM (1987) Fears, phobias and rituals. Oxford University Press, Oxford New York
19. Torgerson S (1983) Genetic factors in anxiety disorders. Arch Gen Psychiatry 40:1086–1089
20. Liebowitz MR, Gorman JM, et al (1985) Lactate provocation of panic attacks. Arch Gen Psychiatry 42:709–719
21. Reiman EM, Raichle ME, Robins E, et al (1986) The application of positron emission tomography in the study of panic disorder. Am J Psychiatry 143:469–477
22. Klein DF, Ross DC, Cohen P (1987) Panic and avoidance in agoraphobia: application to path analysis of treatment studies. Arch Gen Psychiatry 44:377–385
23. Mavissakalian M, Michelson L (1986) Two-year follow-up of exposure and imipramine treatment of agoraphobia. Am J Psychiatry 143:1106–1112
24. Swinson RP, Pecknold JC, Kirby ME (1987) Benzodiazepine dependence. J Affective Disorders 13:109–118
25. Klein E, Uhde T, Post RM (1986) Preliminary evidence for the utility of carbamazepine in alprazolam withdrawal. Am J Psychiatry 143:235–236

Parental Psychological Distress: Prevention and Treatment

S. Fanconi and M. Lebert

Introduction

In our modern industrial society the death of an infant is an uncommon event. In the past centuries there was a ritualized pattern of mourning behavior, but in the last 50 years death has moved from the home to the hospital. As a result, the traditions developed to ensure a biological mourning reaction have been in part lost [1]. With the development of modern hospitals the care of sick, severely ill, and dying infants has been concentrated in intensive care units, where the emphasis has been mainly on the infant and its illness [2]. Increasing regionalization of newborn care means that physicians caring for sick infants often have not had prior contact with the families. Responsibility for communicating to the parents the fact that the infant is dying is often ill-defined and may reflect poor coordination between the referring hospital and the ICU staff.

A stillbirth or neonatal death is a stressful experience for both family and medical staff. Although it is accepted that one of the physician's roles is to advise parents about the death of their child, disappointment and feelings of failure on the part of the family and the medical staff make communication particularly difficult [3]. Since physicians cannot change the reality of the tragic situation, they frequently feel unable to lessen the parental suffering. However, understanding the nature of the stress as experienced by the family, and appreciating that there are characteristic ways in which parents can cope with the situation, should enable physicians to offer helpful support [4].

Grief Reactions of Parents

Some investigators have suggested that the parents' reactions to neonatal loss are proportionate to the closeness of the relationship prior to death. It is important to realize that in some women affectional ties to their babies will begin or accelerate with the development of fetal movement. By the end of the second trimester, the majority of women who initially rejected pregnancy have accepted it. In this period a woman usually begins to have dreams about how her baby will be like. At this time there is further acceptance of pregnancy. Unplanned and unwanted pregnancies seem more acceptable [1]. The father's attitude has received little attention, but affection ties are usually also developing before birth.

Intense mourning reactions after a neonatal death last for periods of 4 to 6 or even 12 months, similar to those observed after the loss of an older close family member. But in this situation the nonfulfillment of a wish-fantasy plays a more important role [2]. The main reactions are grief, apathy, feelings of emptiness and inadequacy. 2 aspects seem to be of specific importance for understanding the reactions of the mother in this emotional catastrophe: 1. the object loss and 2. the challenge of the mother's sexual identification [5].

According to Kennel [1] 5 reactions can be summarized as pathognomonic of grief:
1. Somatic distress;
2. Preoccupation with the image of the deceased;
3. Guilt;
4. Hostile reactions; and
5. Loss of the usual patterns of conduct.

At first the full reaction may be delayed or there may be a period of blunting; some parents act as if nothing had happened. But Lindemann [6] observed that the clinical signs of acute grief in adults are remarkably uniform. Sensations of somatic distress occur in waves and last from 20 to 60 min; a feeling of thightness in the throat, choking, shortness of breath, the need of sighing, complaints about a lack of strength, exhaustion, an empty and lonely feeling, a sense of unreality, and a feeling of increased emotional distance from other people are characteristic. The deceased child is often imagined to be present, and the mother behaves as if he was still alive. A feeling of guilt often torments the mother because of an imagined personal failure. Additionally there may be a loss of warmth in relationships with other people with a tendency to respond with irritability and anger. The activity through the day shows remarkable changes [2], and may even suggest a change in the personality of the grieving person. The intensity of these mourning reactions begins to decline after 1–6 weeks and, according to Parkes et al. [3], is minimal by 6 months. But for several years brief periods of yearning will regularly return when the deceased is remembered.

Harmon et al. [7] studied maternal grieving after neonatal loss in the intensive care unit and found that most mothers described the death of their infant as having a major impact on their functioning. At 3 months after the event, 80% and 74% after 9 months said their life was different as a direct result of the loss. Only 23% of the mothers felt that things were going reasonably well. About three-fourths emphasized that the period from 2 to 4 months was the most difficult. After 3 months, 68% of the mothers were still feeling angry at health professionals for their infant's death, but by 9 months only 37% were feeling angry. There were also positive effects: about 50% described the relationship to their husband as being closer as a result of the loss. Surprisingly, only 10% described marital difficulties.

Husbands' reactions have received little attention. Their situation is obviously different: they hardly have any direct relationship with the baby during pregnancy. After its delivery they are rarely involved in the care of the baby, and the loss is usually not related to guilt and personal failure. Kennel et al. [2] report that several husbands grieved as long or even longer than their wives, particularly if they were involved in the medical care of the baby during its stay in the ICU. While in the nursery the father is physically closer to the baby than his wife, and he also is more aware of the details of the baby's ongoing care.

A stillbirth represents a special problem because there is a sense of loss without the feeling of having lost somebody in particular. There is an added sense of unreality, as there are no real experiences with the baby to remember [8]. It is the nature of stillbirth that leads us to avoid the subject. Stillbirth is a nonevent in which there is guilt and shame with no tangible person to mourn. A stillborn is someone who did not exist, a nonperson, often without a name [8].

Mourning is an ongoing process during which the conscious and unconscious works on coming to an understanding with the memories, thoughts, and feelings about the dead person. During mourning we digest our memories and feelings about the deceased and free ourselves from the identification. With failed mourning the identification can persist and result in long-term psychological disturbances in parents and surviving children.

Cullberg [5] observed that 19 of 56 mothers, studied 1 to 2 years after the death of their newborn infant, had developed severe psychiatric disorders, such as psychosis, anxiety attacks, phobias, obsessive thoughts and deep depression. It would be interesting to know if rooming-in and admission of the parents to the ICU has improved this situation.

The symptoms of pathologic mourning include:

1. overactivity without a sense of loss,
2. acquisition of symptoms belonging to the deceased,
3. psychosomatic reactions,
4. alterations in relationships with others,
5. exaggerated hostility,
6. repression of hostility,
7. loss of normal patterns of social interaction,
8. activities detrimental to economic and social existence, and
9. agitated depression.

The recognition of abnormal mourning in parents and the creation of an atmosphere that facilitates normal grief may minimize the psychological consequences of death [1].

Other Children

To the surviving children the idea of death and stillbirth is incomprehensible and frightening. Yet they usually are left without help with their grief [8]. They sometimes feel overwhelmed and somehow guilty or responsible for the sadness of their parents. It is thus important to explain to the children that the parents are sad because of the loss of the baby, not because they are angry at them. The parents should let them know and feel how good it is to have them nearby [1]. Older children in this situation are frequently neglected. It should be explained to them why the sick baby is so important and receives all the attention. When death is approaching, they are left alone with their fear, instead of being allowed to mourn with the rest of the family. The optimation of the dead child by the parents does not give the surviving children the chance to compete with the ideal child. This situation leads frequently to later psychologic problems [9]. Parents should be prepared for the fact that children react to the loss of a sibling in different ways: they may continue to behave as before, without strong evidence of sadness. They may even ask to get another child to replace the lost sibling. This behavior represents the need to deflect the impact of the loss, in order to avoid being emotionally overwhelmed by depression and anxiety [10].

Subsequent Pregnancy

Rowe et al. [3] in a follow-up of 26 families who experienced perinatal death, found that the only factor associated with morbid grief reaction was either the presence of a surviving twin or a new pregnancy less than 5 months after the death. The grieving process of the father in this situation is another unexplored area. The increased risk both for the next infant and for the parents should temper physicians' enthusiam for encouraging families to have another baby [3]. Whether the presence of an early subsequent infant in the home interferes with the grieving process or whether it is a reflection of the severity of the parents' grief is an open question. Many women seek a second or third pregnancy, hoping to forget the loss of the index baby (Ersatzkind). Adequate mourning is of upmost importance, and only after successful termination of this process, should the next pregnancy be initiated. If the parents are unable to get through their grief reaction, future children will be affected by this loss [1]. Children born before or after an index baby can have severe emotional difficulties. Many mothers have mothering problems with the child born subsequently [8].

Reactions on Diagnosis

The communication of diagnosis is a critical, and for many parents unforgetable event. The majority wants to know the reality, many have foreseen what will happen, but others cannot accept the approaching death. Phases of hope and dispair, negation and acceptance of the diagnosis come in waves. Both, father and mother should be present when the diagnosis is explained, but in this situation, the parents will not understand what is happening. They mourn in anticipation or negate the diagnosis. Only after crying or motionless dispair, will they begin to understand what is really happening. The cause of the disease, guilt and fear trouble the parents. They either find help in each other or have to master the crisis alone, in isolation. Hostility, depression, overactivity may follow. They have to deal with the separation from the child, with uncertainty about the outcome, with a feeling of menace, with fear from diagnostic and therapeutic interventions and with the confrontation with unknown people and procedures [9]. This leads inevitably to considerable emotional alterations within the family unit. The initial phases of awareness of the disease are accompanied by reactions of shock and alarm. Emotional arousal usually persists and there is profound anxiety of separation from the loved one. An evaluation of parental distress [11] demonstrated that women scored higher than men on all subscales of psychological distress, except hostility. It was difficult for the authors to decide wether this was due to a stronger reaction to disease-related stress in women, or to their closer emotional involvement with the child. Whether and how the distress influences the ability to cope with the "disease problem" is difficult to say, but the authors suggest that the arousal of emotional distress may be an inherent part of the normal processes of adjustment. Reactions of shock and generalized alarm are deriving from fear to lose a loved one [12]. In this situation the parents always blame themselves for not having paid attention to the early signs of the disease. It is important to realize when talking about the diagnosis and the possible death, that the parents feel guilty and that the majority readily accept assurance that they did not neglect their child. Parents may become anxious and confused whenever they perceive divergent facts or opinions regarding the child's condition, even if the differences are negligible or imaginary. The parents perceive minor and major variations in degrees of pessimism or optimism among doctors. Seeking information can be an attempt to learn as much as possible about the disease in order to better cope with the situation, but a sudden upsurge of questions often indicate increased anxiety or a conflict. Parents may or may not wish to be with their children in critical situations. The majority however feels better when allowed to stay with their dying child. Friedman et al. [4] analyzed behavior on parents anticipating the death of a child with leukemia and found that parents in such critical situations behave in a surprisingly similar way: there is a typical defence pattern, a mechanism of coping with any threat to the psychological stability that enables them to function effectively, to tolerate the stressful situation without disruptive anxiety or depression. The fact of having a child with a fatal disease will lead to conflicts and feelings of guilt. The shock of learning the diagnosis and the associated lack of emotional experience in similar situations (isolation of affect) protects the parents from intolerable emotional response and enables them to talk realistically about their child's condition and prognosis. The apparent intellectual recognition of a painful event is not associated with an intolerable emotional response. The parents may appear "strong" and "cold" with a lack of sincere concern. Often the parents are aware of this paucity of emotional feelings, and explain it by not wanting to break down. Sometimes they verbalize their confusion and guilt over not feeling worse. Parents frequently ask for many details. This serves as a defence function by allowing them, as well as the doctors to avoid the more general, but more tragic and threatening aspects of the case. Discussing details frequently does not really help and probably generates more anxiety than it dissipates.

Another defence, less ubiquitous than isolation of affect is the mechanism of denial: the parents deny the seriousness of the illness and prognosis, they do not understand the importance of the various procedures, and therefore are prone to hostility. Motor activity is another coping function and serves to physically remove the parents from the threatening situation, and gives them something else to do. The defensive activity, if in an optimal range, protects the parents from the emotionally overwhelming situation of having a child with a fatal disease. Deviation from this range interferes with optimal participation in the care of the child. On the other hand, lack of defensive activity reduces the parents' ability to care effectively for the child. Most parents of children with leukemia constructed an explanation for the disease which was a composite of scientific facts, elements from the parent's experiences, and fantasies. This synthesis sometimes seemed to reflect parental self-blame [4]. It appears that guilt sometimes was less anxiety-provoking than the total lack of causes for the fatal disease. It is possible that guilt may have a defence function. Religion can be of help in accepting the fact that the child is dying; some parents have a tendency to accept the illness as God's will, but others doubt their previously unquestioned religious faith. Hope is of general clinical importance, but hope does not necessarily interfere with effective behavior, unless it is extreme and is not compatible with intellectual acceptance of reality. The persistence of hope does not usually require the need to intellectually deny reality, as it usually differentiates hope from defense patterns that may distort reality. As disease progresses there is usually a corresponding curtailment of hope. They no longer make long-range plans and they live on a day-to-day basis. This gradual dissipating of hope is inversely related to anticipatory grief. The grief process is usually precipitated by acute critical episodes. There is a process of resigning oneself to the inevitable outcome. The parents begin to feel "detached„ from the child [4].

Death and severe disease is always a shock, no matter what preparation. The doctor should be prepared tho accept the initial reaction of surprise, bitterness, anger and resentment as the beginning of the grieving process, and not as a personal reaction to him [10].

Reactions of Physicians and Staff

Stillbirth and neonatal death evoke a sense of guilt in the staff [5]. Doctors have a tendency to feel personally responsible for the unhappiness of the family. Being aware of this, he will not have the need to apologize and will be able to speak in a clear and direct manner. In this situation staff members handle anxiety in different ways:

1. avoidance of the situation,
2. projection of personal feelings in form of aggressive or accusing behavior,
3. denial [5].

Physicians tend to treat physical symptoms only and avoid discussing the baby's death [3]. Frequently the physician wonders if another treatment would have been successful. "Loss" is difficult to accept [1]. Tears and nonverbal messages of anger that normally accompany true grief and mourning from the parents and feelings of disappointment from the nurses make it difficult for the medical staff to function easily in this situation. Parents are extremely sensitive to what doctors say and do not say. The facial expression, signs of approval or disapproval are given hidden meanings. Frequently parents are critical because they received information only during the infant's hospitalisation, and nobody contacted them about autopsy information. Possibly the follow-up looks unimportant in the excitement of an intensive care unit [3]. Concern about laboratory details have a defence function by allowing doctors and parents to avoid the more tragic and general aspects. It is important to realize that parents are surrounded by disbelief: friends and family members question the ability of the doctor, and might suggest to seek additional medical opinions [4]. Frequently the doctor is experienced as a friend or ally, and the child's death appears as being his failure. The parents may be initially disappointed and angry at him. The death of a patient also evokes feelings of defeat and discomfort in the physician. He usually reviews critically the case in order to reassure himself and to learn as much as possible from the experience. If guilt and self-criticism interfere with his performance, it is much more difficult to handle the situation with the parents.

Interventions

Kincey [3] has demonstrated a relationship between patient' satisfaction and their level of understanding the information given. Knowledge of the normal reaction of parents handling their baby's death is of upmost importance. Parents should be encouraged to touch and hold their babies. The infant's identity can best be established if the parents are able to look, touch and hold their child. Some parents hate the idea of seeing the dead or dying child. One should explain to them that most parents have similar reactions, but later on appreciated the fact that they were present at that time. The mourning process is particularly prolonged and difficult to resolve when the parents did not see the child. A photograph of the dead baby can be very helpful for parents who were not able to see it [8]. These photographs, even if there are visible anomalies, help to make the baby real, a prerequisite of normal grief. The physician should show the dead baby or the photographs and point out the baby's perfect features in addition to its problems. Photographs should be taken even if the parents do not wish to see the baby. Parents imagine they have given birth to a monster. Death without a body that has been seen seems unreal. It is important to increase the staff awareness of the complex issues regarding the care of a dying child. The involvement with families should be encouraged as well as the staff follow-up [7]. Training should emphasize the handling of life as well as the handling of death. The birth of a malformed baby, whether alive or dead results in feelings of loss. The parents have been bereaved of the perfect baby they expected. The death of a child in the intensive care unit is an unnatural death. The hope for survival is frequently followed by disappointment, and physicians should be able to help the parents so that mourning, in its acute form, is complete. Professional skill combined with empathy are essential in this situation.

References

1. Kennel JH, Klaus MH (1976) Caring for parents of an infant who dies. In: Klaus MH, Kennel JH (eds) Maternal-infant bonding. The CV Mosby Company, Saint Louis, pp 209–239
2. Kennell JH, Slyter H, Klaus MH (1970) The mourning response of parents to the death of a newborn infant. N Engl J Med 283:344–349
3. Rowe J, Clyman R, Green C, et al (1978) Follow-up of families who experience a perinatal death. Pediatrics 62:166–170
4. Friedman SB, Chodoff P, Mason JW, et al (1963) Behavioral observations on parents anticipating the death of a child. Pediatrics 32:610–625
5. Cullberg J (1972) Mental reactions of women to perinatal death. In: Morris N (ed) Proceedings of the third international congress of psychosomatic medicine in obstetrics and gynaecology. Karger, New York, pp 326–329
6. Lindemann E (1944) Symptomatology and management of acute grief. Am J Psychiatry 101:141–148
7. Harmon RJ, Glicken AD, Siegel RE (1984) Neonatal loss in the intensive care nursery: Effects of maternal grieving and a program for intervention. J Am Acad Child Psychiatr 23,1:68–71
8. Lewis E (1979) Mourning by the family after a stillbirth or neonatal death. Arch Dis Child 54:303–306
9. Pichler E, Richter R, Jürgenssen AO (1982) Konzept zur Ganzheitsbetreuung von Familien leukämie- und tumor-kranker Kinder, basierend auf Gesprächen mit Eltern. Onkologie 5(4):178–185
10. Solnit AJ, Green M (1959) Psychologic considerations in the management of deaths on pediatric hospital services. Pediatrics 24:106–112
11. Magni G, Carli M, De Leo D, et al (1986) Longitudinal evaluations of psychological distress in parents of children with malignancies. Acta Paediatr Scand 75:283–288

Imaging in the Critically Ill

Interpretation of Pulmonary Vascular Congestion

A. F. Turner

Introduction

The concepts of interpretation of a chest radiograph taken on a patient in the upright position and full inspiration are different from the concepts of interpretation of the supine chest radiograph of a critically ill or injured patient.

Critically ill and injured patients are difficult to radiograph. In the intensive care unit, it is the subtle radiographic variations that may warn one of life-threatening changes in the patients condition. Therefore excellent radiographs are in order to identify such findings.

Technical Factors

High Kilovoltage chest radiographs are best suited for the optimal detection of pulmonary disease. Radiographs taken at 150 KVp allow excellent detection of small densities and give a very low false positive reading. For nodule detection, the accuracy was 61% for 120 KVp grid technique as opposed to 27% detection rate for a 70 KVp non-grid technique. When one considers KVp, there is a considerable difference between single phase and constant potential equipment. With constant potential equipment such as the new portable battery powered units, a 100 KVp setting gives a true 96 KVp radiograph, while a 100 KVp setting on single phase portable gives a true 64 KVp radiograph [1].

Technical factors such as the patient's position, KVp and mA must be recorded. Similarly, knowledge of the type of mechanical ventilation, peak pressure, peak expiratory pressure and phase of ventilation at the time of filming are essential for accurate interpretation.

Labelling of a radiograph is important and should always include left or right markers, the patient's name with the date and time of the radiograph. Proper time-dated radiographs are important since the most important radiograph is the most recent for purposes of comparison. Radiographs should be marked as portable, supine, or prone. Pleural effusions obscure the lung bases on a supine radiograph, while a prone radiograph would allow evaluation of the lung bases.

Analyzing chest radiographs of patients in both upright and recumbent patients requires an excellent knowledge of anatomy, physiology, cardiopulmonary hemodynamics and a clear concept of clinical medicine.

Pulmonary Vascular Congestion

In considering pulmonary vascular congestion, one may assess variations in pulmonary vascularity and the distribution of extravascular lung water. Pulmonary vascularity may be assessed with knowledge of the three basic patterns of pulmonary blood flow; normal, redistribution and increased pulmonary blood flow.

Normal Blood Flow

The pulmonary circulation, being a low-pressure system, remains quite gravity-dependent. In the awake patient in the lateral decubitus position, the dependent lung receives relatively more perfusion and ventilation than the nondependent lung, thus the ventilation perfusion ratio of each lung remains approximately constant regardless of position. The increased perfusion of the dependent lung results in increased pulmonary capillary pressure in the dependent lung, with consequent increase in fluid transudation [2]. During anesthesia, the dependent lung continues to receive more perfusion than the upper lung, but the majority of ventilation is switched to the nondependent lung [3–5], this results in a mismatch of ventilation and perfusion. This consideration has to be given to the interpretation of chest radiographs in the ICU in patients who have been given pancuronium as a neuromuscular blocker to induce apnea, in this situation an annotation of the patient's position and time in that position prior to the chest radiograph being taken would be essential to allow an adequate evaluation of the chest radiograph.

Interpretation of normal blood flow in the upright full inspiration radiograph reveals that flow is greater in the lower lung zones than the upper lung zones. The vascular pedicle represented by the superior vena cava, the ascending and descending thoracic aorta and the main pulmonary artery and the main branches of the pulmonary artery are normal. If one observes the pulmonary bronchi "on end" in the hilar regions of the lungs, they are thin, almost blending with the surrounding hilar and pulmonary structures.

In the recumbent chest radiograph, normal vasculature has a homogeneous distribution, however, on a CT scan, the distribution is from anterior to posterior with greater vasculature posteriorly and decreased vascularity anteriorly.

In the upright full inspiration radiography pulmonary vascular redistribution pulmonary blood flow is altered so that flow is diverted from the lower lung zones to the upper lung zones. Early on, there is no significant decrease in pulmonary blood flow, however, as left heart failure ensues, there is a decrease in the total pulmonary blood flow. With decreased cardiac output, the assessment of the pulmonary vascular pattern becomes more difficult.

Pulmonary vascular redistribution has been graded and correlated with the pulmonary venous pressure in the upright full inspiration chest [6] and in the recumbent radiograph [7].

1+ redistribution is present when there is equal perfusion of the upper and lower lung zones. This increased perfusion in the upper zones is due to a shifting of blood from the lower lung zones. There is a true oligemia in the lower lung zones as a result of this shift. The homogeneous distribution of flow should not be confused with the similar appearance in increased pulmonary blood flow. In increased flow there is normal or increased vascularity to the lower lung zone and increased vascularity to the upper lung zone. When 1+ redistribution is present, the pulmonary venous pressure is estimated to be 12 mmHg ± 3 mmHg.

In the supine recumbent radiograph, redistribution of pulmonary vascularity is in an anterior-posterior direction and may be detected on axial computed tomographic slices of the chest. On the recumbent chest radiograph, 1+ pulmonary vascular redistribution cannot be accurately assessed.

2+ redistribution is present when there is greater perfusion of the upper than the lower lung zones. This represents an inversion of the normal blood flow pattern. This pattern may be appreciated on an upright chest radiograph in the critically ill or injured patient, however, it is difficult to assess on the recumbent chest radiograph taken in the intensive care unit. On CT changes may be detected with increased vascularity anteriorly and decreased vascularity posteriorly. The estimated pulmonary venous pressure would be 17 ± 3 mmHg.

3+ redistribution is present when 2+ redistribution is accompanied by interstitial edema. Interstitial edema may be present when one or more of the following are present:

a) perihilar indistinctness,
b) perivascular indistinctness
c) peribronchial indistinctness
d) Kerley B lines – interstitial Kerley B lines are insensitive markers of elevated estravascular lung water in absence of pulmonary vascular engorgement [8]
e) Kerley A lines
f) subpleural edema
g) overall haziness of lower lung zone.

On CT scans interstitial pulmonary edema is readily apparent.

The estimated pulmonary venous pressure in the upright full inspiration radiograph would be 25 ± 5 mmHg. In the recumbent chest radiograph in the ICU, the pulmonary venous pressures are estimated to be 22 ± 5 mmHg.

4+ redistribution is present when interstitial edema is accompanied by alveolar edema. The pulmonary patterns found in alveolar disease are:

1. Acinar nodule – represents consolidation of the functional unit of the lung. Densities measure approximately 5 mm in diameter and are ill-defined. Acinar shadows were originally described by Aschoff in 1924 [9];
2. Secondary pulmonary lobule (rosette) is formed by 3–5 acini. Through the pores of Kohn, adjacent air spaces are quickly involved. Rosettes are ill-defined densities approximately 1–3 cm in size;

3. Homogeneous densities. The coalescence of the acinar nodule and rosettes causes an ill-defined density in the periphery of the lung. The homogeneous densities appear to spread along the subpleural regions of the lung, then centrifugally, surrounding bronchi and bronchioles as they proceed toward the hilum;

4. Nonsegmental distribution is present since segmental boundaries do not impede the passage of fluid or air through the pores of Kohn. The exudate of acute alveolar pneumonia can spread throughout the lobe, totally unimpeded by segmental anatomy;

5. Air bronchogram results from consolidation of the parenchyma with no air displacement in the bronchi. The term "air bronchogram sign" suggested by Felson [10], is highly appropriate. Regardless of etiology, any pathological process associated with an air bronchogram must be anatomically situated within the lung parenchyma;

6. Air terminal bronchiologram is the result of consolidation of the air spaces (alveoli) with no displacement of air in the terminal bronchioles.

This gives an ill-defined mottle to the periphery of the lung. In the recumbent radiograph, alveolar pulmonary edema is clearly identified.

When 4+ redistribution is present, pulmonary venous pressures are usually above 30 mmHg.

Increased Pulmonary Blood Flow

With increased flow, there is uniform distribution of blood flow to both the lower and upper zones of the lungs. The pulmonary volume is usually increased. The vascular pedicle represented by the superior vena cava, the ascending and descending aorta and the main pulmonary artery and the main branches of the pulmonary artery is increased.

Extravascular Lung Water

Pulmonary edema is the result of an increased transpulmonary flux of water and solute and a concomitant insufficiency of lung lymphatic drainage. Although this pathogenetic concept seems well-established, the microcirculatory details of pulmonary edema formation and its ultimate resolution are still poorly understood [11].

Pulmonary edema, the transudation of fluid from the capillaries into the interstitium and subsequently into the alveolar spaces frequently results from increased pressures in the pulmonary veins. Guyton and Linsey [12] reported a biphasic relationship between left atrial pressure and edema accumulation. Little edema accumulated until a left atrial pressure of approximately 24 mm Hg was reached. They interpreted this initial refractory state to represent a "threshold" for edema accumulation caused by protein osmotic forces counteracting hydrostatic gradients (osmotic safety factor). Using sheep, Erdmann et al. [13] obtained a comparable relationship and introduced the concept of the "lymphatic safety factor" to explain the phenomena. Lymphatics would constantly drain the excess liquid from the extravascular space, and edema would only occur once lymphatic flow is overwhelmed. When Guyton and Lindsey [12] decreased plasma protein concentration to half normal by plasmapheresis, they found that fluid transudation to begin above left atrial pressure of approximately 11 mmHg. Rutili et al [14] considered extravascular water volumes at comparable pulmonary capillary pressures obtained with the infusion of crystalloid and dextran and found no differences in edema contributed to the composition of the infusate. It is known from the work of Staub et al. [15] and Gee and Havill [16], that hydrostatic edema tends to accumulate initially in the central interstitium around large bronchi and vessels. This complex interstitial tissue offers significant resistance to fluid movement [17].

Pulmonary edema is usually classified as either "cardiogenic" or "non-cardiogenic". Often the phenomena of "increased permeability" pulmonary edema is made by inference; when pulmonary edema develops in the setting of normal hydrostatic pressure (estimated from pulmonary artery wedge pressure) its pathogenesis is ascribed to non-cardiogenic edema. This distinction, however, ignores that pulmonary edema may arise simultaneously from both cardiac and non-cardiac sources, that therapy itself may alter hydrostatic pressure, or that the "permeability defect" encompasses a wide range of severity that is estimatable only by direct measurement.

In a patient with chronic left heart failure, the pulmonary venous pressures may return to normal, however, pulmonary edema may still be present after four or five days. Thus, the possibility that pulmonary edema in the presence of normal filling pressures may represent resolution of a transient high-pressure edema as opposed to a capillary leak syndrome [18].

Hydrostatic pulmonary edema may occur with only slight elevation of the pulmonary venous pressures in patients with decreased plasma osmolality [12], chronic left heart failure with cardiac dilatation [19] and patients with renal dysfunction [20].

Noncardiac pulmonary edema may result from increased capillary permeability, decreased plasma oncotic pressure, decreased lymphatic or venous drainage, renal failure and overhydration. Overhydration is probably the most common problem faced in the critically ill.

The radiological assessment of extravascular water in patients in the ICU has been shown to be a difficult problem, some authors feel that the chest radiograph can be reasonably accurate in quantitating extravascular lung water [21, 22] and other authors find it an inaccurate method [23, 24] of quantitating extravascular lung water. Thermal-dye techniques were found to give erroneously high values in septic sheep [25]. This finding could be probably due to erythrostasis and leukocyte plugging with uneven perfusion and prolonged transit times due to reduced cardiac output. In the control animals and oleic acid group of the same study lung water measured with thermal-dye technique and correlated to gravimetrically measured lung water ($r=0.70$ and $r=0.93$ respectively), however, in the septic animals the correlation was $r=-0.25$. Several reports have documented reliability and validity of thermal-dye technique for measuring extravascular lung water [26–29]. If one were to separate the septic from the nonseptic patients, there may be a closer correlation of the chest radiograph and the quantitation of extravascular lung water. The following criteria have been used to quantitate extravascular water by Milne [21] with a stated accuracy of 5%.

Criteria for quantitating fluid water are shown in Table 1.

There are four basic patterns of pulmonary edema, that can be interpreted with a reasonable degree of reliability.

1. *Cardiac distribution* is primarily at the lung bases below the level of the hili bilaterally and is associated with pulmonary vascular redistribution.
2. *Renal or overhydration* is usually pericardiac in nature with sparing of the periphery and is usually associated with some prominence of the pulmonary vasculature.
3. *Capillary permeability* is an irregular, patchy type of distribution. Positive pressure is a slow progressive increase in the interstitial markings that have a perihilar or lower lobe distribution, however, is not associated with pulmonary vascular redistribution. Interstitial and alveolar edema ensues unless the problem is corrected.
4. It is not unusual to have edema resulting from one or more etiologies.

There are several other parameters that aid in the classification of pulmonary edema patterns. They are lung volume, peribronchial cuffing, cardiothoracic ratio and cardiac configuration.

Lung volume appears to be small in patients with heart failure, whereas in patients with overhydration edema tends to be somewhat enlarged. Lungs enlarge as they are filled with blood.

Peribronchial cuffing is not common in patients with capillary permeability, whereas in overhydration and cardiac failure it is present in approximately 95% of cases.

Cardiothoracic ratio: Patients with ARDS have a cardiothoracic ratio which is usually normal early in the disease, however, later in the disease process, there may be some cardiac enlargement. Overhydration, renal failure and most cardiac failure patients have an increase in cardiothoracic ratio.

Table 1. Criteria for quantitating lung water

Criteria	Quantity ml/L of lung & TLC
Real sharp vessel margins	25
Normal vessels with no peribronchial cuffing	50
Minimal vascular indistinctness with questionable peribronchial cuffing	60– 70
Minimal interstitial edema with peribronchial cuffing	70–100
Moderate interstitial edema with no alveolar component	90–110
Interstitial edema with an alveolar component present	110–130
Alveolar edema primarily in the lower lobes	130–150
Alveolar edema of the total lung	more than 160

Cardiac configuration: Classical cardiac configurations may give insight into the etiology of cardiac failure. e. g. mitral valve disease with an enlarged left atrial appendage.

Additional problems in interpretation are related to interstitial and alveolar viral and bacterial pneumonia and aspiration pneumonia. Aspiration infiltrates are non specific, occur in the dependent portions of the lungs (posterior segment of the upper lobes, superior and posterior basal segments of lower lobes) may give a clue as to the etiology. Anterior nondependent infiltrates are usually caused by bacterial pneumonias. Knowledge of the position of the patient is very important when assessing aspiration.

Lung infections occur in approximately 10 to 20% of patients in the ICU. These infections are usually atypical clinically and radiographically. Mortality rates of pneumonias developed in the ICU may approach 50%.

Chest radiographs remain the principle diagnostic study in defining the presence and extent of pneumonia.

Mechanical Ventilation

The institution of positive pressure therapy may markedly alter the appearance of the chest radiograph. Because the respirator is usually set to deliver a volume of gas larger than the patient has when breathing spontaneously, the radiograph taken at the peak of forced inspiration reflects larger lung inflation. Areas of atelectasis may reexpand, and interstitial pulmonary water may be driven into the vascular space. It is important to recognize when the patient is removed from the support apparatus that the lungs are no longer "pumped up". With re-institution of PEEP, infiltrates either cleared or diminished in over half the patients studied. Infiltrates disappeared, vessels became sharper and smaller and areas of silhouetting disappeared. These radiographic changes, which reversed when PEEP was removed, appeared to be more marked in patients with diffuse edema rather than other types of pulmonary infiltrates [30]. It is imperative that the radiologist know whether the patient was receiving positive pressure therapy at the time the radiograph was taken.

References

1. Christensen EE, Dietz GW, Murry RC, et al (1977) Effects of kilovoltage on detectability of pulmonary nodules in a chest phantom A J R 128:789–793
2. West JB (1979) Respiratory physiology, 2nd edn. The Williams and Wilkins Co., Baltimore
3. Rehder K et al (1973) Function of each lung in spontaneously breathing man anesthetized with thiopental-meperidine. Anesthesiology 38:320–327
4. Rehder K et al (1972) The function of each lung of anesthetized and paralysed man during mechanical ventilation. Anesthesiology 37:16–26
5. Bindslev L et al (1981) Distribution of inspired gas to each lung in anesthetized human subjects. Acta Anaesthesiol Scand 25:297–302
6. Turner AF, Lau FYK, Jacobson G (1972) A method for the estimation of pulmonary venous and arterial pressures from the routine chest radiograph. A J R 116:97–106

7. McHugh TJ, Forrester JS, Adler L, et al (1972) Pulmonary vascular congestion in acute myocardial infarction; hemodynamic and radiologic correlations. Ann Intern Med 76:29-33

8. Slutsky RA, Olson LK, Costello D, Brown JJ (1984) Extravascular lung water in patients with mitral stenosis: relationship to pulmonary capillary wedge pressure and Kerley B lines. Radiology 153:317-320

9. Aschoff L (1924) Lectures on pathology. Hoeber, New York 10 lung

10. Felson B (1969) Disseminated interstitial diseases of the lung. In: Simon M, Potchen EJ, LeMay M (eds) Frontiers of Pulmonary Radiology. Grune & Stratton, Inc., New York

11. Schuster DP, Mintun MA (1987) Pulmonary circulation, extravascular water, and solute flux as determined by positron emission tomography. Lymphology 20:25-35

12. Guyton AC, Lindsey AW (1959) Effect of elevated left atrial pressure and decreased plasma protein concentration on the development of pulmonary edema. Circ Res 7:617-657

13. Erdmann III AJ, Vaughn TR, Brigham KL, et al (1975) Effect of increased vascular pressure on lung fluid balance in unanesthetized sheep. Circ Res 37:271-284

14. Rutilli G, Parker JC, Taylor AE (1984) Fluid balance in ANTU-injured lungs during crystalloid and colloid infusions. J Appl Physiol 56:993-998

15. Staub NC, Nagano H, Pearce ML (1967) Pulmonary edema in dogs, especially the sequence of fluid accumulation in the lungs. J Appl Physiol 22:227-240

16. Gee MH, Havill AM (1985) The relationship between pulmonary perivascular cuff fluid and lung lymph in dogs with edema. Microvasc Res 19:209-216

17. Unruh HW, Goldberg HS, Oppenheimer L (1985) Pulmonary interstitial compartments and tissue resistance to fluid flux. J Appl Physiol 57:1512-1519

18. Mayers I, Stimpson R, Oppenheimer L (1987) Delayed resolution of high-pressure pulmonary edema or capillary leak. Surgery 101:450-458

19. Grover M, Slutsky RA, Higgins CB, Shabetai R (1983) Extravascular lung water in patients with congestive failure. Difference between patients with acute and chronic myocardial disease. Radiology 147:659-662

20. Slutsky RA, Day R, Murray M (1985) Effect of prolonged renal dysfunction on intravascular and extravascular pulmonary fluid volumes during left atrial hypertension. Proc Soc Exp Biol Med 179:25-31

21. Milne E (1986) Role of the radiologist in the intensive care unit. Lecture pulmonary medicine 1986 - Advances in internal medicine. Pasadena Hilton, Pasadena California

22. Laggner A, Kleinberger G, Sommer G, et al (1985) Bestimmung des extravaskularen Lungenwassergehalts bei Intensivpatienten: Gegenüberstellung mit radiologischen, hämodynamischen und funktionellen Lungenbefunden. Schweiz Med Wochenschr 115:210-213

23. Halperin BD, Feeley TW, Mihm FG, et al (1985) Evaluation of the portable chest roentgenograms for quantitating extravascular lung water in critically ill adults. Chest 88:649-652

24. Haller J, Czembirek H, Salomonowitz E, et al (1985) Die Thoraxbettaufnahme und extravaskulare Lungenwasserbestimmung bei Intensivpatienten. ROFO 142:68-73

25. Andreasson S, Bylock A, Smith L, Risberg B (1986) Extravascular lung water measurement in septic sheep. J Surg Res 40:95-104

26. Hill SL, Elings VB, Lewis FR (1980) Sepsis and the pulmonary capillary dependence of permeability changes on hydrostatic pressure and tissue after septic insult. Crit Care Med 8:225-231

27. Hill SL, Elings VB, Lewis FR (1980) Changes in lungwater and capillary permeability following sepsis and fluid overloads. J Surg Res 28:140-7

28. Holcroft JW, Trunkey DD, Carpenter MF (1978) Excessive fluid administration in resuscitating baboons from haemorrhagic shock, and an assessment of the thermo-dye technic for measuring extravascular lungwater. Ann Surg 135:412-419

29. Oppenheimer L, Elings VB, Lewis FR (1979) Thermal-dye lungwater measurements. Effect of edema and embolization. J Surg Res 26:504-511

30. Zimmerman JE, Goodman LR, Shahvari MBG (1979) Effect of mechanical ventilation and positive endexpiratory pressure (PEEP) on chest radiographs. AJR 133:811-819

The Interpretation of the Portable Chest Film in Intensive Care

K. Hillman

Introduction

Although their quality is less than optimal, the antero-posterior (A-P) chest film made with portable X-ray equipment is one of the most useful tools in critical care medicine. It is a mandatory supplement to the examination of the respiratory system and should be performed daily as a routine on most seriously ill patients. During examination of the daily chest film, progress of the underlying disease is observed and compared, early changes of barotrauma looked for and the position of lines and endotracheal tubes checked. A chest film should also be performed after intrathoracic line placement or intubation, as well as in response to sudden changes in the patient's clinical state, such as fever, hypoxia or increased ventilatory pressures. Many unsuspected abnormalities not detected on clinical examination, are seen on chest films and these often lead to major management changes [1].

However, interpreting A-P chest films taken in less than ideal circumstances on seriously ill patients can be uneasy. The patients are difficult to position and often move while the X-ray is being taken, causing blurring of the film. The A-P projection magnifies the heart and mediastinum and can make interpretation of pulmonary vessel distribution and edema difficult. Commenting on heart size, vessel diameter and vessel distribution is therefore less accurate. Although it is tempting to take a chest film with the patient supine, it is crucial to gain the cooperation of the nursing and radiology staff to take the film with the patient erect. Air-fluid levels, such as effusions or lung abscesses can be visualized only if the patient is erect. Pneumothoraxes and distribution of pulmonary vessels and lung edema can be interpreted with more certainty when the patient is erect. The staff working in Intensive Care can soon learn the art of sitting unconscious patients erect.

Lung shadows on the chest film must always be interpreted together with the clinical examination, pathology information and the rate of change of the shadowing. The first major distinction is between pleural and parenchymal lesions. As well as the typical fluid level found in pleural effusions, pleural shadows tend to veil lung markings, while those in the parenchyma obliterate them. Lung parenchymal shadows are divided into alveolar and interstitial opacities. Alveolar filling processes such as edema, consolidation and hemorrhage produce heterogeneous shadows because large aggregates of fluid filled acini occur, making the individual units unrecognizable. Air bronchograms and obliteration of vascular markings can calso occur. Interstitial shadows are recognized by lines representing thickened connective tissue septa between lobules in the cortex of the lung and less well-defined interstitial planes within the medulla of each lung - the so-called Kerley's lines.

Intraparenchymal Opacities

Cardiogenic Pulmonary Edema

It is comforting to know that there is a good correlation between the estimation of extravascular lung water (EVLW) by the thermal-dye technique and chest X-ray [2-4]. However, there has to be a 35% increase in EVLW before edema is seen on the chest film [2]. Variations in pulmonary artery wedge pressure (PAWP) also correlate well with changes on the chest film [5]. The chest film appearances are normal when the PAWP is less than 12 mmHg. The peripheral vessels dilate, and interstitial edema occurs when the PAWP is between 18 and 22 mmHg and alveolar filling is seen when it is more than 22 mmHg. However, many of the radiological signs of interstitial edema are seen best in chronic rather than acute edema states. Peri-bronchial edema remains a good sign in acute edema [6], but many of the classical signs such as 'bats wings' pattern are inconsistent findings.

Unfortunately the features of an A-P supine film can mimic some of the radiological changes of pulmonary edema, especially upper lobe diversion of pulmonary vessels and peri-bronchial cuffing. A generalized increase in pulmonary blood volume and flow may obliterate the normal gravitational effect and result in distension of upper and lower zone vessels [7]. The patient position, abnormalities of parenchyma and the integrity of the pulmonary vascular bed can all affect the distribution of pulmonary edema. It is common to see atypical patterns of pulmonary edema in patients with chronic lung disease [8].

Adult Respiratory Distress Syndrome (ARDS)

As both cardiogenic pulmonary edema and ARDS result in an increase in EVLW, it is not surprizing that they are indistinguishable on chest X-ray. Both conditions cause pulmonary edema, but for different reasons. Cardiogenic pulmonary edema usually occurs as a result of a failing heart and raised left atrial pressures, where as ARDS occurs in particular clinical circumstances (e.g. sepsis, shock, etc.) in the presence of a normal left atrial pressure. The conditions are clinically differentiated on clinical grounds and by measuring the PAWP.

Because both the clinical and radiographic features of ARDS are not specific, it is important to interpret the films serially. It is the progression of abnormalities that is the hallmark of ARDS [9]. Signs usually first occur between 24-36 hours in the form of a peri-hilar haze, interstitial edema and alveolar filling. There is little change in the primary disease after 36 hours.

Other later occurring radiological features of ARDS, such as cavitation, pulmonary interstitial emphysema (PIE), repeated pneumothoraxes (PT) and scarring [10] may, in fact, be the result of treatment and not part of the normal radiological features of ARDS. They occur as a result of barotrauma and lung damage due to high ventilatory pressures [11]. Other conditions such as expansion of the interstitial space with crystalloid solutions may also be confused with ARDS [12]. When large amounts of crystalloid are used for resuscitation in conditions such as sepsis multi-trauma and diabetic ketoacidosis, pulmonary edema results. This cannot be differentiated clinically nor radiologically from true ARDS. Notable improvement in the radiological appearances of ARDS and many other types of parenchymal abnormalities can occur with positive pressure ventilation and PEEP. This is not necessarily due to re-aeration of atelectatic alveoli and may indicate over-distension of the smaller conducting airways [13] or alveolar rupture [11].

Pneumonia

Pneumonia is a clinico-pathological diagnosis, and there is no definite radiological appearance which marks its presence. This is unfortunate because it is common in Intensive Care and difficult to diagnose and distinguish from other causes of intrapulmonary shadowing. Furthermore, bacteria are often cultured in the sputum of seriously ill patients in the presence of intrapulmonary shadows, but this does not mean the two are related. The association has resulted in misdiagnosis and over-prescribing of antibiotics in Intensive Care. In fact, there is a poor correlation between sputum culture and the actual microbiology of pneumonia [14, 15]. Apart from lobar consolidation, which is strongly indicative of bacterial pneumonia, the chest film is used more to follow the course of treatment in pneumonia rather than as a specific diagnostic indicator.

Aspiration

The sequelae of aspiration depends on the type of material aspirated, its volume, distribution of the material and the host reaction to the aspirated material [9]. Aspiration can be classified according to the type of material aspirated, the distribution of the material or the resulting radiological appearance.

Material aspirated

(a) *Foreign body-particulate matter:* Depending on the position of the patient at the time of aspiration, it is more common to aspirate into the right main bronchus. If radio-opaque, the material can be directly visualized. Otherwise effects of airway obstruction, such as atelectasis, air trapping, mediastinal shift and lobar hyperinflation can be visualized. An inflammatory response, particularly with plant matter and nuts, is seen later with particulate matter. This can eventually result in fibrosis and granuloma formation [16].

(b) *Infected material:* If the patient is recumbent, the apical segments of the right upper and lower lobes are often affected; if the patient is sitting, the right lower lobe is commonly involved. Consolidation occurs slowly over

5–7 days, often accompanied by infected pleural exudate, and may take weeks to clear [17]. Cavitation with or without fluid levels occur within the parenchymal consolidation and empyema may also result.

(c) *Non-toxic liquid aspiration:* It is unusual for this type of aspiration to have sufficient bacterial inoculum to produce infection, nor sufficient volume or particulate size to produce significant airway blockage. Nothing more than a mild chemical pneumonitis usually results. There is a wide spectrum of radiological changes from minimal to mixed (alveolar and interstitial) parenchymal opacities, occasionally with atelectasis and effusions. The distribution is usually bilateral, affecting the lower lobes more than the upper. Radiographic clearing usually occurs within 7–10 days if uncomplicated by infection [18].

(d) *Toxic liquid aspiration:* Mendelson is generally accredited with the first description of aspiration of gastric acid [19]. The radiographic appearance is indistinguishable from pulmonary edema. The toxic liquid "burns" the alveolar surfaces resulting in alveolar capillary membrane leak. It is indistinguishable on chest film from drowning, ARDS, fat embolism and cardiogenic pulmonary edema; except uncommonly when the distribution is lobar or unilateral. However, the radiographic changes develop within 24–36 hours and in the absence of infection (25% incidence) usually disappears within 7–10 days [9].

(e) *Near-drowning:* The radiographic appearance in near-drowning is often similar to toxic liquid aspiration. There is an appearance of pulmonary edema within 36 hours. If there has also been particulate inhalation, there can be atelectasis and if the water is contaminated, consolidation and even cavitation. Despite claims that there is a different radiographic appearance with fresh and salt water drowning [20], others suggest they are indistinguishable [9].

Smoke Inhalation

Inhalation of smoke and toxic gases can cause severe damage to the airways and lung parenchyma. Focal linear opacities may occur within 24 hours after smoke inhalation and usually clear within three days [9]. Focal or patchy alveolar filling can also occur within a few hours and up to three days. The standard chest radiograph is a relatively insensitive means of evaluating pulmonary abnormalities due to smoke inhalation.

Fat Embolism

Clinically and radiographically, fat embolism simulates ARDS. The chest film shows parenchymal opacities consistent with interstitial or alveolar edema, usually occurring within 24 hours and often in association with neurological signs and petechiae following major orthopedic trauma.

Atelectasis and Collapse

Consolidation and collapse often co-exist. It is, however, convenient to consider the two phenomena separately. Pure consolidation shows no loss of volume, while collapse shows loss of volume of a lung or lobe. The most common cause of collapse in Intensive Care is intraluminal obstruction of the airways, particularly by mucous plugging. The radiological signs include the shadow of the collapsed lobe or lobes, the silhouette sign and displacement of structures to take up the space normally occupied by the collapsed lung. The signs of displacement include crowding of the lung markings, elevation of a hemi-diaphragm, and mediastinal shift.

Apart from collapse of a lobe or lung, there can also be collapse of smaller sub-units of the lung – often referred to as atelectasis. These produce many types of shadows, and are often described as triangular line or plate shaped. Following re-expansion of a collapsed lobe, various shaped shadows often remain at the site of residual segmental collapses which are not totally resolved.

Collapse and atelectasis often respond rapidly to maneuvers such as posturing, physiotherapy, suction and deep breathing. The presence or absence of an air bronchogram in association with persistent collapse can give an indication as to whether fiberoptic bronchoscopy is indicated.

Differentiation Between Lung Parenchymal Pathology

This is probably the greatest challenge in the interpretation of chest films in Intensive Care. As there are no absolute radiological differences between pathological processes such as ARDS, fat embolism, pneumonia, smoke inhalation, aspiration and cardiogenic pulmonary edema, the interpretation of the chest film has to be tempered by clinical examination, pathology results and the time period for onset and disappearance of shadows as a result of the natural history and treatment. For example, bronchiole breath sounds are frequently found with pneumonia, but are rare in pulmonary edema. A substantial response to treatment within 24 hours indicates pulmonary edema, not pneumonia. The differentiation between the edema in ARDS and cardiogenic pulmonary edema is made easy these days by assessing cardiac function with pulmonary artery catheterisation, nuclear medicine or ultrasound studies.

The differentiation between pneumonia and ARDS remains difficult. This is not made easier by the fact that there is often multiple lung pathology in Intensive Care. Patients with pneumonia are often septic, and septic patients often have ARDS. Conversely patients with ARDS can develop nosocomial pneumonia. A precise diagnosis of ARDS or nosocomial pneumonia is often difficult. Both groups of patients are often febrile, have a leukocytosis, are hypoxic, with reduced lung volumes and compliance. Often the organism causing the pneumonia is not isolated, even with open lung biopsy. And then, on histology, both ARDS and pneumonia can have hyaline membranes, interstitial fibrosis and changes in the epithelium [21]. In a recent comparison of the two diseases, pathogens were found in the sputum with equal frequency and only a minority of the patients with nosocomial pneumonia responded to antibiotics [22]. If the diseases cannot be defined adequately, then accurate figures on their incidence and outcome are impossible.

If is not surprising, therefore, that the diagnosis and differentiation of ARDS and pneumonia remains one of the greatest challenges in critical care medicine, and one that not only has the chest film not been able to resolve, but one which also stretches our other clinical and investigative resources to their limits. The most reliable radiological guide remains the temporal relationship in the onset of ARDS. Unless patients are admitted to Intensive Care with primary pneumonia, it usually takes several days for it to develop, while ARDS usually occurs within 36 hours of the initial insult.

Clinical ARDS can be differentiated from pulmonary edema associated with cardiac failure by several means [23]. The pattern of cardiac failure begins as interstitial edema, later becoming alveolar, where as ARDS develops as a random alveolar pattern with a tendency to be peripherally located and not in the costophrenic angles. ARDS is not classically associated with septal lines or peribronchial cuffing. The pattern of ARDS usually becomes established within 36 hours and does not change greatly with position. Abrupt deterioration may be due to fluid overload or heart failure. Abrupt improvement is usually related to a change in ventilatory pattern. Effusions are common in cardiac or overhydration pulmonary edema but rare in ARDS.

Pulmonary Embolism

The portable chest X-ray is not an accurate way to detect pulmonary emboli. The chest film can be normal or have a host of non-specific signs such as focal redistribution of blood flow, pulmonary infarction, atelectasis, pleural effusions or a raised hemi-diaphragm. In the presence of other intrapulmonary pathologies these signs are even less valuable. If a pulmonary embolism is suspected, perfusion lung scintigraphy or angiography should be performed. Intravenous digital angiography may be the investigation of the future.

Abdominal Pathology Affecting the Chest X-Ray

The chest X-ray is an excellent reflection of intra-abdominal pathology in Intensive Care. The onset of ARDS or its persistence may be an indication of unresolved intra-abdominal sepsis. A generalized or localised intra-abdominal mass effect can decrease lung volume and push the diaphragm up as well as causing basal atelectasis and later infection. Basal effusions occur in approximately 50% of post-operative patients [24]. Pneumoperitoneum can occur as a result of recent laparotomy, ruptured intra-abdominal viscus or derived from pulmonary barotrauma [25]. It is important to differentiate the cause as different treatment is urgently required for the latter two causes of pneumoperitoneum. Gastric dilatation is often seen as a result of recent resuscitation and positive ventilation with a mask and airway. It can also be encountered following abdominal surgery, sepsis or diabetic ketoacidosis.

Chest Trauma

An urgent upright chest film is crucial in assessing chest trauma. In no other area of medicine can so much important information be gleaned from such limited material [9]. The film must be taken with the patient upright so that effusions, parenchymal damage and pneumothoraces can be visualised. Pulmonary contusion is probably the commonest abnormality seen. It represents edema or blood in the alveoli which may have resulted from direct impact or from a contra-coup injury. They are often seen immediately and usually are represented by maximum shadowing within 24 hours. They begin clearing within 2–3 days and are usually completely cleared within 1–2 weeks [9]. If not, one should suspect superimposed infection, concurrent aspiration, or intrapulmonary hematoma. Pulmonary hematoma usually present as a round opacity that may become visible following clearing of an area of contusion.

The extent of fractured ribs and flail segments should be documented as a guideline for pain management and possible damage to other structures such as the spleen. Although fractured ribs can penetrate lung tissue and cause pneumothoraces, it is very common to have extra-alveolar air formation, including pneumothoraces as a result of blunt lung trauma [11]. Even in the presence of fractured ribs, there can be extra-alveolar air in the form of subcutaneous emphysema (SE) and mediastinal emphysema (ME) as a result of blunt rather than penetrating injury. These patients may not have a pneumothorax and do no need an intercostal drain on the side of the fractured ribs. A fractured sternum is commonly associated with underlying myocardial contusion.

Diaphragmatic rupture, esophageal trauma, pericardial tamponade, aortic rupture and tracheo-bronchial injuries are all rarer but serious complications of chest trauma.

Extra-Alveolar Air

Extra-alveolar air (EAA) should be looked for in ventilated patients in Intensive Care. With excessive intrapulmonary pressures, the alveoli over-distends and bursts, to form pulmonary interstitial edema (PIE) around the pulmonary vessels. The air then migrates towards the lung hila and into the mediastinum to form mediastinal emphysema (ME). From there, with continued intrapulmonary pressure, the gas can form subcutaneous emphysema (SE) or burst through the thin mediastinal pleura to form pneumothoraces (PT) and under high pressures be forced along the aorta or esophagus to form pneumoretroperitoneum (PRP) and pneumoperitoneum (PP) [11]. Each manifestation of EAA can cause serious adverse effects as well as being a marker of further manifestations of EAA. The most common radiological appearance of PIE is generalized irregular radiolucent mottling, particularly in the peri-hilar region, but it can also cause variable sized cysts. It is often difficult to distinguish PIE from the underlying lung pathology. Mediastinal emphysema is important to recognize because as well as causing adverse cardiorespiratory effects, it is the precursor of air elsewhere, especially a PT. Unfortunately, unless it occurs laterally ME may not always be obvious on an A-P film. Mediastinal emphysema can be mistaken for pneumopericardium, which is an extremely rare and usually a terminal event. Subcutaneous emphysema is usually obvious on a portable chest film and can be seen in the superior mediastinum before advancing into the neck and upper chest tissues. Pneumoretroperitoneum is usually located more laterally than PP.

Peripheral Edema

There is a good correlation between the extent of peripheral edema, changes in the thickness of chest wall diameter on chest X-ray and changes in body weight [23]. This is more obvious radiologically and easier to measure than by weighing the patient or clinical assessment. Peripheral edema is now known to have a marked detrimental effect on oxygen consumption in the critically ill [12].

Identifying Cardiorespiratory Support and Monitoring Equipment

It is important to verify the proper placement of the various types of monitoring and support equipment used in seriously ill patients.

Endo- or Nasotracheal Tube (ETT, NTT) and Tracheostomies

Every tracheal intubation should be checked immediately by a chest film. It is important that the tip of the tube is more than 2 cm proximal to the carina and that the cuff is 2 cm distal to the vocal cords to allow for the considerable variation in tube movement with flexing and extension of the head. Approximately 10% of ETT are initially situated in the right main stem bronchus.

Following tracheostomy, the chest film should be checked for evidence of EAA and that the tip of the tube is a least 2 cm proximal to the carina. If the carina cannot be seen clearly on the chest X-ray, its position corresponds to approximately half way around the aortic knob. Neck flexion and extension can cause up to 2 cm movement in the tip of the tube.

Central Venous Catheters

Central venous catheters are commonly employed for monitoring pressure and delivering drugs. A chest film should be taken immediately after placement to confirm correct placement and look for iatrogenic complications such as bleeding, ectopic fluid collection or pneumothoraxes. Correct positioning is important. The tip should be located beyond all peripheral valves but not necessarily within the right atrium. Catheter positions frequently change and should be checked daily.

Infusion of fluid into the mediastinal or pleural space is suggestive of the radiological appearance of intrathoracic bleeding and may even mimic aortic rupture.

Pulmonary Artery Catheter

These catheters are associated with the same complications as central lines as well as other, often more dangerous ones, such as pulmonary embolism or infarction distal to the catheter tip and even pulmonary artery rupture with bleeding. The position of the tip of the catheter may help in the interpretation of wedge pressures and excessive coiling in the heart can predispose to migration and wedging of the catheter.

Intra-aortic Counter Pulsation Balloon (IACB)

The tip of the IACB should be placed just distal to the left subclavian artery. Any further and it may obstruct the bracheocephalic arteries or increase the risk of cerebral embolism. The tip should be at the level of the aortic knob on a upright A-P chest film.

Transvenous Pacemakers (PM)

Depending on where the catheter is inserted, complications similar to central line placement can occur. The tip of the PM should be positioned at the apex of the right ventricle, wedged beneath the trabeculae carneae area to ensure stability as well as direct contact with the endocardium. Aberrant locations include the coronary sinus, right atrium, pulmonary outflow tract and pulmonary artery. Rarely, perforation of the myocardium can occur.

Intercostal Tubes

Most chest tubes have an opaque strip which should demonstrate its position within the pleural cavity. Ensure the proximal drainage hole is within the pleural cavity. Another cause for failure to drain air or fluid is when the tube is in a fissure. This is excluded on lateral chest X-ray [23].

Conclusions

Portable chest films are an essential complement to clinical and pathological information in Intensive Care. Interested intensivists and radiologists can gain invaluable information from these films and develop their own skills by constantly discussing the films together. Not only are the films essential for the assessment of pulmonary pathology but they often provide clues to other aspects of the patient such as their sex, size, as well as mediastinal and cardiac abnormalities. Even information about more distant sites of pathology such as the abdomen can be gleaned from a portable chest film. For example, the patient's level of consciousness and seriousness of the illness can sometimes be gauged by the head oblitering the superior mediastinum – "Hillman's Head Sign". It indicates that the patient has not got the strength or is not conscious enough to hold their own head up after correctly positioning them for an erect portable chest film. In our experience, this is invariably correlated with the presence of an endotracheal tube within 24 hours. The presence of old rib fractures is often associated with alcoholism and this in turn is often associated with the radiological signs of chronic obstructive airways diseases. And so on. Chest films of seriously ill patients are crowded with pathology and always present an interesting challenge.

References

1. Strain DS, Kinasewitz GT, Vereen LE, George RB (1985) Value of routine daily chest x-rays in the medical intensive unit. Crit Care Med 13:534–536
2. Laggner A, Kleinberger G, Haller J, Lenz K, Sommer G, Druml W (1984) Bedside estimation of extravascular lung water in critically ill patients: comparison of the chest radiograph and the thermal dye technique. Intensive Care Med 10:309–313
3. Baudendistel L, Shields JB, Kaminski DL (1982) Comparison of double indicator thermodilution measurements of extravascular lung water (EVLW) with radiographic estimation of lung water in trauma patients. J Trauma 22:983–988
4. Sibbald WJ, Warshawski FJ, Shork AK, Harris J, Lefcoe MS, Holliday RL (1983) Clinical studies of measuring extravascular lung water by the thermal dye technique in critically ill patients. Chest 83:725–731
5. McHugh TJ, Forrester JS, Adler I (1972) Pulmonary vascular congestion in acute myocardial infarction; hemodynamic and radiological considerations. Ann Intern Med 76:29–36
6. Don C, Johnson R (1977) The nature and significance of peribronchial cuffing in pulmonary edema. Radiology 125:577–582
7. Milne ENC (1978) Some new concepts of pulmonary blood flow and volume. Radiol Clin North Am 16:515–536
8. Hublitz VF, Shapiro JH (1969) A typical pulmonary pattern of congestive failure in chronic lung disease. The influence of preexisting diseases on the appearance and distribution of pulmonary edema. Radiology 93:995–1006
9. Putman CE, Goodman L (1983) Imaging in the critically ill or injured. In: Shoemaker WC, Thompson WL (eds) Critical Care: State of the Art. Fullerton: The Society of Critical Care Medicine 4(A):1–63
10. Driedger AA, Sibbald WJ, Lefcoe M, McCallum LJ (1983) Diagnostic imaging in the critically ill. In: Ledingham IMcA, Hanning CD (eds) Recent advances in critical care medicine. Churchill Livingstone, Edinburgh, pp 211–287
11. Hillman K (1985) Pulmonary barotrauma. In: Dobb G (ed) Clinics in Anaesthesiology. W. B. Saunders, London, pp 877–898
12. Twigley AJ, Hillman KM (1985) The end of the crystalloid era? Anaesthesia 40:860–871
13. Swischuk LE (1977) Bubbles in hyaline membrane disease. Differentiation of three types. Radiology 122:471–476
14. Berger R, Arango L (1985) Etiologic diagnosis of bacterial nosocomial pneumonia in seriously ill patients. Crit Care Med 13:833–836

15. French GL, Homi J (1979) Insignificance of colonic bacteria in the sputum of patients in a new ICU. Crit Care Med 7:487-491
16. Bulmer SR, Lamb D, McCormack RJM, Walbarum PR (1978) The aetiology of unresolved pneumonia. Thorax 33:307-314
17. Stevens JM, Lees WR, Mason RR (1983) Radiology. In: Tinker J, Rapin M (eds) Care of the critically ill patient. Springer, Berlin Heidelberg New York Tokyo, pp 963-983
18. Dooner MW, Sirbign ML (1966) Cinefluorographic analysis of pharyngeal swallowing in neuromuscular disorders. Am J Med Sci 251:600-609
19. Mendelson CL (1946) The aspiration of stomach contents into the lungs during obstetric anesthesia. Am J Obstet Gynecol 52:191-199
20. Putman CE, Tummillo A, Myerson D (1975) Drowning: another plunge. AJR 125:543-554
21. Esteban A, Fernandez-Segoviano P, Oliete S, Ruiz-Santana S, Castello J, Cal A de la (1983) Radiographic findings for the adult respiratory distress syndrome in patients with peritonitis. Crit Care Med 11:880-882
22. Johanson Jnr WG (1984) Bacterial infection in ARDS: Pathogenic mechanisms and consequences. In: Shoemaker WC (ed) Critical Care: State of the Art. Fullerton: The Society of Critical Care Medicine 5(H):1-43
23. Milne ENC (1986) A physiological approach to reading critical care unit films. J Thorac Imag 3:60-90
24. Light RW, George RB (1976) Incidence and significance of pleural effusion after abdominal surgery. Chest 69:621-627
25. Hillman KM (1982) Pneumoperitoneum - a review. Crit Care Med 10:476-481

Metabolic Imaging with PET in the Critically Ill Patient with Coronary Artery Disease

C. Nienaber and H. R. Schelbert

Introduction

With positron emission tomography (PET), the non-invasive quantitative assessment of regional myocardial perfusion in blood flow, substrate fluxes and biochemical reaction rates in millimole substrates per minute per gram of myocardium have now become possible with the advent of high temporal and spatial resolution PET scanners [1, 2].

Physiologically active compounds are tagged with positron emitting isotopes of carbon, nitrogen and oxygen which maintain their biochemical properties. The labeled compounds are intravenously administered in tracer amounts (i.e. picomolar quantities). Regional rates of accumulation and uptake or turnover of the tracer in tissue is measured from cross-sectional PET images representing quantitatively local tracer tissue concentrations. From the tissue response to the arterial input function, tracer kinetic models are developed that define the kinetics of a given tracer in tissue to the physiologic process under study, allowing characterization of the tissue kinetics in mathematical terms and therefore calculation of absolute rates of blood flow and metabolism.

The present renaissance of radionuclide studies of the heart are largely due to recent technological developments and the emergence of PET as a new imaging modality with a quantitative capacity [3–5] and the clinical use of new aggressive treatment modalities in the setting of acute myocardial infarction such as thrombolysis and mechanical restoration of coronary blood flow. PET will have a unique place in treatment decision making in acute infarction because of its potential for immediate detection of flow abnormalities and subsequently therapeutic restoration of flow as well as for detection of variable mycardium in the ischemic or post-ischemic target area [6, 7]. The positron emitting isotopes of O-15, C-11, N-13 and F-18 are incorporated in the molecular structure of various biochemical compounds, thus tracing important metabolic substrate pathways without affecting their intrinsic biochemical properties. However, a drawback of positron emitting isotopes is their short half-life, requiring an on-site cyclotron. On the other hand, the short half-life of the isotopes allows serial studies in short intervals with relatively low radiation exposure.

PET Imaging in Myocardial Infarction

The tomographic properties of PET permit an accurate assessment of the spatial extent of myocardial infarction. A series of contiguous cross-sectional images of the myocardium is recorded and the defect size on each image is determined. From the thickness of each slice and the defect size, the mass of infarcted myocardium can be determined. This possiblity has been demonstrated in correlative studies in canine experiments where the tomographic external measurements agreed well with the histochemical sizes of experimentally induced myocardial infarctions determined at postmortem examination [8]. A similarly good agreement has been observed in humans with recent or remote myocardial infarction, where the biochemical estimates of infarct size, i.e., the amount of CK-enzyme released from myocardium, correlated with the size of the myocardial infarction as measured by PET [9, 10]. In these studies, C-11 palmitic acid was used as a tracer of myocardial free fatty acids (FFA) metabolism. Because myocardial FFA oxidation declines or even ceases entirely in infarcted myocardium, failure to extract C-11 palmitic acid by the myocardium is conceivably an accurate indicator of cell viability or residual metabolic activity. Similarly, while the extraction fraction of C-11 palmitic acid remains essentially constant despite cellular injury [11, 12], the initial myocardial concentrations of C-11 activity largely reflect myocardial blood flow. Hence, in most instances of myocardial infarction where a regional flow reduction is the underlying cause, the severity and extent of these regional flow reductions may thus closely correlate with the extent and degree of tissue infarction.

In infarcted or necrotic myocardial tissue, metabolic activity ceases almost entirely. This applies not only to FFA metabolism but also to glycolysis. Using N-13 ammonia as a tracer of regional myocardial perfusion [13, 14], and hence, as an indicator of regional oxygen supply in patients with completed myocardial infarction, uptake of exogenous glucose by the myocardium (as evaluated with FDG: F-18 deoxyglucose), closely paralleled the regional reduction in myocardial oxygen supply [15].

In summary, despite the limited experience with these techniques in myocardial infarction, the studies performed to date indicate that

1. the extent and severity of acute myocardial infarctions can be assessed with a reasonably high degree of accuracy by PET; and
2. that with these metabolic radionuclide techniques myocardial infarction is characterized by an apparent cessation of metabolic activity that closely correlates with the degree and extent of blood flow reduction and oxygen delivery.

Acute Myocardial Infarction

Using N-13 ammonia, F-18 deoxyglucose (FDG) and C-11 palmitate, regional perfusion and metabolic studies in the inital 72 hours after onset of symptoms demonstrate new pathophysiologic information. Figure 1 shows an example of cross-sectional PET imaging following injection of N-13 ammonia and FDG. Blood flow decreases in the anterior wall and the corresponding FDG images show however increased glucose utilization in the same segments. The ECG obtained on the day of PET imaging revealed an extensive anterolateral infarction.

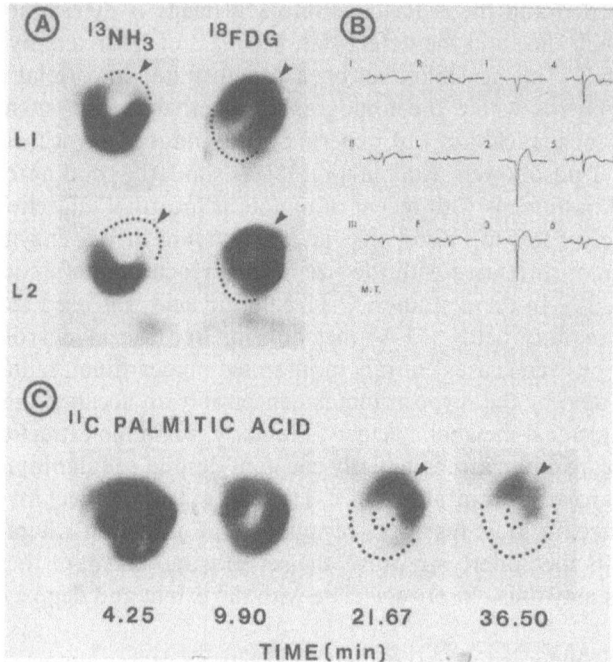

Fig. 1. A Cross-sectional PET images following injection of N-13 ammonia (NH₃) and F-18 deoxyglucose (FDG) in a patient with acute myocardial infarction. Note the decreased blood flow in the anterior wall (arrow). Glucose utilization is enhanced as seen by the increased uptake in the same segments. **B** The electrocardiogram of the same patient is consistent with a transmural anteroseptal infarction. **C** Serial C-11 palmitate study in the same patient shows prolonged clearance of activity from the anterior wall matching the segments with increased glucose utilization

Serial images after C-11 palmitate injection demonstrated prolonged clearance of C-11 in segments with increased FDG uptake. This pattern suggests impaired fatty acid oxidation and enhanced glucose utilization in compromised but viable tissue in "infarcted" myocadium over a prolonged time period despite ECG criteria of transmural infarction and regional akinesis. A regional perfusion defect was documented in all patients with clinical evidence of infarction. However, FDG uptake concordantly decreased in only 50% of the segments and regional wall motion failed to recover over a period of six weeks. In contrast, about 50% of the segments with FDG uptake ("mismatch") showed recovery of function over a period of six weeks. Thus, PET could identify "hibernating myocardium" (Fig. 2). Several aspects of these findings are important because

1. in a considerable subset of patients the metabolic pattern of a "mismatch" indicates ongoing ischemia in the subacute phase of acute infarction;
2. PET correctly identifies irreversible tissue injury in the presence of a concordant decrease in flow and glucose metabolism ("match"); and
3. evidence of viable but compromised tissue in the infarcted area identifies potentially salvageable myocardium.

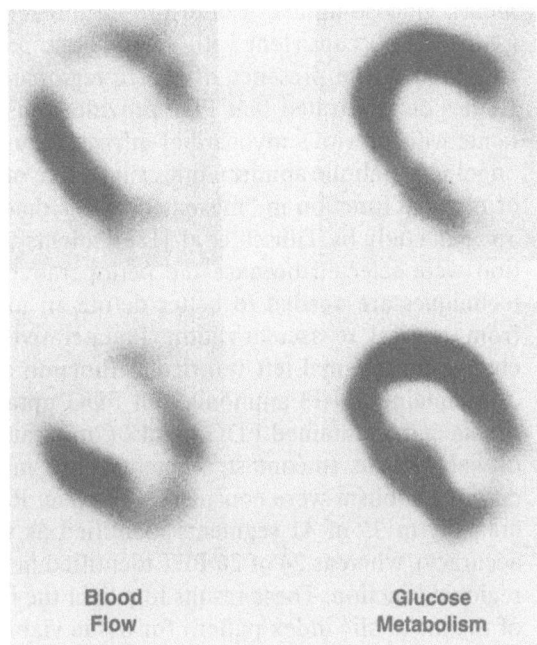

Fig. 2. PET study of a 59 year old man after anterolateral infarction. Diminished perfusion is noted on the N-13 ammonia images (left). However, the FDG study demonstrated well preserved glucose utilization in anterolateral segments, indicating persistent ischemia and reversible damage

Blood
Flow

Glucose
Metabolism

Development and validation of quantitative parameters are currently underway to identify patients who need revascularization to salvage myocardium at risk. Furthermore, PET will aid in defining the efficacy of therapeutic interventions such as thrombolysis and mechanical revascularization (PTCA and bypass surgery). Especially with ultrashort tracers such as Rb-82 (rubidium-82; half-life 75 s), repeat studies before and during or after intravenous injection of thrombolytic agents are feasible that might immediately indicate successful revascularization and tissue reperfusion without the need for angiographic documentation. In conjunction with a metabolic tacer such as FDG, the amount of viable myocardium in the territory of the still occluded or successfully recanalized artery is accessible. This information is crucial in guiding further decision making and patient management in the acute phase.

Metabolic Evaluation in Post-Infarction Patients

Post-infarction complications such as infarct extension, reinfarction, arrhythmias and sudden death tend to occur more often in the first year after an acute event. These complications are limited to residual ischemic areas in "infarcted" tissue [16]. In our laboratory two recent studies were evaluated by PET in order to define the incidence of viable but compromised tissue [18]. Basically, two different metabolic patterns were identified in these patients; about 60% of myocardial segments with a decrease in blood flow demonstrated a matching spatial decreae in glucose utilization. However, in about 40% of flow impaired segments, glucose uptake was disproportionately increased relative to blood flow ("mismatch") consistent with an ischemic pattern of enhanced glucose utilization even in the presence of severe regional wall motion abnormalities. These studies demonstrated that PET provides sensitive tissue characterization in patients with previous myocardial infraction and aids in identifying patients with ongoing metabolic abnormalities suggestive of tissue viability. The final recovery of regional function in "mismatch" areas detected by PET was demonstrated in a recent study by Tillisch et al. [18]. Patients with impaired left ventricular function were selected because the perioperative risk in this subset is higher and techniques are needed to better define an indication for and potential benefit from surgical revascularization. Preoperative PET findings were compared to changes in regional left ventricular function after bypass surgery. The presence of maintained N-13 ammonia and FDG uptake as well as decreased N-13 ammonia and maintained FDG uptake ("mismatch") was considered to be an index of viable tissue. In contast, segments with "matched" decreases in flow and glucose metabolism were considered necrotic. Regional function improve post-operatively in 35 of 41 segments identified as viable (i.e. 85% positive predictive accuracy), whereas 24 of 26 PET identified necrotic segments did not improve in regional function. These results highlight the improved sensitivity and specificity of the metabolic index pattern for tissue viability compared to ECG or thallium scintigraphic indices. Metabolic imaging helps to identify patients who benefits from revascularization and seems to be especially useful in severely impaired left ventricular function. However, some pathophsiologic aspects are still insufficient defined. Is chronically enhanced glucose uptake utilization a metabolic adaptation to decreased oxygen delivery resulting in preferred anaerobic glucose metabolism? Or, is it a reflection of "metabolic stunning" after repetitive ischemic episodes?

Acute Myocardical Ischemia and Unstable Angina

The metabolic abnormalities observed in the human heart with PET reflect alterations described in myocardial ischemia from invasive animal experiments or in vitro studies. In the acute supply-demand imbalance, substrate metabolism is geared towards maintaining high energy phosphate production. As the production of high energy phosphate declines in myocardial ischemia, expenditures of ATP for generation of contractile force and diastolic relaxation are minimized with subsequent cessation of mechanical function. Whatever energy is available is now spent to maintain transmembraneous electrolyte gradients and for support of basic cell function crucial for survival. Thus, it is the amount of energy phosphates that can still be produced through anaerobic or aerobic metabolic pathways that may account for tissue viability. The amount of residual blood flow in acute ischemia may determine at what level the sequence of metabolic alterations stop and whether residual metabolic activity prevents rapid transition to cell necrosis. There is a consensus that β-oxidation of FFA is most sensitive to oxygen deprivation [19]. As blood flow and oxygen supply fall only moderately, the flux of free fatty acid through β-oxidation declines and a disproportionately greater fraction of free fatty acid is diverted into the endogenous lipid pool. Subsequently, tissue clearance rates were markedly prolonged and their biphasic phase was abolished. For example, compared with tissue half-lives of 28.7 minutes in normal myocardium at exercise, the half-lives were significantly longer during stress-induced ischemia (46.4 minutes) and in patients with unstable angina (45.3 minutes) in ischemic segments, indicating the decline in β-oxidation in ischemia [20, 21]. A corresponding example from an experimental study is given in Figure 3.

The metabolic shift with a relative or absolute increase in glycolysis can be similarly demonstrated in experimental and clinical studies [15, 22, 23]. Patients with unstable angina invariably revealed a regional increase in glucose uptake in the ischemic segment or in segments with decreased perfusion independent of chest pain at the time of study. This regional metabolic pattern of myocardial ischemia is demonstrated in Figure 4 in a patient with previous anterior myocardial infarction. Cardiac catheterization several weeks prior to the PET study revealed an apical aneurysm but normal coronary arteries. Nevertheless, the patient was readmitted for recurrent chest pain. As expected, the perfusion image after intravenous N-13 ammonia disclosed an extensive anterior apical perfusion defect. However, the myocardium in the aneurysmatic segment still used glucose as evidenced from the FDG image with increased glucose uptake in the presumably infarcted area. Diminished FDG uptake in the apparently normal myocar-

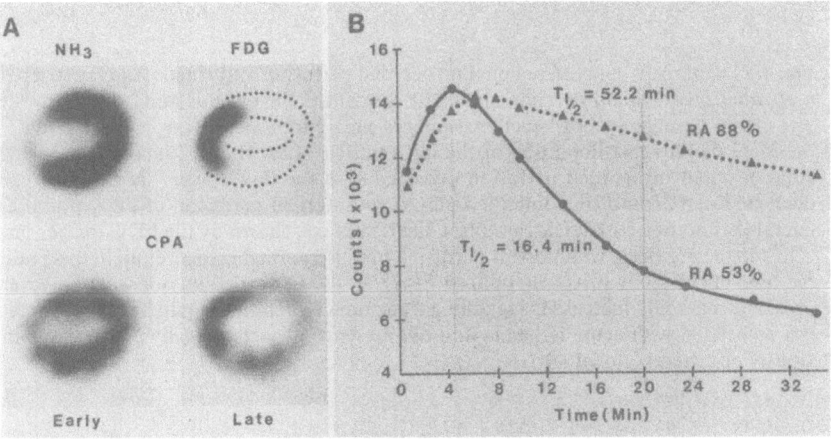

Fig. 3 A, B. Effects of reperfusion on RMBF and metabolism. **A** Cross-sectional images of the heart in a chronic dog model at 24 hours of reperfusion following a 3 hour LAD occlusion. The images were obtained after ^{13}N ammonia (upper left), [1-^{11}C] palmitic acid (right), and FDG (lower left). Blood flow is still decreased in the repefused segment within the anterior wall. However, there is markedly increased FDG uptake in the same segment. The serial images following [1-^{11}C] palmitic acid injection show inital uptake of tracer that parallels blood flow but later images demonstrate the delayed clearance of ^{11}C activity from the reperfusion myocardium suggesting impaired fatty acid oxidation and enhanced glucose utilization. **B** Regional ^{11}C time activity curve after [1-^{11}C] palmitic acid injection from serial images shown in panel A. Note the decreased initial uptake and delayed clearance of ^{11}C activity from the reperfused myocardium (dotted line) as compared to control myocardium (solid line)

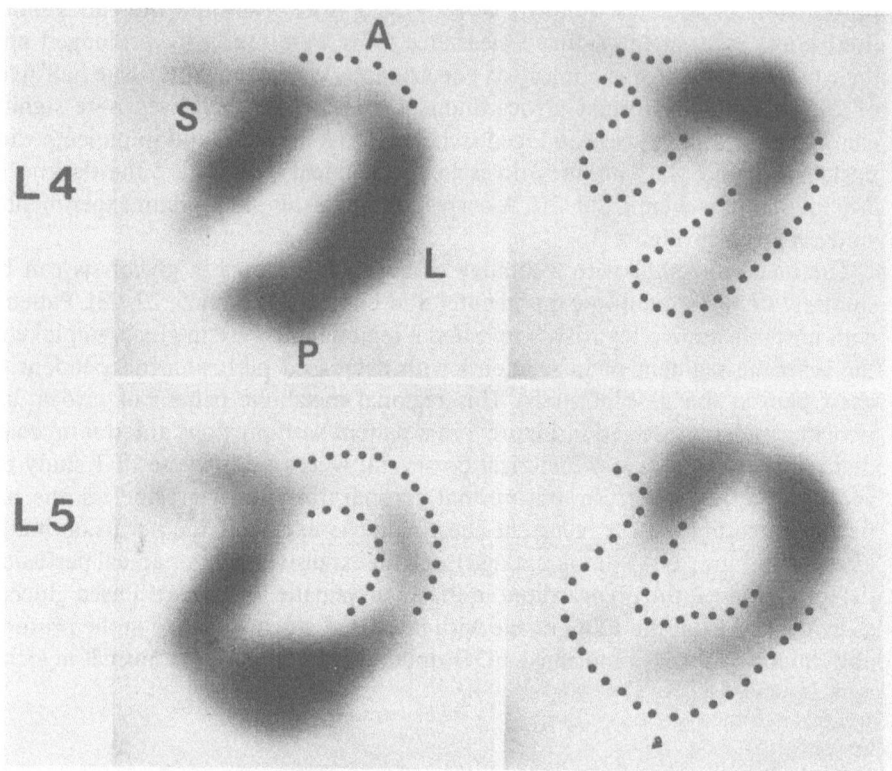

Fig. 4. Comparison between regional myocardial perfusion and glucose uptake in a patient with a previous myocardial infarction and chest pain at the time of the study. The figure shows two sets of two contiguous cross-sectional images slicing transaxially through the middle (L4) and the more diaphragmatic portion of the left ventricle (L5). The two images on the left demonstrate regional myocardial perfusion (assessed with the flow tracer ^{13}N-ammonia) and reveal decreased perfusion of the anterior wall (A) with normal perfusion of the septum (S) and the lateral (L) and posterolateral (P) walls. Glucose uptake, shown by the FDG images on the right, is low in the segments with normal perfusion because normal myocardium in this patient and at the time of the study primarily utilized FFAs. In the ischemic anterior wall, however, glucose uptake is markedly increased, suggesting a regional switch in the pattern of substrate metabolism associated with acute ischemia and the presence of metabolically active tissue in the previously infarcted segment

dium is explained by the dietary state (i.e. after an overnight fast with low serum insulin and glucose but high FFA levels). This results in almost exclusive FFA utilization by normal myocardium, whereas ischemic tissue derives most of its energy through glycolysis. This example demonstrates that despite previous well documented infarction, there is still metabolically active tissue in the infarcted segment, highlighting the unique capabilities of metabolic imaging. Neither perfusion imaging, nor assessment of regional wall motion would permit in vivo demonstration of metabolically active tissue that still may be amenable to therapy.

Summary and Future Aspects

In summary, metabolic and perfusion studies are feasible with PET in the critically ill patient with coronary artery disease (i.e. in the clinical setting of acute ischemic events, acute myocardial infarction as well as in the post-infarction patient). A characteristic "mismatch" pattern of perfusion and regional metabolic activity heralds myocardium at risk for necrosis but is still amenable to successful treatment. In addition, in ischemia the regional decline in FFA oxidation and diversion into slow turnover pools in the cell can now be shown noninvasively. Moreover, demonstration of the predicted shift from β-oxidation of fatty acids to glucose utilization is possible. Finally, inital experience with C-11 acetate may indicate that citric cycle activity can be selectively assessed in the future.

Significant progress will be made with quantification of regional metabolic rates rather than evaluating relative differences between myocardial segments. This would allow nontraumatic quantitative description of the inter-relationship between flow, mechanical function and metabolism to more specifically characterize myocardial ischemia and to assess the success of interventional therapy in the critically ill patient. Since metabolic and histochemical disturbances precede structural myocardial changes, PET identifies ichemic damage in the acute stage (i.e. at a time when the disease process is still amenable to treatment and reversal).

Acknowledgements: The authors would like to thank M. Lee Griswold for preparing and the illustrations and Kerry Engber for her assistance in preparing this manuscript.

References

1. Phelps ME (1977) Emission computed tomography. Semin Nucl Med 7:337–349
2. Wisenberg G, Schelbert HR, Hoffman EJ, et al (1981) In vivo quantitation of regional myocardial blood flow by positron emission computed tomography. Circulation 63:1248–1258
3. Schelbert HR, Henze E, Phelps ME (1980) Emission tomography of the heart. Semin Nucl Med 10:355–361
4. Henze E, Huag SC, Ratib O, et al (1983) Measurements of regional tissue and blood pool indicator concentrations from serial tomographic images of the heart. J Nucl Med 24:987–996
5. Ratib O, Phelps ME, Huang SC, et al (1982) Positron tomography with deoxyglucose for estimating local myocardial glucose metabolism. J Nucl Med 23:577–586
6. Marshall RC, Tillisch JH, Phelps ME, et al (1981) Identification and differentiation of resting myocardial ischemia and infarction in man with positron computed tomography ^{18}F-labeled fluorodeoxyglucose and N-13 ammonia. Circulation 64:766–778
7. Schwaiger M, Schelbert HR, Ellison D, et al (1985) Sustained regional abnormalities in cardiac metabolism after transient ischemia in the chronic dog model. J Am Coll Cardiol 6:336–347
8. Weiss ES, Ahmed SA, Welch MJ, et al (1977) Quantification of infarction in cross sections of canine myocardium in vivo with positron emission transaxial tomography and ^{11}C-palmitate. Circulation 55:66–73
9. Sobel BE, Weiss ES, Welch MJ, et al (1977) Detection of remote myocardial infarction in patients with positron emission transaxial tomography and intravenous ^{11}C-palmitate. Circulation 55:853–857

10. Ter-Pogossian MM, Klein MS, Markham J, et al (1980) Regional assessment of myocardial metabolic integrity in vivo by positron emission tomography with ^{11}C-labeled palmitate. Circulation 61:242–255

11. Schon HR, Schelbert HR, Najavi A, et al (1982) C-11-labeled palmitic acid for the noninvasive evaluation of regional myocardial fatty acid metabolism with positron computed tomography. I. Kinetics of C-11 palmitic acid in normal myocardium. Am Heart J 103:532–547

12. Schon HR, Schelbert HR, Najafi A, et al (1982) C-11 palmitic acid for the noninvasive evaluation of regional myocardial fatty acid metabolism with positron computed tomography. II. Kinetics of C-11 palmitic acid in acutely ischemic myocardium. Am Heart J 103:548–561

13. Schelbert HR, Phelps ME, Hoffman EJ, et al (1979) Regional myocardial perfusion assessed with N-13 labeled ammonia and positron emission computerized axial tomography. Am J Cardiol 43:209–218

14. Schelbert HR, Phelps ME, Huang SC, et al (1981) N-13 ammonia as an indicator of myocardial blood flow: Factors influencing its uptake and retention in myocardium. Circulation 63:1259–1272

15. Schelbert HR, Phelps ME, Selin C, et al (1980) Regional myocardial ischemia assessed by ^{18}F-fluoro-2-deoxyglucose and positron emission computed tomography. In: Kreuzer H, Parmley WW, Rentrop R, et al (eds) Advances in Clinical Cardiology, Vol 1. J Witzstrock, New York, pp 437–449

16. Marmor A, Geltman EM, Schechtman K, et al (1982) Recurrent myocardial infarction: Clinical predictors and prognostic implications. Circulation 66:415–421

17. Schwaiger M, Brunken R, Grover-McKay M, et al (1986) Regional myocardial metabolism in patients with acute myocardial infarction assessed by positron emission tomography. J Am Coll Cardiol 8:800–808

18. Tillisch J, Brunken R, Marshall R, et al (1986) Reversibility of cardiac wall motion abnormalities predicted by positron tomography. N Engl J Med 314:884–888

19. Liedtke AJ (1981) Alterations of carbohydrate and lipid metabolism in the acute ischemic heart. Progr Cardiovasc Dis 23:321–336

20. Van der Wall EE, Heidendal GAK, Den Hollander W, et al (1981) Metabolic myocardial imaging with I-123-labeled heptadecanoic acid in patients with angina pectoris. Eur J Nucl Med 6:391–400

21. Van der Wall EE, Heidendal GAK, Den Hollander W, et al (1981) Myocardial scintigraphy with ^{123}-labeled heptadecanoic acid in patients with unstable angina pectoris. In: Van der Wall EE (ed) Dynamic Myocardial Scintigraphy with ^{123}I-labeled face fatty acids. Rodopi, Amsterdam, pp 93–99

22. Marshall RC, Tillisch JH, Phelps ME, et al (1983) Identification and differentiation of resting myocardial ischemia and infarction with positron computed tomography, F-18 labeled fluorodeoxyglucose, and N-13 ammonia. Circulation 67:766–778

23. Schelbert HR, Henze E, Phelps ME, et al (1982) Assessment of regional myocardial ischemia by positron computed tomography. Am Heart J 103:588–594

The Contribution of Nuclear Medicine in the Care of the Critically Ill Patient

G. A. K. Heidendal

Introduction

It is usually stated that the ciritically ill or traumatized patient should benefit from a spectrum of clinical procedures offered by a multidisciplinary team. Ultrasonography, a non-invasive diagnostic method, is more and more used in intensive care units, being simple, painless and safe. An excellent review of nuclear medicine as another non-invasive diagnostic approach in the care of the critically ill patient was published in 1975 [1]. In this article, Wiener et al. concluded that valuable information is frequently obtained and a significant improvement in the clinical care of critically ill patients results from the optimal use of radionuclide imaging examinations. However there has been until now, no general consensus on what should be the impact of nuclear medicine in the handling of critically ill patients even when mobile scintillation cameras and/or imaging scintillation probes are available. The reasons for this are multiple. Firstly, there are objections intrinsic to the nuclear medicine investigations themselves (diagnostic accuracy, availability of tests 24 hours a day ...). In addition specialists in nuclear medicine are not sufficiently involved in the practice of an intensive care unit and clinicians are often not aware of the possible role that a specific procedure can play in a particular clinical situation. The utilization of radioactive material in an intensive care unit may also form a psychological barrier. One should realize that the amount of irradiation received by personnel in contact with a "radiating patient" in an actual situation is much less than the amount received by natural irradiation.

We will not attempt to provide a complete set of current imaging procedures in nuclear medicine, but rather present investigations which may be valuable in certain critically ill patient care problems.

The Cardiovascular System

An intensive care unit has several conventional technologies to its disposal to monitor rapid changes in the cardiovascular system. However, none of the measured indices of ventricular performance is ideal. Additional functional data such as wall motion of the myocardium or ejection fractions may increase diagnostic accuracy. These data can be obtained non-invasively by ultrasound and nuclear medicine techniques. Echocardiography produces images of the cardiac structures with excellent temporal resolution and this simple, safe and inexpensive technique appears to be the first choice to study the heart. However, a considerable number of critically ill patients cannot be studied satisfactorily with ultrasound due to the mechanical ventilation, non cooperative patients or patients who cannot be positioned properly [2].

Using intravascular radioactive tracers it is possible to visualize the entire heart by analyzing the first transit of the bolus through the central circulation or by applying the equilibrium gated blood pool technique. Both techniques register changes in count rate and as such observe the hemodynamic events occurring throughout the heart. Minicomputer systems have been coupled to mobile gamma cameras and brought directly to the patient's bedside. First pass studies are particularly useful to study the performance of the right ventricle because this technique allows a good temporal and anatomic separation of radioactivity between the right and the left ventricle of the heart. The introduction of a Swan-Ganz catheter in the pulmonary artery prior to a first pass study provides a quick and efficient way to determine left ventricle ejection fractions at the bedside of critically ill patients [3].

A modification of these nuclear medicine techniques is the use of a non-imaging collimated probe, connected with a dedicated microprocessor, instead of a gamma camera. This system has the major advantage of greater mobility and decreased cost. Because there is no visual display of the heart, the positioning of the probe becomes very critical.

Ejection fraction measurements are easily obtained by all these techniques. Ejection fractions are not specific in defining myocardial contractility because they can be altered by changes in loading, both preload and afterload. They have, however, been clinically very useful because the range of normal values is well established and abnormal results are closely related to the prognosis of different cardiac diseases. Parker et al. [2] and Ellrodt et al. [4] applied the gated blood pool scintigraphy using a portable gamma camera in patients with septic shock. These studies showed that significant myocardial depression might occur in septic shock, even in the presence of a normal or elevated cardiac index. The authors did not arrive to the same conclusions concerning the prognostic value of ejection fraction measurements, probably due to differences in the patient population studied. Using the same methodology, Kimchi et al. [5] reported that also right ventricular dysfunction may occur in patients with septic shock. First pass methods are however better suited for the evaluation of right ventricular performance. The ideal tracer for this kind of studies is not available yet, although the high yield of a new Osmium-191/Iridium-191 generator makes it now possible to inject a bolus of a high amount of iridium (physical half-life: 4.9 seconds) so that right and left ventricle performances can now be studied simultaneously and repeatedly without dosimetric problems for the patient or his environment [6].

Right ventricle ejection fractions have been measured with first pass studies in patients with adult respiratory distress syndrome [7] and acute respiratory failure [8]. These studies showed that in these clinical situations right ventricular dysfunction may be caused by an increased afterload due to pulmonary vascular obstruction or hypoxic vasoconstriction.

More than the measurement of absolute values of the ventricle function, the nuclear medicine methods have the great advantage to reliably measure changes in ventricular function with time, which is a necessary condition to evaluate the effects of therapeutic interventions employed in an intensive care unit.

Several radionuclide methods have been proposed for the non-invasive measurements of ventricular volumes [9]. Most of these methods are, however, too complicated or too time-consuming to be applied in critically ill patients. However, one can very well calculate ventricular volumes by combining the conventional thermodilution cardiac output measurements in an intensive care unit with the ejection fraction measurements as mentioned (end-diastolic volume = stroke volume/ejection fraction). A relevant clinical question, may be whether a reduction in ventricular pump function is due to an excess load, a reduced contractility or both. This problem can be solved when volume and ejection fraction measurements are available. The presence of an enlarged left ventricle with relatively preserved left ventricular function suggests volume overload while patients with myocardial failure, in the absence of volume or pressure overload, show ventricular dilatation associated with a significantly reduced ejection fraction.

The so called "Hot Spot" imaging of the heart using technetium-99m stannous pyrophosphate and more recently indium-111 antimyosin has been recommended for the diagnosis of acute myocardial infarction in cases where the ECG or enzyme changes are in doubt. Although it is clear that the majority of patients presenting to the cardiac coronary care unit with acute myocardial infarction do not need cardiac imaging for clinical diagnostic purposes, these radiopharmaceuticals might have a potential application following thoracic trauma or cardiac surgery, when routine studies are often unreliable.

New applications in the prognostic field of acute heart failure may be offered by a recently introduced analog of norepinephrine: radiolabeled metaiodobenzylguanidine (MIBG). The uptake in the heart of this radiopharmaceutical appears to be an index of the functional integrity of the adrenergic system and unusual patterns of innervation of the heart may predispose to arrhythmias [10, 11].

In the late sixties and early seventies a lot of articles appeared on radioisotopic angiography. It is a method to visualize dynamically blood flow through vessels and organs. Although the spatial resolution and therefore the anatomic detail of these radionuclide studies are inferior to most of the competing radiographic and echographic techniques, the nontraumatic nature and the reliability of these examinations still deserves emphasis. The now generally called "scintiangiography" consists of injecting intravenously a bolus of a radioactive tracer, which remains intravascular, and of following its transit by serial 2 to 3 second intervals images, using a probe or camera. Immediately following the dynamic phase of the study, a static blood pool image can be made. This technique has given valuable information in the evaluation of arterial injuries, such as extravasation secondary to arterial leakage [12, 13], arterial graft patency [14] and venous obstruction. The cerebral scintiangiography is on old, well known procedure to confirm suspected brain death. With the use of a mobile scintillation camera and a mobile computer, the procedure can be performed at the bedside. The method evaluates cerebral perfusion, the posterior fossa and brainstem cannot be adequately evaluated. It has, however, been demonstrated, by a number of studies, that in practice there is a correlation between the determination of cerebral death and brainstem death. The data obtained by this technique are not changed by effects of chemical or metabolic states of intoxication, in contrast to other neurologic assessments. Excellent reviews have been recently published on this subjects [15, 16].

There is good reason to believe that newly developed radiopharmaceuticals such as hexamethyl-propyleneamine oxime labelled with technetium-99m (Tc-99m-HM-PAO) could be of particular interest in the diagnosis of brain death, because they also localize in the posterior fossa, which will make it possible to assess the viability of the entire brain [17, 18].

Radionuclide studies currently used for the diagnosis of venous thrombosis involve dynamic flow studies, radionuclide venography, or static blood pool imaging to record a venous obstruction secondary to a thrombosis. Apart from the fact that venography with radionuclides is a rapid, safe and well tolerated test, the major advantages of this technique are its value in the exploration of the pelvic veins, which may be difficult with contrast venography or Doppler flow studies and the possibility to perform a lung scan in patients with an increased risk of pulmonary embolism if human albumin microspheres or macroaggregates are used as radiopharmaceuticals.

Likewise venous stasis may be documented in patients who underwent cardiac studies with bloodpool agents such as red blood cells. The resolution is usually adequate to detect thrombi [19].

Tracers such as radiolabeled fibrinogen localize thrombi positively by incorporation in the actively forming clots. The fibrinogen uptake test may be useful to differentiate active from inactive venous thrombosis when anticoagulation therapy is considered in patients with a history of thrombophlebitis without clear cut clinical findings for acute formation of thrombi. Antifibrin antibodies have recently been labeled to provide "Hot Spot" images of vascular clots. The clinical evaluation is in progress.

The Respiratory System

Pulmonary scintigraphy is a well established procedure and still the most simple non-invasive imaging technique to evaluate patients who are clinically suspected of having lung emboli. Different variations of a fundamentally similar methodological approach have been published many times. The subject has recently been reviewed [20].

In general, pulmonary scintigraphy should be performed within 24 to 48 hours after the onset of clinical suspicion of lung emboli. This does not mean, however, that the test should always be performed on an emergency basis. Therapy with anticoagulants is usually started immediately when there is a strong suspicion for lung emboli and is stopped if the diagnosis is subsequently disapproved. There are of course exceptions to this approach when, for any reason, prophylaxis with anticoagulants is contraindicated. A perfusion scintigram should always be interpreted in the presence of a recently performed chest X-ray. Neglecting this rule should be considered poor medical practice. A significant pulmonary embolus can be ruled out if the perfusion study is normal, so that any further diagnostic work-up can be stopped and an already started therapy can be discontinued. Perfusion scintigraphy is very sensitive but has also a low specificity. An abnormal perfusion study should be followed by ventilation scintigraphy to increase the specificity. Several interpretation schemes have been proposed depending on the size of involved areas, the number of areas, the ventilation-perfusion match and chest X-ray results. The most widely used criteria are those of Biello et al. [21]. Based on these criteria, patients are classified as having an intermediate, high or low probability for lung embolism. Roughly 60, 10 and 28% of the scintigraphies performed are interpreted as "low, high, intermediate probability", respectively. The implications of "intermediate" results are still a matter of controversy.

One should be aware that in critically ill patients ventilation-perfusion mismatches may be seen locally in the presence of a Swan-Ganz catheter [22] or spread throughout the lungs early in the course of fat embolism. On the contrary, the adult respiratory distress syndrome (ARDS) alone will usually show a normal lung scintigraphy or a diffusely sub-segmental defect [23]. There are valuable data because pulmonary emboli are frequently considered in the early course of ARDS. Also in these patients the ventilation-perfusion studies appear to be normal [24].

The value of sequential ventilation-perfusion studies should be stressed. Newly developed abnormal areas in follow-up studies might be suggestive of pulmonary emboli while a stable pattern of more than three weeks duration suggests a low probability of recurrent pulmonary emboli.

It is to be hoped that remaining questions concerning the handling of patients, clinically suspected of having lung emboli, will be answered in the near future by a major multicenter prospective study called PIOPED presently being performed in the United States under the auspices of the national heart, lung and blood institute.

The increased pulmonary protein reflux, as one of the earliest responses to injury, is an important feature in ARDS. Permeability edema has been investigated in animal models and in patients using radioactive labeled albumin, fibrinogen and leukocytes. Sugerman et al. [25] were able to demonstrate pulmonary albumin leakage in patients with ARDS after injecting radioactive labeled human serum albumin and counting the radioactivity externally over the lungs and the heart with a gamma camera connected to a computer system. These preliminary clinical studies suggest that the method is reliable.

Pulmonary accumulation of radioactively labelled leukocytes was demonstrated in three patients with ARDS secondary to systemic sepsis by Powe et al. [26]. At the time of the investigation there was no clinical or laboratory evidence of a primary chest infection. The exact mechanism of this abnormal pulmonary accumulation is unknown.

Another preclinical paper reported the use of radioactive labelled fibrinogen in nine patients with ARDS [27]. In some of these patients, who also received radioactive labelled human albumin, the accumulation of both tracers appeared to be similar suggesting that the fibrinogen uptake was due to leakage from the vascular into the extravascular space rather than to active incorporation into fibrinogen thrombi, known to be present in ARDS.

A variation of the radiolabeled albumin method, using simultaneously blood radioactivity as a reference, has been used by Groeneveld et al. [28] to show evidence of increased soft tissue permeability in porcine septic shock.

The utility of these procedures as a routine procedure in a clinical situation has still to be proven.

Infection

Gallium-67 citrate and indium-111 labeled leukocytes are the two major radiopharmaceuticals actually used in nuclear medicine for the detection of infection. Although several postulates have been put forth to elucidate the localization of gallium citrate, it is generally believed that the accumulation of both substances in infected areas is based on the immediate response of the host to infection: inflammation. Mc Afee and Thakur demonstrated [29] that autologous leukocytes can be labeled efficiently with indium-111 and retain their functional capabilities of host defense against pyogenic infections. As such, these radioactively labelled leukocytes are considered the only specific tracer for the detection of inflammatory lesions. The labeling procedure is however rather time consuming.

Common localizations of infection in the critically ill patient are pulmonary, abdominal and pelvic areas. Gallium scintigraphy or indium-leukocytes studies are not to be routinely used for assessing pulmonary inflammatory diseases. However, the importance of these investigations in the early detection of pneumonia has been stressed in immunocompromised patients [30–32]. Thirty of forty per cent of the chest X-rays have been reported to remain normal even during a fulminant course of pneumocystis carinii pneumonia [33]. Gallium scintigraphy is not only helpful for the diagnosis of pneumonia, but offers in addition the possibility of monitoring treatment. The sensitivity of gallium scintigraphy is more than 90% so that a biopsy may be deferred in high-risk when the study is negative. However, due to the lower specificity (70%), lung biopsy will still be required to confirm the diagnosis if the gallium scintigraphy is positive. A localized gallium uptake, often seen in early disease, may be helpful in looking for the optimal site for bronchoalveolar lavage or transbronchial biopsy. Follow up studies have shown that when gallium scintigraphy becomes negative [34], indium leukocytes scintigraphy can also be very useful in detecting infection of the lung. A sensitivity of 93% and a specificity of 98% has been reported with this test [35].

Acute abdominal abscesses and acalculous cholecystitis are complications which might be examined with nuclear medicine procedures. It is certainly true, that echography or computerized tomography (CT) is the first diagnostic approach if an abscess is to be localized. If, however, the clinical presentation "localized versus multiple abscesses" is as specific as the literature suggests, one may question the use of abdominal CT as the screening test. The great advantage of gallium or indium scintigraphy is the possibility to detect unsuspected septic foci anywhere in the body, especially in patients who cannot be moved from their room [36, 37]. Becaused these studies do not usually provide precise anatomic information, they should only be considered as preliminary procedures to indicate an area for further exploration by CT or echography. Furthermore, these studies can be performed even in patients with large surgical wounds or to detect abscesses in certain areas, particularly the pelvic area, which are difficult to examine by ultrasound or CT.

The overall reliability of these procedures for the detection of acute abdominal infections is about the same as for ultrasonography or CT. A major disadvantage of the use of these radiopharmaceuticals is the delay of 24 to 48 hours in getting results. Furthermore, repeated imaging is often necessary, especially with gallium, because of the uncertainty presented by normal bowel activity. This latter problem could be avoided using indium labeled white blood cells [38, 39].

Severely ill patients, such as those suffering major trauma, are candidates for developing acute acalculous cholecystitis, a diagnosis which may be difficult to ascertain. The physiologic basis of a cholescintigraphy with technetium-99m labeled HIDA (dimethyliminodeacetic acid) is similar to that of an intravenous cholangiogram. It provides a rapid representation of hepatobiliary function and permits gallbladder visualization despite elevated serum albumin or the presence of pancreatitis. Non-filling of the gallbladder in a fasting patient with a good hepatic uptake and excretion of the HIDA through the common bile duct has a high probability of cystic duct obstruction. False positive results have, however, been described especially in patients after recent food intake or on total parenteral nutrition [40].

Controversy exists on which test should be ordered first by the clinician: cholescintigraphy or real-time ultasonography [41, 42]. A practical problem with cholescintigraphy is the necessity to perform late images when the appearance of the tracer within the gallbladder is delayed. The clinician can however exclude the possibility of acute cholecystitis with a very high degree of certainty when cholescintigraphy is normal [43, 44].

Efforts are made to develop new radiopharmaceuticals which are be less expensive, do not require complex in vitro cell labelling and yield more rapid results. Promising results have been recently described with technetium-99m labeled liposomes [45] and radiolabeled anti-granulocytes [46].

Gastro-enterology

Endoscopy is considered the best available technique to identify bleeding lesions in the gastro-intestinal (GI) tract [47]. Selective arteriography and radionuclide scintigraphy are considered when endoscopy fails. Most nuclear medicine departments now use patients own labeled red blood cells for the detection of GI bleeding [48–50]. The advantage of this radiopharmaceutical over Tc-sulfur colloid or arteriography is that red blood cells are normally restricted to and remain in the vascular space, so that a GI bleeding can be investigated over a much longer period of time. This is very valuable because a GI hemorrhage is often an intermittent process.

Red blood cell dog laboratory data showed that the lowest active detectable bleeding rate is 0.05 ml/min which is considerably less than that required for the experimental detection with angiography (0.5 to 1 ml/min). Red blood cell scintigraphy is reported to be more sensitive than angiography for detecting bleeding sites, so that an angiography is likely to be negative if the scintigraphy fails to show a bleeding focus [51].

As scintigraphy allows the possibility of whole body imaging the test is advocated for the initial documentation of the site of active bleeding in order to eventually apply other procedures for a more specific diagnosis [47].

Although the Budd-Chiari syndrome is an uncommon disorder one should keep in mind, that a colloid liver scintigraphy can play an important role in diagnosis. A specific finding is the preservation of even an hypertrophy of the caudal lobe of the liver and non-visualization of the other portions of the liver. A recent well documented article summarizes other patterns associated with the Budd-Chiari syndrome [52].

Traumatology

Posttraumatic abnormalities are usually well evaluated with radiographic procedures. Special nuclear medicine investigations can nevertheless provide valuable additional information in particular clinical situations.

Electrocardiographically gated cardiac scintigraphy, applied to patients with severe blunt chest trauma, revealed a higher frequency of posttraumatic cardiac dysfunction than heretofore recognized and frequently involves the more anteriorly situated right ventricle [53–55]. Infarct avid Tc-99m-pyrophosphate has been reported to be sensitive in the diagnosis of myocardial contusion [56]. Further experimental and clinical evaluation is necessary to determine the significance and prognostic value of these techniques.

Ventilation-perfusion lung scintigraphy with a noble gaz, Xenon-133, has been used to evaluate inhalation lung injury. The scintigraphy appears to be safe, easy and accurate for the early detection of lung involvement, often being abnormal several days before the chest X-ray [57].

The contribution of nuclear medicine in patients with ARDS has been mentioned earlier. Bone scintigraphy is particularly helpful to identify occult fractures which are often difficult to define by radiography, such as rib fractures, carpal or torsal bones, thoracic vertebrae or sternum [58, 59]. This imaging technique has also ben proposed to assess bone healing [60], molunion [61], and the early detection of bone grafment viability [62].

Liver and biliary tract injuries can be investigated using hepatic scintigraphy and cholescintigraphy [59, 63]. Nagle et al. [64] reported the detection of mesenteric bleeding after trauma using liver scintigraphy. Especially, biliary leakage can be very well detected with cholescintigraphy after blunt or penetrating trauma [63], surgical injuries [65] and after liver biopsy [66]. This techniques has a greater sensitivity than contrast studies due to the small amount of radioactive tracer that is necessary for detection. Cholescintigraphy is a functional procedure so that the presence or absence of a communication between an intrahepatic cavity (abscess, cyst) and the biliary system can be documented [63]. This procedure is recommended as a routine, non-invasive imaging procedure, in risk patients [67].

There is certainly no agreement as to where nuclear medicine procedures do fit in for the evaluation of patients with blunt or penetrating urinary tract injury. There is sufficient evidence available to state that, while radiologic procedures and ultrasonography reveal meanly morphologic information, nuclear medicine procedures in general render meanly direct functional information about the renal parenchyma and are very sensitive in disclosing urinary extravasation. A combination of ultrasound and nuclear medicine procedures seems to have the highest yield [68].

Conclusion

In presence of critically ill patients nuclear medicine procedures are often complementary to radiology or ultrasonography. In order to get definitive diagnoses in the most efficient way it becomes necessary to perform different test in a particular sequence. The contribution of nuclear medicine to decision maps will not only be determined by the awareness of the clinician of the information gained by a test, but also by the availability and willingness of a nuclear medicine department to provide excellent service.

References

1. Wiener SN, Weiss PH (1975) Radionuclide imaging in the care of the critically ill patient. Surg Clin North Am 55:729-753
2. Parker MM, Shelhamer JH, Bacharach SL, et al (1984) Profound but reversible myocardial depression in patients with septic shock. Ann Intern Med 100:483-490
3. Van Aswegen A, Otto AC, Herbst CP, et al (1986) Left ventricular function evaluation using radionuclide methods in intensive coronary care unit. Radiology 158:252-253
4. Ellrodt AG, Riedinger MS, Kimchi A, et al (1985) Left ventricular performance in septic shock: reversible segmental and global abnormalities. Am Heart J 110:402-409
5. Kimchi A, Ellrodt AG, Berman DS, et al (1984) Right ventricular performance in septic shock: A combined radionuclide and hemodynamic study. J Am Coll Cardiol 4:945-951
6. Franken PR, Brihaye C, Dobbeleir, et al (1987) Mesure de la fraction d'éjection ventriculaire gauche par la technique du premier passage en utilisant l'iridium 191m. J Biophys Bioméc 11:188-190
7. Snider MT, Rie MA, Bingham JB, Laver J, Urbina A, Strauss HW (1980) Right ventricular performance in ARDS: Radionuclide scintiscan and thermal dilution studies. Am Rev Respir Dis 121:192 (abstr.)
8. Laver MB, Strauss HW, Pohost GM (1979) Right and left ventricular geometry:; adjustments during acute respiratory failure. Crit Care Med 7:509-519
9. Burns RJ, Druck MN, Woodward DS, Houle S, McLaughlin PR (1983) Repeatability of estimates of left-ventricular volume from blood-pool counts: concise communication. J Nucl Med 24:775-781
10. Sisson JC, Shapiro B, Meyers L, et al (1987) Metaiodobenzylguanidine to map scintigraphically the adrenergic nervous system in man. J Nucl Med 28:1625-1636
11. Fagret D, Wolf JE, Comet M (1987) Scintigraphie myocardique à la m-I123 MIBG dans les infarctus du myocarde. Cardiol Nucl/Communications orales 11:59-51

12. Rudavsky AZ, Moss CM (1981) Radionuclide angiography for the evaluation of peripheral vascular injuries. In: Freeman LM, Weismann HS (eds). Nuclear Medicine Annual 1981. Raven Press, New York, pp 315–335

13. Matin P, Glass EC, Villarica J (1979) Peripheral radionuclide angiography. JAMA 242:1781–1784

14. Moss CM, Rudavsky AZ, Veith FJ (1976) Isotope Angiography: Technique, validation and value in the assessment of arterial reconstruction. Ann Surg 184:116–121

15. Brill DR, Schwartz JA, Baxter JA (1985) Variant flow patterns in radionuclide cerebral imaging performed for brain death. Clin Nucl Med 10:346–352

16. Pjura GA, Kim EE (1987) Radionuclide evaluation of brain death. Nucl Med Ann 269–293

17. Holmes RA (1986) A reawakening of interest in radionuclide brain imaging. J Nucl Med 27:299–301

18. Ell PJ, Hocknell JML, JArritt PH, et al (1985) A 99m-Tc- labelled radiotracer for the investigation of cerebral vascular disease. Nucl Med Commun 6:437–441

19. Lisbona R, Rush C, Lepanto L (1987) Technitium-99m red blood cell venography of the lower limb in symptomatic pulmonary embolization. Clin Nucl Med 12:93–98

20. Wellman HN (1986) Pulmonary Thromboembolism: Current status report on the role of nuclear medicine. Semin Nucl Med 16:236–274

21. Biello DR, Mattar AG, McKnight RC, Siegel BA (1979) Ventilation-perfusion studies in suspected pulmonary embolism. AJR 133:1033–1037

22. Siddiqui AR, Wellman HN, Klatte EC, Faris JV (1983) Wedged Swan-Ganz catheter causing ventilation-perfusion mismatch: Case report and review of the literature. Clin Nucl Med 8:597–599

23. Putman CE, Ravin CE (1978) Chapter 5 Adult respiratory distress syndrome: Intensive Care Radiology. The CV Mosby Company. pp 114–123

24. Biersack HJ, Rommelsheim K, Thelen M, Hnermann B, Straaten HG, Winkler C (1976) Szintigraphische Befunde bei progressiver pulmonaler Insuffizienz (Schocklunge). Dtsch Med Wochensch 101:927–929

25. Sugerman HJ, Tatum JL, Burke TS, Strash AM, Glauser FL (1984) Gamma scintigraphic analysis of albumin flux in patients with acute respiratory distress syndrome. Surgery 95:674–682

26. Powe JE, Short A, Sibbald WJ, Driedger AA (1982) Pulmonary accumulation of polymorphonuclear leukocytes in the adult respiratory distress syndrome. Crit Care Med 10:712–718

27. Quinn DA, Carvalho AC, Geller E, et al (1987) 99m-Tc- Fibrinogen scanning in adult respiratory distress syndrome. Am Rev Respir Dis 135:100–106

28. Groeneveld ABJ, Thijs LG (1987) Evidence for increased soft tissue permeability in porcine septic shock. Free Papers Presentation, Intensive Care Symposium, Valkenburg (The Netherlands)

29. McAfee JG, Thakur ML (1976) Survey of radioactive agents for in vitro labeling of phagocytic leucocytes. J Nucl Med 17:480–487

30. Cartier F (1987) Strategy in immunocompromised patients with pulmonary infiltrates. Intensive Care Med 13:87–88

31. Kramer EL, Sanger JJ, Garay SM, et al (1987) Gallium-67 scans of the chest in patients with acquired immunodeficiency syndrome. J Nucl Med 28:1107–1114

32. Mc Mahon H, Bekerman C (1978) The diagnostic significance of gallium lung uptake in patients with normal chest radiographs. Radiology 127:189–193

33. Barron TF, Birnbaum NS, Shane LB, Goldsmith SS, Rosen MJ (1985) Pneumocystis carinii Pneumonia studied by gallium-67 scanning. Radiology 154:791–793

34. Ketchum LE (1985) Aids diagnosis and monitoring improved by radionuclide procedures. Sem Nucl Med 26:1109–1112

35. Segall GM, McDougall IR (1986) Diagnostic value of lung uptake of indium-111 oxine-labeled white blood cells. AJR 147:601–606

36. McDougall IR, Baumert JE, Lantieri RL (1979) Evaluation of 11-In leukocyte whole body scanning. AJR 133:849–854

37. Holland RD, Gooneratne NS, West TE, Selby JB (1980) Gallium-67 scintigraphy in abdominal anaerobic abscesses. Clin Nucl Med 5:393-396
38. Coleman RE, Black RE, Welch DM, Maxwell JG (1980) Indium-111 labeled leukocytes in the evaluation of suspected adominal abscesses. Am J Surg 139:99-104
39. McAfee JG, Samin A (1985) In-111 labeled leukocytes: A review of problems in image interpretation. Radiology 155:221-229
40. Shuman WP, Gibbs P, Rudd TG, et al (1982) PIPIDA scintigraphy for cholecystitis: false positives in alcoholism and total parental nutrition. Am J Radio 138:1-6
41. Fink-Bennett D, Freitas JE, Ripley SD, Bree RL (1985) The sensitivity of hepatobiliary imaging and real-time ultrasonography in the detection of acute cholecystitis. Arch Surg 120:904-906
42. Johnson DG (1983) Diagnosing acute right upper quadrant pain: Tc-99m IDA or ultrasound. J Nucl Med Technol 11:77-80
43. Rosenthal L (1978) Clinical experience with the newer hepatobiliary radiopharmaceuticals. Can J Surg 21:297-300
44. Szlabick RE, Catto JA, Fink-Bennett D, Ventura V (1980) Hepatobiliary scanning in the diagnosis of acute cholecystitis. Arch Surg 115:540-544
45. Morgan JR, Williams LA, Howard CB (1985) Technetium-labelled liposome imaging for deep-seated infection. Br J Radiol 58:35-39
46. Locker JTh, Seybold K, Andres RY, Schubiger PA, Mach JP, Buchegger F (1986) Imaging of inflammatory and infectious lesions after injection of radioiodinated monoclonal anti-granulocytes antibodies. Nucl Med Comm 7:659-670
47. Eastwood GL (1985) Upper gastro-intestinal bleeding. In: Intensive Care Medicine. Rippe JM, Irwin RS, Alpert JS, Dalen JE. Little, Brown and Company, pp 730-735
48. Smith R, Copely DJ, Bolen FH (1987) 99m-Tc- RBC scintigraphy: correlation of gastrointestinal bleeding rates with scintigraphic findings. AJR 148:869-874
49. Gupta S, Luna E, Kingsley S, Prince M, Herrera N (1984) Detection of gastointestinal bleeding by radionuclide scintigraphy. The Am J Gastroent 79:26-31
50. Winzelberg GG, McKusick KA, Froelich JW, Callahan RJ, Strauss HW (1982) Detection of gastrointestinal bleeding with 99m-tc-labeled red blood cells. Sem Nucl Med 12:139-146
51. McKusick KA, Froelich J, Callahan RJ, Winzelberg GG, Strauss HW (1981) Tc-99m red blood cells for detection of gastrointestinal bleeding: experience with 80 patients. AJR 137:1113-1118
52. Picard M, Carrier L, Chartrand R, et al (1987) Budd-Chiari Syndrome: Typical and atypical scintigraphic aspects. J Nucl Med 38:803-809
53. Harley DP, Mena I, Miranda R, Nelson RJ (1983) Myocardial dysfunction following blunt chest trauma. Arch Surg 118:1384-1387
54. Sutherland GR, Driedger AA, Holliday RL, Cheung HW, Sibbald WJ (1983) Frequency of myocardial injury after blunt chest trauma as evaluated by radionuclide angiography. Am J Cardiol 52:1099-1103
55. Rosenbaum RC, Johnston GS (1986) Posttraumatic cardiac dysfunction: assessment with radionuclide ventriculography. Radiology 160:91-94
56. Lopez-Majano V, Sansi PS, Colter R (1985) Nuclear medicine in the diagnosis of cardiac contusion. Eur J Nucl Med 11:290-294
57. Shall GL, McDonald HD, Carr LB, Capozzi A (1978) Xenon ventilation-perfusion lung scans: the early diagnosis of inhalation injury. JAMA 240:2441-2445
58. Milstein D, Nusynowitz ML, Lull RJ (1974) Radionuclide diagnosis in chest disease resulting from trauma. Sem Nucl Med 4:339-355
59. Sty JR, Starshak RJ, Hubbard AM (1983) Radionuclide evaluation in childhood injuries. Sem Nucl Med 13:258-281
60. Wahner HW (1976) Radionuclide in the diagnosis of fracture healing. J Nucl Med 21:931
61. Matin P (1983) Bone scintigraphy in the diagnosis and management of traumatic injury. Sem Nucl Med 13:104-122
62. Velasco JG, Bega A, Leisorek A (1976) The early detection of free bone graft viability with 99mTc: A preliminary report. Br J Plast Surg 29:344
63. Weissmann HS, Byun KJC, Freeman LM (1983) Role of Tc-99m IDA scintigraphy in the evaluation of hepatobiliary trauma. Sem Nucl Med 13:199-222

64. Nagle CE, Freitas JE, Murphy JW, Howard RS (1984) Abdominal and pelvic imaging as part of liver-spleen scintigraphy for the detection of mesenteric bleeding in trauma. A case report. Clin Nucl Med 9:684–686
65. Weissmann HS, Ghedman ML, Wilk OJ (1982) Evaluation of the postoperative patient with 99m-Tc-HIDA cholescintigraphy. Sem Nucl Med 12:27–52
66. Gryn R, Tytyat GN, Van der Schoot JB, Van Royen EA (1984) Bile leakage after liver biopsy and its diagnosis by HIDA scan. Dutch J Med 27:408–411
67. Creutzig H, Gratz K, Brolsch C (1982) Diagnosis of bile leak by cholescintigraphy. J Nucl Med 23:73
68. Rosenthal L, Ammann W (1983) Renal trauma. Sem Nucl Med 13:238–244

Computed Tomography of Head and Abdominal Trauma

A. F. Turner

Introduction

Trauma is the third leading cause of death in the United States behind stroke and cancer and it is the leading cause of death in the age group from 1 to 44 years. Men between the ages of 45 and 64 die more commonly from trauma than from stroke [1].

The head is the most commonly injured part of the body in multiply injured patients, and at autopsy 75% of road accident victims will have brain injury [2].

First priority must be given to the ABC's; that is, airway, breathing and circulation. Since it is estimated that 7% of trauma patients die of asphyxiation, establishment of an airway is given the same priority as the control of hemorrhage. Radiographs are obtained only when the patient's condition is stable.

Due to the dire consequences of cervical cord injury, X-rays of the cervical spine are necessary prior to moving the patient in the following circumstances; all patients

a) who are unconscious
b) who have a history of or clincial findings suggesting cervical injury
c) who have facial or skull injuries.

It is important to recognize that a lateral cervical radiograph that does not include the seventh segment is an inadequate examination and that the patient should be managed as he would had he suffered such a fracture.

Computed tomography is the eminent procedure. It is easy, fast and allows an excellent examination of the bone structures. Computed tomography is capable of identifying small amounts of intracranial air.

Scanning technique should provide a high resolution scan without motion. Routine sections are taken at 10 mm contiguous thoughout the head. Five mm contiguous sections are necessary to define abnormalities of the posterior fossa, orbits, craniovertebral junction, floor of the anterior cranial fossa, base or paranasal sinuses. Direct coronal images may be necessary to identify convexity lesions. If direct coronal images are not possible, then reformatted images may provide similar information. Special bone reconstruction algorithms can aid in depicting fine bony detail [3].

Intravenous contrast is not needed in acute injury, however, intravenous contrast administration may be useful in the post-traumatic period to assess the presence of isodense subdural hematomas, secondary infections, and capsule detection in chronic extracerebral collections.

Intracranial Extracerebral Collections

Subdural Hematoma

Acute subdural hematoma usually results from traumatic tearing of the veins bridging the space between the dura and the brain surface [4, 5]. Fractures may or may not be present. An acute subdural hematoma is crescentic in shape [6], because it occupies a crescent-shaped potential space between the brain surface and the dura. There is no mechanical barrier to its spread, and it can cover most or all of the hemisphere. It can be deceiving as to size on a single computed tomographic slice.

Initially an acute subdural is hyperdense, however, in patients that are very anemic, it may have a density less than or equal to that of normal brain. The degree of shift reflects the magnitude of mass effect.

Over time, the acutely crescentic shape evolves into a straight-edge collection and finally becomes biconvex. Maturation of the subdural hematoma reveals that hyperdensity gives way to isodensity and finally hypodensity. If there is a sudden increase in density, one has to consider the possibility of rebleed, however, an infectious process can result in increased density.

Contrast enhancement may be of value, thickened membrane and dura suggest the presence of infection. The membrane and dura should not change in a rebleed. Subacute subdurals are isodense. It is essential when reviewing subacute collections to observe the size of the sulci. If the sulci are smaller on one side compared to the other, this is suggestive evidence of an isodense subdural.

Subacute for computed tomography represents 8 to 10 days, while subacute for magnetic resonance imaging represents 72 hours or more.

Some chronic subdurals can accumulate slowly under low pressure, but present as an apoplectic event [7]. Contrast enhancement fails to opacify an intracerebral mass, but identifies the subdural membrane. Comparison of scans immediately after infusion of contrast medium and six hours later, reveal enhancement of the chronic subdural: blood iodine ratio is 20:1.

Epidural Hematoma

Epidural hematoma results from traumatic disruption of a meningeal artery with bleeding between the dura and the skull [8]. Because the dura is firmly attached to the inner table, there is not potential epidural space. Time is required to tears the dura from the inner table.

Epidural tends to be localized. It is a lenticular shaped collection, the edges of the collection are the attachment of the dura to the inner table. The collection is usually hyperdense, unless the patient is severely anemic. It frequently appears larger than a subdural hematoma, but in the majority of cases is just the opposite. Because the collection is epidural, it can cross points of attachment of the falx and tentorium.

If an epidural is not enlarging, is not life-threatening and not producing neurological deficit, it may be treated conservatively. As the epidural becomes decreases in density, contrast scans may be necessary for follow-up. The shape changes from biconvex to crescentic prior to complete absorption as a result decrease in amount of fluid and reexpansion of the underlying brain.

Intraparenchymal Hemorrhage

The coup-contracoup injury is well known, and represents the moving skull coming to an abrupt stop, but the enclosed brain continues to move for another moment. The brain then comes to an equally abrupt stop against the inner table. That portion of the brain 180 degree away from the impact site is cavitated from being pulled suddenly from its dura, but on recoil is caused to strike it with great force. Both coup and contracoup injuries can be associated with hemorrhage, however, the contracoup is more frequent.

Shearing forces are the result of asymmetric pressure to the brain and are exerted on the white matter and deep gray matter [8]. The most frequent areas are the thalamus, corpus collosum and subcortical gray-white matter interface. Shearing injury produces areas of parenchymal hemorrhage which are round, discrete, well-marginated areas of increased density. Although small areas of apparent involvement, they may have a poor prognosis. One should always look for mass effect, these areas may represent areas of potential delayed hemorrhage.

Intraventricular Hemorrhage: Traumatic intraventricular hemorrhage can result from extension of intraparenchymal hemorrhage [10] since the ependymal surface does not offer a significant barrier to extension of bleeding or from shearing of the subependymal veins.

The CT appearance is straightforward with dense blood seen in one or more of the ventricles and usually conforming to the ventricular shape. When blood enters the aquaduct of Sylvius, obstructive hydrocephalus almost follows. This causes dilatation of the lateral ventricles which if not relieved can result in a rapid increase in intracranial pressure and ultimately in brain death. If ventricular enlargement occurs early without blood in the ventricles or contralateral ventricular enlargement points to tentorial herniation.

Early chronic changes include infection, ischemic infarct and hydrocephalus. Late chronic changes include both focal and diffuse atrophy, gliosis and hydrocephalus.

Brain stem injury: Computed tomography of the brain stem is useless. Brain stem injury needs magnetic resonance imaging, especially after 72 hours and when the patient is stable.

Ventricular enlargement with edema-like density of the surrounding brain represents gliosis, with cerebral edema the ventricles are usually compressed.

CT of Abdominal Trauma

It is realized that the degree and severity of the trauma and the risk to the patient's life will determine whether the patients is resuscitated in the operating room or the emergency room. Fischer [11] stated "mortality from blunt abdominal trauma decreased from 30% to 18% when we began evaluating and resuscitating severely traumatized patients in the operating room rather than in the emergency room".

Evaluation of renal function in order to preclude the possibility of unknowingly removing the patient's only functioning kidney can be obtained in surgery with a single radiograph of the abdomen following the intravenous injection of a double dose of contrast medium. This is usually sufficient to appraise the function of the kidney on the injured side and to determine function of the contralateral kidney.

Computed tomography provides a clear and anatomical presentation of the abdominal organs and permits accurate assessment of the extent of injury. In the upper abdomen, it allows assessment of spleen, liver, pancreas and retroperitoneal structures simultaneously.

Spleen

Rupture of the spleen is the most common serious intraabdominal injury associated with blunt abdominal trauma [12]. While most injuries follow severe abdominal trauma, splenic rupture or subcapsular hematomas may follow minimal or apparently inconsequential abdominal trauma. Delayed rupture of the spleen is a well documented syndrome consisting of rupture of the spleen occurring more than 48 hours following the traumatic episode. Delayed rupture accounts for up to 30% of splenic injuries [13]. During the latent period it is postulated that blood collects from a small subcapsular or intrasplenic tear and with increasing volume, the hematoma breaks through its capsular restraint resulting in all the clinical signs of an acute surgical abdomen and shock. Delayed rupture of the spleen carries a ten-fold greater mortality than does acute rupture of the spleen. Fifty percent of delayed ruptures occur in the first week following trauma [14]. This increased mortality is presumably due to the fact that it is unsuspected and therefore unrecognized. Its existence reflects the difficulty in making the diagnosis of subcapsular splenic rupture at the time of the initial trauma. Mortality without surgery is 90%.

Computed tomography is an excellent non invasive modality for identifying splenic trauma, it is both sensitive and specific for various types splenic injuries. Extensive splenic rupture is usually associated with free intraperitoneal fluid (blood). Where available, computed tomography has replaced angiography in the diagnosis of possible splenic rupture or hematoma [15, 17]. Experimentally produced hematomas [18, 19] are initially isodense with the splenic tissue. Following intravenous injection of contast medium, the spleen shows an increase in attenuation while the hematoma does not. It is essential to use intravenous contrast media in splenic trauma. It is imperative to opacify the loops of bowel adjacent to the spleen with oral 3% iodine contrast media. CT scans more than one week following the trauma reveal a lower CT number within the hematoma than within the parent organ. Subcapsular hematomas have concentric low density areas that flatten or produce a concave imprint on the spleen. Hematomas can be larger than the spleen itself. Fractured spleens have blurred margins or no margins can be identified, and the fractured spleen may be associated with free intraperitoneal fluid (blood). Sometimes the fracture plane of the spleen is identified.

Liver

Although less frequent than spleen or kidney, hepatic injury is more significant in terms of mortality. Blunt trauma to the liver is usually associated with injury to other intra-abdominal organs as well as to the head, chest and extremities [20]. Approximately 50% of patients have fractures of the right lower ribs. Because of the severe consequences of hepatic damage and associated injuries, these patients are commonly in profound shock when initially seen and are usually not able to tolerate the time and manipulation required to have a detailed radiologic evaluation of the abdomen.

Computed tomography of the liver is capable of detecting hepatic abnormalities with a high degree of accuracy. The exact site and extent of the hepatic injury can be determined. Subcapsular hematomas are low density concentric areas that flatten or produce a concave imprint on the liver. Intrahepatic hematomas are rounded or lobulated areas of decreased density. Contrast medium allows easier detection by enhancing the liver and not the hematoma. There may be layering of sediment in the dependent portions of these low density areas. These areas may increase, but usually decrease in size and can be followed by computed tomography or ultrasound. Increase in size or enlarging subcapsular hematomas may be the result of unrecognized bile leak, or continous bleeding due to the presence of bile interfering with the clotting mechanism. Hepatic necrosis and bile pseudocysts have been reported [21]. Small intraparenchymal or subcapsular hematomas of the liver can be managed conservatively [22]. Subphrenic collections of fluid and intraabdominal collections of fluid can be detected. Dilated bile ducts suggest extra hepatic or intrahepatic biliary obstruction. Computed tomography is an excellent tool in following these lesions.

Pancreas

The head and uncinate process of the pancreas lie directly over the upper lumbar spine. Pancreatic injury occurs when the driver is thrust against the steering wheel or when a child falls on the handle bar of a bicycle [23]. Pancreatic injury is usually associated with injury to other organs and carries a 20% mortality rate [24]. Mild contusion without disruption of the parenchyma causes transient elevation of the white blood cell count and the serum amylase. Pancreatic laceration allows secretions and blood to leak into the retroperitoneal tissues.

Computed tomography's ability to totally visualize the pancreas has been well demonstrated. CT scanning should be considered the imaging modality of choice in the evaluation of pancreatic trauma. Diffuse or focal enlargement of the pancreas with no changes are found in traumatic pancreatitis. Repeat scans after an interval of time may reveal pseudocysts which appear as regions of decreased density which may increase or decrease in size with time. With pancreatic laceration, diffuse hemorrhagic pancreatitis is identified by mass dislacement with areas of varying attenuation and non visualization of the pancreas. Contrast enhancement of the pancreatic tissue may facilitate its visualization and is recommended in pancreatic injury. CT scanning can be utilized to follow the course of pancreatic injury and to attempt to detect formation of a pancreatic abscess. Ill defined areas of low attenuation without a rind and the presence of gas are diagnostic of abscess formation. It is not possible to distinguish infected from noninfected pseudocysts or other pancreatic fluid collections by other CT criteria. Diagnostic percutaneous needle aspiration is indicated in patients with pancreatic pseudocyst or fluid collection with persistent fever or leukocytosis [25].

Intestinal Injury

Bowel disruption due to blunt abdominal trauma is not rare. The most common cause of intestinal disruption is the automobile accident [26]. Griswold and Collier [27] noted that 16.2% of patients operated on four blunt abdominal trauma had sustained intestinal injury. Reports from the Charity Hospital in New Orleans showed an increase in bowel injuries from 9.3% in the years 1951–1966 to 15.3% in the years 1967–1973 [28, 29].

The various mechanisms of bowel disruption are:

a) direct, crushing impingement of the bowel against the unyielding vertebral column [30, 31],
b) a tearing or shearing force due to deceleration in areas where the bowel or the mesentery are relatively fixed [30], and
c) a sudden increase of intraluminal pressure transmitted to fluid and air filled loops of intestine especially the duodenum [32].

The duodenum's fixed position directly over the spine renders it especially susceptible to injury. With intramural hematoma of the duodenum, the abdominal pain subsides and the patient has a symptom-free period of 12 to 24 hours, then vomiting occurs and persists, simulating a high intestinal obstruction [33]. Peritoneal lavage, free air and serum amylase studies are unreliable for the diagnosis of duodenal injury [26]. If no other visceral injury coexists with intramural hematoma of the duodenum, conservative therapy with gastric suction and intravenous feedings are recommended [34]. Within two weeks the mucosal changes diminish and by one month the duodenum has regained its normal appearance [35]. Retroperitoneal perforation of the duodenum may have a latent period with few signs or symptoms [36]. The onset of continuous abdominal pain accompanied by back pain suggests the possibility of retroperitoneal laceration [37]. Delay in diagnosis of duodenal perforation for more than 24 hours yields mortality rates as high as 65% [38].

Although some authors have noted the duodenum more commonly injured than jejunum [39], the majority of authors have found that the jejunum and ileum are most commonly injured [26, 29].

Computed tomography is of value in assessing the retroperitoneal space. Retroperitoneal hematomas have vague and misleading signs and symptoms and therefore exploratory is often performed on the assumption that the source of blood loss is intraperitoneal [30]. Computed tomography would avert unnecessary laparotomies in these patients. The diagnosis of retroperitoneal duodenal rupture and sequelae may be enhanced by CT with its ability to detect very small amounts of retroperitoneal gas and extravasated contrast medium not detected on conventional radiographs of the abdomen. It is felt by some that retroperitoneal hematomas around the duodenum must be explored [26]. However, with the increasing use of computed tomography, concepts regarding the management of these patients may change in the future.

Kidney

Renal injury is frequently encountered in abdominal injuries. It is often associated with injuries of the spleen, liver and pancreas. Examination of the urine is imperative in all cases of blunt abdominal trauma since hematuria is the hallmark of injury. Since hematuria was not present in 27% of patients with significant renal injuries [40] and not present in 27% of patients with renal artery thrombosis [41], hematuria cannot be used as the sole criterion for intravenous pyelography. The anterior pararenal space is bounded anteriorly by the posterior layer of abdominal peritoneum and extends posteriorly to the anterior renal fascia. The anterior pararenal space contains pancreas, duodenum, ascending and descending colon and the splenic and hepatic arteries. The pararenal space contains the kidneys, adrenal glands and great abdominal vessels [42]. The posterior pararenal space contains fatty tissue. The posterior pararenal space is the most frequent site for spontaneous extraperitoneal bleeding in patients with bleeding disorders.

Computed tomography is excellent for imaging the kidneys, the perirenal, pararenal and retroperitoneal regions [43]. Urograms were normal in four cases in which computed tomography demonstrated small to moderate sized intra- and extrarenal hematomas [21]. Imcomplete laceration or intrarenal hematomas are clearly seen as areas of decreased density when contrast medium is infused. Complete laceration is demonstrated by separation of the renal poles. Subcapsular hematomas appear as lentiform fluid collections confined by the high density renal capsule. Avulsion of the renal vascular pedicle is identified by a very prominent ring like enhancement of the renal capsule with the renal cortex exhibiting a low density. Bolus infusion of contrast further enhances the capsule, with no significant increase in the renal parenchymal density. This anatomically is due to capsular collaterals attempting to perfuse the renal cortex. Perirenal hematomas are low to medium densities confined by Gerota's fascia. In some cases of excessive renal bleeding the blood can dissect into the anterior para-renal space which contains the ascending and descending colon. Blood can dissect lateral to the ascending or descending colon and displace the colon medially. Since computed tomography can differentiate between incomplete and complete laceration, it can be extremely helpful in patient management. In one series, computed tomography directed three patients to surgery with complete lacerations and ten patients to conservative therapy with incomplete lacerations [21]. A computed tomography scan can often provide rapid information that might not be obtained by urography, ultrasonography or arteriography [21, 43]. Computed tomography of the "Page kidney" demonstrated a large mass in the left renal bed on the non-contrast scan and with contrast showed a kidney surrounded by an avascular zone [44].

Pelvis

As much as two liters of blood can be sequestered in the extraperitoneal space without clinical symptoms. Life threatening pelvic hemorrhage can result from rupture of the internal iliac vessels or its branches. The injuries are usually due to pelvic fractures and dislocations which can also result in disruption of the urinary bladder, the urethra and sometimes bowel.

Computed tomography allows excellent visualization of the pelvic structures and can be utilized to diagnose fractures, dislocations and pelvic hematomas. Computed tomography offers advantages in imaging fractures, particularly those of the acetabulum [45–48].

References

1. Frazee JG (1986) Head trauma. J Emerg Med Clin North Am 4:859–874
2. U.S. Department of Health, Education and Welfare; Facts of Life and Death (1974) Publication number (HRS) 74–1222. National Center for Health Statistics Rockville, Maryland
3. Levine RS, Grossman RI (1985) Head and facial trauma. J Emerg Med Clin NA 3:447–473
4. Slager UT (1970) Mechanical trauma and the effects of space occupying lesions. In: Basic Neuropathology. Williams and Wilkins Co, Baltimore, pp 67–68
5. Ingvar S, Ask-Upmark E (1938) Contributions to the knowledge of subdural hematomas. Acta Med Scand 94:225–240
6. Norman O (1956) Angiographic differentiation between acute and chronic subdural and extradural haematomas. Acta Radiol 46:371–378
7. Horton JA (1985) Cranical Trauma. In: Lachaw RE (ed) Computed Tomography of Head, Neck and Spine. Year Book Publishers, Chicago pp 55–69
8. Ford LE, McLaurin RL (1963) Mechanisms of extradural hematomas. J Neurosurg 20:760–769
9. Zimmerman RA, Bilaniuk LT, Genneralli T (1978) Computed tomography of the cerebral white matter. Radiology 127:393–396
10. Cardobes CD, de la Fuente M, Lobato RD, et al (1983) Intraventricular hemorrhage in severe head injury. J Neurosurg 58:217–222

11. Fischer RP, Beverlin BC, Engrav LH, Benjamin CI, Perry JF Jr (1978) Diagnostic peritoneal lavage. Am J Surg 136:701–712
12. Terry JF, Self MM, Howard JM (1956) Injuries of the spleen: a report of 102 patients and a review of the literature. Surgery 40:615–619
13. Sizer JS, Wayne ER, Frederick PL (1966) Delayed rupture of the spleen. Arch Surg 92:362–366
14. Harris JH (1975) In: Harris JH, Harris WH (eds) The radiology of emergency medicine. Williams and Wilkins Co, Baltimore, pp 290
15. Bird D, Kelly MJ, Baird RN (1979) Spontaneous rupture of normal spleen. Diagnosis by computerized tomography. Br J Surg 66:598–603
16. Druy EM, Rubin BE (1979) Computed tomography in the evaluation of abdominal trauma. J Comput Assist Tomogr 3:40–45
17. Mall JC, Kaiser JA (1980) CT diagnosis of splenic laceration. A J R 134:265–269
18. Moss AA et al (1979) Computet tomography of splenic subcapsular hematomas: an experimental study in dogs. Invest Radiol 14:60–67
19. Korobkin M et al (1978) Computed tomography of subcapsular splenic hematoma: clinical and experimental studies. Radiology 129:411–415
20. Kindling PH, Wilson RF, Walt AJ (1969) Hepatic trauma with particular reference to blunt injury. J Trama 9:17–22
21. Federle MP, Goldberg HI, Kaiser JA, et al (1981) Evaluation of abdominal trauma by computed tomography. Radiology 138:637–641
22. Lucas CE, Walt AJ (1970) Critical decisions in liver trauma. Experience based on 604 cases. Arch Surg 101:277–283
23. Otherson HB, Moore FT, Boles ET (1968) Traumatic pancreatitis and pseudocyst in childhood. J Trauma 8:535–539
24. Donovan AJ, Turrill F, Berne CJ (1972) Injuries to the pancreas from blunt trauma. Surg Clin North Am 52:649–653
25. Federle MP, Jeffery RB, Crass RA, Dalsem VV (1981) Computed tomography of pancreatic abscesses. A J R 136:879–881
26. Shuck JM, Lowe RJ (1978) Intenstinal disruption due to blunt abdominal trauma. Am J Surg 136:668–671
27. Griswold RA, Collier HS (1961) Blunt abdominal trauma. Int Abstr Surg 112:309–314
28. DiVicenti FC, Rives JD, Laborde EJ, et al (1968) Blunt abdominal trauma. J Trauma 8:1004–1008
29. Davis JJ, Cohn I Jr, Nance FC (1975) Diagnosis and management of blunt abdominal trauma. Ann Surg 183:672–679
30. Orloff MJ, Charters AC (1972) Injuries of the small bowel and mesentery and retroperitoneal hematoma. Surg Clin North Am 52:729–733
31. Snyder CJ (1972) Bowel Injuries from automobile seatbelts. Am J Surg 123:312–317
32. Williams RD, Yurko AA (1972) Controversial aspects of diagnosis and management of blunt abdominal trauma. Am J Surg 111:477–482
33. Davis DR, Thomas CY (1961) Intramural hematoma of duodenum and jejunum, cause of high intestinal obstruction: report of three cases due to trauma. Ann Surg 153:394–398
34. Sanidad P, Miller HL (1970) Small bowel submucosal hematoma: a conservative attitude. S Afr Med J 44:811–816
35. McCort JJ (1966) In: Radiologic examination in blunt abdominal trauma. WB Saunders Co, Philadelphia
36. Wilson TS, Costopoulos LB (1971) Retroperitoneal injury to duodenum by blunt trauma: report of eight cases. Canad J Surg 14:114–117
37. Resnicoff SA, Morton JH, Block AL (1967) Retroperitoneal rupture of the duodenum due to blunt trauma. Surg Gynecol Obstet 125:77–84
38. Federle MP, Crass RA, Jeffery RB, Trunkey DD (1982) Computed tomography in blunt abdominal trauma. Arch Surg 117:645–650
39. Cerise EJ, Scully JH Jr (1970) Blunt trauma to the small intestine. J Trauma 10:46–51
40. Carlton CE (1978) Injuries of the kidney and ureter. In: Harrison JH, Gittes RF, Permutter AD, et al (eds) Campbell's Urology Edition 4. WB Saunders Co, Philadelphia, pp 881–905

41. Barlow B, Gandhi R (1980) Renal Artery Thrombosis following Blunt Trauma. J Trauma 20:614–618
42. Meyers MA (1976) Dynamic Radiology of the Abdomen. Springer, Berlin Heidelberg New York, pp 113–194
43. Schaner EG, Balow JE, Doppman JL (1977) Computed Tomography in diagnosis of subcapsular and perirenal hematoma. AJR 129:83–89
44. Takahashi M, Tamakawa Y, Shibata A, Fukushima Y (1977) Computed tomography of "page" kidney – a case report. J Comput Assist Tomogr 1:344–346
45. Canale ST, Manugian AH (1979) Irreducible traumatic dislocation of hip. J Bone Joint Surg 61A:7–12
46. Gilula LA, Murphy WA, Tailor LC, et al (1979) Computed tomography of the osseus pelvis. Radiology 132:107–111
47. Lasda NA, Levinsohn EM, Yuan HA, et al (1978) Computed tomography in disorders of the hip. J Bone Joint Surg 60A:1099–1105
48. Shirkhoda A, Brashear HR, Staab EV (1980) Computed tomography of acetabular fractures. Radiology 134:683–687

Renal Failure:
Prevention and Treatment

Role of Endothelial Injury in the Pathogenesis of Acute Renal Failure

G. H. Neild

Introduction

Acute renal failure in a sick patient is principally a consequence of renal ischemia, with the renal tubule being most vulnerable. This ischemic injury results in "acute tubular necrosis" (ATN), a reversible condition, except when the ischemia is so profound that tubular infarction ("cortical necrosis") occurs. While the cause of oliguria and ATN is relatively uncontroversial, the mechanism by which these are sustained is less clear. However, for the purpose of this chapter we are principally concerned with measures which will prevent or minimize acute renal failure, and so require an understanding of the mechanisms leading to ATN.

How Does Normal Glomerular Filtration Occur?

The glomerular circulation is not truly capillary as no metabolism occurs. The glomerular capillary can be considered as a hemi-arteriole since on one side it is covered by mesangial cells, which are derived from smooth muscle. The glomerular basement membrane (GBM) is freely permeable to crystalloids and filtration across the membrane is proportional to the hydrostatic pressure inside the capillary. (The hemodynamics of the glomerulus are in all way analogous to a hemofiltration system). The hydrostatic pressure inside the glomerulus is regulated by the two capacitance vessels, the afferent and efferent arterioles. For filtration to occur the hydrostatic pressure has to exceed the sum of the capillary oncotic pressure and the opposing tubular fluid pressure in Bowman's space. When renal blood flow is decreased hydrostatic pressure may be maintained by an increase in efferent arteriolar tone relative to afferent tone. If the hydrostatic pressure falls below a critical level filtration will cease even though blood still flows through the glomerular capillary circulation.

The tone in the arterioles is influenced by several vasoactive system – sympathetic nervous system, renin-angiotensin, prostaglandins and thromboxanes [1]. The potential role of vascular paracrine mediators such as neuropeptides and endothelium-derived relaxant factor (EDRF) are still being explored. The rate of filtration, i.e. glomerular filtration rate (GFR), also depends on the total capillary surface area available for filtration and the rate of plasma flow. Vasoconstrictors such as angiotensin, not only increase arteriolar tone but cause mesangial cell contraction thus reducing effective capillary surface area [2].

Thus, glomerular ultrafiltration is controlled by arteriolar tone, which in turn is regulated by the nephron's own computer – the juxta-glomerular apparatus (JGA). The concept of "tubulo-glomerular feedback" has evolved whereby the specialized part of the distal convoluted tubule (the macula densa) adjacent to the JGA senses the ionic composition of the tubular fluid and from this signal (probably chloride ion concentration) regulates ultrafiltration [2, 3].

Why Does Oliguria Occur in ARF?

There are two components to this question. Firstly why does oliguria occur and secondly how is it sustained? We are principally concerned with the first question.

There are many factors that may lead to ATN, but, as in so many conditions, there is a final common pathway. Thurau and his colleagues have proposed the most likely sequence of events [3]. The renal tubule is particularly sensitive to ischemia. Much of its large oxygen consumption is concerned with the active reabsorption of salt and water by the loop of Henle. Under normal circumstances the tubular fluid at the junction of the ascending limb of the loop of Henle and the DCT is hypotonic. As tubular damage progresses the ability to reabsorb salt and water fails and the tonicity of the tubular fluid at the macula densa rises. It is this signal that changes arteriolar tone to the point at which ultrafiltration may cease altogether [3, 4]. The reason why oliguria persists, particularly when renal blood flow is restored, is less certain. It may be partly related to intraluminal tubular obstruction, partly related to a back leak of tubular fluid through the injured tubules into the renal interstitium [4–6].

Mechanisms of Tubular Injury

Ischemia

Tubular cells have a large oxygen consumption and concomitantly rich blood supply via peritubular capillaries and the medullary vasa rectae. If this capillary circulation is compromised tubular ischemia will occur.

The part of the nephron most susceptible to ischemia appears to be the thick ascending limb of the loop of Henle and the distal segment of the proximal tubule [5, 7, 8]. As a consequence of ischemia, cells become depleted of energy stores (ADP, ATP), they swell, become more permeable to sodium, and there is a rise in intracellular calcium. Cell swelling may contribute to both an increase in vascular resistance in adjacent capillaries and tubular obstruction [5, 7]. Treatment aimed at reducing cellular injury will be discussed later. Pathological changes include loss of the epithelial cell brush border, cell necrosis, casts in the loop of Henle, and nucleated erythrocytes and inflammatory cells in vasa rectae.

Direct Tubular Toxicity

Tubular injury may also be the result of a direct toxic insult as occurs with carbon tetrachloride poisoning. In some examples, both in man and experimental models, such as aminoglycoside poisoning, it is likely that both ischemia and toxicity play a role [5].

Experimental Models of ATN

Models of ischemic injury include temporary renal artery occlusion, intra-renal infusion of norepinephrine, and intramuscular injection of glycerol. Models of toxicity include administration of uranyl nitrate, and mercuric chloride. These models will be discussed.

Renal Ischemia

Pre-renal Failure (Physiological Ischemia)

The commonest causes of decreased renal perfusion include volume contraction, severe heart failure, arrhythmias, sepsis, hepatorenal failure [9, 10]. Hypovolemia may be readily treated and this "prerenal failure" can be reversed.

The immediate increase in renal vascular resistance in response to hypovolemia and heart failure is mediated by massive sympathetic activity with secondary activation of the renin-antiogensin system. Although renal blood flow is decreased, glomerular filtration (GFR) may be preserved initally by a disproportionate rise in efferent arteriolar tone, which is mediated in particular by angiotensin. In addition the increased tone in the pre-glomerular vessels is offset by local, renal production of vasodilatory prostaglandins. For these reasons the use of either angiotensin-converting enzyme inhibitors or inhibitors of cyclo-oxygenase may cause a precipitous decline in GFR and sometimes oliguria.

If hypovolemia is not corrected the decreased renal perfusion will lead to ATN and established renal failure. The major causes of ATN are hypoperfusion, nephrotoxins, sepsis and rhabdomyolysis, often with several factors occurring together. In approximately 60% of cases this will occur in a surgical setting [9, 10].

Relationship to GFR

In experimental models of ischemia there is a reduction in renal blood flow by more than 50% with a rise in renal vascular resistance. Once ATN is established, renal blood flow may return to normal and the reduction in GFR is out of proportion to the blood flow. Correction of blood flow during the initial phase of injury will lead to recovery of GFR, but if correction occurs after 24–48 hours GFR dose not recover. In models of toxic injury renal blood flow is often, but not consistently, decreased and volume expansion and vasodilation do not cause a rise in GFR [5].

In ATN there is evidence in man of reduced blood flow particularly to the cortex. Blood flow is reduced by 25–50% of normal, and GFR is disproportionaly decreased. It is likely that this disproportionate and sustained reduction in GFR is due to reduction in the effective capillary surface area (Kf). Direct measurements of Kf by micro-puncture and other techniques have confirmed this in several models of ATN [5, 10, 11].

Regional Variations in Renal Perfusion

At first renal hypoperfusion leads to a relative reduction in flow to the outer cortex (physiological hypoperfusion). However when medullary blood flow is reduced ischemic damage to the local tubules occurs [7, 8, 12]. This leads to severe impairment of urinary concentrating ability and sodium reabsorption, with the consequences on page 662.

In renal sections, the dark zone at the outer medulla seen in ATN is due to intense vascular congestion. Using colloidal carbon or silicon rubber, obstruction of the vasculature in the deep cortex and outer medulla is found in experimental models. In established ATN, there is a reduction in medullary blood flow of greater than 50% (shown by microsphere techniques, hydrogen clearance, Rb extraction) even when blood flow to the outer cortex is restored. This regional impairment may be reduced in some experimental circumstances by clonidine, but not by heparin. The precise role played by endothelial and epithelial cell swelling, rheological, humoral and neural factors is unclear [reviewed by 5].

How in Renal Ischemia Sustained?

In ATN the mechanism of continued reduction in renal blood flow is unknown. It has been suggested that endothelial swelling prevents recovery ("no re-flow" phenomenum). However endothelial swelling is patchy and transient [13], with the exception in the cortico-medullary area were it is consistent and persists [7].

In experimental ATN, loss of renal autoregulation occurs [14, 15]. This may have two consequences: firstly, there may not be the expected compensatory vasodilation following the initial ischemia, and secondly the kidney will not be protected from subsequent falls in perfusion pressure. This may explain the observation in man that active tubular necrosis continues for some days after the inital insult.

Locally produced vasoconstrictors such as thromboxane may add a further insult to a compromised microcirculation.

Finally, in these models, vascular pathology in capacitance vessels in the form of focal and segmental arteriolar necrosis is seen. This is probably a consequence of the initial severe vasospasm, but may contribute to any continuing reduction in blood flow [13–15].

Is Endothelial Injury Involved?

There are several ways in which one might expect endothelial injury to play a role.

a) Ischemia may damage the capillary endothelium. This might cause endothelial swelling and capillary obstruction. However, as discussed previously there is very little evidence for this except in the medullary vessels.
b) Endothelial damage may cause platelet aggregation and thrombosis to occur. It is possible that this may also occur in the glomerular as well as the tubular circulation. Unfortunately, platelets can only be identified by electron microscopy and, if they are involved, they are likely to have degranulated and be unrecognizable. Similar fibrin may be very difficult to identify as the fibrinolytic capacity of the endothelium is so large that fibrin persists only when the system is overwhelmed. In attempting to address this question Mason and her colleagues found that neither aspirin nor heparin were able to modify medullary vascular obstruction [12]. However both pathological and functional aspects of this injury were prevented by either raising perfusion pressure or lowering blood hematocrit [12].
c) Sepsis may trigger off localized intravascular coagulation leading to occlusion of the capillary microcirculation and secondary endothelial damage. Models of endotoxin shock can produce renal failure and thrombosis in the renal microcirculation. However, there is little information regarding the renal microcirculation and sepsis in either man or experimental models.
d) It has been suggested that alterations in the morphology of glomerular endothelium, in particular a reduction in the size and number of fenestrations, may play a role in the maintenance of reduced GFR [5, 10]. Significant changes have been reported in a number of models, but some of these changes may be artefactual, since very careful studies in other models have shown no abnormalities [16].

Therapeutic Approaches to the Prevention of ATN

There is no single protection maneuver which is universally effective.

Volume Loading

Hypovolemia makes the kidney more susceptible to ATN, and volume expansion protects. It has been known for many years that chronic saline loading will reduce or prevent ATN in many experimental models of ATN [4, 5, 10]. Volume expansion will suppress the renin-angiotensin system. Very high levels of renin may commonly be found in the initial stages of acute renal failure, and as discussed earlier it would seem likely that this system should play a key role. Nevertheless, inhibitors of this system have been singularly unsuccessful in attenuating ATN. Mannitol may also be effective in this way.

Solute Diuresis

Saline infusions and mannitol may also protect by maintaining a solute diuresis. It is more difficult to understand the mechanism here unless the diuresis reduces the possibility of tubular obstruction. Related to this is some evidence that frusemide may protect. Observations in the isolated perfused kidney have suggested that reduction in active transport and O_2 demand in the thick ascending limb protects the tubule from anoxia [5].

Vasodilators

There is some evidence that vasodilators may help prevent the onset of ATN. Mannitol has a vasodilator effect on the kidney, mediated by vasodilatory prostaglandins and independent of volume expansion. Dopamine in lose doses has also been shown to have some protective effect in experimental models. Saline may also have an effect in this way.

Cyto-protection

There is very little consistent evidence that drugs such as mannitol have an effect through reducing cell swelling. A number of means of protecting cells have been tried: these include ATP-$MgCl_2$, inosine, calcium-channel blockers, DMSO. Enthusiastic reports have suggested some benefit from them all [5, 10].

Conclusions

It now appears that pathological reduction in medullary blood flow plays a critical role in the intiation of ATN following ischemia. There have been no recent established advances in the prevention of ATN. Measures which keep the patient's blood volume expanded and maintain a diuresis are likely to help protect. Recent experimental work suggests that a low hematocrit may reduce the medullary pathology.

References

1. Heller J (1987) Effect of vasoactive mediators on renal haemodynamics. Nephrol Dial Transplant 2:197–204
2. Brenner BM, Dworkin LD, Ichikawa I (1986) Glomerular Ultrafiltration. In: Brenner BM, Rector FC (eds) The Kidney, 3rd ed. Saunders, Philadelphia, pp 124–144
3. Thurau K, Boylan JW (1976) Acute renal success. The unexpected logic of oliguria in acute renal failure. Am J Med 61:308–315
4. Levinsky NG (1977) Pathophysiology of acute renal failure. N Engl J Med 296:1453–1458
5. Brezis M, Rosen S, Epstein FH (1986) Acute Renal Failure. In: Brenner BM, Rector FC (eds) The Kidney, 3rd ed. Saunders, Philadelphia, pp 735–799

6. Myers BD, Moran SM (1986) Hemodynamically mediated acute renal failure. N Engl J Med 314:97–105
7. Frega NS, Dibona DR, Guertler B, Leaf A (1976) Ischemic renal injury. Kidney Intern 10:S17–S25
8. Mason J, Torhorst J, Welsch J (1984) Role of the medullary perfusion defect in the pathogenesis of ischemic renal failure. Kidney Intern 26:283–293
9. Hou SH, Bushinsky DA, Wish JB, Cohen JJ, Harrington JT (1983) Hospital acquired renal insufficiency: a prospective study. Am J Med 74:243–252
10. Gross PA, Anderson RJ (1985) Acute renal failure and toxic nephropathy. In: Klahr S, Massry SG (eds) Contemporary Nephrology. Plenum, New York, p 447
11. Williams RH, Thomas CE, Navar LG, Evan AP (1981) Hemodynamic and single nephron function during the maintenance phase of ischemic acute renal failure in the dog. Kidney Intern 19:503–515
12. Mason J, Welsch J, Torhorst J (1987) The contribution of vascular obstruction to the functional defect that follows renal ischemia. Kidney Intern 31:65–71
13. Kashgarian M, Siegel NJ, Ries AL, DiMeola HJ, Hayslett JP (1976) Hemodynamic aspects in development and recovery phases of experimental postischemic acute renal failure. Kidney Intern 10:S160–S168
14. Adams PL, Adams FF, Bell PD, Navar LG (1980) Impaired renal blood flow autoregulation in ischemic acute renal failure. Kidney Intern 18:68–76
15. Matthys E, Patton MK, Osgood RW, Venkatachalam MA, Stein JH (1983) Alterations in vascular function and morphology in acute ischemia renal failure. Kidney Intern 23:717–724
16. Bulger RE, Eknoyan G, Purcell DJ, Dobyan DC (1983) Endothelial characteristics of glomerular capillaries in normal, mercuric chloride-induced and gentamicin-induced acute renal failure in the rat. J Clin Invest 72:128–141

Value of Diagnostic Investigations in Acute Renal Failure

R. L. Lins, M. Coutenye, and M. E. De Broe

Introduction

Acute renal failure (ARF) may be defined as an abrupt decline in renal function, sufficient to result in an elevation of serum creatinine above 2 mg/dl (177 µmol/l) or, in patients with preexisting chronic renal failure, an increase in serum creatinine by 50% of the baseline value. This renal failure may be of the oliguric or non-oliguric type. Although acute renal failure is easy to recognize, it is often confused with its main cause, which is inaccurately described as acute tubular necrosis (ATN) or acute vasomotor nephropathy. This is mainly due to the fact that the exact pathophysiologic mechanism of this condition is still poorly understood, despite great experimental efforts in this field.

It is however very important to classify the patient as early as possible after the onset of the acute renal failure in one of the etiologic categories, because this has immediate consequences for the further management.

Causes of Acute Renal Failure

The syndrome may evolve from transient diminished renal blood flow (i.e. prerenal ARF) from a sudden renal insult (i.e. intrinsic renal ARF) or from obstruction to urine flow (i.e. postrenal ARF). The most important causes are listed in Table 1. The first step is localization of the site of damage and once the disease is classified to one of the three areas, the specific treatment is usually quite apparent.

For intrarenal events it is most useful to identify the anatomical element primarily affected. Consequently a nephrobiopsy is the only reliable method for this purpose. In a series of 96 consecutive patients with severe ARF, defined as a sudden increase in creatinine to more than 4 mg/dl, who were admitted to the Renal Unit between 1/1/80 and 31/12/82 we noted an incidence of prerenal ARF in 4%, intrinsic renal ARF in 79% and postrenal ARF in 17% of cases.

Table 1. Causes of acute renal failure

Prerenal:	*Renal hypoperfusion*
	– Reduced cardiac output
	– cardiogenic shock
	– congestive heart failure
	– cardiac tamponade
	– Volume depletion
	– hemorrhage
	– gastrointestinal losses
	– sequestration (pancreatitis, burns, peritonitis ...)
Postrenal:	*Obstructive nephropathy*
	– Ureteral obstruction
	– stones, papillary necrosis, blood clots, tumor
	– retroperitoneal fibrosis, surgical ligation
	– Bladder obstruction
	– prostatic hypertrophy, cervix cancer
	– urethral obstruction
Renal:	*Glomerular-vascular*
	– glomerulonephritis
	– accelerated hypertension
	– hemolytic uremic syndrome
	– vasculitis
	– amyloidosis
	– pregnancy nephropathy
	– cholesterol emboli
	Interstitial
	– drugs
	– hypercalcemia, hypokalemia
	Acute tubular necrosis
	– shock
	– nephrotoxins: aminoglycosides, radiocontrast material, cisplatinum, heavy metals, poisons
	– pigments: myoglobin, hemoglobin
	Tubular obstruction
	– proteins: multiple myeloma, amyloidosis
	– crystals: uric acid, Ca-oxalate

Medical History and Physical Examination

The medical history can help us to find some etiological factors that may have contributed to the ARF. A recent history of events potentially responsible for a reduction in effective arterial blood volume, due to external losses, internal redistribution of heart failure must draw our attention to possible prerenal ARF. The presence of nephrotoxic substances such as drugs, intravenous contrast media or certain circulation poteins points toward acute tubular necrosis or acute interstitial nephritis [1]. A history of urinary tract obstruction or prostatism suggest postrenal failure.

Physical examination may show signs of dehydration or fluid retention: one of the most useful tools for the nephrologist in assessing and following the patient with ARF is a patient scale. Dermal involvement may be suggestive for allergic causes like in drug-induced acute interstitial nephritis or for multisystem diseases as in different forms of vasculitis. A tentative diagnosis of postrenal ARF may be derived from evaluation of bladder distention, prostatic examination in man and pelvic examination in women.

Urine Examination

Urine Volume

Non-oliguric renal failure is defined as an urine output greater than 500 ml/24 h. It occurs in at least 40% of cases of ARF [2]. A volume of 100 to 400 ml/24 h is called oliguria. This distinction is clinically relevant since the mortality rate is 50% in oliguric patients and only 26% in patients with non-oliguric ARF [3]. We define anuria as a 24-h urine volume less than 50 ml. Complete anuria occurs rarely and is caused by lower urinary tract obstruction, sometimes by acute glomerulonephritis and very rarely by bilateral renal artery occlusion or by cortical necrosis [4].

Urinary Indices

Normal tubules, stimulated by hypovolemia, reabsorb solute-free water and sodium elaborating sodium-free urine that is more highly concentrated than plasma. Kidneys suffering intrinsic damage cannot adequately process the glomerular filtrate, causing the production of a small volume of sodium-rich urine, the concentration of which remains close of that of plasma. This has been attributed in ATN to a decreased sensitivity of collecting tubules to antidiuretic hormone [5]. Based on these assumptions urinary diagnostic indices were found to discriminate in most cases between prerenal and renal values (Table 2) [6].

Although 80% of oliguric patients can be classified based on the urinary osmolality, 10% of patients with ATN and 10% of patients with prerenal ARF have however unexpected values [6]. For urinary sodium excretion there is also a large degree of overlap so that intermediary values yield little diagnostic aid. The fractional excretion of sodium (FE_{Na}) and the renal failure index (RFI) have been offered as more precise indices of renal tubule sodium reabsorption, and it

Table 2. Urinary indices in acute renal failure

	Prerenal	Renal
Urinary osmolality (mOsm/kg)	> 500	< 350
Urine/plasma osmolality	> 1.2	< 1.2
Urinary sodium (mEq/l)	< 20	> 40
Urine/plasma urea	> 8	< 3
RFI = $(U_{Na})/(U/P$ creatinine)	< 1	> 4
FE_{Na}(%) = $(U/P_{Na})/(U/P_{krea} \times 100)$	< 1	> 3

has been suggested that they are more likely to effectivily separate prerenal from intrinsic renal ARF [7]. The tendency to loose sodium despite salt depletion in ATN has been attributed to an impaired sodium reabsorption particularly of the proximal tubule [5]. Fractional excretion of filtered sodium (FE_{Na}) has been found to be less than 1.0% in 94% of patients with prerenal ARF. The renal failure index (RFI) is less than 1.0% in 85% of patients with prerenal ARF, while no patients with ATN had a RFI of less than 1.98% [6]. There are however also exceptions to these rules. A significant number of patients with otherwise classic oliguric and non-oliguric ARF have FE_{Na} and RFI consistent with prerenal ARF. This was demonstrated in patients with extensive burns, nephrotic syndrome and heart failure, after cardiac surgery, with renal allograft rejection, rhabdomyolysis, ARF due to converting enzyme inhibitors and contrast-induced ARF [8]. This was also demonstrated in non-oliguric ARF with sodium-acid states, such as cirrhosis with ascites. This could be explained by augmented angiotensin II generation due to renal hypoperfusion, resulting in diminished peritubular capillary pressure leading to enhanced proximal solute and water reabsorption [8]. Another potential efferent factor is distal tubular overreabsorption due to secondary hyperaldosteronism. It becomes even more complicated when prerenal ARF occurs in a non-oliguric form with RFI below 1%. This has ben attributed to a concentrating defect. Intrinsic renal values associated with prerenal failure are described in elderly patients and in hypertension [4]. Anderson and colleagues [9] have found that urinary chloride concentration provided a more sensitive and equally specific parameter when compared with urinary sodium concentration in distinguishing between prerenal azotemia and acute tubular necrosis. These results await further confirmation. The ratios of urinary to plasma creatinine and urinary to plasma creatinine and urea show also an important diagnostic overlap.

There are also conditions where urinary diagnostic indices cannot separate unequivocally between prerenal and renal values, like in acute glomerulonephritis where they can be similar to the values observed in prerenal ARF, because of normal tubular function [6]. In most patients with acute interstitial nephritis the indices are of the renal type except if there is a concomitant important proteinuria. In these rare cases described with the use of non-steroidal anti-inflammatory drugs urinary sodium is low [10].

Postrenal causes of ARF can also be associated with indices similar to those of prerenal ARF early in the course of obstruction. With continued obstruction the indices mimic these of intrinsic renal disease. It is also important that these urinary indices are meaningless for diagnosing prerenal ARF if tubular concentrating mechanisms and sodium reabsorption are reduced for other reasons: chronic uremia and the use of diuretics before the collection of the urine sample on admission.

In conclusion, the utility of urinary indices in the differential diagnosis of ARF must be interpreted in conjunction with clinical, physical and additional laboratory investigations. Physicians do well not to slavishly follow the numbers if they do not fit with their clinical assessment. With these restrictions in mind the indices are a valuable tool in the early diagnosis and management of patients with ARF.

Urinary Sediment

Microscopic and chemical urine analysis affords inexpensive but valuable information in the differential diagnosis of intrinsic renal ARF [11]. Granular, dirty brown casts and epithelial cellular casts are described as characteristic elements of ATN. Free erythrocytes and red blood cell casts denote the presence of acute glomerulonephritis or vasculitis, and are frequently associated with proteinuria greater than 1 g/24 hours. Since red blood cells (RBC) may gain access to the urine at any level of the urinary tract, differentiating glomerular from postrenal hematuria would be welcomed. Using phase microscopy distorted RBC suggestive of glomerular hematuria could be distinguished. A sensitivity of 80% and a specificity of 90% were noted [12]. Mild proteinuria, microscopic hematuria and leukocyturia with marked eosinophiluria are characteristic for acute interstitial nephritis. In the series of Galpin et al [13] eosinophils accounted for one-third of the white blood cells (WBC) in the urinary sediment of patients with methicillin-induced nephropathy, but the absence of eosinophils has no discriminatory value. The use of the Hansel's stain instead of the classical Wright stain substantially improves the recognition of eosiniphiluria. Indeed a prevalence of 10 in 11 patients with acute interstitial nephritis and none in 30 patients with acute tubular necrosis was found [14]. Numerous leukocytes with casts are suggestive of pyelonephritis. These cellular findings are obviously meaningless for diagnostic purposes in the presence of an indwelling bladder catheter [4].

Chemical testing like a positive reaction with orthotoluidine dipstick – in the absence of red blood cells in the sediment – indicates the presence of myoglobin as seen in rhabdomyolysis, or of hemoglobin as seen in acute hemolytic anemias.

Laboratory Pitfalls

It should be pointed out that in some conditions serum creatinine becomes less reliable as index of renal function. Both cimetidine, trimethoprim and quinidine-like drugs may cause a slight increase in serum creatinine without changing glomerular filtration rate due to competitive inhibition of creatinine secretion by the proximal tubules [15].

Serum values of urea are influenced by protein intake or by the catabolic state of the patient. They are particularly misleading in the case of gastro-intestinal hemorrhage due to the enhanced production of ureum from the blood present in the gut, which causes a disproportionate increase in urea even in the absence of renal failure. The opposite occurs in cases of renal failure in combination with liver failure.

The serum values of amylase are bad indices for acute pancreatitis unless serum levels exceed 10 times the upper limit of normal and hyperlipasemia has no diagnostic value at all, as we showed recently in a series of 42 consecutive patients with ARF [16].

Hemodynamic Evaluation

Although the vast majority of patients with prerenal ARF may be identified by the clinical and laboratory investigations already outlined, there are some whose volume status cannot be clearly quantified. In these settings central venous pressure and pulmonary capillary wedge pressure are invaluable guides to therapy. Such clinical settings are: hypoalbuminemic, edematous patients, overdiurized patients with chronic heart failure, elderly azotemic patients with compromised cardiac status, hypovolemic cirrhotics. However, since infection is the most common cause of death in ARF, catheters have not to be used unless absolutely indicated.

Radiological Studies

Radiological examinations are often invaluable for determining whether obstructive uropathy is present, for differentiating acute from chronic disease, and for assessing the patency of renal arteries and veins.

Tomography of Kidneys

Tomography without contrast media still remains an important tool in the differential diagnosis of ARF. It is used to determine kidney size and shape and to identify radiopaque stones. Shrunken kidneys are an early clue to chronic renal damage and swollen kidneys are suggestive for acute obstruction or acute interstitial nephritis. These X-ray films are also useful as a guide to perform renal biopsy.

Intravenous Urography

Radiocontrast media can induce intrinsic ARF in patients with pre-existing renal failure. Intravenous urography is useful to determine kidney size and to exclude obstruction, but this information can be obtained either without contrast, or by echography. This procedure has a limited place in ARF.

Antegrade Percutaneous Techniques

These techniques allow for localization of the exact site of obstruction while avoiding the need for general anesthesia in patients who are commonly infected and hemodynamically unstable. Following drainage by a nephrostomy catheter and improvement in renal function, patients are better suited for more invasive diagnostic and therapeutic procedures. Reported success rate is 95 to 98% [17]. Mortality from percutaneous nephrostomy is less than 0.2% while surgical nephrostomy has a mortality rate of 6% in different series [11].

Retrograde Pyelography

Due to the development of newer techniques, the use of retrograde pyelography has greatly diminished. It is still helpful in defining sites of obstruction and its immediate relief when visualization is minimal with ultrasonography or computerized axial tomography. Complications have become less frequent but introduction of bacteria into the urinary tract, ureteral trauma and allergic reactions can still occur.

Computerized Axial Tomography

At present it would appear that ultrasound tomographies provide sufficient informtion to make CT scanning unnecessary in most cases of ARF. However, the examination has given reliable information regarding the presence of renal tissue, kidney size, hydronephrosis and evaluation of renal cortical thickness in order to exclude chronical renal failure.

Arteriography

Renal arteriography offers little diagnostic or prognostic value in the evaluation of the parenchymal lesions in ARF. Its limited role – and more recently that of digital substraction angiography –, can be considered in the demonstration of renal artery occlusion.

Ultrasonography

Renal echography provides the most important contribution to ARF among recent medical imaging technology. It is a safe, reliable and widely available technique to immediately exclude urinary tract obstruction. Dilatation of the urinary tract is detectable within 24 to 36 hours after the onset of obstruction. It has a 98% sensitivity and a 74% specificity [18].

The echogram is also useful for evaluating the renal cortex, perirenal collections and ureteral calculi, which may all be important in defining the etiology of ARF.

Radionuclide Studies

Although there are important advances in the use of these techniques in renal disease, they are not sufficiently precise for routine use in the evaluation of ARF. Several attempts have been made to correlate these tests to individual disorders but they are not ready for clinical use. Their major indication relates to the assessment of vascular perfusion of the kidney.

Renal Biopsy

There is still some controversy among nephrologists as to the proper approach to using renal biopsy as a tool in ARF. In selected patients it can provide important information that can influence diagnosis, prognosis, and therapy.

In large series renal biopsy has been performed in 12 to 28% of patients with ARF [19–22]. Biopsies are not performed in cases of prerenal or postrenal ARF. Possible indications for renal biopsy in patients with intrinsic ARF include:

1. no obvious etiology;
2. ARF lasting more than two to three weeks;
3. evidence for glomerular disease e.g. from the urinary sediment;
4. evidence for systemic disease, e.g. vasculitis;
5. possible interstitial nephritis due to drugs, especially in patients who require continuous therapy with the alleged drug;
6. acute renal failure after transplantation.

In an unselected series of 91 patients with ARF, who were all biopsied, acute tubulo-interstitial nephritis was found in 62%, with only 4% of acute interstitial nephritis, and glomerulonephritis in 20% [23]. In most series renal biopsy was only performed in selected patients. The reported incidences are 16 to 43% for tubulo-interstitial disease, 11 to 15% for acute interstitial nephritis, 24 to 52% for glomerulonephritis, and 16 to 25% for acute vascular lesions [19–22]. Most clinical diagnosis agreed with the histopathological findings.

In a retrospective analysis of 183 biopsies performed in our departement between 1/1/78 and 31/12/86 the incidences were: ATN 15%, acute interstitial nephritis 8%, acute glomerulonephritis 13%, acute rejection 28%. The correlation between clinical diagnosis and anatomopathological findings was 62,9%. If we exclude posttransplant biopsies (mostly rejection), that account for 38% of cases, the correlation is only 53%. The importance of renal biopsy for diagnosis can be derived from calculations of sensitivity and of specificity of clinical diagnosis in three series, including our own (Table 3) [21, 23]. These results show that there

Table 3. Sensitivity and specificity of clinical diagnosis of ARF, compared with histological findings

	Mustonen et al. [23] (n = 91)		Richet et al. [21] (n = 178)		present series (n = 183)	
	sens. %	spec. %	sens. %	spec. %	sens. %	spec. %
All bopsies	69	81	73	71	67	62
Glomerular	56	67	93	57	42	53
Tubulo-interstitial	77	86	46	89	81	47
Interstitial			75	55	29	31
Vascular			82	93		
Systemic disease	75	75			71	67
Rejection					85	92

are important rates of false positive and false negative diagnosis making biopsy worthwhile in these cases.

Renal biopsy is also valuable in determining shortterm prognosis [23]. Also longterm prognosis can be predicted from histopathological findings [24]. In a series of 227 biopsies, Bonomini found normal renal function in 75% of cases after one year and 67% after 5 years in patients with acute interstitial nephritis. Among patients with ARF of glomerular origin these figures were 41 and 29%, respectively. Progression to endstage renal disease was noted in only 8% of patients with acute interstitial nephritis, but in 47% of acute glomerulonephritis. Attempts have been made to make clinicopathological correlates based on more quantitative, histomorphometric methods. Interstitial volume is directly correlated with the most recent available serum creatinine concentration and inversely related with prognosis [25].

Solez et al. [20] have demonstrated that the extent of tubular cell necrosis correlated with the duration of renal failure in patients with non-oliguric but not with oliguric renal failure. The histologic changes in acute glomerulonephritis correlate possibly better with prognosis than in ATN [11].

Biopsy findings influenced treatment in 19 to 22% of cases [21, 23], which influenced outcome in 58% of cases in one series [23]. In 62% of our biopsies diagnosis directly influence the further management of the patients.

Major complications are rare [21] and are not different from those in chronic renal failure. Even in patients with bleeding diathesis biopsy, guided by echography, can be performed safely after temporary correction of coagulation.

Conclusion

Given the range of conditions that can result in ARF and their different therapeutic implications, it is important to establish an accurate diagnosis. Initially one should distinguish prerenal, renal and postrenal causes, followed by investigations to find a more specific etiology.

The renal biopsy contributes substantially to the choice of a specific treatment for systemic disease, some forms of glomerulonephritis and acute interstitial nephritis. Further investigations will be needed to find clinicopathological correlations and to define the exact role of diagnostic procedures as renal biopsy in the diagnosis, prognosis and therapy of acute renal failure.

References

1. Kleinknecht D, Landais P, Goldfarb B (1968) Les insuffisances rénales aiguës associées à des médicaments ou à des produits iodés. Néphrologie 7:41-46
2. Anderson RJ, Schrier RW (1980) Clinical spectrum of oliguric and nonoliguric acute renal failure. In: Brenner BM, Stein JH (eds) Acute Renal Failure. Churchill Livingstone, New York, pp 1-16
3. Anderson RJ, Linas SL, Berns AS, et al (1977) Nonoliguric acute renal failure. N Engl J Med 296:1134-1138

4. Andreucci VE, Federico S, Memoli B, Usberti M (1985) Clinical diagnosis of acute renal failure. In: Andreucci VE (ed) Acute Renal Failure. Martinus Nijhoff Publishing, Boston, pp 189–200
5. Hanley MJ, Davidson K (1981) Prior mannitol and furosemide infusion in a model of ischemic acute renal failure. Am J Physiol 241:F556–564
6. Miller TR (1978) Urinary diagnostic indices in acute renal failure. Ann Intern Med 89:47–50
7. Espinel CH, Gregory AW (1980) Differential diagnosis of acute renal failure. Clin Nephrol 13:73–77
8. Zarich S, Leslie ST, Fang LST, Diamond JR (1985) Fractional excretion of sodium. – Exceptions to its diagnostic value. Arch Intern Med 145:108–112
9. Anderson RJ, Gabow PA, Gross PA (1984) Urinary chloride concentration in acute renal failure. Miner Electroyte Metab 10:92–97
10. Lins RL, Verpooten GA, De Clerck DS, De Broe ME (1986) Urinary indices in acute interstitial nephritis. Clin Nephrol 26:131–133
11. Rudnick MR, Bastl CP, Elfinbein IB, Narins RG (1983) The Differential Diagnosis of Acute Renal Failure. In: Brenner BM, Lazarus JM (eds) Acute Renal Failure. WB Saunders Company, Philadelphia, pp 176–222
12. Bouffet E, Laville M, Zanettini MC, Pellet H, Buenerd A, Traeger J (1984) Le sédiment urinaire dans l'insuffisance rénale aiguë. Presse Medical 13:2307–2310
13. Galpin JE, Shinaberger JH, Stanley TM, et al (1978) Acute interstitial nephritis due to methicillin. Am J Med 65:756–765
14. Nolan CR, Anger MS, Kelleher SP (1986) Eosinophiluria – A new method of detection and definition of the clinical spectrum. N Engl J Med 315:1516–1521
15. Muther RS (1983) Drug interference with renal function tests. Am J Kidney Dis 3:118–120
16. Zachée P, Lins RL (1985) Serum amylase and lipase values in acute renal failure. Clin Chemistry 31:1237
17. Stables DP (1982) Percutaneous nephrostomy: Techniques, indications, and results. Urol Clin N Am 9:15–29
18. Ellenbogen PH, Scheibl FW, Talner LB, Leopold GR (1978) Sensitivity of gray scale ultrasound in detecting urinary tract obstruction. AJR 130:731–740
19. Wilson DM, Turner DR, Cameron JS, Ogg CS, Brown CB, Chantler C (1976) Value of renal biopsy in acute intrinsic renal failure. Br Med J II,459–461
20. Solez K, Morel-Maroger L, Srear J-D (1979) The morfology of "Acute Tubular Necrosis" in man: Analysis of 57 renal biopsies and a comparison with the glycerol model. Medicine 58:362–376
21. Richet G, Duhoux P, Morel-Maroger L, Kourilsky O, Kanfer A, Sraer JD (1982) Biopsy as a guide in the treatment of 'medical' acute renal failure. In: Eliahou HE (ed) Acute Renal Failure. John Libbey, London, pp 200–206
22. Tanter Y, Dubot P, Mousson C, et al (1987) Acute renal failure due to glomerulonephritis in patients over 60. Interest of renal biopsy. Kidney Int 32:426
23. Mustonen J, Pasternack A, Helin H, Pystynen S, Tuominen T (1984) Renal biopsy in acute renal failure. Am J Nephrol 4:27–31
24. Bonomini V, Stefoni S, Vangelista A (1984) Long-term patient and renal prognosis in acute renal failure. Nephron 36:169–172
25. Bohle A, Mackensen-Haen S, Grund KE, Christ H, Knopfle E, Schellhorn S (1979) Shock Kidney. Path Res Pract 165:212–220

Ventilation and the Kidney

H. J. Priebe

Introduction

Respiratory support is amongst the most frequently employed therapeutic as well as prophylactic aids in anesthesia and intensive care. It is therefore important to be aware that respiratory support may impair renal function. The reason for this is essentially twofold:

a) patients requiring mechanical ventilation frequently suffer from underlying diseases that by themselves predispose to the development of renal insufficiency; and

b) ventilation per se predisposes to renal dysfunction. Ventilation should therefore be viewed as an additional risk factor for the development of acute renal failure.

Acute respiratory insufficiency is frequently associated with increased extravascular lung water. Mobilization of water may therefore become essential for improvement in gas exchange. If excretory renal function is impaired, respiratory function may worsen. As this will in turn necessitate more aggressive respiratory support, a viscious cycle may well be triggered. Mortality in patients with acute respiratory insufficiency is in the order of 20–40%. If additionally acute renal failure develops, mortality rises to 60–80%. Thus, overall mortality can be reduced only by effective prevention. This requires detailed knowledge of the interactions between ventilation and renal function.

Renal Effects of Ventilation

Since the first report by Drury in 1947 [1], the renal effects of various modes of ventilation have been examined in numerous human and experimental studies [see 2 and 3]. In particular, the renal effects of three modes of respiratory support have been studied: those of spontaneous respiration with continuous positive airway pressure (CPAP), those of intermittent positive pressure ventilation (IPPV), and those of mechanical ventilation with positive end-expiratory pressure (PEEP), i.e. continuous positive pressure ventilation (CPPV).

IPPV and CPAP tend to reduce renal blood flow (RBF), glomerular filtration rate (GFR), and urine output. The effects on urinary sodium excretion ($U_{Na}\dot{V}$), free water (C_{H_2O}) and osmolar clearance (C_{osm}) are somewhat inconsistent [3]. Of the various modes of respiratory support, CPPV has the most adverse effects on the kidney, and almost uniformly reduces RBF, GFR, $U_{Na}\dot{V}$, C_{osm} and urine output [3].

The results are difficult to compare because of substantial differences in study design. Different modes of ventilation have been evaluated in both the human and the experimental animal, with normal or diseased hearts and lungs, and awake or anesthetized. Temperature, hematocrit, serum oncotic pressure, intravascular volume, arterial blood gases and pH have rarely been controlled. However, all of these variables may affect renal function either directly or indirectly by modifying the response of the cardiovascular system of ventilation. Thus despite the multitude of existing data it will be very difficult if not impossible to predict the renal effects of ventilation in the individual patient.

Cardiovascular Effects of Ventilation

Renal function and hemodynamics are largely determined by systemic factors. Consequently, the extent to which renal function will be affected depends in part on changes in cardiovascular dynamics in response to institution of respiratory support. The extent of these alterations will, in turn, depend on mode of ventilation, lung compliance, blood volume and cardiac function.

Ventilation may affect the cardiovascular system in a variety of ways: it may alter cardiac output, systemic arterial pressure, pulse pressure, effective intervascular volume, and renal and hepatic venous pressures. Most studies demonstrating altered renal function during mechanical ventilation found simultaneous *decreases in cardiac output*. This would suggest a cause-and-effect relationship between reduced cardiac output and impaired renal function. However, the effect of the decrease in cardiac output per se on renal function is difficult to establish because of simultaneous changes in arterial pressure, pulse pressure, filling pressure and effective intravascular volume. Volume expansion during CPPV may completely restore renal function even though cardiac output remains depressed [4]. This would suggest that CPPV impairs renal function primarily by its *adverse effects on effective intravascular volume or renal perfusion pressure*, rather than its effect on cardiac output.

The increase in intrathoracic pressure following the institution of CPPV will result in an increase in inferior vena caval pressure. This, in turn, will cause *elevations in hepatic and renal venous pressures*. It has been suggested that both, per se, may interfere with renal function and intrarenal hemodynamics [5–7]. However, some of the observed changes are probably related to simultaneous impairment of cardiac output or arterial pressure [8]. It is, therefore, rather unlikely that elevated hepatic or renal venous pressures per se significantly contribute to renal dysfunction during ventilation. They may, however, play a contributory role when systemic arterial pressure falls during mechanical ventilation, thus reducing effective organ perfusion pressures.

Total *renal blood flow* is mostly reduced during respiratory support [3, 4]. In addition, redistribution of intrarenal blood flow during CPPV has been postulated [9], but could not be confirmed using the radioactive microsphere technique [4]. It is unlikely that redistribution of intrarenal blood flow plays a significant role in the pathogenesis of renal dysfunction during respiratory support.

Neural Effects of Ventilation

Low-pressure stretch receptors in cardiac atria and pulmonary veins sense changes in filling pressures and intrathoracic blood volume. The role of these *low-pressure cardiopulmonary receptors* in modulating renal function and hemodynamics during respiratory support remains controversial. In general, they may affect renal sympathetic nerve activity [10], renal vasomotor tone [11] and rening release [12]. However, denervation of the cardiopulmonary receptors prior to institution of PEEP does not necessarily ameliorate renal dysfunction [13].

In contrast, it has been reported that denervation of aortic arch and carotid sinus prevents changes in renal function in response to PEEP [13]. This would suggest that *systemic baroreceptors* play a crucial role in initiating renal dysfunction during CPPV. An inverse relationship exists between carotid sinus pressure and renal sympathetic nerve activity [14]. Unrelated to changes in renal perfusion pressure, an increase in renal sympathetic nerve activity can markedly reduce renal blood flow, GFR, urinary sodium excretion, and urine output [15].

The *renal nervers* constitute the efferent part of the reflex arc that originates at the low- and high-pressure receptors. In accordance with the previously cited work, renal denervation also prevents changes in renal function and hemodynamics in response to CPPV [16]. This clearly indicates that the renal nerves participate in the mediation of antidiuresis and antinatriuresis during CPPV.

The relative importance of low- vs high-pressure receptors in modulating renal function and intrarenal hemodynamics during ventilation in humans remains to be established. In the nonhuman primate, only combined sinoaortic denervation and vagotomy completely abolishes all changes in renal sympathetic nerve activity induced by changes in blood volume or systemic arterial pressure [17].

Humoral Effects of Ventilation

It has repeatedly been postulated that elevated levels of *antidiuretic hormone* (ADH) play an important role in the development of antidiuresis during respiratory support. ADH levels are mostly increased during CPPV, but they may remain unchanged [18] or even decrease during IPPV and CPAP [see 3]. More importantly, however, and contrary to what would be expected, free water clearance (C_{H_2O}) frequently remains unchanged despite elevated ADH levels [19, 29]. This would argue against a primary role of ADH in the pathogenesis of reduced urine output.

ADH release is regulated by osmotic and nonosmotic stimuli. Since plasma osmolality is rarely increased during CPPV, stimulation of osmoreceptors as the primary cause for enhanced ADH release can be ruled out in most cases. Low-pressure receptors in the left atrium and pulmonary veins, as well as high-pressure receptors in carotid sinus and possibly aortic arch also modulate ADH release. They respond to changes in blood volume [21], arterial pressure and possibly pulse pressure [22]. In fact most data indicate that increased ADH levels during CPPV are the result of changes in systemic hemodynamics [23]. This would best explain why elevated ADH levels during CPPV are not associated with reduced C_{H_2O}. Since ADH even within physiologic concentrations can act as a vasoconstrictior [24], it may well help to counteract hemodynamic alterations during respiratory support.

It should also be remembered that ADH is not required to produce a concentrated urine or a decrease in C_{H_2O}. Any condition associated with a severely depressed GFR may result in a maximally concentrated urine and a decrease in C_{H_2O} with subsequent hyponatremia and fluid retention [25, 26].

Plasma *renin* activity and plasma *aldosterone* levels may increase during CPPV [27]. This is probably related to renal nerve stimulation, or reductions in renal perfusion pressure and glomerular filtration. The positive correlation between plasma renin activity and plasma aldosterone levels would suggest that aldosterone levels are elevated secondary to an increased release of renin and *angiotensin*.

It has recently been suggested that the antidiuretic and antinatriuretic effects of PEEP may in part be mediated by a decrease in *atrial natriuretic peptide* [28].

Therapeutic Implications

Reduced excretory function must be viewed as a compensatory mechanism by which the kidney tries to restore effective intravascular volume. This may reverse some of the initial cardiovascular and renal effects. However, improvement in renal function during CPPV by mere volume expansion may take longer than two days and is expected to be associated with clinically relevant fluid and sodium retention [29]. In addition, improvement in renal function by gradual volume expansion may well be dependent on simultaneous augmentation of cardiac output. Such a response to volume expansion during CPPV is not necessarily to be expected in patients with underlying cardiopulmonary problems.

Renal dysfunction during ventilation may resemble prerenal failure. Since prerenal failure predisposes to the development or acute renal failure, it must be corrected as quickly as possible. *Adequate filling pressures, cardiac output and perfusion pressures* are essential. Experimental evidence would suggest that higher than normal cardiac filling pressures may be even more important than restoration of cardiac output [4].

A clinical dilemma frequently arises because what is therapeutically optimal for the kidney is not necessarily optimal for other organ systems. In fact many times therapeutic requirements will oppose each other. Ventilation may become necessary because of combined pulmonary and cardiac insufficiency. In such a situation, neither aggressive volume expansion nor liberal augmentation of systemic pressure are feasible as means of protecting the kidney. Therefore, no therapeutic recommendations can be made that would suit every clinical situation. The initial therapeutic priority will clearly be determined by that particular life-supporting organ whose function is critically impaired. If oxygenation is so severely impaired that life is threatened, then every effort must be made to improve oxygenation even if this further impairs renal function. On the other hand, if respiratory function is not a crucial problem, it may at times be reasonable to accept transient worsening in pulmonary function in order to protect the kidney. The reasoning is that mortality from combined respiratory and acute renal failure is much higher than that from isolated respiratory insufficiency caused by fluid overload.

Prophylaxis starts with choosing that mode of ventilation that is least likely to depress cardiac performance. If severe impairment of oxygenation requires fluid restriction and low cardiac filling pressures, pharmacological means of protecting the kidney should be considered early on. The detrimental effects of CPPV on renal function in patients with acute respiratory failure could all be corrected by *dopamine* at a mean dose of 5 ± 0.5 $\mu g \cdot kg^{-1} \cdot min^{-1}$ [30]. Irrespective of whether dopamine at this dose improved renal function by either its benefical effects on cardiac performance or its direct effects on the kidney, it is a valuable alternative to volume expansion. Because of its specific renal effects, low-dose dopamine ($0.5-2$ $\mu g \cdot kg^{-1} \cdot min^{-1}$) may benefit renal function at a dose that will rarely effect the cardiovascular system.

If renal function deteriorates even further, a *combination* of low-dose *dopamine plus furosemide* may be tried. A synergism between dopamine and furosemide in renal insufficiency has been described [31, 32]. If such an approach is chosen, meticulous attention to replacement of urine losses becomes essential. It must be remembered that the symptomatic treatment of oliguria by diuretics alone will not necessarily improve excretory renal function. On the contrary, it may even worsen renal function.

References

1. Drury DR, Henry JP, Goodman J (1947) Effects of continuous pressure breathing on kidney function. J Clin Invest 26:945–951
2. Berry AJ (1981) Respiratory support and renal function. Anesthesiology 55:655–667
3. Priebe H-J, Hedley-Whyte J (1984) Respiratory support and renal function. Int Anesth Clinics 22:203–226
4. Priebe H-J, Heimann JC, Hedley-Whyte J (1981) Mechanisms of renal dysfunction during positive end-expiratory pressure ventilation. J Appl Physiol 50:643–649
5. Levy M (1974) Renal function in dogs with acute selective hepatic venous outflow block. Am J Physiol 227:1074–1083
6. Schmid HE Jr (1972) Renal autoregulation and renin release during changes in renal perfusion pressure. Am J Physiol 222:1132–1237
7. Abe Y, Kishimoto T, Yamamoto K, et al (1973) Intrarenal distribution of blood flow during ureteral and venous pressure elevation. Am J Physiol 224:746–751
8. Priebe H-J, Heimann JC, Hedley-Whyte J (1980) Effects of renal and hepatic venous congestion on renal function in the presence of low and normal cardiac output in dogs. Circ Res 47:883–890
9. Hall SV, Johnson EE, Hedley-Whyte J (1974) Renal hemodynamics and function with continuous positive pressure ventilation in dogs. Anesthesiology 41:452–461
10. Clement DL, Pelletier CL, Shepherd JT (1972) Role of vagal afferents in the control of renal sympathetic nerve activity in the rabbit. Circ Res 31:824–830

11. Kahl FR, Flint JF, Szidon JP (1974) Influence of left atrial distention on renal vasomotor tone. Am J Physiol 226:240–246

12. Zehr JE, Hasbargen JA, Kurz KD (1976) Reflex suppression of renin secretion during distention of cardiopulmonary receptors in dogs. Circ Res 38:232–239

13. Fewell JE, Bond GC (1980) Role of sinoaortic baroreceptors in initiating the renal response to continuous positive-pressure ventilation in the dog. Anesthesiology 52:408–413

14. Kezdi P, Geller E (1968) Baroreceptor control of post ganglionic sympathetic nerve discharge. Am J Physiol 214:427–435

15. Schrier RW (1974) Effects of adrenergic nervous system and catecholamines on systemic and renal hemodynamics, sodium and water excretion and renin secretion. Kidney Int 6:291–306

16. Fewell JE, Bond GC (1979) Renal denervation eliminates the renal response to continuous positive pressure ventilation. Proc Soc Exp Biol Med 161:574–578

17. Echtenkamp SF, Zucker IH, Gilmore JP (1980) Characterization of high and low pressure baroreceptor influences on renal nerve activity in the primate "Macaca fascicularis". Circ Res 46:726–730

18. Payen DM, Farge D, Beloucif S, et al (1987) No involvement of antidiuretic hormone in acute antidiuresis during PEEP ventilation in humans. Anesthesiology 66:17–23

19. Kumar A, Pontoppidan H, Baratz RA, et al (1974) Inappropriate response to increased plasma ADH during mechanical ventilation in acute respiratory failure. Anesthesiology 40:215–221

20. Hemmer M, Viquerat CE, Suter PM, et al (1980) Urinary antidiuretic hormone excretion during mechanical ventilation and weaning in man. Anesthesiology 52:395–400

21. Share L (1976) Role of cardiovascular receptors in the control of ADH release. Cardiology 61 (Suppl 1):51–64

22. Share L, Levy MN (1966) Carotid sinus pulse pressure, a determinant of plasma antidiuretic hormone concentration. Am J Physiol 211:721–724

23. Bark H, Le Roith D, Nyska M, et al (1980) Elevations in plasma ADH levels during PEEP ventilation in the dog: mechanisms involved. Am J Physiol 239:E474–E481

24. Montani JP, Liard JF, Schoun J, et al (1980) Hemodynamic effects of exogenous and endogenous vasopressin at low plasma concentrations in conscious dogs. Circ Res 47:346–355

25. Harrington AR (1972) Hyponatremia due to sodium depletion in the absence of vasopressin. Am J Physiol 222:768–774

26. Renkin EM, Robinson RR (1974) Glomerular filtration. N Engl J Med 290:785–792

27. Annat G, Viale JP, Xuan BB, et al (1983) Effect of PEEP ventilation on renal function, plasma renin, aldosterone, neurophysins and urinary ADH, and prostaglandins. Anesthesiology 58:136–141

28. Kharasch ED, Yeo K-T, Laposky L, et al (1987) Atrial natriuretic peptide and the renal effects of PEEP ventilation Anesthesiology 67 (Suppl):A330 (Abstract)

29. Berry AJ, Geer RT, Marshall C, et al (1984) The effect of long-term controlled mechanical ventilation with positive end-expiratory pressure on renal function in dogs. Anesthesiology 61:406–415

30. Hemmer M, Suter PM (1979) Treatment of cardiac and renal effects of PEEP with dopamine in patients with acute respiratory failure, Anesthesiology 50:399–403

31. Lindner A, Cutler RE, Goodman G (1979) Synergism of dopamine plus furosemide in preventing acute renal failure in the dog. Kidney Int 16:158–166

32. Lindner A (1983) Synergism of dopamine and furosemide in diureticresistant, oliguric acute renal failure. Nephron 33:121–126

Dopamine Agonists in Intensive Care Medicine: From Receptors to Clinical Applications

L. I. Goldberg

Introduction

Dopamine is one of the most commonly used drugs in intensive care medicine. The catecholamine has multiple clinical applications because of its diverse pharmacological effects resulting from activation of several different receptors [1, 2]. More recently, new compounds have been investigated with different spectra of receptor activity and clinical applications than dopamine. The purpose of this chapter is to review the pharmacological effects of dopamine and other drugs acting on dopamine receptors and to summarize current and potential clinical applications in critical care medicine.

Table 1 lists the actions of dopamine on different receptors in the cardiovascular system and the expected pharmacological response. Table 2 compares the

Table 1. Receptors and cardiovascular and renal actions of dopamine

Receptor	Action
DA_1	Vasodilation in the renal, mesenteric, coronary, and cerebral vascular beds; diuresis, natriuresis
DA_2	Inhibition of release of norepinephrine from sympathetic nerve terminals
$Beta_1$	Increase in cardiac contractility and heart rate
$Beta_2$	Little or no activity
$Alpha_1$	Vasoconstriction
$Alpha_2$	Vasoconstriction and inhibition of norepinephrine released from sympathetic nerve terminals

Table 2. Spectra of receptor activity of dopamine and dopamine agonists

Compound	
Dopamine	DA_1, DA_2, $beta_1$, $alpha_1$, $alpha_2$
Propylbutyl DA	DA_1, DA_2; weak alpha, no beta
Dopexamine	$beta_2$, DA_1, DA_2; weak or no $beta_1$; no alpha[a]
Fenoldopam	DA_1
Bromocriptine, Hydergine	DA_2

[a] Also inhibits norepinephrine uptake in sympathetic nerves.

actions of dopamine and several dopamine agonists which have had clinical study.

Dopamine

Diverse cardiovascular and renal effects are produced by different doses of dopamine [1–5]. Because of individual variations in receptor response and clinical conditions, it is not possible to predict the infusion rate required in a critically ill patient and the infusion rate must be carefully regulated with close observation of the patient.

At infusion rates of 0.5 to 1.5 µg/kg/min, dopamine acts predominantly on DA_1 and DA_2 receptors [2–7]. DA_1 receptors are located on arterial smooth muscle cells and this action causes vasodilation, predominantly in the renal, mesenteric, cerebral, and coronary vascular beds. Sodium and urine excretion usually increase. The natriuresis may be due entirely to renal vascular effects, DA_1 receptors located on renal tubules may also be involved [8–11].

DA_2 receptors are located on postganglionic sympathetic nerves and possibly on autonomic ganglia [6, 7]. Activation of these receptors results in inhibition of norepinephrine release from sympathetic nerves causing vasodilation and reduction in heart rate. DA_2 receptors are also located in the area postrema and in the pituitary. Activation of DA_2 receptors can cause nausea and vomiting and may decrease prolactin levels [6, 7].

At infusion rates of 2–4 µg/kg/min dopamine activates beta$_1$-adrenoceptors which result in increased cardiac contractile force and heart rate [3, 5, 12]. Dopamine also has an indirect action to stimulate beta$_1$ receptors by causing release of norepinephrine from cardiac sympathetic nerves. At this infusion rate dopamine usually increases cardiac output with little effect on blood pressure or heart rate [12]. Greater increase in renal blood flow and sodium excretion usually occurs.

At higher dose ranges, the action of dopamine on alpha$_1$- and alpha$_2$-adrenoceptors becomes apparent and blood pressure increases [3, 5, 12, 13]. Because of diverse effects produced by activation of DA_1 and DA_2 receptors and postsynaptic alpha$_1$- and alpha$_2$-adrenoceptors, the infusion rate of dopamine required to elevate diastolic blood pressure exhibits marked individual variations. Increase in blood pressure has been observed with infusion rates as low as 2 µg/kg/min to greater than 10 µg/kg/min in normal subjects [14]. In critically ill patients infusion rates of 50 µg/kg/min and greater have been used to increase blood pressure.

In recent years low infusion rates of dopamine have been used to increase renal perfusion and urinary and sodium excretion, especially in patients who are refractory to diuretics [5, 11, 15–17].

Higher infusion rates of dopamine are used to increase cardiac output and renal blood flow in patients with congestive heart failure [2, 3, 12]. The infusion rate must be carefully titrated to avoid increase in afterload and elevation of pulmonary wedge pressure. Combined use of dopamine and vasodilators atenuates the vasoconstricting actions of dopamine without reducing the cardiac stimulation and renal vasodilator effects. Sodium nitroprusside and nitroglycerin are frequently used with dopamine since they act on both the arterial and venous circulations, and have a transient effect [18–20]. The vasoconstricting effects of dopamine also may be reduced by administration of alpha-adrenoceptor blocking agents, but currently available drugs are not as easily titrated [13]. When dopamine is administered with a vasodilator or alpha-adrenoceptor antagonist, infusion rates must be carefully adjusted to prevent excessive hypotension.

The combined use of dopamine and dobutamine also has been found to be more beneficial in some patients [21]. Norepinephrine may be added to dopamine infusions if greater vasoconstriction is needed [22].

When high doses of dopamine are administered, or the amine has been administered for a prolonged period to time, it may be difficult to wean the patient from the drug. Withdrawal can be accomplished by increasing the reduced in vascular volume resulting from prolonged vasoconstriction and/or persistent diuresis. In others it may be necessary to add dobutamine prior to discontinuing dopamine therapy. Levodopa, which is decarboxylated to dopamine also has been used to wean patients from intravenously administered dopamine [3]. Levodopa must be gradually administered to prevent nausea and vomiting. In the treatment of congestive heart failure, levodopa is administered in an initial dose of 250 mg four times a day and gradually increased to 1–1.5 grams four times a day [24]. Pyridoxine, 50 mg, should be administered with levodopa to increase peripheral decarboxylation.

Administration of large doses of dopamine antagonists such as chlorpromazine, haloperidol, and metoclopramide, could attenuate the renal effects of dopamine. Dopamine must be cautiously administered to patients who have received beta-adrenoceptor blocking agents since the alpha-adrenoceptor vasoconstrictor effects could not be balanced by cardiac stimulation. Dopamine is metabolized by monoamine oxidase, and the initial dose of dopamine should be reduced to at least one-tenth in patients who have received monoamine oxidase inhibitors within 2 to 3 weeks prior to dopamine administration.

Propylbutyldopamine

Propylbutyldopamine differs from dopamine in that it acts on DA_1 and DA_2 receptors without action of $beta_1$- and alpha-adrenoceptors. Thus, more pronounced reductions in peripheral resistance can be obtained with propylbutyldopamine than with dopamine, especially in patients who exhibit exaggerated sympathetic nervous system activity. Fennell et al. [25] infused propylbutyldopamine at rates of 20 to 40 µg/kg/min to three normal volunteers. Renal blood flow approximately doubled. Heart rate increased slightly and blood pressure was not altered. In 11 patients with congestive heart failure i.v. infusion of propylbutyldopamine at 5, 10, and 20 µg/kg/min, caused dose-dependent reductions in mean arterial pressure. Left ventricular filling pressures and pulmonary systemic vascular resistances decreased, cardiac index increased without changes in either stroke work index or heart rate [25].

Taylor et al. [26] administered propylbutyldopamine to 7 patients with essentialhypertension at an infusion rate of 20 µg/kg/min. Mean arterial pressure was lowered by an average of 18 mm Hg. The reduction in blood pressure was accompanied by pronounced increments in renal plasma flow.

The dosage of propylbutyldopamine is limited by the occurrence of nausea and vomiting at higher doses. This effect was not observed with an infusion rate of 20 µg/kg/min, but did occur in a few volunteers and patients with infusion rates of 40 µg/kg/min.

Rapid onset and short duration of action make propylbutyldopamine suitable for intensive care use. The compound should be useful in treating patients in whom the vasoconstrictor and cardiac stimulating actions of dopamine are undesirable. Potential use in the critical care environment includes treatment of congestive heart failure and hypertensive emergencies. The drug has possible advantages over beta-adrenergic blocking agents in the treatment of acute myocardial infarction since the $beta_1$-adrenoceptor is not blocked by propylbutyldopamine, permitting use of $beta_1$-adrenoceptor agonists, if necessary.

Dopexamine

Dopexamine differs from dopamine in having a potent action on $beta_2$-adrenoceptors in addition to dopamine receptor activity [27, 28]. Unlike dopamine, dopexamine does not activate $alpha_1$- and $alpha_2$-adrenoceptors and exhibits little $beta_1$-adrenoceptor activity. The $beta_2$-adrenoceptor action of the drug causes decreased peripheral resistance and reflex increae in heart rate. The DA_1 action results in increase in renal blood flow.

Dopexamine has been administered to a large number of patients with chronic heart failure. Dawson et al. [29] administered dopexamine intravenously to 10 patients with severe congestive heart failure at rates of 1, 3, and 6 µg/kg/min. These investigators observed dose-related increments in cardiac index, stroke volume index, and heart rate, and reductions in systemic vascular resistance and pulmonary vascular resistance.

Svensson et al. [30] administered dopexamine at infusion rates ranging from 0.5 ro 4 µg/kg/min, in 8 patients with congestive heart failure. Cardiac outpout increased in these patients, but the maximum effect was reached at different dose ranges. In four cases the dose was 1 µg/kg/min, in three cases it was 2 µg/kg/min, and in one case it was 4 µg/kg/min. Systemic vascular resistance decreased by 30%. Heart rate increased by 14% at the time of maximum cardiac output measurement, and there were no effects on systemic and pulmonary arterial blood pressures.

Colardyn et al. [31]. infused dopexamine to a maximum rate of 6 µg/kg/min to 12 patients with severe heart failure. Dopexamine was then infused at the dose which produced "optimal improvement" for up to 48 hours. Cardiac index and reductions in systemic vascular and pumonary vascular resistances were found to persist for the duration of the study. These investigators did not observe a significant increment in heart rate.

Jackson et al. [32] reported that dopexamine produced dose-related increments in cardiac index with infusion rates of 0.5, 1, and 2 µg/kg/min and found that the changes were similar to those observed with infusion rates of dopamine of 2.5, 5, and 10 µg/kg/min.

Bonnier et al. [33] compared dopexamine and dobutamine in a randomized cross-over study in 12 patients with chronic congestive heart failure. Dopexamine infused at 2 µg/kg/min produced similar increments in cardiac index as dobutamine infused at 10 µg/kg/min. Reductions in pulmonary artery capillary wedge pressure were similar with both drugs, but systemic vascular resistance was reduced to a greater extent by dopexamine.

Fung et al. [34] infused dopexamine at 0.5, 1, 2, 4, and 6 µg/kg/min for 10 minutes to 10 patients with congestive heart failure. Cardiac index increased from 2.5 to 4.5 l/min/m². Mean blood pressure, mean capillary wedge pressure, systemic and pulmonary vascular resistances significantly decreased; whereas, heart rate increased from 92 to 110 beats/min.

The question which remains unanswered is whether the beneficial effects observed in patients in congestive heart failure are secondary to vasodilation and reflex cardiac stimulation or whether dopexamine possesses a substantial positive inotropic action. A positive inotropic effect was suggested by Jaski et al. [35] who analyzed the effects of infusions of dopexamine, 2 µg/kg/min, for 10 minutes in 10 patients undergoing cardiac catheterization for presumed coronary artery disease. Heart rate and cardiac index progressively increased during the infusion. At the end of the infusion cardiac index had increased by 61% and heart rate by 39%. Systemic vascular resistance had decreased by 33%. Pulmonary vascular resistance remained unchanged. Increases in dP/dt paralleled the increase in heart rate. In a second phase of the study the results of dopexamine were compared during similar increments in heart rate by atrial pacing and there was a greater increase in dP/dt at the same heart rate with dopexamine. It was not possible, however, to eliminate a baroreceptor-mediated increase in dP/dt since peripheral resistance decreased only with dopexamine. Tan et al. [36] studied 10 patients with low output ischemic cardiac failure and infused dopexamine at rates of 0.5 to 6 µg/kg/min. Heart rate and cardiac index increased and systemic vascular resistance decreased. Using a newly-developed analytical technique, these investigators suggested that 8 of the 10 patients demonstrated clear-cut positive inotropism when infused with dopexamine below 2 µg/kg/min.

These results in patients are in marked contrast to results observed in experimental animals [27, 28, 37] which demonstrated that dopexamine exhibits very weak direct positive inotropic actions. Two mechanisms have been suggested for the differences in the clinical and animal studies. One possibility is that dopexamine increases heart rate and cardiac contractile force by direct action on myocardial $beta_2$-adrenoceptors which may have a greater influence in patients with congestive heart failure in whom $beta_1$-adrenoceptors are found to be reduced in number [35]. Another possible mechanism which has been found to occur with therapeutic doses of dopexamine is prevention of uptake of norepinephrine as a sympathetic neuron [37]. Patients with congestive heart failure have high levels of circulating norepinephrine, and prevention of uptake may increase norepinephrine levels at the beta$_1$-adrenoceptor, resulting in a positive inotropic effect.

Two preliminary clinical studies have described the renal effects of dopexamine. Foulds et al. [38] reported that dopexamine infused at 3 µg/kg/min for 15 minutes increased renal blood flow from 504 ml/min to 605 ml/min while increasing cardiac output from 5.9 to 6.7 l/min. There was a small but significant reduction in renal vascular resistance. Tan et al. [39] studied 10 patients with congestive heart failure and measured the hemodynamic and renal effects of infusions of dopexamine ranging from 0.5 to 4 µg/kg/min for successive 20 minute periods to 10 patients with congestive heart failure. Improvement in renal function was seen at 4 µg/kg/min in five patients with increase in urine flow from 0.7 to 2.9 ml/min, creatinine clearance from 34–66 ml/min, and fractional excretion of sodium by 0.5 to 1 percent. Two of the 5 patients who did not respond had normal renal function, two were anuric, and one had pre-existent irreversible renal impairment. Cardiac index increased from 1.6 to 2.5 ml/min and systemic vascular resistance decreased in this study.

Dopexamine has a rapid onset of action and short duration. It could have potential use in critical care medicine in patients with myocardial failure. It has greater vasodilating actions than dopamine and dobutamine, and could be substituted for these drugs or a combination of these agents with vasodilators. Hypotension may limit its usage in some patients [34]. Tremor has been reported in a few patients, presumably due to a beta$_2$-adrenoceptor mechanism [29]

Fenoldopam

Fenoldopam is a selective DA$_1$ agonist which produces pronounced increments in renal blood flow. Carey et al. [40] reported that a single dose of 100 mg to 10 hypertensive patients with average supine blood pressure and heart rate of 156/105 mm Hg and 76 beats/min, respectively, decreased supine blood pressure to 141/89 mm Hg at 90 minutes. Heart rate increased to 91 beats/min. Renal blood flow increased from 371 to a peak of 659 ml/min. Urine volume, urinary sodium excretion, and fractional sodium excretion increased significantly, but glomerular filtration rate was not significantly increased. Single doses of 50 and 100 mg of fenoldopam were administered to 14 hypertensive patients by Ventura et al. [41]. Mean arterial pressure decreased from 174 to 94 mm Hg after one hour. Heart rate increased from 70 to 84 beats/min and cardiac index from 2.9 to 4.2 ml/min/m^2. Hemodynamic studies by these investigators indicated that the reduction in pressure was due to decreased pheripheral resistance. Because of the limited bioavailability of fenoldopam, studies of prolonged administration have not been conducted.

An intravenous form of fenoldopam has become availabe for study. Investigations in our center demonstrated that fenoldopam is an extremely potent and effective antihypertensive agent when administered by this route [42]. Fenoldopam reduced blood pressure in a dose-dependent fashion at infusion rates between 0.025 and 0.5 µg/kg/min and the antihypertensive effect was sustained during 2 hour infusions. Ten patients studied during free-water diuresis, fenoldopam increased renal plasma flow by 42%, glomerular filtration rate by 6%, and sodium excretion by 202%. Mean arterial pressure was lowered by 12%. In the dose ranging studies heart rate increased in parallel with the reduction of blood pressure from 60 to 82 beats/min. Plasma norepinephrine levels doubled from an average of 1.6 to 3.37 nmol/l.

Fenoldopam also has been studied in the treatment of congestive heart failure. Young et al. [43] administered single oral doses of 50, 100, and 200 mg of fenoldopam to 10 patients with severe congestive heart failure. Peak efficacy was noted 30 minutes to 1 hour after the 200 mg dose was administered. Cardiac index increased significantly from 2.2 to 3.1 l/min/m^2. There were no significant changes in heart rate. Mean arterial pressure decreased from 96 to 83 mm Hg and there was a significant reduction in systemic vascular resistance. A slight reduction in pulmonary capillary wedge pressure and pulmonary artery pressure was observed. Significant adverse effects were not reported.

These studies suggest that intravenously administered fenoldopam may be useful in critical care medicine in the treatment of severe and malignant hypertension. A potential advantage of fenoldopam is that it can enhance renal blood flow and sodium and water excretion since these patients frequently present with renal dysfunction. Other potential uses are in the treatment of congestive heart failure and as an alternative to dopamine to improve renal perfusion and to increase urine and sodium excretion in patients refractory to diuretics. Fenoldopam also may be useful when added to drugs such as dobutamine to increase renal perfusion pressure [44, 45]. As with dopexamine, the dose will have to be carefully regulated to prevent hypotension.

Acknowledgements: This research reported in this paper was supported by NIH grant GM-22220, and grants from Smith Kline and French Laboratories and Fisons Corporation. I would like to thank Ms. Patricia Gomben for secretarial assistance.

References

1. Goldberg LI (1972) Cardiovcascular and renal actions of dopamine: Potential clinical applications. Pharmacol Rev 241:1–29
2. Goldberg LI, Rajfer SI (1985) Applications in clinical cardiology. Circulation 72:245–248
3. Beregovich J, Bianchi C, Rubler S, Lomnitz E, Cagin N, Levitt B (1974) Dose-related hemodynamic and renal effects of dopamine in congestive heart failure. Am Heart J 87:550–557
4. Levinson PD, Goldstein DS, Munson PJ, Gill JR Jr, Keiser HR (1985) Endocrine, renal, and hemodynamic responses to graded dopamine infusions in normal men. J Clin Endocrin Metab 60:821–826
5. D'Orio V, El Allaf D, Juchmes J, Marcelle R (1986) The use of low doses of dopamine in intensive care medicine. Arch Int Physiol Biochim 92:S11–S20
6. Goldberg LI, Volkman PH, Kohli JD (1978) A comparison of the vascular dopamine receptor with other dopamine receptors. Ann Rev Pharmacol Toxicol 18:57–79
7. Goldberg LI, Kohli JD (1983) Differentiation of dopamine receptors in the periphery. In: Kaiser C, Kebabian JW (eds) In: Dopamine Receptors. Amer Chem Soc Symposium Series #224, pp 101–113

8. Felder RA, Blecher M, Calcagno PL, Jose PA (1984) Dopamine receptors in trhe proximal tubule of the rabbit. Am J Physiol 247:F499–F505

9. Bello-Reuss E, Higashi Y, Kanega Y (1982) Dopamine decreases fluid reabsorption in straight portions of rabbit proximal tubule. Am J Physiol 242:F634–F640

10. Hilberman M, Maseda J, Stinson EB, et al (1984) The diuretic properties of dopamine in patients after open-heart operation. Anesthesiology 61:489–494

11. Parker S, Carlon GC, Isaacs M, Howland WS, Kahn RC (1981) Dopamine administration in oliguria and oliguric renal failure. Crit Care Med 9:630–632

12. McDonald RH Jr, Goldberg LI, McNay JL, Tuttle EP (1964) Effects of dopamine in man: Augmentation of sodium excretion, glomerular filtration rate and renal plasma flow. J Clin Invest 43:1116–1124

13. MacCannell KL, McNay JL, Meyer MB, Goldberg LI (1966) The use of dopamine in the treatment of hypotension and shock. New Eng J Med 275:1389–1398

14. Horwitz D, Fox SM, Goldberg LI (1962) Effects of dopamine in man. Circ Res 10:237–243

15. Henderson IS, Beattie TJ, Kennedy AC (1980) Dopamine hydrochloride in oliguric states. Lancet 2:827–828

16. Lindner A (1983) Synergism of dopamine and furosemide in diuretic-resistant, oliguric acute renal failure. Nephron 33:121–126

17. Mann HJ, Fuhs DW, Hemstrom CA (1986) Acute renal failure. Drug Intelligence and Clinical Pharmacy 20:421–438

18. Miller RR, Awan NA, Joye JA, et al (1977) Combined dopamine and nitroprusside therapy in congestive heart failure. Circulation 55:881–884

19. Keung EC, Ribner HS, Schwartz W, Sonnenblick EH, LeJemtel TH (1980) Effects of combined dopamine and nitroprusside therapy in patients with severe pump failure and hypotension complicating acute myocardial infarction. J Cardiovasc Pharmacol 2:113–119

20. Loeb HS, Ostrenga JP, Gaul W, et al (1983) Beneficial effects of dopamine combined with intravenous nitroglycerin on hemodynamics in patients with severe left ventricular failure. Circulation 68:813–820

21. Richard C, Ricome JL, Rimailho JA, Bottineau G, Auzepy P (1983) Combined hemodynamic effects of dopamine and dobutamine in cardiogenic shock. Circulation 67:620–626

22. Schaer GL, Fink MP, Parrillo JE (1985) Norepinephrine alone versus norepinephrine plus low-dose dopamine: Enhanced renal blood flow with combination pressor therapy. Crit Care Med 13:492–496

23. Goldberg LI, Hsieh YY, Resnekov L (1977) Newer catecholamines for treatment of heart failure and shock. An update on dopamine and a first look at dobutamine. Prog Cardiovasc Dis 4:327–340

24. Rajfer SI, Anton AH, Rossen J, Goldberg LI (1984) Beneficial hemodynamic effects of oral levodopa in heart failure: Relationship to the generation of dopamine. Engl J Med 310:1357–1362

25. Fennell WH, Taylor AA, Young JB, et al (1983) Propylbutyldopamine: hemodynamic effects in conscious dogs, normal human volunteers, and patients with heart failure. Circulation 67:829–836

26. Taylor AA, Fennell WH, Feldman MB, Brandon TA, Ginos JZ, Mitchell JR (1983) Activation of peripheral dopamine presynaptic receptors lowers blood pressure and heart rate in dogs. Hypertension 5:226–234

27. Brown RA, Dixon J, Farmer JB, et al (1985) Dopexamine: A novel agonist at peripheral dopamine receptors and beta$_2$-adrenoceptors. Br J Pharmacol 85:599–608

28. Brown RA, Farmer JB, Hall JC, Humphries RQ, O'Connor SE, Smith GW (1985) The effects of dopexamine on the cardiovasclar system of the dog. Br J Pharmacol 85:609–619

29. Dawson JR, Thompson DS, Signy M, et al (1985) Acute haemodynamic and metabolic effects of dopexamine, a new dopaminergic receptor agonist, in patients with chronic heart failure. Br Heart J 54:313–320

30. Svensson G, Sjogren A, Erhardt L (1986) Short-term haemodynamic effects of dopexamine in patients with chronic congestive heart failure. Eur Heart J 7:697–703

31. Colardyn F, Clement DL (1986) Acute and long-term haemodynamic effects of dopexamine hydrochloride in patients with chronic cardiac failure. Abstracts of X World Congress of Cardiology, Washington, DC, September, p 346 #1980

32. Jackson N, Frais M, Sharma SK, Reynolds G, Taylor SH (1986) A dose response haemodynamic study of dopexamine vs dopamine in ischaemic left ventricular failure. Abstract of X World Congress of Cardiology, Washington, DC, September, p 400 #2302

33. Bonnier JJRM (1986) Dopexamine hydrochloride, haemodynamic effects in haemochronic cardiac failure, a comparison with dobutamine. Abstracts of X World Congress of Cardiology, Washington, DC, September, p 188 #1076

34. Fung AY, Lal P, Pitt B, Walton JA Jr (1986) Acute hemodynamic effects of dopexamine in patients with congestive heart failure. Abstracts of X World Congress of Cardiology, Washington, DC, September, p 188 #1074

35. Jaski BE, Wijns W, Foulds R, Serruys PW (1986) The haemodynamic and myocardial effects of dopexamine: A new beta$_2$-adrenoceptor and dopaminergic agonist. Brit J Clin Pharmacol 21:393–400

36. Tan LB, Littler WA, Murray G (1987) Beneficial haemodynamic effects of intravenous dopexamine in patients with low-output heart failure. J Cardiovasc Pharmacol 10:280–286

37. Bass AS, Kohli JD, Lubbers N, Goldberg LI (1987) Mechanisms mediating the positive inotropic and chronotropic changes induced by dopexamine in the anesthetized dog. J Pharmacol Exp Ther 242:940–944

38. Foulds RA, Magrini F, Zanchetti A (1986) The renovascular effects of dopexamine hydrochloride, a dopaminergic and beta$_2$ adrenergic agonist. Abstracts of X World Congress on Cardiology, Washington, DC, September, p 201 #1151

39. Tan LB, Smith SA, Murray RG, Littler WA (1986) Renal response to dopexamine infusion in low output heart failure. Clin Sci 71 (Suppl 15):56P #155

40. Carey RM, Stote RM, Dubb JW, Townsend LW, Rose CE Jr, Kaiser DL (1984) Selective peripheral dopamine-1 receptor stimulation with fenoldopam in human essential hypertension. J Clin Invest 74:2198–2207

41. Ventura HO, Messerli FH, Frohlich ED, et al (1984) Immediate hemodynamic effects of a dopamine-receptor agonist (fenoldopam) in patients with essential hypertension. Circulation 69:1142–1145

42. Murphy MB, McCoy CE, Weber RR, Frederickson ED, Douglas FL, Goldberg LI (1987) Augmentation of renal blood flow and sodium excretion in hypertensive patients during blood pressure reduction by intravenous administration of the dopamine$_1$ agonist, fenoldopam. Circulation 76:1312–1318

43. Young JB, Leon CA, Pratt CM, Suarez JM, Aronoff RD, Roberts R (1985) Hemodynamic effects of an oral dopamine receptor agonist (fenoldopam) in patients with congestive heart failure. J Am Coll Cardiol 6:792–796

44. Lass NA, Goldberg LI, Lubbers N, Glock D (1986) Cardiac and renal vascular effects of the selective DA$_1$ agonist, fenoldopam, alone and combined with dobutamine. Clin Res 34:638A

45. Lass NA, Bakris GL, Glock D, Goldberg LI (1987) Alpha-adrenoceptor contribution to renal vascular effects of low-dose dopamine. Clin Res 35:644A

Anticoagulation for Extracorporeal System

M. E. Sinclair

Introduction

Blood, in the intact organism, is kept in a fluid state by the maintainance of an adequate blood flow, and rapid hepatic clearance of the coagulation factors following activation and fibrinolysis. There are also circulating serine protease inhibitors, such as antithrombin III (AT III), that prevent the spontaneous activation of certain factors in the coagulation cascade. During extracorporeal circulation, such as hemodialysis or cardiopulmonary bypass, the intrinsic pathway of the coagulation cascade is activated by the contact of the blood with a "foreign surface". Once the cascade has been activated, it is necessary to use some form of anticoagulation to prevent clotting in the extracorporeal circuit.

The Blood Coagulation Cascade

An outline of the stages in the familiar coagulation cascade is shown in Figure 1. The intrinsic coagulation pathway is initiated by the interaction of factor XII (Hageman factor), factor XI, prekallikrein and high molecular weight kininogen (HMW-kininogen). The optimal activation of factor XII requires prekallikrein, HMW-kininogen and an activating (anionic) surface. Once the intrinsic system is activated, the cascade will be sequentially activated resulting in clot formation. It is this system that is activated by the extracorporeal circulation of blood.

The extrinsic coagulation mechanism requires a tissue factor which gains access to the blood only when tissue is damaged and is initiated by the formation of a complex of the tissue factor with factor VII. This pathway is *not* activated by extracorporeal circulation per se but in the critically ill patient may already be activated through other causes.

The final stage of both pathways is via factor V and requires both platelets and calcium. Platelet adhesion to an injured vessel is a critical early step in the extrinsic pathway. The contact of platelets to a "foreign surface" also leads to activation, with aggregation and activation of prothrombinase on the platelet surface [1]. To form a stable clot platelets are essential. The coagulation sequence culminates, once activated, in the conversion of soluble circulating fibrinogen into a network of fibrin at a site of injury, or on a "foreign surface", which provides stability to the hemostatic plug or platelets.

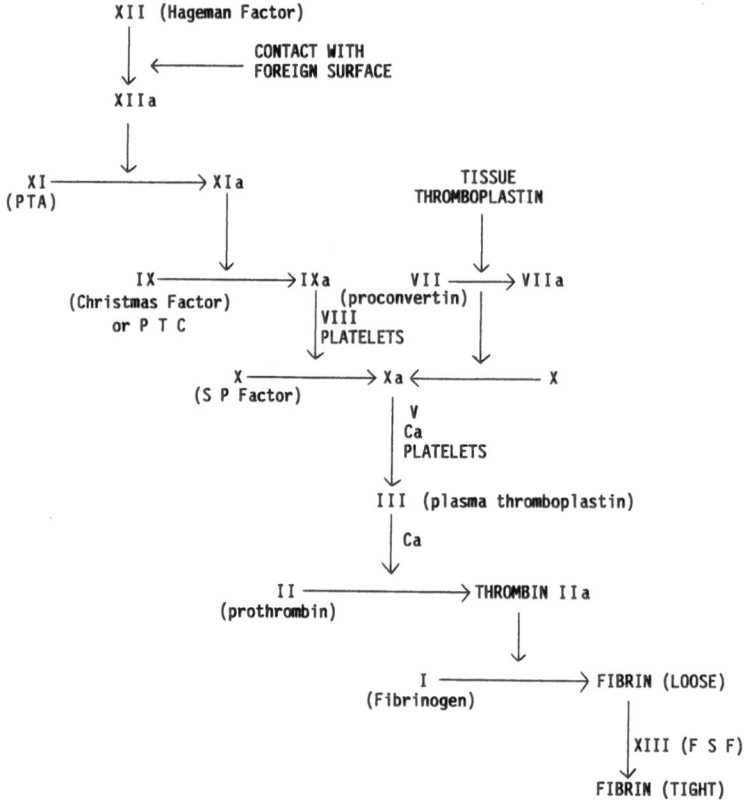

Fig. 1. Simplified analysis of stages of blood coagulation

To maintain fluid blood in an extracorporeal circuit we can "block" the coagulation system at a variety of places:

1. Various factors can be blocked (Heparins, ancrod, gabexate mesilate etc.)
2. Platelet activation can be blocked (prostacyclin)
3. Contact activation can be blocked (Heparin-bonded circuit)

Standard Heparin (SH)

Heparin is the standard anticoagulant by which others are judged. Heparin acts by accelerating the binding of AT III, a naturally occurring serine protease inhibitor, to thrombin thus inhibiting its activation. AT III also acts on factors Xa, IXa, XIa and XIIa. Thus, in conditions where the level of AT III may be decreased, such as major trauma or infection, heparin becomes less effective. Heparin can also affect the platelets, leading to a drop in platelet count of between 20% to 40%, and has been found to cause release of platelet factor 4 in vivo possibly inducing aggregation [2, 3]. It is not surprising, therefore, that troublesome bleeding has been reported in up to 25% of patients receiving it [4]. Heparin, when used as the anticoagulant for extracorporeal CO_2 removal in man using a veno-venous system, is associated with a mean blood loss by hemorrhage of 1.5 litres per day [5].

It has long been known that natural heparin is not a homogenous substance but consists of glycosaminoglycans in a wide range of differing molecular sizes and of different affinity to AT III. For this reason, differences in heparin's anti-coagulant action has has been found depending on the source of the product. By fractionation of natural heparin various low molecular weight heparins (LMWH) have been produced and studied in vivo.

Low Molecular Weight Heparins (LMWH)

The rationale for the use of LMWH is that they have high anti-Xa activity in spite of decreased antithrombin effect [6]. It was assumed that the anti-Xa effect would be of considerable importance because of its antithrombotic effect. In addition platelet function might be less affected by LMWHs than by SH [7]. These properties of LMWH could make them particularly suitable for use in ex-tacorporeal systems utilizing a membrane (hemodialysis, cardiopulmonar bypass) since these systems have a large foreign surface area and therefore favor the contact activation of the blood.

In man successful cardiopulmonary bypass with LMWH has been reported although, despite the short period of bypass, excessive bleeding occurred which was judged unacceptable by the authors [8]. Incomplete anti-Xa activity neutral-ization by protamine either in vitro or in vivo has been reported for different LMWH fractions [9].

A study using LMWH as the anticoagulant for extracorporeal CO_2 removal in dogs has demonstrated that, despite high anti-Xa activity, clots were discovered in the blood reservoir [10]. This would indicate that the inhibition of thrombin is mandatory to prevent the clotting of blood once contact activation has oc-curred.

While the efficacy of LMWH in the prophylaxis of venous thrombosis seems to be firmly established further experiments are needed to determine the dose regimens of the different LMWHs for anticoagulation during extracorporeal cir-culation. The inability to reverse completely the effects with protamine is also a severe drawback to their use.

Ancrod

Ancrod is an anticoagulant derived from Malayan pit viper venom. Its properties were discovered by the observation that people bitten by the viper had blood that did not clot (for up to two weeks!) and yet they did not have any bleeding problems [11]. Ancrod acts by rapidly converting fibrinogen to a loose form of fibrin that is then quickly cleared by the fibrinolytic system. This leads to defi-brinogenation and occurs with no change in the other clotting factors [12]. Ini-tially platelet levels fall due to circulating fibrinogen degradation products but after this early effect platelet number return to normal with a decrease in aggregation, a possible advantage during extracorporeal circulation [13]. Ancrod has been successfully used for hemodialysis, in man, with no adverse effects and, in many studies, the incidence of hemorrhage is lower when compared with heparin [12, 14].

In a recent study, using acrod as the anticoagulant for extracorporeal CO_2 removal in dogs, it was found that despite ancrod per se having no effect on the clotting factors, the level of factors II and V fell during the bypass period (Sinclair ME, Schweizer A, Reber G et al. 1987). This would indicate that contact activation is taking place with activation and consumption of the factors in the coagulation cascade and that hemorrhage may become a problem during long term use such as during extracorporeal CO_2 removal in man. Further studies are needed for longer periods of bypass to assess if ancrod offers any substantial advantage over heparin for this particular use.

Gabexate Mesilate (FOY)

FOY is a serine protease inhibitor with a half-life of 80 seconds. It acts at the same sites as AT III and has the same effects but, unlike heparin, is not dependent on AT III for its action. FOY has been used in sheep as the anticoagulant for extracorporeal circulation and appears to work [15]. If the circuit is the right length then systemic anticoagulation is avoided. The problems are that it is very expensive and difficult to use and the long term effects on the clotting system have yet to be ascertained.

Prostacyclin

Prostacyclin is a potent inhibitor of platelet activation so that its use during dialysis leads to preservation of platelet numbers with no change in β-thromboglobulin levels, although leukocyte aggregation and pulmonary microembolization still occurs [16]. Prostacyclin allows the use of heparin to be reduced or even avoided completely during dialysis [17, 18]. It would also appear to reduce the risk of serious hemorrhage [16]. However the use of prostacyclin at the typical dose of 5 ng/kg/min can cause serious hypotension due to vasodilatation. The short half-life allows rapid resolution of any side effects if the infusion is stopped.

Heparin Bonded Circuits

Since it is contact activation that causes blood to clot in an extracorporeal system, it would seem logical that if this activation could somehow be avoided we would not need systemic anticoagulation with all the attendant drawbacks such as hemorrhage. Heparin can be bound to artificial surfaces rendering the surface non thrombogenic and thus inhibiting contact activation [19]. The use of this technique has already been shown to allow extracorporeal circulation to take place without systemic anticoagulation [20]. Studies are in progress to assess the use of such systems for hemodialysis, cardiopulmonary bypass and also extracorporeal CO_2 removal.

However it is clear that in patients in whom the extrinsic pathway is activated (critically ill patients) some form of conventional anticoagulation may still be necessary to block the coagulation cascade.

Conclusions

Despite the many drawbacks associated with its use, heparin remains the most effective and commonly used anticoagulation for extracorporeal systems. Prostacyclin is being increasingly used for hemodialysis and filtration with good results and further studies are currently in progress on the use of FOY and ancrod, especially in the field of long term erxtracorporeal circulation as used for CO_2 removal. Over the next few years I feel that the use of heparin bonded circuits and membranes will obviate the need for "whole patient" anticoagulation except for in the critically ill thus reducing hemorrhage: the most frequent and serious side effect of all of these drugs.

References

1. Nichols WL, Gerrard JM, Didisheim P (1981) Platelet structure, biochemistry and physiology. In: Poller L (ed) Recent Advances in Blood Coagulation 3- Churchill Livingstone, Edinburgh London Melbourne New York, pp 1–39
2. Ansell J, Slepchuk N Jr, Kumar R, Lopez A, Southard L, Deykin D (1980) Heparin induced thrombocytopenia: a prospective study. Thromb Haemostas 43:61–65
3. Rao AK, Holt JC, Pranee J, Niewiarowki S (1981) Release of platelet factor 4 in vivo after heparin injection. Thromb Haemostas 46:204 (Abstract)
4. Morabia A (1986) Heparin doses and major bleedings. Lancet 1:1278–1279
5. Gattinoni L, Pesenti A, Mascheroni D, et al (1986) Low frequency positive pressure ventilation with extracorporeal CO_2 removal in acute respiratory failure. JAMA 25:881–886
6. Carter CJ, Kelton JG, Hirsch J, Gent M (1986) Relation between the anti thrombotic and the anticoagulant effects of low molecular weight heparin. Thromb Res 21:169–174
7. Carter CJ, Kelton JG, Hirsch J, Cerskus A, Santos AV, Gent M (1982) The releationship between the hemorrhagic and the antithrombotic properties of low molecular weight heparin in rabbits. Blood 59:1239–1245
8. Massonet-Castel S, Pelissier E, Dreyfuss G, et al (1984) Low molecular weight heparin in extracorporeal circulation. Lancet 1:1182–1183
9. Harenberg J, Gnasso A, de Vries JX, Augustin J (1985) Inhibition of low molecular weight heparin by protamine chloride in vivo. Thromb Res 38:11–20
10. De Moerloose P, Schweizer A, Reber G, Sinclair M, Bouvier CA, Gardaz JP (1987) Comparison between a low molecular weight and standard heparin for anticoagulation during extracorporeal CO_2 removal in the dog. Thromb Res (in press)
11. Editorial (1968) A new approach to anticoagulant therapy. Lancet 1:513
12. Bell WR (1982) Defibrinogenating enzymes. In: Colman RW (ed) Hemostasis and Thrombosis. Lippincott, Philadelphia, pp 1013–1027
13. Latello ZS (1983) Retrospective study on complications and adverse effects of treatment with thrombin-like enzymes. A multicentre trial. Thromb Haemostas 50:604–609

14. Hall GH, Holman HM, Webster ADB (1970) Anticoagulation by ancrod for haemodialysis. Br Med J 4:591–593
15. Oedekoven B, Bey R, Mottaghy K, Schmid-Schonbein H (1984) Gabexate Mesilate (FOY) as an anticoagulant in extracorporeal circulation in dogs and sheep. Thromb Haemostas 52:329–332
16. Richards NT, Mansell MA (1986) Developments in dialysis for renal failure. Br J Hosp Med 35:190–192
17. Turney JH, Williams LC, Fewell MR, Parsons V, Weston MJ (1980) Platelet protection and heparin sparing with prostacyclin during regular dialysis therapy. Lancet 11:224–226
18. Zusman RM, Rubin RH, Cato AE, Cocchetto DM, Crow JW, Tolkoff-Rubin N (1981) Haemodialysis using prostacyclin instead of heparin as the sole antithrombotic agent. N Engl J Med 304:934–939
19. Larm O, Larsson R, Olsson P (1983) A new non-thrombogenic surface prepared by selective covalent binding of heparin via a modified reducing terminal residue. Biomat Med Dev Art Org 11:161–173
20. Inacio J, Bindslev L, Nilsson E, Gouda I, Olsson P (1986) Extracorporeal elimination of carbon dioxide using a surface heparinized vein-to-vein bypass system. Life Support Syst 4 Suppl 1:84–92

Metabolic and Nutritional Problems

Management of Hypotonic Hyponatremia

G. Decaux and S. Brimioulle

Introduction

The management of hypotonic hyponatremia depends on its cause and its severity. The cases of hyponatremia with decreased, increased and normal extracellular fluid (ECF) volumes will be examined, followed by a brief mention concerning severe hyponatremia.

Hypotonic Hyponatremia with Decreased ECF Volume

Coexistence of hyponatremia, hypotonicity, and ECF volume depletion implies the presence of either (1) both solute and water deficits, with the solute deficit being of greater magnitude, or (2) an isolated solute deficit. Hypovolemic hyponatremia usually occurs when renal or extrarenal losses of electrolyte-containing fluids are replaced with electrolyte-free water. Even if water intake is sufficient to restore total body water, the ECF (and intravascular) volume will still be diminished, since extracellular sodium content is decreased and less water is retained in the ECF. Associated losses of intracellular solute (potassium) will affect the magnitude of ECF depletion, since relative volumes of ICF and ECF are determined by their respective solute contents.

Clinical signs are usually related to volume depletion. Urinary sodium excretion depends on whether the source of the loss is renal or extrarenal. Patients with extrarenal sodium losses and normal kidneys will conserve sodium in an attempt to reexpand ECF volume (urine sodium usually <20 mEq/L). Urine osmolality will be high because of the volume stimulus to antidiuretic hormone (ADH) release, and because of the enhanced reabsorption of water in the collecting duct under conditions of diminished urine flow. A dissocation between urinary sodium and chloride can be initially observed in metabolic alkalosis from vomiting, since sodium is excreted with bicarbonate and not with chloride. Special attention is also required in case of diuretic administration: shortly after cessation of the treatment, urine sodium concentration decreases below 20 mEq/L although the losses occurred via the kidney. Initial therapy of the hyponatremic volume-depleted patient should be directed at restoration of intravascular volume. Volume expansion with isotonic saline (or sometimes simply the provision of a high-sodium diet) is usually sufficient to produce a water diuresis and restore body fluid tonicity to normal.

Hypotonic Hyponatremia with Increased ECF Volume

Coexistenc of hyponatremia, hypotonicity, and ECF volume expansion implies an increase in total body water greater than the increase in total body sodium. The clinical hallmark is peripheral edema; other findings may include pulmonary edema, oliguria, prerenal azotemia and very low urinary sodium excretion. Patients behave as if their intravascular volume were decreased, although it is normal or increased. The "decreased effective arterial blood volume" results in sodium and water retention by the kidney. Ingested water is retained, and hypotonic hyponatremia ensues. The treatment of hyponatremia, even if primarily due to diuretics, consists in restriction of water intake. This corrects hyponatremia, but is slow to take effects. In patients with oliguric acute renal failure, effects of uremia and hyperkalemia usually predominate over those of hyponatremia, and hemodialysis can be effective to rapidly correct the electrolytes disorders.

In patients with hyponatremia associated to congestive heart failure, the association of furosemide and captopril has been shown useful [1, 2]. Angiotensin converting enzyme (ACE) inhibition improves renal plasma flow and glomerular filtration rate (GFR), and significant diuresis and natriuresis can be achieved without inducing azotemia. These effects are not obtained with captopril alone. ACE inhibition enhances the renal effect of furosemide by either increasing the distal delivery of solute or increasing the delivery of furosemide to its site of action. Titration of the ACE inhibitor is recommended to minimize hypotension, and furosemide is mandatory in patients with azotemia [1, 2]. Water retention in patients with hyponatremic cardiac failure has been treated with demeclocycline, in the same way as inappropriate secretion of ADH. This treatment, however, greatly increases the risk of renal dysfunction, and is better avoided. Recently, one case has been reported of a patient with hyponatremia and congestive heart failure successfully treated with urea [3].

In cirrhotic patients with ascites and hyponatremia, administration of diuretics often worsens hyponatremia. Usual treatment is water restriction, but it is uneasy for the patient and corrects hyponatremia only slowly. Demeclocycline can correct hyponatremia, but also cause renal dysfunction [4]. We studied the effect of urea (30–90 g/day) in addition to diuretics in hyponatremic cirrhotic patients. Intermittent urea administration proved useful in patients with ascites resistant to diuretics and with low or normal blood urea level [5].

Hypotonic Hyponatremia with Normal ECF

Most typical in this category is the syndrome of inappropriate ADH secretion (SIADH). Comparable syndromes can occur in severe hypothyroidism and in glucocorticoid insufficiency, and are best treated with hormonal replacement.

Treatment of hyponatremia associated with the SIADH should be directed primarily to the correction of the underlying disease. If this is not possible, or if SIADH results in clinical symptoms, more specific correction of the hyponatremia is required.

Conventional management consists in water intake restriction, which is also required as the last diagnostic criteria of SIADH [6]. Further treatment is needed if water restriction (down to 400 ml/day) is not efficient, or if complete correction of hyponatremia must be achieved (ex: neurosurgical patients with intracranial hypertension). Further treatment can also be considered if water restriction is not tolerated by the patient, or not accepted by the physician (ex: when substantial enteral or parenteral nutrition is required).

Phenytoin administration has been suggested for SIADH associated with neurological disease [7], but it proved usually inefficient in our experience (unpublished data). Lithium has been discarded because of its multiple side effects [8]. Three other regimens have been found useful, whatever the underlying disease associated with SIADH: demeclocycline, loop diuretics, and urea. Current development of ADH antagonists suggests potential use for SIADH in the future, but specific V2-antagonists are not yet available for clinical use [9].

Demeclocycline (600–1200 mg/day) inhibits cyclic adenosine monophosphate synthesis and action in the renal tubule, resulting in a nephrogenic diabetes insipidus [8, 10]. Demeclocycline can cause photosensitivity, gastro-intestinal symptoms, bacterial selection, and renal failure [11]. Effects on hyponatremia only appear after 5 to 7 days, whereas they are immediate with the other two agents.

Urea and ascending-limb diuretics can be used for chronic treatment, but also to quickly correct symptomatic hyponatremia [12-14]. Urea increases the osmotic load to be eliminated daily in the urine. For instance, if a patient usually eliminates 700 mOsm daily from nutritional and endogenous catabolism, 30 g of urea (500 mOsm) will increase urine output from 900 to 1500 ml/day if urine osmolality is 800 mOsm/kg H_2O. Moreover, the osmotic diuresis due to urea contains little sodium as long as natremia remains below 130 mEq/L [12]. If water intake is 1500 to 2000 ml per day, 30 g urea once or 15 g twice a day is a typical dose, diluted in 100 ml water and given with antacid. Urea is usually well tolerated, especially if taken with a meal. Taste can be improved with fruit syrup. Urea does not require special attention to sodium intake, and does not cause potassium depletion.

The aim of ascending-limb diuretic treatment is to recover water balance by increasing diuresis, while maintaining an adequate sodium intake to compensate urinary losses. The choice of the diuretic is important: ascending-limb diuretics (ethacrynic acid, furosemide) increase diuresis and decrease kidney's concentrating ability, whereas thiazides worsen hyponatremia in SIADH. Potassium losses must be compensated with potassium chloride, or prevented with potassium-sparing diuretics). Daily doses of 40 mg of furosemide or 50 mg ethacrynic acid, with 3 g of sodium chloride and 50 mg triamterene will balance most patients [15]. Diuretics do not have gastrointestinal side effects, and allow higher water intake than urea (2000 to 2500 ml/day) [15].

Ascending-limb diuretics should be preferred when urine osmolality is high (>900 mOsm/kg H_2O) and creatinine clearance is preserved, though higher doses of urea (ex: 60 g/day) would also be efficient. Urea is a better choice when urine osmolality is lower (400-600 mOsm/kg H_2O) and creatinine clearance is lower (40-60 ml/min), as commonly seen in elderly patients. We keep demeclocycline for the few patients whose urine osmolality is high and who refuse restriction of water intake to about 2500 ml; indeed, demeclocycline brings a large iso- or hypotonic diuresis, which allows a higher water intake.

A risk of hypernatremic dehydration exists with the three treatments when water intake is restricted; this is avoided when thirst's center functions normally and access to water is free [15].

Severe Hyponatremia

Clinical symptoms are usually mild when hyponatremia is moderate (>125 mEq/L) and develops over several days. In contrast, rapid and severe hyponatremia can result in cerebral edema and water intoxication with intracranial hypertension, coma and seizures [16]. Irreversible neurological damage has been observed after severe and prolonged hyponatremia [17]. Aggressive treatment is thus recommended in symptomatic patients until natremia reaches 125 mEq/L. Treatment includes hypertonic saline, without or with furosemide [18–19], or high doses of urea [20].

Some controversy raised concerning the optimal rate of natremia correction in patients with severe hyponatremia (<110 mEq/L). Several investigators attributed central pontine myelinolysis to rapid correction of hyponatremia in animals [21] and in humans [22–23]. Recent studies, however, showed that slow correction is associated with higher morbidity and mortality [24], and that rapid correction can reduce mortality and prevent from central nervous system damage [25, 26]. Neurological complications seem to be due to complete normalization of hyponatremia, or to overcorrection to hypernatremia, rather than to the rapid correction. We studied the effects of rapid correction of hyponatremia with urea in patients with SIADH [20]. Natremia increased by 1.1 mEq/L/hr and osmolality increased by 6 mOsm/kg H_2O/hr, but no neurological complication was observed. These results have now been confirmed in many patients. It may thus be recommended that severe symptomatic hyponatremia be corrected at the rate of 1–2 mEq/L/hr up to 125 mEq/L.

References

1. Dzau VJ, Hollenberg NK (1984) Renal response to captopril in severe heart failure: role of furosemide in natriuresis and reversal of hyponatremia. Ann Intern Med 100:777–781
2. Packer M, Medina N, Yushak M (1984) Correction of dilutional hyponatremia in severe chronic heart failure by converting-enzyme inhibition. Ann Intern Med 100:782–788
3. Cauchie P, Vincken W, Decaux G (1987) Urea treatment for water retention in hyponatremic congestive heart failure. Int J Cadiol 17:102–104
4. Carrilho F, Bosh J, Arroyo V, Mas A, Viver J, Rodes J (1977) Renal failure associated with demeclocycline in cirrhosis. Ann Intern Med 87:195–197
5. Decaux G, Mols P, Cauchie P, Flamion B, Delwiche F (1986) Treatment of hyponatremic cirrhosis with ascites resistant to diuretics by urea. Nephron 44:337–343
6. Bartter FC, Schwartz WB (1967) The syndrome of inappropriate secretion of antidiuretic hormone (SIADH). Am J Med 42:790–806

7. Tanay A, Yust I, Peresecenschi G, Abramov AL, Aviram A (1979) Long-term treatment of the syndrome of inappropriate antidiuretic hormone secretion with phenytoin. Ann Intern Med 90:50–52
8. Forrest JN, Cox M, Hong C, Morrison G, Bia M, Singer I (1978) Superiority of demeclocycline over lithium in the treatment of chronic syndrome of inappropriate secretion of antidiuretic hormone. N Engl J Med 298:173–177
9. Hofbauer KG, Mah SC (1987) Vasopressin antagonists: present and future. Kidney Int 32 (suppl):S76–S82
10. Singer L, Rotenberg D (1973) Demeclocycline induced nephrogenic diabetes insipidus: in vitro and in vivo studies. Ann Intern Med 79:679–683
11. Miller PD, Linas SL, Scrier RW (1980) Plasma demeclocycline levels and nephrotoxicity. JAMA 243:2513–2515
12. Decaux G, Brimioulle S, Genette F, Mockel J (1980) Treatment of the syndrome of inappropriate secretion of antidiuretic hormone with urea. Am J Med 69:99–106
13. Decaux G, Genette Fr (1981) Urea for long-term treatment of the syndrome of inappropriate secretion of antidiuretic hormone. Br Med J 283:1081–1083
14. Decaux G, Waterlot Y, Genette Fr, Hallemans R, Demanet JC (1982) Inappropriate secretion of antidiuretic hormone treated by furosemide. Br Med J 285:89–90
15. Decaux G (1983) Treatment of the syndrome of inappropriate secretion of antidiuretic hormone by long loop diuretics. Nephron 35:82–88
16. Decaux G, Szypoer M, Grivegnée A (1983) Cerebral ventricular volume during hyponatremia. J Neurol Neurosurg Psychiatry 46:443–445
17. Ashraf N, Locksley R, Arieff A (1981) Thiazide-induced hyponatremia associated with death or neurologic damage in outpatients. Am J Med 70:1163–1168
18. Hatman D, Rossier B, Zohlman R, Schrier R (1973) Rapid correction of hyponatremia in the syndrome of inappropriate secretion of antidiuretic hormone: an alternative treatment to hypertonic saline. Ann Intern Med 78:870–875
19. Ayus JC, Krothapalli RK, Arieff AI (1982) Rapid correction of severe hyponatremia with intravenous hypertonic saline solution. Am J Med 72:43–48
20. Decaux G, Unger J, Brimioulle S, Mockel J (1982) Hyponatremia in the syndrome of inappropriate secretion of antidiuretic hormone: rapid correction with urea, sodium chloride, and water restriction therapy. JAMA 247:471–474
21. Kleinschmidt-De Masters BK, Norenberg MD (1981) Rapid correction of hyponatremia causes demyelinization: relation to central pontine myelinolysis. Science 211:1068–1070
22. Loreno R (1983) Central pontine myelinolysis following rapid correction of hyponatremia. Ann Neurol 13:232–242
23. Sterns RH, Riggs JE, Schichet SS (1986) Osmotic demyelination following correction of hyponatremia. N Engl J Med 314:1535–1541
24. Dubois GD, Arieff AI (1984) Symptomatic hyponatremia: the case for rapid correction. In: Narins RS (ed) Controversies in nephrology and hypertension. Churchill-Livingstone, New York, pp 393–407
25. Ayus JC, Krothapalli R, Armstrong DL (1985) Rapid correction of severe hyponatremia in the rat: Histopathological changes in the brain. Am J Physiol 248:F711–F719
26. Ayus JC, Krothapalli RK, Arieff AI (1987) Treatment of symptomatic hyponatremia and its relation to brain damage: A prospective study. N Engl J Med 317:1190–1195

Acute Diabetic Emergencies

K. Hillman

Introduction

Diabetes is a family of metabolic derangements which have hyperglycemia in common. Approximately 5% of the population is diabetic and because patients are surviving longer and having children, the incidence is increasing. There are two main types of diabetes: type I or insulin dependent diabetes mellitus (IDDM) and type II or non-insulin dependent diabetes mellitus (NIDDM).

Type I accounts for about 20% of all diabetics and is usually heralded by an abrupt onset in childhood or adolescence and involves destruction of the B-cells in the pancreas resulting in an absolute deficiency of insulin.

Type II occurs in about 80% of all diabetics and is as a result of a relative lack of insulin. The plasma insulin is normal or even high but ineffective due mainly to insulin resistance. It usually develops insidiously in patients who are obese and over the age of 40. These patients are often controlled by weight reduction and oral hypoglycemics.

Diabetic emergencies present in three main forms:

1. euglycemic ketoacidosis (normal to slightly high blood sugar and acidotic)
2. hyperosmolar hyperglycemic nonketotic coma (HHNKC) (high blood sugar and little or no acidosis) are at extreme ends of a wide spectrum of presentation.
3. Diabetic ketoacidosis (DKA) is marked by both acidosis and hyperglycemia and includes the majority of presentations.

Type I diabetics mostly suffer DKA, while type II diabetics may present with or without acidosis. Patients with HHNKC are usually much older than those with DKA. The onset of HHNKC is over days to weeks whereas patients with DKA usually develop over days. Euglycemic ketoacidosis is classically seen in young type I diabetics and the onset is rapid.

Pathogenesis

The decreased or absent insulin in DKA results in [1–3]:

1. Proteolysis – which causes hyperamino-acidemia, a negative nitrogen balance and wasting.

2. Glycogenolysis and gluconeogenesis resulting in hyperglycemia and glycosuria.
3. Lipolysis which releases free fatty acids (FFA) which are converted to ketones in the liver.

While insulin deficiency results in severe DKA, patients with HHNKC have sufficient insulin to inhibit ketone body formation but not enough to prevent hyperglycemia. Hyperosmolar hyperglycemic nonketotic coma has three separate components for its development – a lack of insulin, renal impairment and cerebral impairment [4, 5].

The relative lack of insulin leads to hyperglycemia, glycosuria and hyperosmolality. The hyperglycemia is itself made worse by a reduced glomerular filtration rate (GFR) and impairment of glucose excretion. This renal impairment may be related in part to the old age of these patients. The hyperosmolality and dehydration is exacerbated by decreased fluid intake because the thirst mechanism is reduced by cerebral impairment.

Stress hormones such as epinephrine, norepinephrine, cortisol, growth hormone and glucagon are released in patients with both DKA and HHNKC. These in turn exacerbate the hyperglycemia and peripheral resistance to insulin.

Diabetic Ketoacidosis

Precipitating Factors

Approximately one-third of cases are in newly discovered diabetics. There may be a specific cause in other cases such as infection, myocardial infarction, cerebrovascular accident or thromboembolic disorders [1, 3, 6, 7]. Poor diabetic education and undetermined factors account for over half of all cases.

Clinical Manifestations

Although the word coma is associated with DKA and HHNKC, it may not be a feature at presentation. In DKA only about 10% of cases are actually unconscious and at least 20% have no clouding of consciousness [7]. Patients may present with vomiting, thirst, polyuria, weakness, air hunger, altered sensorium and abdominal pain.

The patients are often tachycardic, dehydrated, often with signs of poor perfusion and postural hypotension indicating hypovolemia [8]. They have rapid deep (Kussmaul) respiration and their breath has a sweetly fruity odour (like Juicy Fruit chewing gum).

Laboratory Investigations

Blood glucose averages 30 mmol/l on admission but varies widely and probably reflects the amount of fluid lost and the ability of the kidneys to excrete glucose, as much as excessive production.

Blood urea, nitrogen and creatinine are usually elevated, reflecting dehydration and prerenal failure but they may be an element of chronic renal insufficiency.

Hematocrit and hemoglobin are usually high and proportional to the degree of dehydration

White cells: a leukocytosis (15–90 000/cc) with left shift does not necessarily indicate infection.

Sodium is low or normal. Spurious result can occur with hypertriglyceridemia.

Potassium is low, normal or high (often high).

Blood gases: pH often less than 7.1 with bicarbonate less than 10 mmol/l and very low $PaCO_2$.

Triglycerides: marked elevation of serum triglycerides may be detected in the form of lactescent serum. This reverses with insulin therapy.

Plasma ketones and blood lactate should always be measured.

Treatment

Patients with DKA are hyperglycemic, acidotic and dehydrated. The mainstay of treatment is the correction of the hyperglycemia with insulin and rehydration with fluids.

Fluids: Fluid is mainly lost in the urine as the result of an osmotic diuresis due to the glycosuria. Vomiting, pyrexia and hyperventilation may also contribute. Hypovolemia and decreased interstitial space is made worse once treatment commences, as water is driven into the cells by insulin and glucose. The average water loss is between 5 and 10 litres and the average sodium loss is 400–700 mmol [9]. Although fluid loss as a result of an osmotic diuresis is isotonic, sodium only accounts for a concentration of approximately 50–70 mmol/l [10]. Other ions and, of course, glucose account for the remainder of the osmolality. Approximately half of the fluid is lost from the extracellular space and half from the intracellular space [11]. It would thus seem logical to replace these losses with fluid that has a similar sodium concentration to that which is lost [12, 13]. This would represent a hypotonic solution with respect to sodium. This kind of hypotonic solution is distributed to the three body fluid compartments – the intravascular, the interstitial and the intracellular space. However, the rate at which the hypotonic solution would correct the hypovolemia is not rapid enough to adequately resuscitate the patient. Isotonic saline is often used to overcome this disadvantage [2, 6, 14]. However, isotonic saline is mainly distributed to the interstitial rather than the intravascular space and is inefficient at correcting the immediate problem of hypovolemia or shock [15]. It is important to titrate intravascular fluid against specific end points such as pulse rate, blood pressure, central venous pressure (CVP) and pulmonary artery wedge pressure (PAWP). This is less satisfactory with a fluid such as isotonic saline which is distributed mainly to the interstitial space compared to a colloid which is largely confined to the intravascular space. The volume of isotonic saline needed to correct the hypovolemia would invariably mean an overexpansion of the interstitial space which causes pulmonary and peripheral edema [16]. Pulmonary edema causes hypoxia while peripheral edema seriously impairs oxygen consumption [15]. Moreover isotonic saline does not provide free water for replacing the intracellular fluid losses. Isotonic saline is thus inappropriate and inefficient for correcting hypovolemia and does not address the problem of intracellular losses. A more logical fluid regime would involve correcting the shock or hypovolemia rapidly with a colloid solution and simultaneously replacing the intracellular losses with 5% dextrose [17]. Electrolyte losses such as sodium, potassium, phosphate and magnesium could be replaced as necessary instead of as part of a fixed fluid composition.

It is an important principle in treating the critically ill that shock or hypovolemia is treated rapidly and efficiently. It is equally important that apart from rapid correction of hypovolemia, the fluid losses in the other spaces should be slowly corrected [11, 17, 18]. This enables the body's water to be slowly distributed according to inherent osmotic forces. Cell size and electrolyte concentration can slowly adjust without rapid and detrimental changes.

Electrolytes

Sodium: Sodium is initially diluted by water moving out of the cells in response to the osmotic pressure generated by extracellular glucose. Thus hyponatremia is almost invariable in the early stages of DKA. Concurrently, however, there is a relatively hypotonic solution lost in the urine. This would normally cause hypernatremia, which in fact occurs in the latter stages of DKA as water losses from the urine are greater than water gains from the intracellular space. Thus the patient with DKA may present with a low, normal or high plasma sodium. To confuse matters further a spurious hyponatremia may occur as a result of the high triglyceride levels sometimes found in DKA. As glucose and water under the influence of insulin move back into the cell, the plasma sodium returns to normal and the urine losses are greatly diminished [11]. Sodium retention accompanies insulin treatment of DKA [11]. The average sodium losses would be partly or wholly replaced by the sodium content in most colloids (approximately 140 mmol/l) if that solution was used to correct hypovolemia. Additional sodium expands the interstitial space causing pulmonary, peripheral and even cerebral edema [11].

Potassium: There are probably even greater losses of potassium than sodium in DKA [14]. However, up to a third of patients present with significant hyperkalemia. This is related to the metabolic acidosis causing hydrogen ions to move intracellularly in exchange for potassium. Other mechanisms include glucagon, dehydration, renal impairment, increased metabolism and cell breakdown as well as the lack of insulin to promote cellular uptake of potassium [19]. Although some proposed regimens advocate immediate potassium administration, on the basis of the high initial incidence of hyperkalemia, it should be administered according to measured levels. The rate of administration usually varies from 5–40 mmol/hr and continual ECG monitoring is essential during this time.

Phosphate: While initial phosphate levels in DKA can be normal or high, the losses can be as high as 320 mmol/l [2, 3]. Average losses are approximately 1 mmol/kg weight. However, hypophosphatemia becomes common as the phosphate moves intracellularly once therapy has commenced. Hypophosphatemia has been increasingly shown to be common in the seriously ill and it is frequently accompanied by complications such as respiratory paralysis and failure, decreased level of consciousness, generalized muscle weakness, impaired cardiac function and tissue hypoxia as a result of decreased 2,3-diphosphoglycerate (2,3-DPG). Phosphate should be measured initially and at least once per day during the acute period and replaced accordingly. While some studies have suggested that phosphate has no effect on the course of DKA [2] it does not make sense that DKA is singled out as the only condition where hypophosphatemia is not detrimental. Indeed, acute respiratory failure in DKA has been reported when hypophosphatemia has been overlooked [20].

Magnesium: Like phosphate, increasing attention has been focussed on hypomagnesium and its complications in Intensive Care. Magnesium is another important intracellular ion depleted during DKA. It should be measured on admission and at least once daily. Hypomagnesemia is common during an osmotic diuresis and has been associated with asystole during DKA [21]. Between 10–80 mmol of magnesium is often needed to restore normal levels.

Insulin: Hyperglycemia and ketoacidosis results from lack of insulin. However, the commencement of insulin therapy is not the most urgent aspect of therapy in DKA. Like any other seriously ill patient, they should be assessed and resuscitated first. This mean securing the airway, guaranteeing adequate oxygenation and correcting the shock.

Insulin has been administered in many ways for the treatment of DKA. Increasingly, a continuous low dose intravenous infusion is used as it is effective, and easily manageable [1–3, 6]. Usually 2 to 10 U/hr of soluble short-acting insulin is effective. Carrier solutions to prevent adsorption are not necessary as the rate of insulin is titrated against a known and easily measured end-point – the blood glucose. Although the infusion rate varies between patients and insulin resistance is common in DKA. However, the infusion rate is fairly constant in any given patient. Each patient must therefore be carefully evaluated and the correct infusion rate tailored to their needs. Occasionally insulin resistance is high due to antibodies, stress hormones or intracellular defects [2]. In these cases the insulin needs to be increased. There is no danger in high levels of insulin as the maximal response occurs when a finite number of receptors are occupied, regardless of the amount of insulin needed to achieve that occupancy.

It is crucial to assess the infusion rate for each individual patient and to adjust it so that *the blood sugar is bought down slowly and smoothly over at least 24 hours.* The blood sugar should be measured hourly and the rate adjusted accordingly. Insulin does not simply decrease blood glucose, it drives glucose and potassium into cells accompanied by water. Rapid movement of glucose, ions and water encourages cellular swelling and edema. The body needs time and free water to slowly adjust to a new osmotic environment.

Bicarbonate: Most patients with DKA are seriously acidotic as a result of over-production of acetoacetic and β-hydroxybutyric acids. Acidosis supposedly impairs myocardial contractility, decreases sensitivity of fat and muscle to insulin and decreases respiratory drive. However, most experts would now recommend that bicarbonate is not given unless the pH is intially below 6.9 or persistently below 7.1 [1–3, 7, 22]. Once treatment has commenced, hydrogen ions are metabolised as ketone bodies, neutralizated by endogenous bicarbonate or excreted in the urine.

Bicarbonate therapy may be harmful in the treatment of DKA because it can cause paradoxical central nervous system acidosis, intracellular acidosis in the peripheral tissues, hypokalemia, increased oxygen affinity with hemoglobin and contributes to sodium and osmolar loads with possible edema formation.

General measures:
1. Protection of airway – intubation and nasogastric tube if necessary.
2. Low dose heparin – prophylaxis for thromboembolic complications.
3. Monitoring
   - continuous ECG.
   - urinary catheter and hourly measurement in presence of hypotension
   - CVP and/or PAWP if necessary.
4. Antibiotics – if indicated.

Complications

Cerebral edema: Cerebral edema probably occurs in all patients with DKA, although in most cases it is subclinical [12, 23, 24]. However, in some it becomes clinically evident; in which case it is associated with a mortality approaching 90%. The development of cerebral edema is associated with the treatment of DKA, not the disease itself. There have been many postulated causes including increased cerebral blood flow, damaged capillary endothelial cells and the presence of intracellular idiogenic osmoles which cause cellular swelling. However, the swelling appears to be pericellular rather than cellular [24]. Fein's group has described subclinical cerebral and pulmonary edema in patients resuscitated with crystalloid therapy [23] and suggested it was related to expansion of the interstitial space due to a decreased colloid osmotic pressure (COP). Another explanation is that because of the proportional distribution of isotonic saline, the crystalloid itself could be responsible for interstitial fluid expansion causing pulmonary and cerebral edema [11].

Pulmonary edema: Pulmonary edema or ARDS has also been described in DKA. The cause may be related to decreased COP, altered capillary permeability, disseminated intravascular coagulopathy (DIC) coexisting myocardial infarction or excessive crystalloid therapy [11].

Shock: May be due simply to hypovolemia. However, severe acidosis, myocardial infarction, septicemia, bleeding, hypokalemia, hypophosphatemia, adrenal insufficiency and hypomagnesemia should be excluded.

Vascular thrombosis: Many features of DKA predispose to thrombosis – dehydration hypovolemia, increased blood viscosity and underlying atherosclerosis. Low dose heparin should be routinely used unless otherwise contraindicated.

Hyperosmolar, Hyperglycemic, Non-ketotic Coma (HHNKC)

The principles of treatment are the same as for DKA, however, the mortality is much higher and remains between 40% and 70% [4, 11]. The patients are usually more elderly, with a greater degree of dehydration and hypovolemia and have a higher incidence of coma. It is even more important to avoid isotonic saline in these patients as they are often hypernatremic and always hyperosmolar. Judicious use of low dose continuous insulin infusion to slowly reduce blood sugar over 48–96 hours is essential. The hypovolemia should be rapidly corrected with aggressive use of colloids and hypotonic solutions such as 5% dextrose should be administered simultaneously in order to slowly correct the water losses. Elecrolyte abnormalities (Ca^{2+}, K^+, PO_4^{2-}, Mg^{2+}) should all be measured regularly and corrected as necessary. Patients often remain semi-conscious for up to 5 days. The airway should always be maintained and vigorous physiotherapy used to prevent basal lung collapse and pneumonia.

Outcome

The mortality of diabetic emergencies is determined by the age, state of consciousness and the presence or absence of co-existing conditions such as myocardial infarction, sepsis and pancreatitis. The mortality for DKA remains between 1% and 20% [1, 6, 7] and up to 50% for HHNKC [4, 5, 8]. These figures have not changed appreciably in recent years and may even be higher in units

Table 1. Management of diabetic emergencies

1. Correct hypovolemia and shock. Titrate colloid against intravascular measurements.
2. Investigate and treat concurrent illness, e.g. infection, myocardial infarction.
3. Simultaneously correct water losses *slowly* (100–200 mls/hour over 24–96 hours.
4. Slowly reduce blood sugar with continuous insulin infusion over at least 24 hours and at a rate not exceeding 5 mmol/h.
5. Regularly measure serum potassium and replace at an hourly rate (5–40 mmol/h) to maintain normokalemia.
6. Regularly measure Mg^{2+}, PO_4^{2-} and Ca^{2+} and replace as necessary.
7. Avoid bicarbonate unless pH below 6.9 or persistently below 7.1.

who do not have a special interest in diabetic emergencies [6]. It is therefore crucial to resuscitate these patients rapidly and monitor them carefully during their stay in Intensive Care.

References

1. Keller U (1986) Diabetic ketoacidosis: current views on pathogenesis and treatment. Diabetologia 29:71-77
2. Foster DW, McGarry JD (1983) The metabolic derangements and treatment of diabetic ketoacidosis. N Engl J Med 309:159-169
3. Kreisberg MD (1978) Diabetic ketoacidosis: new concepts and trends in pathogenesis and treatment. Ann Intern Med 88:681-695
4. Arieff AI, Carroll HJ (1972) Nonketotic hyperosmolar coma with hyperglycemia: clinical features, pathophysiology, renal function, acid-base balance, plasma-cerebrospinal fluid equilibria and the effects of therapy in 37 cases. Medicine 51:73-94
5. Gerich JE, Martin MM, Recant L (1971) Clinical and metabolic characteristics of hyperosmolar nonketotic coma. Diabetes 20:228-231
6. Griffith DNW, Yudkin JS (1986) Diabetic ketoacidosis. Br J Hosp Med Feb: 82-87
7. Alberti KGM, Hockaday TD (1973) Diabetic coma: a reappraisal after five years. Clin Endocrinol Metab 6:421-427
8. Gale EAM, Dornan TL, Tattersall R (1976) Diabetic coma and precoma in the elderly. Presented to the British Diabetic Association Autumn Meeting, Guildford
9. Atchley DW, Loeb RF, Richards DW Jr, Benedict EM, Driscoll ME (1933) On diabetic acidosis: a detailed study of the electrolyte balance following the withdrawal and re-establishment of insulin therapy. J Clin Invest 12:297-302
10. Gennari ER, Kassirer JP (1974) Osmotic diuresis. N Eng J Med 291:714-720
11. Hillman K (1987) Fluid resuscitation in diabetic emergencies - a reappraisal. Intensive Care Med 13:4-8
12. Kleeman CR, Liberma B (1972) Diabetic acidosis and coma. In: Maxwell MH, Kleeman CR (eds) Clinical disorders of fluid and electrolyte metabolism. McGraw-Hill, pp 971-975
13. Waldhausl W, Kleinberger G (1980) Acute treatment of diabetic coma. In: Podolsky S, Viswanathan M (eds) Secondary diabetes: the spectrum of the diabetic syndromes. Raven Press, New York, pp 215-219
14. Johnson DG, Alberti KGMM (1980) Diabetic emergencies: practical aspects of the management of diabetic ketoacidosis and diabetes during surgery. Clin Endocrinol Metab 9:437-460
15. Twigley AJ, Hillman (1985) The end of the crystalloid era? Anaesthesia 40:860-871
16. Hillman K (1987) Fluid replancement in the critically ill. Medicine International 2:1567-1572
17. Hillman KM (1983) Resuscitation in diabetic ketoacidosis. Crit Care Med 11:53-54
18. Swales JD (1987) Dangers in treating hyponatremia. B Med J 294:261-262
19. Anonymous (1986) Hyperkalemia in diabetic ketoacidosis. Lancet ii:845-846
20. Hasselstrom L, Wiberley PD, Nielsen VG (1986) Hypophosphatemia and acute respiratory failure in a diabetic patient. Intensive Care Med 12:429-431
21. McMullen JK (1977) Asystole and hypomagnesaemia during recovery from diabetic ketoacidosis. Br Med J 1:690-694
22. Morris LR, Murphy MB, Kitabchi AE (1986) Bicarbonate therapy in severe diabetic ketoacidosis. Ann Intern Med 105:836-840
23. Fein IA, Rackow ER, Sprung CL, Grodman R (1982) Relation of colloid osmotic pressure to arterial hypoxemia and cerebral edema during crystalloid volume loading of patients with diabetic ketoacidosis. Ann Intern Med 96:570-575
24. Winegrad AI, Kern EFO, Simmons DA (1985) Cerebral edema in diabetic ketoacidosis. N Engl J Med 312:1184-1185

Nutritional Assessment of Critically Ill Patients

A. Van Gossum

Introduction

The two main goals of nutritional assessment of a patient are: first, to detect patients requiring a nutritional support and second to use the nutritional status as a prognostic factor. Nevertheless, the more seriously ill is the patient, the more difficult is the assessment of nutritional status. Indeed, in such clinical conditions, other factors such as surgical stress, ongoing sepsis or therapeutic management are likely to interfere with the nutritional assessment itself.

Methods of Nutritional Assessment

Nutritional status can be assessed by different methods that can be classified as subjective, objective or functional. The validity of the subjective assessment of nutritional status has been pointed out by the team headed by K. N. Jeejeebhoy in Toronto [1]. Subjective evaluation performed by different investigators is well reproducible and highly correlated with objective methods [2]. However, a subjective approach cannot easily detect latent malnutrition and this is especially true in acutely ill patients. For these patients, medical history is often unobtainable or incomplete; physical examination is perturbated by the acuteness of the disease or the therapeutical management such as mechanical ventilation or postoperative status. Most of the short-term fluctuations in weight can also be explained by changes in the water content of the body.

Objective methods attempt to assess the composition of different compartments of the body. Anthropometric measurements evaluate either fat store or muscular proteins content. These methods are simple but have many sources of errors: the distribution of subcutaneous varies with age, sex, race, presence of edema or subcutaneous emphysema, site of measurement and tables of references [3].

The 24 hour creatinine excretion in urine is dependent on the muscle mass, provided that renal function is normal. Moreover, it has been demonstrated that creatinine excretion can be influenced by ongoing sepsis, trauma, steroid therapy or thermal injury [4]. Similar criticisms are valuable for measurement of 3-methylhistine urine, which is formed by the methylation of histidine and excreted unchanged in the urine [5]. The technique of evaluation of visceral proteins relies on the serum concentration of proteins synthetized by the liver. The assumption is that a fall in the serum concentration of these proteins is a consequence of a nutrition related decrease in protein synthesis. However, the plasma levels of any protein are the result of a balance between synthesis and catabolism. In the presence of abnormal losses (protein-losing enteropathy, nephropathy) or liver disease, the abnormal plasma level may not be due to malnutrition and consequently may not respond to increased nutritional support [6]. It is also worth mentioning that protein levels may be influenced by water balance and that many critically ill patients receive blood or blood products, which can influence their plasma proteins levels.

Moreover, interpretation of plasma proteins levels must take in consideration the half-life of proteins which can vary from 20 days for albumin to a few hours for fibronectin [7]. On the other hand, in case of sepsis, synthesis of acute-phase proteins predominates over synthesis of structural proteins such as albumin [8].

Malnutrition is a main cause of secondary immunodeficiency. The most common form of in vivo testing of immune competence is the measurement of delayed cutaneous hypersensitivity (DCH) to known antigens. However, a multitude of factors including infection, metabolic and systemic disorders (uremia, sarcoidosis), malignancy, chemo and radiotherapy, drugs, general anesthesia, surgery and zinc deficiency have all been reported as potentially affecting DCH. All of these must therefore be taken into account before attributing abnormalities of skin testing to malnutrition alone [9, 10]. Muscle is the main component of the human lean body mass and muscle wasting is prominent in severe malnutrition. Therefore, muscle mass is a good reflect of the nutritional status. Different methods have been settled to assess muscle function. Klidjian et al. [11] proposed to detect severe malnutrition by measuring the hand-grip strength using a dynamometer. Hand-grip dynamometry has been shown to be an useful screening test of patients at risk. Unfortunately, this method requires active participation of the patient, so that it is often unfeasible in critically ill patients.

Jeejeebhoy et al. [12] proposed another technique for investigation of the effect of nutrition on muscle function. Supramaximal ulnar nerve stimulation is performed with square wave pulses for 60–70 microseconds at frequencies increasing from 10, 20 to 50 Hz, for one to two seconds at a time, and the force of contraction is recorded. Then the maximal rate of muscle relaxation is observed during a one to two second 20 Hz stimulation. In hypocalorically fed and fasted humans, the F10/F20 and F10/F50 ratios are higher than in normal subjects and the muscle relaxation rate is significantly lower. Alterations of muscle performance could be due to an increase in the intracellular concentration of calcium [13].

Neither renal failure per se, nor peritoneal dialysis, nor hemodialysis changed the F10/F50 ratio or the maximal relaxation rate. The same is true for chronic obstructive lung disease. Patients studied in the recovery room immediately after laparotomy also had normal F10/F50; F10/F20 ratios and maximal relaxation rate. Severe sepsis in patients with adequate nutritional support was associated with a slight rise in F10/F50 ratio but with a normal maximal relaxation rate. The changes were considerably less than in patients with a caloric intake less than 90% of their measured resting metabolic rate [14].

Assessment of Nutritional Status as a Prognostic Index

While nutritional status has been thought to influence morbidity and mortality of acutely ill patients, no single nutritional parameter is likely to be a valuable prognostic factor. Only subjective clinical assessment and serum albumin levels could detect patients at risk to develop postoperative complications [15].

Validity of muscle function testing must be confirmed in further studies. Many authors have tried to select parameters in order to propose a prognostic index. The most popular index has been proposed by Mullen et al. [16] who used a computer based stepwise regression procedure. The comparison between nutritional assessment determinations at admission in complicated and uncomplicated surgical patients indicated that 4 parameters (albumin, total proteins, transferrin, and DCH) had predictive significance and allowed to calculate a "prognostic nutritional index" using a linear predictive model. This formula was modified and simplified by Simms et al. [17]. Ingenbleek and Carpentier (personal communication) recently proposed a new prognostic inflammatory and nutritional index for scoring critically ill patients, which is based on the determination of the two sensitive acute phase reactants (orosomucoid and CRP).

An alternative approach to the interpretation of multivariable nutritonal assessment has been developed by Nazari et al. [18]. In this approach, four patterns of nutritonal depletion have been defined by cluster analysis of 11 anthropometric, biochemical and immunological parameters. Classification of patients into one of these four clusters may provide a useful means to assess the risk of nutrition-related operative complications. However, it takes several days to obtain values of all the parameters included in this analysis.

In a recent provocative study, Pettigrew et al. [19] claimed that operative performance is the main factor in the development of postoperative complications. In their hands, immediate postoperative assessment was superior to any preoperative method including nutritional assessment for selection of high risk patients. This original approach should be assessed in future studies of outcome.

On the other hand, response to total parenteral nutrition (TPN) could also have a prognostic value. Starker et al. [20] observed that critically ill patients who developed hypoalbuminemia and hyponatremia, and gained weight after one week on TPN regimen had an uncontrolled sepsis and a very poor prognosis. In a study performed on 18 patients with severe acute pancreatitis receiving lipids with TPN, persistent hypertriglyceridemia, hyperglycemia, hypoalbuminemia with higher insulin requirements were observed in fatalities in comparison with survivors [21].

In conclusion, nutritional assessment in the critically ill patients is not easy. Interpretation of nutritional parameters must take into account other factors such as sepsis, surgical stress, and therapeutical management which could influence the outcome of the patient. The decision to start a nutritional support has to be based not only on the initial nutritional assessment but also on the estimation of the period of time during which the patient will be unable to eat. Nutritional approach of the critically ill patient must be dynamic and prospective.

References

1. Baker JP, Detsky AS, Weeson DE, et al (1982) Nutritional assessment: a comparison of clinical judgement and objective measurements. N Engl J Med 306:969–972
2. Detsky A, Mc Laughlin J, Baker J, et al (1987) What is subjective global assessment of nutritional status. JPEN 11:8–13
3. Heymsfield SB, Mc Manus CB, Seitz SB (1984) Anthropemetric assessment of adult protein energy malnutrition. In: Nutritional assessment. Oxford, Blackwell Scientific Publications 27
4. Heymsfield SB, Arteaga C, Mc Manus C, Smith J, Moffit S (1983) Measurement of muscle mass in humans: validity of the 24 hours urinary creatinine method. Am J Clin Nutr 37:478–494
5. Long CL, Birkham RH, Geiger JW (1981) Urinary excretion of 3-methylhistidine: an assessment of muscle protein catabolism in adult normal subjects and during malnutrition, sepsis and skeletal trauma. Metabolism 30:765–72
6. Young G, Chem C, Hill G (1978) Assessment of protein-caloric malnutrition in surgical patients from plasma proteins and anthropometric measurements. Am J Clin Nutr 31:429–435
7. Howard L, Dillon B, Saba T, Hofmann S, Cho E (1984) Decreased plasma fibronectin during starvation in man. JPEN 8:237–244
8. Dominioni L, Dionigi R, Zanello M, et al (1987) Sepsis score and acute-phase protein response as predictors of outcome in septic surgical patients. Arch Surg 122:141–146
9. Chandra RK (1981) Immunocompetence as a functional index of nutritional status. Brit Med Bull 37:89–94
10. Forse RA, Christou N, Meakins JL, Mc Lean L, Shizgal HM (1984) Reliability of skin testing as a measure of nutritional state. Arch Surg 116:1284–1288
11. Klidjian AM, Archer TJ, Foster KJ, Karran SJ (1982) Detection of dangerous malnutrition. JPEN 6:118–121
12. Russel D, Leiter L, Whitwell J, Marliss E, Jeejeebhoy KN (1983) Skeletal muscle function during hypocaloric diets and fasting: a comparison with standard nutritional assessment parameters. Am J Clin Nutr 37:133–138
13. Jeejeebhoy KN (1986) Muscle function and nutrition. GUT 27:25–39
14. Brough W, Horne G, Irving, Jeejeebhoy KN. A study of malnutrition, sepsis, trauma, steriod administration and surgery on muscle function. Br Med J (in press)
15. Starker PM, Gump FE, Askanazi J, et al (1982) Serum albumin levels as an index of nutritional support. Surgery 91:194–199
16. Buzby GP, Mullen JL, Mathews DC, et al (1980) Prognostic nutritional index in gastrointestinal surgery. Am J Surg 138:160–167
17. Simms JM, Smith JA, Woods HF (1982) A modified prognostic index based upon nutritional measurements. Clinical nutrition 1:71–79
18. Nazari S, Dionigi R, Comodi I, Dionigi P, Campani M (1982) Preoperative prediction and quantification of septic risk caused by malnutrition. Arch Surg 117:266–274
19. Pettigrew R, Burns H, Carter D (1987) Evaluating surgical risk: the importance of technical factors in determining outcome. Br J Surg 74:791–794
20. Starker PM, Lasala PA, Askanazi J, Gump FE, Forse RA, Kinney JM (1983) The response to TPN. A form of nutritional assessment. Ann Surg 198:720–724
21. Van Gossum A, Lemoyne M, Gregg P, Jeejeebhoy K. Lipid associated TPN in patients with acute severe pancreatitis. JPEN (in press)

Special Amino-Acid Formulas in Intensive Care Medicine

P. B. Soeters and M. P. von Meyenfeldt

Introduction

Tailoring of the amino-acid (AA) composition of parenteral nutrition to specific needs may be relevant especially when handling of nitrogen is disturbed like in renal failure, hepatic failure, sepsis and severe trauma. Specifically the addition of extra branched chain amino acids (BCAA) to the AA mixture may for theoretical reasons be of benefit in patients with hepatic failure or in patients suffering from severe sepsis or trauma. We will discuss the rationale for BCAA enrichment of the nutritional regime and review the results of trials in which BCAA enrichment was employed.

Physiology of BCAA

The essential AA leucine, isoleucine, valine are called BCAA because they have a branched carbon chain. The liver lacks BCAA transaminase which catalyzes the first step in the degradation of BCAA. Therefore, BCAA are degraded in peripheral tissues, predominantly muscle and adipose tissue. All other essential AA (phenylalanine, methionine, lysine, threonine and tryptophan) are degraded in the liver. Twenty different AA are biologically active in man, but the three BCAA together constitute 20% of all body proteins.

Alternative Energy Source

BCAA can furnish fuel in peripheral tissues. It has been hypothesized that this predominantly occurs under circumstances where ordinary fuel like carbohydrate and fat are lacking. During severe stress, trauma or sepsis glucose intolerance and diminished lipolysis have been claimed to limit the utilization of fat and glucoses as fuel sources. Due to the ability of the peripheral tissues to degrade BCAA these AA might then serve as alternative energy source. Although BCAA (and most other AA) are degraded to a greater degree during severe disease states the hypothesis has no firm ground:

1. Although well documented during trauma/sepsis glucose intolerance implies that more insulin is needed to metabolize the same amount of glucose and

that the maximal capacity to burn glucose is diminished. It does not imply that glucose can not be utilized at all.

2. Although hyperinsulinemia may inhibit lipolysis, reports in the literature have revealed that fat can be well degraded during severe trauma/sepsis and utilized to cover energy needs [11].

3. If indeed BCAA serve as alternative fuel source not more than approximately 5% of total energy requirements can be covered by the degradation of BCAA.

4. Other hypotheses have been put forward to explain accelerated peripheral proteolysis in severe disease states. Peripheral proteolysis may serve to furnish AA that can be used in the liver for protein synthesis which is crucial in the defense against trauma/sepsis/stress [2].

Effects on Protein Synthesis

BCAA and specifically leucine stimulate protein synthesis *in vitro* [3]. In addition BCKA (branched chain keto acids result after transamination of BCAA: the first step in the degradation of BCAA) inhibit BCAA degradation, equally in vitro. No convincing evidence has been put forward however that better protein sparing can be achieved *in vivo* after inclusion of extra BCAA in the nutritional regimen.

Normalization of Plasma AA Profile

It has been hypothesized that a distorted plasma AA profile (low plasma BCAA; high plasma aromatic AA) may be responsible for hepatic encephalopathy [4]. The neutral AA (BCAA and aromatic amino acids) share a common transport system into the brain so that a distorted plasma AA profile is reflected in the brain. There the aromatic amino acids (AAA) serve as precursors for neurotransmitters so that increased AAA transport into the brain may distort the neurotransmitter profile and lead to encephalopathy. BCAA enrichment of the diet might reverse this chain of events: normalize abnormal plasma AA profiles and improve hepatic encephalopathy [5].

In addition metabolic changes in severe sepsis/trauma or hepatic failure might include an amino acid pattern which is less optimal for protein synthesis. Normalization of the plasma AA profile may also normalize the composition of body AA pools and improve the precursor pattern for protein synthesis and consequently nitrogen balance [6].

Effect on Ammonium Levels

Infusion of ammonium salts results in a depression of plasma BCAA levels [7]. On the other hand infusion of BCAA has been suggested to decrease plasma ammonia levels. BCAA might furnish the amino group with which alpha-ketoglutarate forms glutamin acid which in peripheral tissues (adipose tissue, muscle) can take up ammonia, resulting in the formation of non-toxic glutamine.

BCAA Enrichment in Hepatic Failure and Hepatic Encephalopathy

Twenty anecdotal or randomized series have been presented as oral presentation, in abstract form or as full publication. Only the five studies, that have employed a randomized set up, and that have appeared as complete publications in the literature will be reviewed [8–12] (Table 1). In all studies chronic liver patients are described suffering from acute deterioration of mental state. The duration of these studies amounted to 7–10 days. The aims of nutritional repletion and BCAA enrichment in patients with hepatic failure are:

1. Improvement of liver function, morbidity, mortality;
2. Nutritional repletion;
3. Improvement of hepatic encephalopathy.

The published trials are listed in Table 1. The form of nutritonal support is different in every study.

Morbidity and Mortality (Table 2)

In most studies morbidity is not mentioned. Mortality is not significantly different between control groups and the groups receiving BCAA enrichment, except in the US multicenter study where survival is significantly improved in the BCAA enriched group. This suggests that BCAA enrichment not only repletes liver patients nutritionally thereby exerting a beneficial modulating effect on the result of primary treatment but also acts as pharmacological treatment, waking patients up, thereby reducing complications secondary to the comatose state, or even ameliorating hepatic function. There is no indication in the study however that this is the case, nor is there in the other studies which do not confirm improved survival. Therefore there is no conclusive evidence that BCAA enrichment has a beneficial effect on survival in chronic liver patients suffering from acute deterioration of mental state.

Nutritional Repletion

It is not to be expected that improvement of nutritonal parameters (plasma proteins, immunological data and anthropometric) can be obtained within 10 days. In most studies they are not mentioned and only nitrogen balances are recorded. The US multicenter trial records a clear improvement in nitrogen balance in the group receiving BCAA ($+0.8$ g N/24 h in BCAA treated group versus -8.6 g N/24 h in control group). All other studies either do not mention nitrogen balance [8, 9, 11], or do not show a benefit [10]. Only in the study of Michel et al. [10]

Table 1

Authors (year)	Nutritional treatment Groups BCAA (%)		Nutritional regime AA	Glucose (calories)	Fat (calories)
Rossi Fanelli (1982)	1) Lactulose	+ Dextrose 20%	–	1600/24 h	–
	2) BCAA	+ Dextrose 20%	56 g/day	1600/24 h	–
Wahren (1983)	1) Glucose/fat	+ Dextrose 5%	–	20 Cal/kg/24 h	15/kg/day
	2) Glucose/fat	+ Dextrose 5% BCAA	40 g/day	20 Cal/kg/24 h	15/kg/day
Fiaccadori (1984)	1) Lactulose	+ Dextrose 30%	–	2500/24 h	–
	2) AA (BCAA 45%)	+ Dextrose 30% AA (BCAA 45%)	0.8–1 g/kg/day	2500/24 h	–
	3) Lactulose	+ Dextrose 30%	0.8–1 g/kg/day	2500/24 h	–
Michel (1985)	1) Glucose/fat	+ Conv. AA (BCAA 20%)	60 g/day	1060/24 h	540/day
	2) Glucose/fat	+ AA (BCAA 45%)	60 g/day	1060/24 h	540/day
Cerra (1985)	1) Neomycin	+ Dextrose 25%	–	27 Cal/kg/24 h	–
	2) AA (BCAA 38%)	+ Dextrose 25%	1.1 g/kg/day	27 Cal/kg/24 h	–

Table 2. Effects of BCAA enrichment on recovery and mortality in hepatic encephalopathy

Author	Recovery (%)		Mortality (%)	
	Control	BCAA	Control	BCAA
Rossi Fanelli	47	70	29	23
Wahren	48	56	20	40
Fiaccadori	62	94	?	?
Michel	25	35	25	30
Cerra	17	53	55	17

a control group received isonitrogenous amounts of AA of conventional composition.

Hepatic Encephalopathy (Table 2)

BCAA enrichment does not worsen hepatic encephalopathy. Arousal was as fast or faster and in a larger proportion of patients in the BCAA treated groups than in control groups receiving conventional treatment (generally 20–25% dextrose + neomycin/lactulose). BCAA enrichment allows the administration of 0.6–1.1 g AA/kg/24 h. In only one study however a control group received isonitrogenous amounts of a conventional AA mixture, and no differences were observed between the two AA mixtures [10]. It should therefore be concluded that parenteral AA mixtures, administered up to 1.1 g AA/kg/24 h allow a wake-up response which is at least as good as conventional treatment (hypertonic dextrose, neomycin/lactulose). It is not certain however that this is due to the BCAA content of the AA mixture.

Conclusions

There is no conclusive evidence that BCAA enrichment improves survival from acute hepatic encephalopathy, and nutritional state in chronic hepatic failure. Parenteral administration of BCAA enriched glucose – AA mixutres improves mental state as well or better than conventional types of treatment. It further allows administration of amounts of AA up to 1.1 g/kg/24 h. The studies do not provide evidence that this is specifically due to the BCAA content of the mixtures.

BCAA Enrichment in Sepsis/Trauma

The aims of BCAA enrichment are twofold:
1. Improvement of morbidity and mortality;
2. Nutritional repletion.
   In this review only prospective randomized trials will be considered (Table 3).

Most studies deal with patients with severe stress and/or sepsis related to polytrauma or major operations. The number of patients in all studies is relatively
small with the exception of the recent study of Cerra and the Maastricht study.
Protein intake varied from 1 to 2 g/kg/day. Non-protein calories were given as
glucose only (30–35 Cal/kg/day) or in combination with fat (15–50% of non-
protein calories).

Table 3. Results of prospective and randomized studies

Author (year)	Group characteristics	No. of patients	Duration (days)	AA composition
Blinded studies				
Cerra (1983)	polytrauma post-surg.	32	7	Standard TPN with BCAA 0.16 – 0.3 – 0.5 – 0.7 g/kg/day (16%, 20%, 50%, 50%)
Cerra (1982)	polytrauma post-surg.	15	7	Standard AA-solution BCAA 15.5%–50%
Nuwer (1983)	post-surg.	19	7	Standard AA-solution with BCAA 24%–45%
Cerra (1984)	post-surg. sepsis polytrauma	23	7	Standard AA-solution BCAA 24%–45%
Unblinded studies				
Lundholm (1986)	polytrauma post-surg.	12	10	Standard AA-solution with BCAA 15%–100%-EAA
Bower (1986)	post-surg. sepsis polytrauma	37	10	Standard AA-solution BCAA 25%–45% val. –45% Leu
Cerra (1987)	post-surg. sepsis	87	7	Standard AA-solution 18% BCAA enriched 50%

Table 4. Prospective blinded, randomized study of Maastricht

Author	Group characteristics	No. of patients	Duration (days)	AA composition
von Meyenfeldt Maastricht 1986	trauma sepsis stress	101	7	Standard TPN with BCAA 18%–50% (0.19–0.56 g/kg/day)

Author	Metabolism		Clinical state
von Meyenfeldt Maastricht 1986	N-balance: Cum. balance: Urinary 3-MH:	↑ ↑BCAA 50% moderate stress ↓BCAA 50% severe stress ↓both groups	No diff. morbidity (renal, resp., circ., hepatic) No diff. mortality

Morbidity and Mortality (Table 4)

In the study which assessed clinical outcome no difference in outcome between treatment groups was observed.

Nutritional Repletion (Table 5)

It is difficult to improve nutritional state within 7–10 days. Moreover it is difficult to measure it because most established parameters react slowly, and can also be

Table 5. Results of prospective randomized studies

Author (year)	Metabolism		Clinical state
Blinded studies			
Cerra (1983)	N-balance:	↑ + all groups ↑↑ + 0.5 and 0.7 BCAA (sign.)	Not studied
	Cum. N-balance:	↑with increasing BCAA-concentration	
	Urinary 3-MH excr.:	↓All groups	
Cerra (1982)	N-balance:	↑↑ + BCAA 50% ↑ + BCAA 15.5% N.S.	Not studied
	3-MH excretion:	↓both groups	
Nuwer (1983)	N-balance: Urinary 3-MH excr.: Abs. Lymph. Count: D.C.H. reaction:	↑↑ + BCAA 45% (sign.) not changed both groups ↑↑BCAA 45% (sign.) ↑↑BCAA 45% (sign.)	Not studied
Cerra (1984)	N-balance:	↑↑ + BCAA 45% ↑BCAA 24% N.S.	Not studied
	3-MH excretion: Plasma transferrine: Abs. Lymph. Count: D.C.H reaction:	↓BCAA 24%–45% ↑↑ ⎤ ↑↑ ⎟ BCAA 45% (sign.) ↑↑ ⎦	
Unblinded studies			
Lundholm (1986)	N-balance:	– all groups ↑standard group N.S.	Not studied
	When N from blood-products is taken into account:	N-equilibrium all groups	
Bower (1986)	N-balance: 3-MH excretion: Albumin: Transferrin Pre-albumin: Ret.-bind. protein: Insulin need:	↑↑BCAA 45% groups ↓all groups ↓in BCAA 45% (val↑) ↑ ↑in BCAA 45% (leu↑) ↑ ↓in BCAA 45% (leu↑)	
Cerra (1987)	N-balance: Plasma proteins Better nitrogen retention	↑BCAA group unchanged in BCAA groups	Not studied

influenced by the disease itself. Recovery from illness achieved by non-nutritional means may therefore also result in improvement of parameters generally used for nutritional assessment. Assessment of nutritional status has therefore been limited to measurement of short half-life plasma proteins synthesized by the liver, and of nitrogen balance and 3-methylhistidine excretion (see Chapter by A. Van Gossum in this book).

All authors except Lundhol et al. [14] report an improved nitrogen balance (or a tendency towards improvement) when BCAA-containing solutions are used. The urinary 3-methylhistidine excretion, which is considered as a parameter for muscle degradation, decreases in most studies. Differences in urinary 3-methylhistidine excretion between the various BCAA solutions are not found, suggesting that muscle proteolysis is not influenced. In the earlier studies, immune function was investigated by Cerra and co-workers who [17, 18] found a significant increase in absolute lymphocyte count and delayed cutaneous hypersensitivity in the group of patients receiving BCAA enriched nutrition. Cerra et al. [17] and Bower et al. [19] found a significant increase in plasma proteins with short half-lives like transferrin and prealbumin. In these studies relatively few patients were included and little information was furnished regarding the clinical charcteristics. It is therefore impossible to ascertain whether the improvements observed were due to BCAA enrichment or rather the result of clinical differences between groups. In the larger studies [20, and Masstricht study], no improvement in plasma proteins and lymphocyte counts was found.

Conclusion

There is a theoretical rationale to add extra BCAA to the AA part of parenteral or enteral nutritional regimes in patients with hepatic failure, or sepsis/trauma. In this chapter available prospective randomized studies are reviewed employing parenteral BCAA enrichment in both patient groups mentioned above. Although a BCAA enriched AA composition in the nutritional regimen may be of higher biological and nutritional value under circumstances of severe disease and liver failure the duration of the studies does not allow major changes to become visible. Nutritional assessment is strongly influenced by the primary non nutritional treatment of the disease itself. This also explains why it is difficult to demonstrate a clinical improvement of morbidity and mortality: nutritional repletion as a secondary treatment modality can only have a modulating effect on outcome, and most likely only after longer time periods. However, some studies suggest that in trauma/stress nitrogen balances are improved. In liver disease AA administration up to 1.1 g/kg/24 h can relieve hepatic encephalopathy at least as well or better as conventional treatment (glucose 20–25%, neomycin, lactulose). It is not certain that this is specifically the result of the BCAA content.

References

1. Carpentier YA, Askanazi J, Elwyn DH, Kinney JL (1979) Effects of hypercaloric glucose infusion on lipid metabolism in injury and sepsis. J Trauma 9:649-653
2. Clowes GHA, George BC, Villee CA, et al. (1983) Muscle proteolysis induced by a circulating peptide in patients with sepsis or trauma. N Engl J Med 308:545-548
3. Buse MG, Reid SS (1975) Leucine, a possible regulator of protein turnover in muscle. J Clin Invest 56:1250
4. Fischer JE, Baldessarini RJ (1971) False neurotransmitters and hepatic coma. Lancet 2:75-78
5. Fischer JE, Rosen HM, Ebeid AM, James JH, Keane JM, Soeters PB (1976) The effect of normalization of plasma amino acids on hepatic encephalopathy in man. Surgery 80:77-91
6. Soeters PB (1984) Amino acid metabolism in liver disease: nutritional aspects. In: Holm, Kasper (eds) Metabolism and nutrition in liver disease. MTP Press Ltd, pp 57-66
7. Leweling H, Holm E, Staedt U, Striebel J-P, Tschepe A (1984) Intra- and extracellular amino acid concentrations in ammoniuminfused rats. Evidence that hyperammonemia reduces BCAA levels. In: Kleinberger, Ferenci, Riederer, Thaler (eds) Advances in hepatic encephalopathy and urea cycle diseases. Karger, Vienna, pp 552-555
8. Rossi-Fanelli F, Riggio O, Cangiano C, et al (1982) Branched chain amino acids vs lactulose in the treatment of hepatic coma: A controlled study. Dig Dis Sci 27:929-935
9. Fiaccadori F, Ghinelli F, Pedretti G, et al (1985) Branched-chain enriched amino acid solutions in the treatment of hepatic encephalopathy: a controlled trial. Ital J Gastroenterol 17:5
10. Michel H, Pomier-Layrargues G, Duhamel O, Lacombe B, Cuilleret G, Bellet H (1984) Intravenous infusion of ordinary and modified amino acid solutions in the management of hepatic encephalopathy. In: Capocaccia, Fischer, Rossi-Fanelli (eds) Hepatic encephalopathy in chronic liver disease. Plenum Press, New York, pp 323-333
11. Wahren J, Denis J, Desurmont P, Erickson SJ, et al (1983) Is intravenous administration of branched chain amino acids effective in the treatment of hepatic encephalopathy? A multicenter study. Hepatology 3:475-480
12. Cerra FB, Cheung NK, Fischer JE, et al (1985) Disease-specific amino acid infusion (FO80) in hepatic encephalopathy: a prospective, randomized, double-blind, controlled trial. JPEN 9:288-295
13. Freund H, Hoover HC Jr, Atamian S, Fischer JE (1979) Infusion of the branched chain amino acids in postoperative patients. Ann Surg 190:18-23
14. Lundholm K, Bennegard K, Wickström I, Lindmark L (1986) Is it possible to evaluate the efficacy of amino acid solutions after major surgical procedures or accidental injuries?. Evaluation in a randomized and prospective study. JPEN 10:29-33
15. Cerra FB, Upson D, Angelico R, et al (1982) Branched chains support postoperative protein synthesis. Surgery 92:192-198
16. Cerra FB, Mazaski J, Teasley K, et al (1983) Nitrogen solution in critically ill patients is proportional to the branched chain amino acid load. Crit Care Med 11:775-778
17. Cerra FB, Mazaski J, Chute E, et al (1984) Branched chain metabolic support. Ann Surg 199:286-291
18. Nuwer N, Cerra FB, Shronts E, Lysne J, Feasley K, Konstantinides F (1983) Does modified amino acid total parenteral nutrition alter immune response in high level surgical stress? JPEN 7:521-524
19. Bower R, Muggia-Sullam M, Vallgren S, et al (1986) Branched chain amino acid enriched solutions in the septic patient. Ann Surg 203:13-20
20. Cerra F, Blackburn G, Hirsch J, Mullen K, Luther W (1987) The effect of stress level, amino acid formula, and nitrogen dose on nitrogen retention in traumatic and septic stress. Ann Surg 204:282-287

Aspects of the Gastrointestinal Tract in Intensive Care

K. Hillman

Introduction

Because treatment of the seriously ill often involved artificial ventilation, the specialty of Intensive Care was initially biased towards the study of respiratory pathology, then cardiac function and how the cardiorespiratory system interacted in acute illness. As the specialty of caring for the seriously ill has become more complex, increasing attention is being focussed on other organs, including the gastrointestinal tract (GIT) and abdomen. In this review some aspects of this area will be covered. Rather than concentrate on disorders such as pancreatitis and fulminant hepatic failure I have chosen some of the less prominent but nevertheless important areas of the GIT. The intensivist should examine and understand the GIT and abdomen as meticulously as other more "glorious" organs such as the heart and lungs.

The Mouth and Sinuses

The mouth and sinuses are often overlooked in the seriously ill. They can often be the source of pathology, especially infection. When teeth infection and abscesses occur, they can be easily overlooked especially when an endotracheal tube is in place. Similarly, bleeding and infection can result from blind oropharyngeal suction or instrumentation. The mouth should be inspected regularly by the attending medical team. Similarly, the sinuses can be the source of serious infection which is difficult to diagnose [1]. Sinusitis is predisposed to by foreign bodies in the nose such as nasogastric tubes and nasotracheal tubes which impede sinus drainage and encourage infection. As with lesions in the mouth, these infections would normally be associated with symptoms such as pain and as such, often masked in the critically ill. If suspected, skull X-ray and CT scan are helpful in defining fluid levels in the sinuses. Like any other suspected source of sepsis, it should then be aggressively drained.

Ileus and Enteral Feeding

The question of whether the GIT is working or not often confronts intensivists. Among other reasons, it is important in assessing whether the patient can tolerate enteral feeding. Most authorities would suggest that enteral feeding is preferable to parenteral feeding. The lack of bowel sounds does not correlate well with ileus or decreased GIT function [2]. Enteral nutrition is contraindicated after recent major surgery, in the presence of gross abdominal distension or in the presence of significant volumes of gastric aspirate (more than 400 ml in 24 hours.). However, enteral feeding has been used successfully in the presence of "ileus" and sepsis [3] and within 24 hours. of major abdominal surgery [4]. Full strength feed should be started in small quantities initially. Nasoduodenal or nasojejunal tubes may be preferable to nasogastric tubes as gastroparesis or atony is relatively common in the seriously ill even in the presence of a normally functioning small bowel.

The Stomach as a Source of Infection

Endogenous infection in the seriously ill is far more common than exogenous infection. Nosocomial or hospital acquired infection is one of the major problems in Intensive Care and most of these infections are endogenous. The organisms responsible for infection are mainly derived from the gastrointestinal tract.

Because acute stress ulceration is a potentially lethal problem in the seriously ill, attempts are usually made to raise the stomach pH [5]. This is usually achieved by antacids or H_2-receptor antagonists. Unfortunately, by alkalinizing the stomach, a first line of defense against bacteria is compromised. Microorganisms, especially coliforms, rapidly colonize the alkalinized gastric contents of the seriously ill [6]. It would seem logical to attack this potential cause of endogenous infection at its source rather than wait for systemic absorption of either the micro-organism or its endotoxin, or aspiration of the infected contents past the endotracheal tube to cause pneumonia [7-9]. Rather than attempt to eradicate all micro-organisms in the gut, which would in any case be highly unlikely, a technique of selective decontamination of the digestive tract (SDD) has been developed [9]. The proponents of this approach suggest that there is a beneficial effect of anaerobic flora in resisting colonization by aerobes in the GIT: SDD aims at selective elimination of the aerobic gram-negative bacilli and yeasts, leaving the anaerobic flora unaffected. Strict microbiological surveillance of the feces, oropharynx and nasogastric contents are necessary, as well as more routine microbiological monitoring in order to assess the effectiveness of the regimen and prevent emergence of other species such as gram positive organisms. In initial studies the results have proven to be very successful with few complications. However, the technique is costly, time consuming and is ideologically opposite to the view of defining an infection and prescribing the appropriate antibiotic. However, the more conventional approach to nosocominal infection still results in a high incidence and is associated with a disappointing mortality rate [10].

We eagerly await further developments. In the meantime it must be remembered that the gastric contents are contaminated. It should be handled carefully by the staff and respected as a potentially lethal source of endogenous infection.

Acute Abdominal Disorders in the Critically Ill [11]

In the critically ill, sedated and sometimes paralyzed patients with no symptoms, suspicion and diagnosis of intra-abdominal catastrophes can be difficult. It is important to include a thorough examination of the abdomen at least daily on all seriously ill patients.

The abdomen can contain an occult source of sepsis with systemic features of septicemia. Postoperative complications such as a leaking anastomosis, abscess or wound infection can also occur. Patients receiving peritoneal dialysis or who have ascites can develop peritonitis. Splanchnic hypoperfusion as a result of cardiorespiratory dysfunction or abdominal tamponade can result in mesenteric artery insufficiency with diffuse areas of ischemia or infarcted bowel [12]. Intestinal pseudo-obstruction is relatively common in the seriously ill [13]. The abdomen is tense and tympanic, gastric feeding is poorly tolerated and the large bowel does not function. There is no specific site of obstruction and it may be related to an electrolyte disorder or drugs such as opiates, anticholinergics or sedatives.

Acute gastric dilatation is common after CPR and is also seen sometimes in association with diabetic ketoacidosis.

Concurrent abdominal disorders can occur coincidentally in the seriously ill. These include perforated peptic ulcer, appendicitis, cholecystitis, volvulus or complications of a coexisting disease such as diverticulitis, Crohn's disease or ulcerative colitis.

Abdominal Effects of Artificial Ventilation

What happens in the chest can aso affect the abdomen. We now know that positive pressure applied to the chest is not as innocuous as initially thought. Positive intrathoracic pressure decreases venous return and cardiac output. As well as decreasing arterial blood flow, venous flow is impeded. The result is that blood flow to many extrathoracic organs is impeded. These include the brain, liver, kidneys and mesenteric supply. High intrathoracic pressures decrease regional blood flow and may have implications in the development of multi organ failure (MOF) [14].

Positive pressure ventilation can also disrupt alveoli and cause barotrauma [15]. The gas moves along the adventitia of the pulmonary alveoli to the mediastinum. From there, with high enough pressures, gas can move along the oesophagus and aorta into the abdomen to form pneumoretroperitoneum and pneumoperitoneum. Gas may also move in the adventitia of the mesenteric vessels to cause pneumatosis cystoides intestinalis coli. Thus free gas in the diaphragm may have its origins in the chest rather than from an abdominal viscus. This has important diagnostic and therapeutic implications.

Acalculus Cholecystitis

Although rare, a calculus cholecystitis is likely to occur in seriously ill patients in association with trauma, burns as well as postoperatively [16, 17]. Although the etiology is unknown, factors such as hypotension, massive transfusion, septicemia, fat embolism, parenteral nutrition, positive pressure ventilation and lack of enteral feeding have all been implicated. The cystic duct may become obstructed secondary to inspissated bile causing gall bladder ischemia with necrosis and infection. It has also been suggested that the gallbladder may be the site of hematogenous spread of infection.

Patients may present with right upper quadrant tenderness, generalized peritonitis, an occult source of infection and MOF. There are no specific laboratory findings. Because these patients usually cannot complain of symptoms and there are other possible sources of infection, the diagnosis is elusive and often delayed. Because the gallbladder by this stage is commonly gangrenous or perforated there is a high mortality. Ultrasound can show a thickened gallbladder wall, an enlarged gallbladder or a pericholecystic collection [16]. CT – scan and radionuclide scans may also be useful. Laparotomy may be necessary for definitive diagnosis as well as being obligatory for treatment. Early suspicion and aggressive surgery are crucial for the outcome of acalculus cholecystitis.

"ICU Jaundice"

Many patients with previously normal liver function become jaundice while acutely ill, especially during septicemia and shock. The jaundice involves a mild to moderate rise in bilirubin (usually <50 μmol/l) and is hepatocellular in origin [18]. The mechanism is unknown but predisposing factors include hypoxia, hypotension, raised intrathoracic pressure with decreased liver blood flow and the direct effect of endotoxins. Hemolysis of transfused blood and resorption from hematomas can also contribute to the jaundice. The management is aimed at providing optimum physiological conditions for liver function – i.e. rapid resuscitation as well as avoiding hypotension and hypoxia. Avoid high intrathoracic pressures and encourage spontaneous respiration. The underlying problem, especially sepsis should be treated aggressively.

Intra-abdominal Tamponade

Girth measurements are often performed in Intensive Care for suspected intra-abdominal bleeding or acute fluid collection. The compliance of the intra-abdominal cavity is very unpredictable. There is little relationship between intra-abdominal volume and external circumstance of the abdominal wall [19]. Observer error and position of the patient make these measurements even less useful. There is no place for abdominal girth measurement in clinical medicine. A more reliable assessment can be made by palpating the abdomen and assessing its tenseness. An even more accurate reflection of intra-abdominal pressure can be made by measuring the pressure in the bladder via a urinary catheter. This can be achieved in a similar fashion to measuring CVP with a water column manometer.

Oliguria can occur with abdominal pressures greater than 15 mmHg and anuria with pressures greater than 30 mmHg. Raised intraabdominal pressure can impede venous and arterial blood flow as well as obstruct the ureters [20]. This can cause renal failure and ischemia of the GIT and other intra-abdominal organs as well as severe disturbances of left ventricular function.

Diarrhea

It is fitting that in this brief review that as we began at the mouth, we finish at the other end. Diarrhea is a common occurrence in Intensive Care [21]. It adds to the problems of nursing care, complicates the patient's fluid and electrolyte balance and may worsen the nutritional state. The incidence is approximately 40% in seriously ill patients who are admitted for more than 48 hours.

Nasogastric feeds, alkinization of the stomach, low albumin and antibiotics have all been associated with diarrhea. It may be a manifestation of general hypoactivity and malfunction of the GIT and part of MOF associated with many conditions in Intensive Care.

It has been suggested, but never proven, that commencing enteral feeding in a diluted form, reduces the incidence of diarrhea. Antibiotics, especially broad spectrum ones, should be used cautiously and for a limited time as they predispose to gut flora changes and diarrhea. Clostridium difficile is not common in Intensive Care despite widespread antibiotic usage. However, in persistent or severe diarrhea it should always be excluded.

A gram stain and culture should also be performed. In particular antibiotic associated methicillin resistant Staphylococcus aureus diarrhea should be suspected [22]. It is diagnosed by a distinctive gram-stain appearance of fecal smears and treated with vancomycin. It is particularly prone to cross infection and patients should be isolated early. Diarrhea can be an early presenting sign of any form of infection, particularly septicemia and toxic shock syndrome.

References

1. Grindlidnger GA, Niehoff J, Hughes SL, Humphrey MA, Simpson G (1987) Acute paranasal sinusitis related to nasotracheal intubation of head-injured patients. Crit Care Med 15:214–218
2. Shelly MP, Church JJ (1987) Bowel sounds during intermittent positive pressure ventilation. Anaesthesia 42:207–209
3. Cerra FB, Shrouts FP, Konstantinides NN, et al (1985) Enteral feeding in sepsis: a perspective, randomized double-blind trial. Surgery 98:632–639
4. Sagar S, Harland P, Shields R (1979) Early postoperative feeding with elemental diet. BR Med J 1:293–295
5. Hillman K (1985) Acute stress ulceration. Anaesth Intensive Care 13:230–240
6. Hillman KM, Riordan T, O'Farrel SM, Tabaqchali S (1982) Colonization of the gastric contents in critically ill patients. Crit Care Med 10:444–447
7. van Uffelen R, van Saene HKF, Fidler V, Lowenberg A (1984) Oropharyngeal flora as a source of bacteria colonizing the lower airways in patients on artificial ventilation
8. Stoutenbeek CP, van Saene HKF, Miranda DR, Zandstra DF (1984) The effect of selective decontamination of the digestive tract on colonisation and infection rate in multiple trauma patients. Intensive Care Med 10:185–192

9. van Uffelen R, Rommes JH, van Saene HKF (1987) Preventing lower airway colonization and infection in mechanically ventilated patients. Crit Care Med 15:99–102
10. Kerver AJH, Rommes JH, Mevissen-Verhage EAE, et al (1987) Colonization and infection in surgical intensive care patients – a prospective study. Intensive Care Med 13:347–351
11. Worthley LIG (1985) Acute abdominal disorders in the paralysed patient. Anaesth Intensive Care 13:263–271
12. Aranha GV, Goldberg NB (1981) Surgical problems in patients on ventilators. Crit Care Med 9:478–480
13. Editorial (1979) Intestinal pseudo-obstruction. Lancet 1:535–536
14. Dorinsky PM, Hamlin RB, Gadek JE (1987) Alterations in regional blood flow during positive end-expiratory pressure ventilation. Crit Care Med 15:106–113
15. Hillman KM (1985) Pulmonary barotrauma. Clin Anaesthesiology 3:877–897
16. Johnson LB (1987) The importance of early diagnosis of acute acalculus cholecystitis. Surg Gynecol Obstet 164:197–203
17. Savino JA, Scalea TM, Del Guerico LRM (1985) Factors encouraging larparotomy in acalculous cholecystitis. Crit Care Med 13:377–380
18. Murray WR, MacSween RNM (1983) In: Ledingham I McA, Hamming CD (eds) Recent advances in critical care medicine, 2nd edn. Churchill Livingstone, Edinburgh, pp 143–159
19. Aitken RJ, Clifford PC (1985) Girth measurement is not a reliable investigation for the detection of intra-abdominal fluid. Ann R Coll Surg Engl 67:241–242
20. Richards WO, Scovill W, Baekhyo S, Reed W (1983) Acute renal failure associated with increased intra-abdominal pressure. Ann Surg 197:183–187
21. Kelly TWJ, Patrick MR, Hillman KM (1983) Study of diarrhea in critically ill patients. Crit Care Med 11:7–9

Respiratory Support:
Old and New Techniques

Methods of Increasing FRC
in Acute Respiratory Failure

G. Lazarus and M. Sold

Introduction

The goal of respiratory therapy to increase functional residual capacity (FRC) is not only to improve oxygenation, so important this effect may be, but to reestablish pertinent and normal ventilation of all regions of the lung. In acute respiratory failure (ARF), ventilation is endangered by destabilization of alveoli [1, 2]. Apart from interstitial edema the clinical picture will be determined by the pathophysiological consequences of increased pulmonary retraction and decreased lung volume leading to reduced compliance, hypoventilation, shunting, and hypoxemia. In addition fluid balance is disturbed and extravasation will increase further [3] (Fig. 1). Respiratory therapy at increased FRC does not influence the initial or the causative mechanisms of ARF, but it will confine their influence on pulmonary volume and therefore mechanics and gas exchange because it counteracts volume loss and prevents it becoming a causative factor per se. From that point of view ventilation with increased FRC is a struggle against progressive pulmonary retraction. The improvement of gas exchange that usually results is important and a useful monitor of successful therapy, however it is not indispensable for justification of ventilatory patterns with increased FRC.

Ventilatory Patterns

To increase FRC means to elevate the end-expiratory alveolar pressure. Basically two methods are available:
1. incorporation of an expiratory threshold resistor (PEEP ventilation in its original sense),

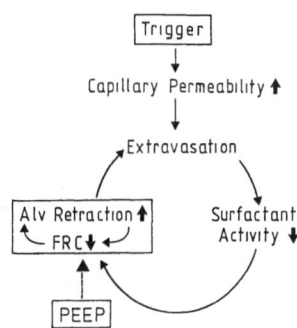

Fig. 1. Role of ventilation with increased FRC (PEEP) in the treatment of ARF

2. premature termination of expiration by beginning the inspiration at a positive alveoloathmospheric pressure gradient and an expiratory flow greater than zero (IRV, HFPPV). Moreover the term FRC becomes a semantic problem in the case of ventilatory patterns that keep the lung in a predominant inspiratory position (high I/E-ratio, APRV).

Positive end-expiratory pressure (PEEP) was the original [4] and still is the most often used means of increasing FRC. Its effects on respiratory mechanics and gas exchange and its hemodynamic side effects have been widely studied. Most authors used the PEEP level for reference, but only few quantified the corresponding change in pulmonary volume (5–7). However, improvement of gas exchange depends upon the increase in FRC [5], the rise in intrathoracic pressure upon alveolar pressure *and* lung compliance (which again means lung volume), and the rise in pulmonary vascular resistance (PVR) upon the state of inflation [8]; thus the effects and side effects of ventilation with PEEP can be attributed to volume at least as well as to pressure [5, 7]. One may therefore anticipate that each increase in FRC by whatever technical means has comparable consequences when referred to the actual lung volume.

Inversed ratio ventilation (IRV) with an I/E ratio greater than 1/1 was first used in infants [9] and later also for therapy of adult respiratory distress syndrome [10, 11]. It is not yet clear whether prolonged inspiration of further increase in FRC is the predominant factor for improvement of gas exchange. When expiratory time is too short to achieve a pressure equilibrium between alveoli and the upper airways and expiration is still incomplete, an intrinsic PEEP is created that exceeds the external end-expiratory pressure [12]. In obstructive lung disease characterized by high time constants this often happens accidentally [13]. If retraction prevails, as in ARF, expiratory time constants are short, so that expiratory time must be markedly reduced by a high I/E ratio and/or higher frequency to increase FRC. The effect of a shortened expiratory time on FRC can be seen from the following observations:

a) persisting expiratory flow at end-expiration,
b) rise of end-*in*spiratory pressure plateau at constant tidal volume (VT) or
c) decrease in VT at constant end-*in*spiratory pressure.

In the latter case the increase in FRC can be quantified from the reduction of VT. An upper pressure limit in IRV has the additional advantage of preventing inadequate end-inspiratory hyperinflation even of obstructive "slow" compartments.

Airway pressure release ventilation (APRV) was presented by Downs in this series last year [14] and is the subject of a study by Rasanen in this book. Starting at individual pressure plateaus up to a high level of positive end-expiratory pressure, CO_2 elimination is improved by intermittent pressure release [15]. As the patient is allowed to breathe spontaneously at the selected pressure plateau, this breathing pattern shares elements of IRV and CPAP as well.

A further type of ventilation at an increased FRC owing to an extreme reduction in expiratory time is *high frequency ventilation* [16]. The airway pressure remains positive and lung volume is enhanced (Fig. 2). The increase in lung volume is determined by the driving pressure and the I/E ratio and barely by the frequency [16]. Its quantification is possible off line by passive exhalation [16], or on line using transthoracic electrical impedence instead of volume [17]. When monitoring intratracheal pressure one has to bear in mind that it may underestimate peripheral airway and alveolar pressure [18, 19].

Distribution of the Increase in FRC

At FRC, the upper and lower parts of the lung are located at different points of their individual pressure-volume relationship due to a transpulmonary pressure difference of 7.5 cm H_2O [20] (Fig. 3). In fact, increasing P_{aw} by 10 cm H_2O will change the transpulmonary pressure by about 7 cm H_2O and raise overall lung volume. However, the dependent parts of the lungs will expand to a volume that was already reached by the upper parts before. Starting at this PEEP level the added ventilation will be more evenly distributed; but ventilation of the base of the lung will only improve at the cost of overinflation of the apex, shifting perfusion towards the base [21, 22]. Thus regional overinflation usually occurs even if respiration takes place at the steepest (linear) part of the cumulative PV-curve of the respiratory system which indicates optimal compliance [23]. An optimal increase in FRC is attained when even the dependent and/or stiffer regions are saved from progressive volume loss and on the other hand the unavoidable regional overinflation does not prevail which would compromise hemodynamics [8]. If success is only incomplete the vicious circle of decreased lung volume and increased retraction will continue in the primarily affected and/or dependent areas (Fig. 3). Their re-expansion will then afford an even more drastic overin-

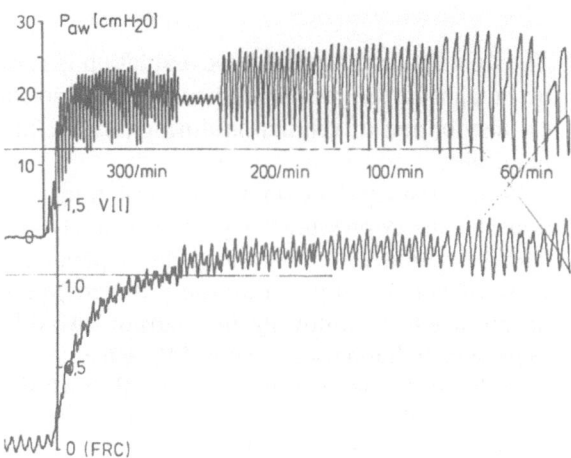

Fig. 2. Increase in lung volume, derived from transthoracic electrical impedance *(lower curve)* with rising tracheal pressure *(upper curve)* during HFJV. Note that mean lung volume is not influenced by frequency

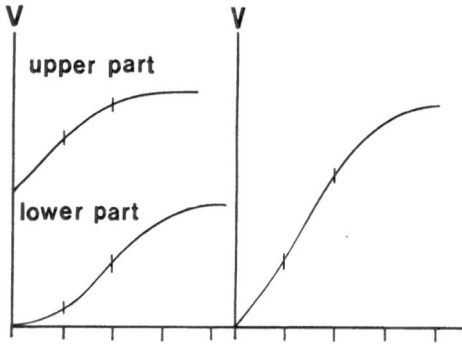

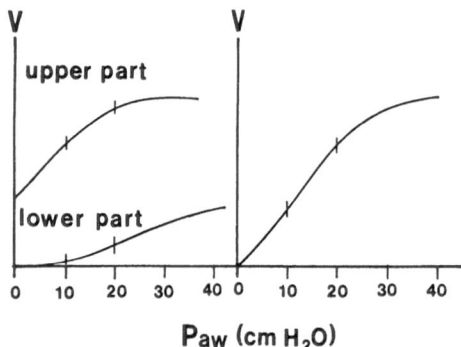

Fig. 3. Influence of increasing airway pressure (P_{aw}) on the upper and lower part of a supine lung with equal *(upper left)* and different *(lower left)* elastical properties. – Corresponding total PV-curves *(right)*

flation of the viable compartments. In extreme cases an "adverse PEEP effect" is created: Despite PEEP, PaO_2 deteriorates due to a shift of perfusion into regions that are still barely ventilated [24].

Effects of Positioning

The fight against regional hypoventilation is supported if the retractive area can be brought into a non-dependent, exposed position [25]. Thus the unphysiological distribution of ventilation during positive pressure ventilation is used therapeutically.

From existing data on the vertical transpulmonary pressure gradient [20], transpulmonary pressure is higher by 5 cm H_2O for the non-dependent lung in the lateral position as compared to the dependent lung. Therefore to achieve the same effect in the supine position, a unilateral restriction (due to aspiration, contusion or edema following reexpansion) would have to be ventilated with the same transpulmonary pressure difference i.e. with a PEEP 7.5 cm H_2O higher than that of the unaffected lung. In other words the lateral position is an effective means of *side-different* ventilation which does not necessarily require *side-separate* ventilation of the lungs.

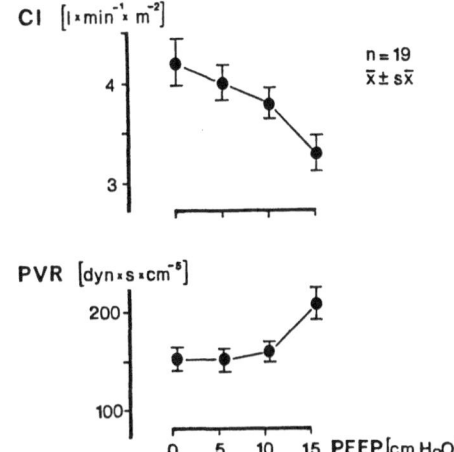

Fig. 4. Change of cardic index (CI) and pulmonary vascular resistance (PVR) with increasing PEEP levels

Limitations of Increasing FRC, Interrelationship FRC – VT

The complex consequences of positive pressure ventilation, especially of ventilation with increased FRC, on overall cardiac performance and hemodynamics are reduced in the clinical setting. They include changes in cardiac output and PVR which do not necessarily run parallel. As may be inferred from Figure 4, increasing PEEP up to 10 cm H_2O results in a linear, moderate and acceptable reduction of cardiac index whilst PVR does not change. Raising PEEP further leads to a disproportionate decrease of cardiac index that is no longer acceptable and to a brisk rise in PVR. In fact if the rise in PVR is the hemodynamic correlate of hyperinflation [8], it must depend more upon the end-*in*spiratory lung volume which is the sum of FRC and VT than upon PEEP or FRC alone.

To test this hypothesis, 17 patients with ARF were ventilated with increasing PEEP and known VT after the expiratory quasi-static pressure-volume curve had been registered [26]. Then the position of end-inspiratory volume in respect to total inspiratory capacity (IC) was recorded at different levels of PEEP to measure the fraction of IC that was "consumed" at end-inspiration (Fig. 5) A definite rise of PVR was not observed before end-inspiratory volume had reached the

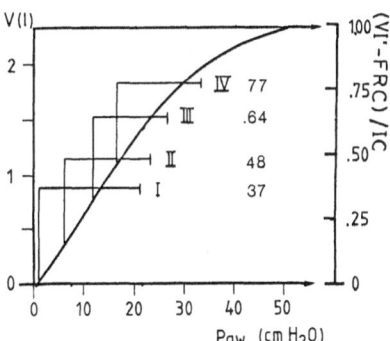

Fig. 5. Volume and pressure excursions with increasing PEEP along the individual quasi-static expiratory PV-curve taken from an original registration. (VI' – FRC)/IC is the fraction of IC consumed at end-inspiration. (From [7])

upper third of IC i.e. the flattening part of the PV-curve. A close parabolic correlation was found between the rise of PVR and the fractional end-inspiratory
consumption of IC almost mirroring the concomitant decrease in compliance
(Fig. 6). Thus the strong interrelation between hemodynamics and pulmonary
mechanics during increases of PEEP levels was confirmed [27].

The same procedure was repeated during high frequency jet ventilation
(HFJV) i.e. at a VT close to zero in 5 other patients (Fig. 7) [17]. The methodological problem of precise measurement of lung volume was avoided by registration of transthoracic electrical impedance instead of volume, both being li-

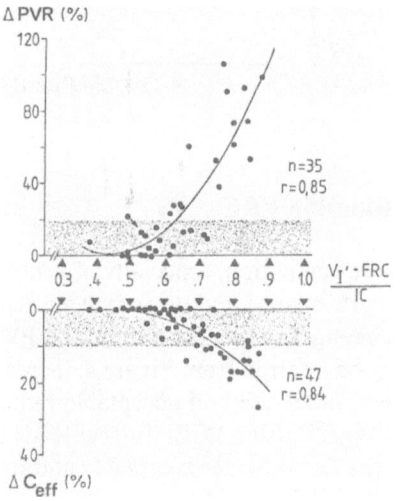

Fig. 6. Changes in PVR and effective static compliance (C_{eff}) with increasingly consumed fraction at end-inspiration. (For (VI' – FRC)/IC see
Fig. 5). The compliance curve (below) incorporates data from 17 patients, the PVR curve
(above) from 12 patients (5 patients without he-
modynamical response were excluded). (From
[7])

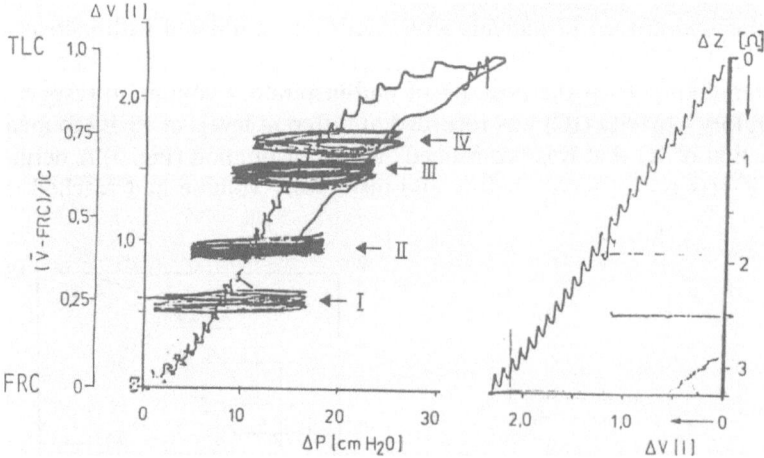

Fig. 7. Tracheal pressure-impedance (PZ-) loops during HFJV at different stages of lung inflation, displayed at the individual quasi-static expiratory PZ-curve. Left scale: occupied fraction
of IC. The right curve shows the linearity between Z and V. (From [17]).
$\bar{V}$ = mean lung volume during HFJV

nearly correlated. Tracheal pressure-impedance (PZ-) loops were displayed on the background of an expiratory pressure-impedance curve that had been registered beforehand. By changing driving pressure and I/E ratio, lung volume was gradually increased so that the discs came to rest at several heights of the curve and IC.

Again PVR did not rise noticeably before the upper third of the PZ- (or PV-) curve had been reached. The correlation between volume position and PVR increase resulted in nearly the same shape of curve as it was obtained in the above study for the end-*inspiratory* volume using conventional PEEP ventilation (Fig. 8). Therefore, with respect to hyperinflation-related side effects, a ventilatory pattern "without" a tidal volume can be placed at the same lung volume where conventional ventilatory excursions must end. Thus the VT is a volume reserve to augment FRC beyond best PEEP.

Clinical Strategy of Increasing FRC in ARF

An effective increase in FRC without overinflating the lungs should avoid the upper third of the IC but use the lower two thirds. Within this range the lower VT the higher the FRC can be set. The initially chosen ventilatory pattern will favorably use the middle third of the available volume distance between uninfluenced FRC and TLC (Fig. 9, vector a). This is achieved in most cases at PEEP of 10–12 cm H_2O and VT of about 700 ml thus confirming the clinical experience [26]. This respiratory pattern corresponds well with the best PEEP with regard to compliance [27]. However, it may not be good enough when gas exchange and chest X-ray

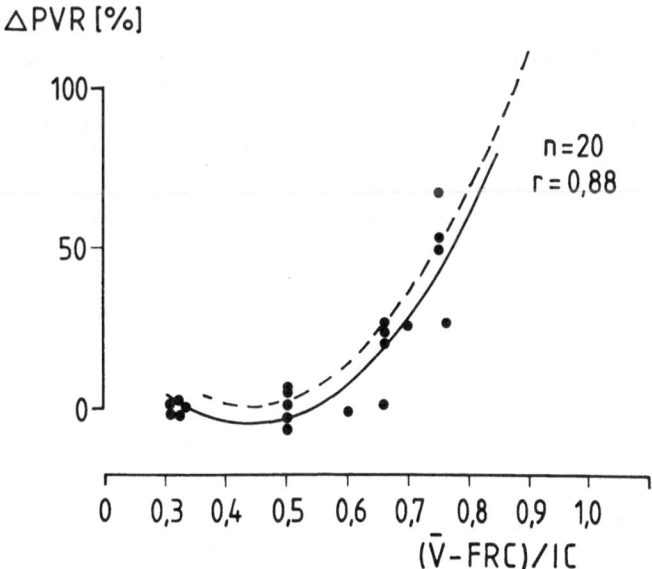

Fig. 8. Relative changes in PVR with increasing use of IC during HFJV. The broken line is transferred from Fig. 6 for comparison. (From [17])
$\bar{V}$ = mean volume during HFJV

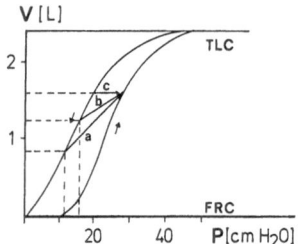

Fig. 9. Pressure-volume vectors between ex- and inspiratory static PV-curve representing ventilation *a)* within the middle third of IC ("best PEEP"): *b)* with further augmented FRC and an equivalent reduction of VT; *c)* "without" VT, end-inspiratory volume always remaining constant. Note that decreased steepness (compliance) of vector b is determined by the low VT rather than by overdistention

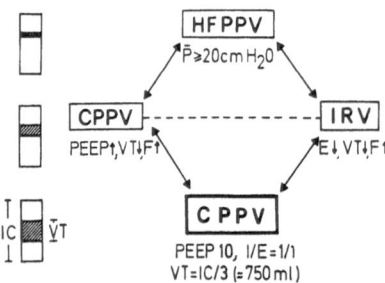

Fig. 10. Strategy of escalating controlled ventilation with increased FRC in severe ARF. The columns on the left indicate the position of VT within the inspiratory capacity (IC)
E = expiratory time, F = frequency

are considered. In this situation FRC can further be raised whilst reducing VT and increasing respiratory rate (Fig. 9, vector b). The interrelationship between VT and FRC needs no further consideration, if the end-*in*spiratory lung volume is fixed by use of an upper pressure limit. Each subsequent increase in FRC with PEEP, IRV or both will then automatically lead to an equivalent reduction of VT. The endpoint of this strategy is a ventilation "without" volume excursion (Fig. 9, vector c) e.g. by means of HFV, at a high lung volume and a mean tracheal pressure of at least 20 cm H_2O. The aim of this strategy is to win rapidly the fight against retraction in order to return to a standard ventilatory pattern with PEEP of 10 cm H_2O and an acceptable FiO_2 (below 0.40) as soon as possible (Fig. 10).

References

1. Baum M, Benzer H, Blümel G, Bolcic J, Irsigler K, Tölle W (1971) Die Bedeutung der Oberflächenspannung beim experimentellen posttraumatischen Syndrom. Z Exper Chir 4:359–378
2. Lachmann B (1987) The role of pulmonary surfactant in the pathogenesis and therapy of ARDS. In: Vincent JL (ed) Update in Intensive Care and Emergency Medicine, vol 3. Springer, Berlin Heidelberg New York London Paris Tokyo, pp 132–134
3. Cruyton AC, Moffatt DS, Adair TA (1980) Role of alveolar surface tension in transepithelial movement of fluid. In: Robertson B, van Golde LMG, Batenburg JJ (eds) Pulmonary surfactant. Elsevier, Amsterdam, pp 171–185

4. Ashbaugh DG, Petty TL, Bigelow DB, Harris TM (1969) Continuous positive-pressure breathing (CPPB) in adult respiratory distress syndrome. J Thorac Cardiovasc Surg 57:31-41
5. Falke KJ, Pontoppidan H, Kumar A, Leith DE, Geffin B, Laver MB (1972) Ventilation with end-expiratory pressure in acute lung disease. J Clin Invest 51:2315-2323
6. Holzapfel L, Robert D, Perrin F, Blauc PL, Palmier B, Guerin C (1983) Static pressure-volume curves and effect of positive end-expiratory pressure on gas exchange in adult respiratory distress syndrome. Crit Care Med 11:591-597
7. Lazarus G (1983) Endinspiratory lung volume as the limiting factor of ventilation with PEEP. Anaesthesist 32:582-590
8. Whittenberger JD, McGregor M, Berglund E, Borst HG (1960) Influence of state of inflation of the lungs on pulmonary vascular resistance. J Appl Physiol 15:858-864
9. Reynolds EOR (1975) Management on hyaline membrane disease. Br Med Bull 31:18-24
10. Baum M, Benzer H, Mutz N, Pauser G, Tonczar L (1980) Inversed ratio ventilation (IRV). Anaesthesist 29:592-596
11. Lachmann B, Haendly B, Schulz H, Jonson B (1980) Improved arterial oxygenation, CO_2 elimination, compliance and decreased barotrauma following changes of volume-generated PEEP ventilation with inspiratory/expiratory I/E-ratio of 1:2 to pressure-generated ventilation with I/E-ratio of 4:1 in patients with severe adult respiratory distress syndrome (ARDS). Intensive Care Med 6:64
12. Rossi A, Gottfried FB, Zocchi L (1985) Measurement of static compliance of the total respiratory system in patients with acute respiratory failure during mechanical ventilation: the effect of intrinsic positive end-expiratory pressure. Am Rev Respir Dis 131:672-677
13. Milic-Emili J, Gottfried SB, Rossi A (1987) Dynamic hyperinflation: intrinsic PEEP and its ramifications in patients with respiratory failure. In: Vincent JL (ed) Update in Intensive Care and Emergency Medicine, vol 3. Springer, Berlin Heidelberg New York London Paris Tokyo, pp 192-198
14. Downs JB, Stock MC, Rasanen J (1987) Airway pressure release ventilation (APRV): a new approach to the management of acute lung injury. In: Vincent JL (ed) Update in Intensive Care and Emergency Medicine, vol 3. Springer, Berlin Heidelberg New York London Paris Tokyo, pp 228-233
15. Kirby RR, Downs JB, Civetta JM, Modell JH, Dannemiller FJ, Klein EF et al. (1975) High level positive end-expiratory pressure (PEEP) in acute respiratory insufficiency. Chest 67:156-169
16. Rouby J, Fusciardi J, Bourgain JL, Viars P (1983) Highfrequency jet ventilation in postoperative respiratory failure: determinants of oxygenation. Anesthesiology 59:281-287
17. Lazarus G, Rothhammer A, Lazarus W, Weis KH (1986) Hemodynamic side-effects of high-frequency jet ventilation (HFJV) as a function of lung volume. Anaesthesist 35:24-29
18. Beamer WC, Prough DS, Royster RL, Johnston WE, Johnson JC (1984) High-frequency jet ventilation produces auto-PEEP. Crit Care Med 12:734-737
19. Sutton JE, Glass DD (1984) Airway pressure gradient during high-frequency ventilation. Crit Care Med 12:774-776
20. Milic-Emili J (1977) Ventilation. In: West JB (ed) Regional differences in the lung. Academic Press, New York, pp 167-199
21. Hughes JMB, Glazier JB, Maloney JE, West JB (1968) Effect of lung volume on the distribution of pulmonary blood flow in man. Resp Physiol 4:58-72
22. Landmark SJ, Knopp TJ, Rehder K, Sessler AD (1977) Regional pulmonary perfusion and V/Q in awake and anesthetized-paralyzed man. J Appl Physiol 43:993-1000
23. Hopping FG, Hildebrandt J (1977) Mechanical properties of the lung. In: West JB (ed) Bioengineering aspects of the lung. Dekker, New York, pp 83-162
24. Kanarek DJ, Shannon DC (1975) Adverse effect of PEEP on pulmonary perfusion and arterial oxygenation. Am Rev Resp Dis 112:457-459
25. Prokocimer P, Garbino J, Wolff M, Regnier B (1983) Influence of posture on gas exchange in artificially ventilated patients with local lung disease. Intensive Care Med 9:69-72
26. Lazarus G (1985) PEEP ventilation without hyperinflation of the lung. A primary ventilatory pattern derived from expiratory pressure-volume curves. Anaesthesist 34:59-64
27. Suter PM, Fairley HB, Isenberg MD (1975) Optimum endexpiratory airway pressure in patients with acute pulmonary failure. N Engl J Med 288:284-289

Thoraco-Pulmonary Pressure/Volume Relationship During Mechanical Ventilation

S. Benito and J. Mancebo

Introduction

The anatomic and functional disposition of the pleura, the rib cage and the respiratory muscles, allow modifications to be produced in the thorax which in turn, induce variations in lung volume. The result is breathing.

For flow to exist a pressure difference must be previously generated. In spontaneous respiration, the contraction of inspiratory muscles creates a pressure change that is transmitted to the lung. Muscular pressure higher than lung elastic pressure, will be useful in generating flow. During mechanical ventilation the contractions applied to the respiratory system are not of muscular origin but created by the application of a positive pressure in the trachea of the mechanically ventilated patient.

In the lung, the pressure increase is proportional to the volume increase. The term compliance refers to the quotient between the increments of volume and pressure ($\Delta V/\Delta P$). Pulmonary compliance measurement depends on the amount of the insufflated volume and the velocity of volume change. When there is a long pause with zero flow after a volume change, the airway pressure (Paw) and alveolar pressure are equilibrated, and static compliance is obtained. The same change in pulmonary volume generates lower pressure in deflation than in inflation and this phenomenon is known as hysteresis. The difference also depends on the volume, the greater the volume increase, the greater the hysteresis. The specific compliance is the ratio of compliance to functional residual capacity (FRC).

Measurement of Pressure-Volume Relationship in Patients with Mechanical Ventilation

Monitoring the elastic properties of the lung in patients with acute respiratory failure (ARF) under mechanical ventilation has been dealt with by several authors. Falke et al. [1] registered pressure-volume (P–V) curves in dynamic conditions and found a reduced compliance in ARF patients. Suter et al. [2] calculated "quasi-static" compliance by dividing the tidal volume (V_T) by the Paw difference between end-inspiratory hold and end-expiration, with an inspiratory hold with zero flow of 1 to 1.5 second. Bone [3], increasing the V_T and the positive end-expiratory pressure (PEEP), studied the pulmonary distensibility in a wide range of the inspiratory capacity. Jonson et al. [4] designed a compliance calculator to be incorporated in a mechanical ventilator.

To calculate quasi-static thoracopulmonary compliance during mechanical ventilation, some requisites to normalize the obtained values have been recommended, such as V_T 12-15 mL/kg weight and inspiratory hold 1.2-1.5 second. Additionally, the PEEP level must be taken into account as PEEP changes the initial pulmonary volume and also modifies compliance measurement [5].

In order to normalize the measurement of pulmonary distensibility in intubated patients, Janney, in 1959, reported a system called the supersyringe method [6]. This consists of a large calibrated syringe with which a known gas volume may be introduced in a stepwise manner, and the different pressures that are generated in the lung may be measured in static conditions either during inflation or deflation.

Some years later, Créteil's group reported a modified system [7]. This procedure basically consists of tracing the P-V relationship in static conditions from FRC to total pulmonary capacity during inflation and deflation. The patients are supine, sedated and paralyzed. PEEP is removed if present, and the initial FiO_2 level is increased 30%. The bronchial secretions are carefully suctioned and the cuff of the endotracheal tube is tested for leaks. A sigh twice the tidal volume is applied and the patient is disconnected from the ventilator at the end of a respiratory cycle. The syringe is then attached to the tracheal tube. A differential pressure transducer is connected to the proximal end of the tracheal tube so as to obtain the Paw signal. The volume signal is obtained by means of a potentiometer which transforms the displacement of the syringe plunger into volume. Both the Paw and the volume signals are incorporated in a X–Y plotter. The chest is inflated successively by 150–200 mL increments, with a 3 second period between successive inflations to allow the patient's airway pressure to stabilize. The total insufflated volume is 25 mL/kg, but if a Paw of 40 cm H_2O is reached, deflation starts immediately [8]. The lung is deflated by slow syringe aspiration in the same way as insufflation, until the Paw is zero.

Pulmonary insufflation of a known volume of gas can be performed by means of a constant gas-flow generator. This flow can be delivered by the ventilator, with an appropriate modification, or by a special designed device [9]. If a constant and slow flow can be assured, without changes with respect to pressure, time measurement is proportional to the insufflated volume. The rest of the procedure is similar to that reported above.

Parameters Derived from the P-V Curve

Thoracopulmonary Compliance

A linear segment of about 0.5 to 1 liter above the FRC appears in the deflation of the P-V curve (Fig. 1), and this is the segment in which we calculate the static thoracopulmonary compliance. Values of static thoracopulmonary compliance measured either in the linear segment of the deflation or in the linear segment of the inflation of the P-V curve, show an excellent correlation with the quasi-static

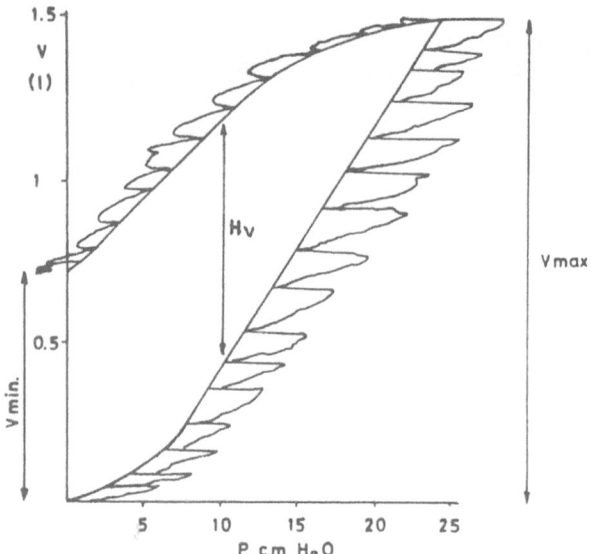

Fig. 1. Inflation and deflation of a P–V curve. Hv is the volume hysteresis at a pressure of 10 cm H_2O. Vmin is the unrecovered volume

compliance values measured with a V_T 12–15 mL/kg and inspiratory hold of 1.2–1.5 seconds [10] although the absolute values of compliance are higher when calculated from the P–V curve (Fig. 2). Pulmonary compliance is not an isolated concept, but provides information regarding the pulmonary volumes. It is well

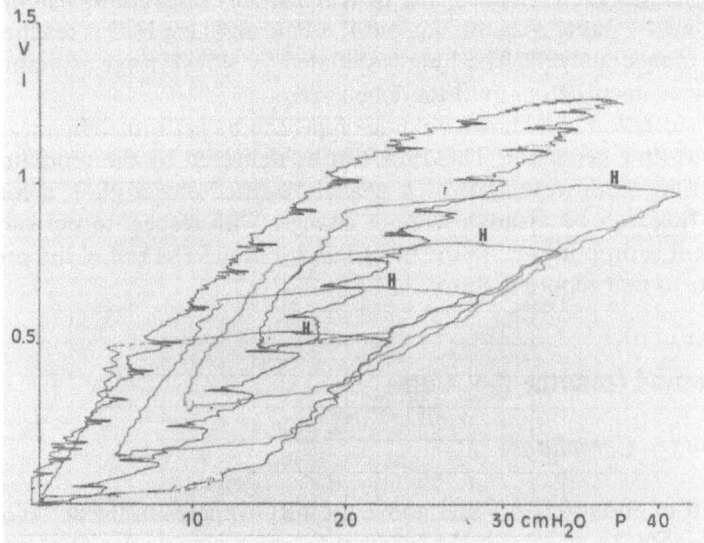

Fig. 2. Static P–V curve and superimposed P–V curves obtained in quasi-static conditions during mechanical ventilation and different PEEP levels. H is the inspiratory hold with zero flow and is used to calculate quasi-static compliance

known that in healthy subjects there is an excellent correlation between compliance and FRC, and we have found a good correlation between these parameters in patients with ARF (Fig. 3).

Hysteresis

This is expressed either as the surface within the P-V curve, or as the index between this surface and the surface of the rectangle which includes the P-V curve. The mechanisms involved in producing hysteresis are related to the lung tissue characteristics, the surfactant activity and the number of open lung units at the beginning of the inspiration [11]. Surface measurement is complex in the clinical setting and more simple indexes have been recommended, such as those proposed by Hillman et al. [12] which define the volume hysteresis (Hv) (Fig. 1), i.e.: the volume difference between inspiration and expiration at a determined pressure.

Gas Trapping

When P-V curves are performed in patients with ARF, there is an unrecovered gas volume at the end of deflation (Fig. 1). This is the volume trapped by the

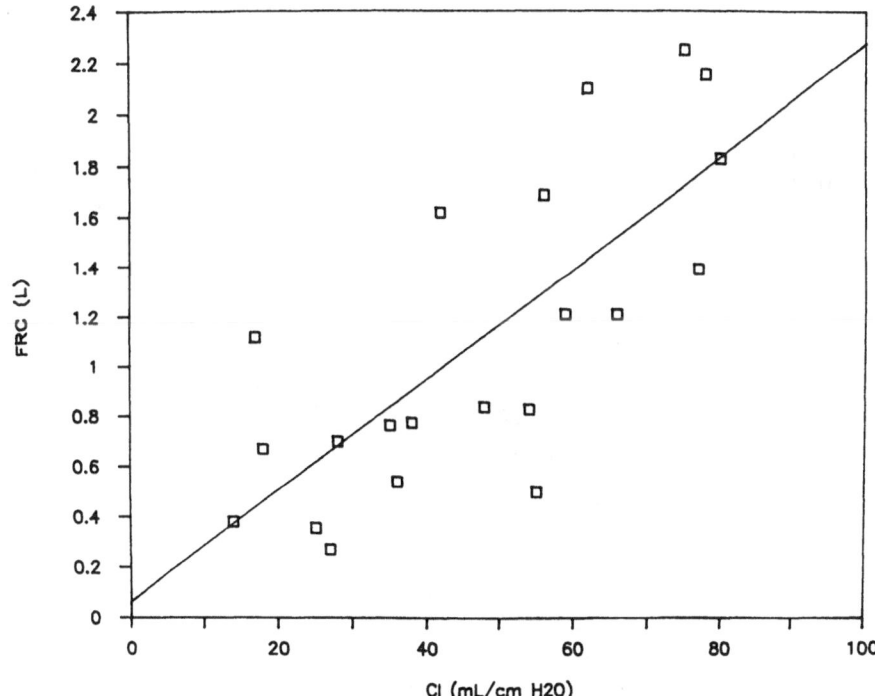

Fig. 3. Correlation between FRC and static thoracopulmonary compliance measured on the inflation of the P-V curve (Cl) in 22 patients with ARF. Regression equation: FRC (L) = 61.69 + 22.14 Cl(mL/cm H_2O). r = 0.75; F = 25:12, p < 0.001

closing of lung units. Frazer et al. [13]have studied this point and developed an index which is the quotient between the unrecovered volume and the total insufflated volume (Vmin/Vmax). In this experimental work they found that values close to 0.3 or higher were correlated to pulmonary edema.

Total Lung Capacity (TLC)

The measurement of TLC in sedated and paralyzed patients under mechanical ventilation is difficult. To estimate TLC different values such as the volume generated by a transpulmonary pressure of 30 cm H_2O or the volume corresponding to 12–14 mL per gram of lung weight have been suggested [14]. We usually estimate the TLC as the volume generated by a transthoracic pressure of 40 cm H_2O plus the FRC from which we start the insufflation with the syringe.

Inflection

One of the most clinically important parameters to be considered in the P–V curve is the appearance of an inflection in the beginning of inspiration and at low pulmonary volumes (Fig. 4). This initial inflection is an opening mechanism, that is to say, a mechanism which produces alveolar recruitment and which

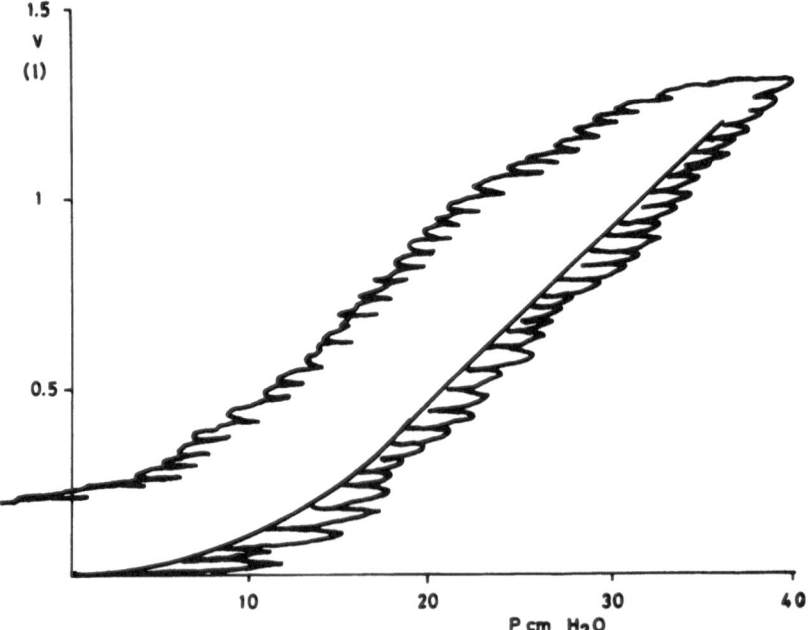

Fig. 4. P–V curve with an initial inflection point at a pressure of 14 cm H_2O

crosses from a low distendible zone to a high distensible zone. This has been demonstrated both experimentally and clinically [15-18].

Methodological Problems

With the P–V curve technique the volume is measured by means of the displacement of the plunger while the continuous flow technique volume is proportional to the duration of flow. Obviously the most important problem is volume loss as it is not directly measured. During inflation leaks may be detected from the pressure increments. Variations in the temperature and humidity of the insufflated gas, compression and decompression of gas, and the O_2 and CO_2 exchange during the maneuver are physiologic phenomena which may modify the deflation and the parameters thus derived such as compliance, hysteresis and unrecovered volume. This has been recently studied by Gattinoni et al. [19]. The clearance of CO_2 from the mixed venous blood to the lung decreases as does the respiratory quotient to values close to 0.3, ten seconds after a breath-holding maneuver is begun [20]. The problem is to define when such a holding in inflation or deflation exists. Recently Dall'Ava et al. [21] studied the phenomenon of volume loss and their results were related to gas exchange and the duration of the maneuver. They recommended that this maneuver should last less than 90 seconds.

Another shortcoming of this technique is the slight pulmonary involvement especially when there is unilateral lung disease, as the contralateral healthy lung tissue maintains its mechanical properties (Fig. 5).

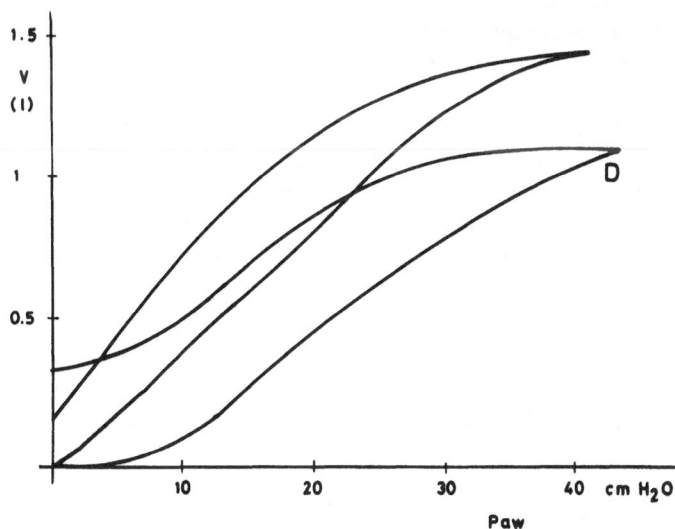

Fig. 5. Unilateral lung disease. P–V curve of the right diseased lung (D) with an initial inflection at a pressure of 12 cm H_2O, decreased compliance, increased hysteresis and trapped gas. The other P–V curve of both lungs appears normal in the same patient

Clinical Application

Monitoring pulmonary compliance in patients with ARF provides information of diagnostic, evolutive, therapeutic and prognostic interest. While the study in static conditions gives information about the lung tissue status, the dynamic characteristics provide information about the resistive properties of the lung. Lung diseases such as pneumonia, atelectasis or pulmonary edema, which increase lung recoil or decrease lung volume, will decrease static compliance. Dynamic measurements reflect compliance and flow restrictive properties of the airways, and the dynamic characteristics are frequently affected by bronchoconstriction and excess secretions in the airways [22].

The point of most therapeutic interest is probably the morphology of the P–V curve in its initial inflation segment, i.e. the presence or the absence or inflection. This pattern of inflection, with increased hysteresis and normal or decreased compliance, corresponds to initial and intermediate stages of the adult respiratory distress syndrome (ARDS) and is correlated to the presence of alveolar and alveolo-interstitial opacities on the chest X-ray film [16].

The presence of inflection allows optimal mechanical ventilation and PEEP utilization. An adequate PEEP level would be that equal to the inflection pressure (Pi) as it would produce alveolar recruitment. Suter et al. [2] indicated a PEEP level which corresponds to the highest O_2 transport, the highest $P\bar{v}O_2$, the highest compliance, and the lowest dead space. The fact that compliance increased progressively up to this PEEP level and then decreased above it agrees with the presence of an inflection at low lung volumes. PEEP levels higher than Pi would lead to a V_T displacement to a lung zone with unfavorable P–V relationships, i.e. with low compliance and this would produce overdistension phenomena.

Other authors studying P–V curves with an initial inflection showed that a PEEP level equal to Pi led to an optimal gas exchange [15–18, 23] and higher PEEP levels led to overdistension, as evidenced by an increment in the arterial minus end-tidal carbon dioxide gradient [23].

The study of the P–V curve also provides prognostic information. The pattern of low compliance, without inflection or increased hysteresis corresponds to the end-stage ARDS and predominant interstitial opacities in the chest X-ray film. In the study of Matamis et al. [16], 5 of the 6 patients who presented this morphologic pattern died. Series dealing with a greater number of patients demonstrate that diminished static compliance and advanced age are important prognostic factors of mortality in patients with severe ARF [24]. This is important because some of these patients who are not responding to conventional mechanical ventilation and who present a very low pulmonary compliance, may respond favorably with techniques of respiratory support not currently available such as the low frequency positive-pressure ventilation with extracorporel CO_2 removal [25].

The measurement of pulmonary compliance in ARF patients is an adjunct to conventional diagnostic parameters and the study of the P–V relationship may help in defining the stage and the prognosis of the disease. The inflection pressure, when it appears, is an important morphologic element which allows to optimize mechanical ventilation with PEEP.

References

1. Falke K, Pontoppidan H, Kumar A, Leith DE, Geffin B, Laver MB (1972) Ventilation with end-expiratory pressure in acute lung disease. J Clin Invest 51:2315-2323
2. Suter PM, Fairley HB, Isenberg MD (1975) Optimum end-expiratory airway pressure in patients with acute pulmonary failure. N Engl J Med 292:284-289
3. Bone RC (1976) Diagnosis of causes for acute respiratory distress by pressure volume curves. Chest 70:740-746
4. Jonson B, Nordström L, Olsson SG, Akerback D (1975) Monitoring of ventilation and lung mechanics during automatic ventilation. A new device. Bull Eur Physiopathol Respir 11:729-743
5. Suter PM, Fairley HB, Isenberg MD (1978) Effect of tidal volume and positive end-expiratory pressure on compliance during mechanical ventilation. Chest 173:158-162
6. Janney CD (1959) Super-syringe. Anesthesiology 20:709-711
7. Harf A, Lemaire F, Lorino H, Atlan G (1975) Etude de la mécanique ventilatoire: application à la ventilation artificielle. Bull Eur Physiopathol Respir 11:709-728
8. Benito S, Lemaire F, Mankikian B, Harf A (1985) Total respiratory compliance as a function of lung volume in patients with mechanical ventilation. Intensive Care Med 11:76-79
9. Mankikian B, Lemaire F, Benito S, et al (1983) New device for measurement of pulmonary pressure volume curves in patients on mechanical ventilation. Crit Care Med 11:897-901
10. Mancebo J, Calaf N, Benito S (1985) Pulmonary compliance measurement in acute respiratory failure. Crit Care Med 13:589-591
11. Radford EP (1964) Static mechanical properties of mammalian lungs. In: Fenn WO, Rahn H (eds) Handbook of Physiology. Sect 3, vol 1, 1st edn. American Physiological Society, Washington DC, pp 429-449
12. Hillman DR, Finucane KE (1983) The effect of hyperventilation on lung elasticity in healthy subjects. Respir Physiol 54:295-305
13. Frazer DG, Stengel PW, Weber KC (1979) The effect of pulmonary edema on gas trapping in excised rat lungs. Respir Physiol 38:325-333
14. Hoppin FG, Hildebrandt J (1977) Mechanical properties of the lung. In: West JB (ed) Bioengineering aspects of the lung. 1st edn. Marcel Dekker, New York, pp 83-162
15. Lemaire F, Harf A, Simonneau G, Matamis D, Rivara D, Atlan G (1981) Echanges gazeux, courbe statique pression-volume pulmonaire et ventilation en pression positive de fin d'expiration. Ann Anesth Franc 5:435-441
16. Matamis D, Lemaire F, Harf A, Brun-Buisson C, Ansquer JC, Atlan G (1984) Total respiratory pressure-volume curves in the adult respiratory distress syndrome. Chest 86:58-66
17. Pesenti A, Marcolin R, Prato P, Borelli M, Riboni A, Gattinoni L (1985) Mean airway pressure vs positive end-expiratory pressure during mechanical ventilation. Crit Care Med 13:34-37
18. Mancebo J, Benito S, Calaf N, Caviedes I, Blanch L (1986) Presión positiva espiratoria y presión de apertura en la insuficiencia respiratoria aguda. Med Intensiva 10:24-27
19. Gattinoni L, Mascheroni D, Basilico E, Foti G, Pesenti A, Avalli L (1987) Volume/pressure curve of total respiratory system in paralysed patients: artefacts and correction factors. Intensive Care Med 13:19-25
20. Mithoefer JC (1965) Breath holding. In: Fenn WO, Rahn H (eds) Handbook of Physiology. Sect 3, vol II, 1st edn. American Physiological Society, Washington DC, pp 1011-1025
21. Dall'Ava J, Armangadis A, Brunet F, Dhainaut JF, Lockhart A (1986) Indirect spirometry improves the understanding of total respiratory pressure-volume curves in ventilated patients. Bull Eur Physiopathol Respir 22:140s (Abstract)
22. Bone RC (1976) Compliance and dynamic characteristics curves in acute respiratory failure. Crit Care Med 4:173-179

23. Blanch L, Fernández R, Benito S, Mancebo J, Net A (1987) Effect of PEEP on the arterial minus end-tidal carbon dioxide gradient. Chest 92:451–454
24. Mancebo J, Benito S, Martín M, Net A (1988) Value of static pulmonary compliance in predicting mortality in patients with acute respiratory failure. Intensive Care Med 14 (in press)
25. Gattinoni L, Pesenti A, Caspani ML, et al (1984) The role of total static lung compliance in the management of severe ARDS unresponsive to conventional treatment. Intensive Care Med 10:121–126

Mechanical Ventilation in Cardiogenic and Septic Shock

C. Roussos

Hypoxemic or hypercapnic respiratory failure has traditionally been the main cause of mechanical ventilation. Although respiratory failure is a frequent complication of shock, the use of mechanical ventilation has been instituted only when severe gas exchange abnormalities occurred. We maintain that mechanical ventilation should be instituted early in the course of shock for two reasons:

1. to put the respiratory muscles at rest, and thereby avoid respiratory muscle fatigue, and
2. to free blood from the working respiratory muscles. The blood can, in turn, supply vital organs.

Our thesis is supported by several recent experimental findings in animals and patients [1–4]. In shock the respiratory muscles are impeded in their performance. On the one hand there is hyperventilation, while the lungs are stiff and the airway resistance high, all of which increase the work of breathing and therefore the energy demands. On the other hand, there is a limited amount of blood available. Thus, it is inescapable that either the respiratory muscles will not receive the amount of blood they need, leading to anaerobic metabolism; or the respiratory muscles will receive adequate blood, depriving the rest of the body of blood and oxygen.

Figure 1 depicts the relation of minute ventilation to oxygen consumption at different degrees of lung disease (right quadrant). On the left quadrant, the relationship of blood flow to oxygen consumption is shown, as predicted by the Fick equation: [$\dot{V}O_2 = \dot{Q}(Ca\text{-}Cv)O_2$] (where $\dot{Q}$ = blood flow, $\dot{V}O_2$ = oxygen consumption, $(Ca\text{-}Cv)O_2$ = arterial-venous oxygen content difference) at different degrees of $(Ca\text{-}Cv)O_2$ difference. Low $(Ca\text{-}Cv)O_2$ (i.e. 2.5 vol %) is common in septic shock, whereas high $(Ca\text{-}Cv)O_2$ (ie. 10–15 vol %) is common in cardiogenic shock.

Clearly, if the respiratory muscles need 200–300 ml O_2/min, a value not unreasonable under conditions of high work of breathing with severe lung disease, the amount of blood that must be directed to the respiratory muscles is excessively high, relative to the blood flow available. In keeping with this we have shown that in animal models of cardiogenic and septic shock, up to 20% of cardiac output may be directed to the respiratory muscles [3, 5] when animals breath spontaneously, while only 3% of cardiac output is directed to the same musculature when the animals are mechanically ventilated (Fig. 2).

The re-distribution of blood flow has its effects on anaerobic metabolism and lactate production. It may be predicted that as the respiratory muscles do not

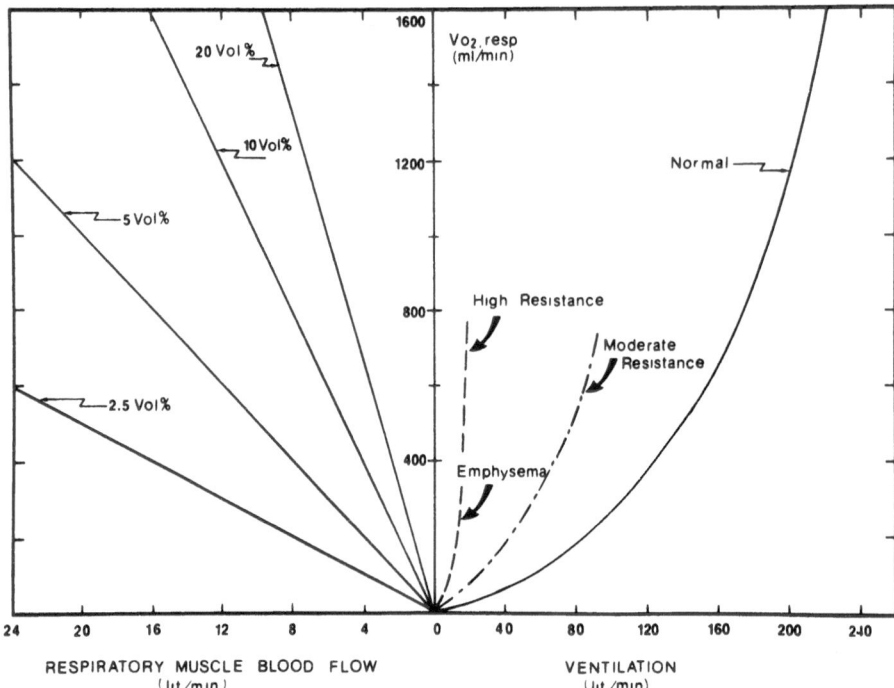

Fig. 1. The left-hand panel plots the oxygen cost of breathing ($\dot{V}O_2$ resp) against respiratory-muscle blood flow for various values of CaO_2-$C\bar{v}O_2$, and is the graphic solution of the Fick equation $\dot{V}O_2$resp $= \dot{Q}(CaO_2$-$C\bar{v}O_2)$

work, in view of the limited supply of oxygen, lactate production will be reduced. Indeed, in the experiments on cardiogenic shock, we have found [4] that blood lactate is substantially reduced when animals are ventilated (Fig. 3).

It follows that since the severity of lactic acidosis in shock bears a prognostic value [6–8], maintaining these muscles in the aerobic state has obvious advantages. Finally, by placing the respiratory muscles at rest, respiratory muscle fatigue is avoided, ventilatory failure is prevented and mortality is reduced [1], (Fig. 4).

To summarize, placing respiratory muscles at rest in patients with shock has strong a theoretical and experimental basis, both to avoid the complications of respiratory failure and to improve the prognosis of the syndrome. Presently the most widely accepted method of minimizing respiratory muscle activity and reducing respiratory muscle oxygen requirements [9–11] is through the institution of mechanical ventilation. However, does such an approach have only beneficial effects in view of the fact that positive pressure ventilation may impair circulation?

Mechanical ventilation raises the thoracic pressure. For many years the effect of positive pressure ventilation on cardiovascular function has remained unclear and only recently has the subject been elucidated [12, 13]. Traditionally it has been accepted that mechanical ventilation and PEEP are detrimental in shock

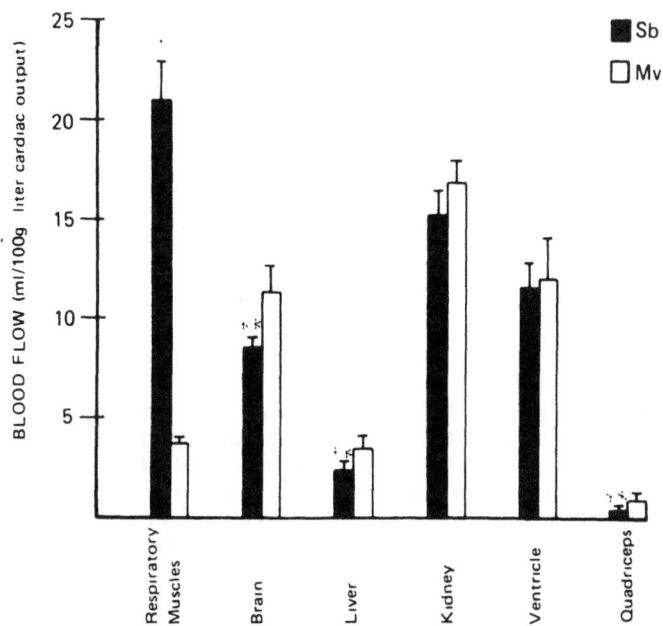

Fig. 2. Comparison of the fractional distribution of cardiac output during tamponade in the two groups of dogs. Solid columns represent the spontaneously breathing (Sb) dogs; open columns, the mechanically ventilated (Mv) animals. Bars represent standard error. Note that while the respiratory muscles received a significantly greater portion of the cardiac output in the Sb group, the brain, liver and quadriceps muscles received significantly less. (From [3])

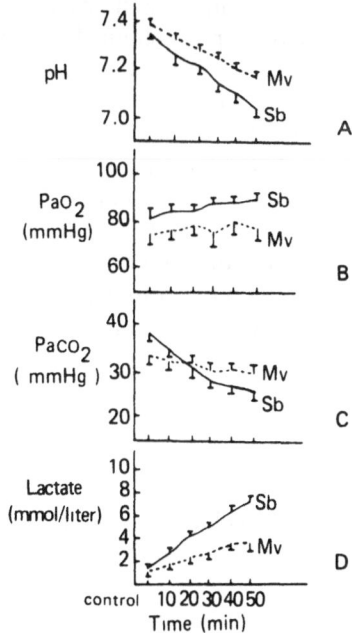

Fig. 3. Evolution of arterial pH (panel A), blood gases (panels B, C), and lactate (panel D) during the course of low cardiac output state in the two groups of dogs, one breathing spontaneously (Sb) and another mechanically ventilated (Mv). Note that while arterial PO_2 and PCO_2 were not significantly different between the two groups, pH was significantly lower ($p < 0.001$) and lactate significantly higher ($p > 0.005$) in the Sb group at any time during the hypotensive period. (From [3])

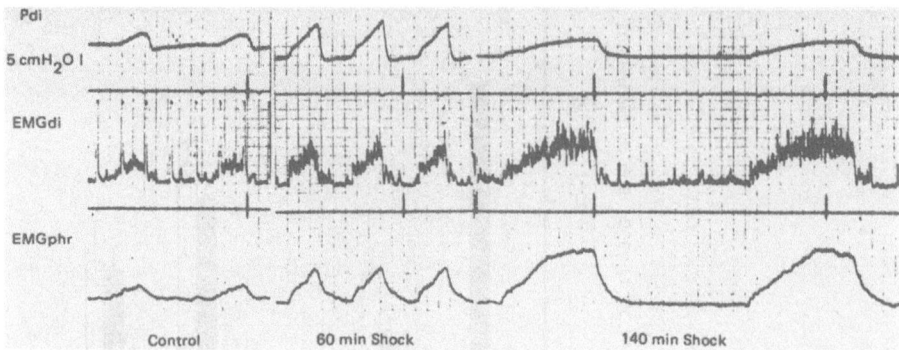

Fig. 4. Typical record of one dog showing evolution during cardiogenic shock of transdiaphragmatic pressure (Pdi) (top trace), electrical integrated activity of diaphragm (Edi) (middle trace), and electrical integrated activity of phrenic nerve (Ephr) (bottom trace). Left panel, during control; middle panel, 60 min after onset of cardiogenic shock; right panel, 140 min after onset of cardiogenic shock prior to death of animal. Decrease in size of electrocardiographic artifact on Edi trace is a consequence of injection of saline into pericardium. (From [1])

[14]. Several experimental findings have supported this attitude. Although there is no intention to review the subject at great length here, it is worth mentioning a few findings. In brief, due to a decrease in cardiac output in many instances, it was suggested that there was a fall in right ventricular, and eventually left ventricular preload [15]. Others have suggested the existence of cardiopressive humoral reflexes [6], or the activity of neural reflexes mediated via stretch receptors [17]. However, all these conclusions have been challenged [18–20].

Firstly, there is the notion by Bjork et al. [11] that the observed decrease in cardiac output with the institution of mechanical ventilation may represent a beneficial physiological response to the decreased oxygen demand of the respiratory muscles that do not continue to work. In contrast to the decrease in cardiac output observed in healthy animals or humans, there is accumulated evidence that in patients or animals with heart failure, institution of mechanical ventilation may improve hemodynamics. Beach et al. [21] have reported a deterioration in hemodynamic stability in post-operative patients during discontinuation of mechanical ventilation, unrelated to blood gas changes. There is also evidence that intermittent elevation of intrathoracic pressure may benefit patients with congestive heart failure. Although the mechanism is unclear, the prevailing explanation is that mechanical ventilation decreases ventricular afterload [12, 13]. Along these lines are the experiments of Pinsky et al. [22, 23], in animals subjected to heart failure induced by propranolol. In these studies it was shown that during positive pressure ventilation, in concert with thoracic binding (rib cage and abdomen), there was a significant increase in the cardiac output. Consistent with this are the findings of Prewitt et al. [24], who found a decrease in ventricular end-systolic volume during mechanical ventilation, and Grace et al. [25] who reported an increase in cardiac output in patients with cardiovascular dysfunction when ventilated with PEEP. The mechanism of such an effect is not completely clear but we hypothesize that in raising the intrathoracic pressure, the left ventricular afterload is reduced and thus cardiac output improves.

The significance of intrathoracic positive pressure fluctuations in maintaining the circulatory flow has been mostly shown during new-cardiopulmonary resuscitation. After the original observations that adequate blood flow can be maintained by raising the intrathoracic pressure [26, 29], our recent experiments have clearly demonstrated that carotid blood flow is maintained by ventilating the animals. In order to achieve high intrathoracic pressure, however, both the rib cage and abdomen were surrounded by a rigid cast [30].

Thus, based on our work and others, cardiogenic shock should be managed by judiciously using mechanical ventilation early in the course of the disease. Such an approach offers several practical and theoretical advantages. Apart from correcting the blood gas abnormalities due to lung disease, it avoids respiratory muscle fatigue and thus ventilatory failure. In addition, putting the respiratory muscles at rest results in an increase of blood flow and oxygen availability to other vital organs.

The experience in septic shock is not large yet, but from animal models of septic shock evidence is accumulating that mechanical ventilation has beneficial effects similar to those achieved in cardiogenic shock [2, 5].

References

1. Aubier M, Trippenbach T, Roussos Ch (1981) Respiratory muscle fatigue during cardiogenic shock. J Appl Physiol 51:499–508
2. Hussain SNA, Simkus G, Roussos Ch (1985) Ventilatory muscle fatigue, the cause of respiratory failure in septic shock. J Appl Physiol 58:2033–2040
3. Viires N, Sillye G, Aubier M, Rassidakis A, Roussos Ch (1983) Regional bood flow distribution in dog during induced hypotension and low cardiac output. Spontaneous breathing versus artificial ventilation. J Clin Invest 72:935–947
4. Aubier M, Viires N, Sillye G, Mozes R, Roussos Ch (1982) Respiratory muscle contribution to lactic acidosis in low cardiac output. Am Rev Respir Dis 126:642–652
5. Hussain S, Roussos Ch (1985) Distribution of respiratory muscle and organ blood flow during endotoxin shock in dogs. J Appl Physiol 59:1802–1808
6. Peretz DI, McGregor M, Dossetor JB (1964) Lactic acidosis: a clinically significant aspect of shock. Can Med Assoc J 90:673–675
7. Vincent JL, Dufaye P, Berré J, Leeman M, Degaute JP, Kahn RJ (1983) Serial lactate determinations during circulatory shock. Crit Care Med 11:449–451
8. Blair E, Cowley A, Tait MK (1965) Refractory septic shock in man: role of lactate and pyruvate metabolism in prognosis. Ann Surg 31:537–540
9. Field S, Kelly SM, Macklem PT (1982) The oxygen cost of breathing in patients with cardiorespiratory disease. Am Rev Respir Dis 126:9–13
10. Burzstein S, Taitelman U, DeMyttenaere S, et al (1978) Reduced oxygen consumption in catabolic states with mechanical ventilation. Crit Care Med 6:162–168
11. Bjork VO, Grenvik A, Holmdahl MH, Westerholm CJ (1964) Cardiac output and oxygen consumption during respiratory treatment. Acta Anaesth Scand (supp) 15:158–160
12. Robotham JL, Scharf SM (1983) Effects of positive and negative pressure ventilation on cardiac performance. Clin Chest Med 4:161–187
13. Luce JM (1984) The cardiovascular effects of mechanical ventilation and positive end expiratory pressure. JAMA 252:807–811
14. Ashbaugh CG, Petty TL (1973) Positive end-expiratory pressure physiology, indications and contraindications. J Thor Cardiovas Surg 65:165

15. Qvist J, Pontoppidan H, Wilson RS, Lowenstein E, Laver MB (1975) Hemodynamic responses to mechanical ventilation with PEEP. Anaesthesiology 42:45-55
16. Grindlinger GA, Manny J, Justice R, Dunham, Shepro D, Heshtman HB (1979) Presence of negative inotropic agents in caning plasma during positive end-expiratory pressure. Circ Res 45:460-467
17. Click G, Weschler AS, Epstein SE (1969) Reflex cardiovascular depression produced by stimulation of pulmonary stretch receptors in the dog. J Clin Invest 48:467-473
18. Marthru M (1985) Mechanical breath; non-pharmacologic support for a failing heart? Chest 85:1
19. Ellman H, Dembin H (1982) Lack of adverse hemodynamic effects of PEEP in patients with acute respiratory failure. Crit Care Med 10:706-711
20. Calvin JE, Driedser AA, Sibbald WJ (1981) Positive end-expiratory pressure does not depress left ventricular function in patients with edema. Am Rev Respir Dis 124:121-128
21. Beach T, Millen E, Grenvik A (1973) Hemodynamic response to discontinuation of mechanical ventilation. Crit Care Med 1:85-90
22. Pinsky MR, Summer WR (1983) Cardiac augmentation by phasic high intrathoracic pressure support in man. Chest 84:370-375
23. Pinsky MR, Summer WR, Wise RH, et al (1983) Augmentation of cardiac function by elevation of intrathoracic pressure. J Appl Physiol 54:950-955
24. Prewitt RM, Oppenheimer L, Sutherland JB, Wood LDH (1981) Effect of positive end-expiratory pressure on left ventricular mechanics in patients with hypoxemic respiratory failure. Anaesthesiology 55:409-415
25. Crace MR, Greenham DM (1982) Cardiac performance in response to PEEP in patients with cardiac dysfunction. Crit Care Med 10:358-360
26. Criley JM, Balfuss Ah, Vissel GL (1976) Cough-induced cardiac compression: self-administered form of cardiopulmonary resuscitation. JAMA 236:1246-1250
27. Chandra N, Weisfeldt ML, Tsitlik J, et al (1981) Augmentation of carotid flow during cardiopulmonary resuscitation by ventilation at high airway pressure with chest compression. Am J Cardiol 48:1053-1063
28. Rosborough JP, Nieman JT, Griley JM, et al (1981) Lower abdominal compression with synchronized ventilation; a CPR modality. Circulation 64 (suppl 4):303 (Abstract)
29. Niemann JT, Rosborough JP, Niskanen RA, Criley JM (1984) Circulatory support during cardiac arrest using a pneumatic vest and abdominal binder with simultaneous high-pressure airway inflation. Ann Emerg Med 13:270-277
30. Passerini L, Wise RA, Roussos Ch (1985) Maintenance of circulation during CPR with mechanical ventilation. Clin Invest Med 8:R164

Intermittent Mandatory Ventilation: Revisited

K. J. Falke

Introduction

Intermittent mandatory ventilation (IMV) was introduced as a weaning technique by Downs in 1973 [1]. It allows the patients to breathe spontaneously inbetween or simultaneous with mandatory breaths delivered from the mechanical ventilator. This was first accomplished by connecting a continuous flow CPAP system to the inspiratory line of the ventilator.

However, most of these early IMV/CPAP-devices did not allow synchronization of mandatory with spontaneous breaths. If continuous flow IMV circuits are properly used airway pressure swings between ex- and inspiration are small, hence, a trigger mechanism dependent upon an inspiratory airway pressure drop tends to fail. In addition there is consensus among experienced clinicians that synchronization of mechanical with spontaneous breaths is not needed if the ventilator includes a well functioning high-pressure relieve valve. Nevertheless, most manufacturers felt that synchronized IMV (SIMV) was a necessity, so that most commercially available ventilators have incorporated a demand valve system allowing SIMV.

Demand valve systems have the inherent problem that they require additional work by the patient to overcome resistance imposed by the ventilator and its circuit. The first is the effort to initiate (trigger) the gas flow and the second may be due to an inadequate flow supplied by the demand valve not matching the patients inspiratory flow requirements. The first ventilators with demand valve systems, such as the Siemens Servo B and the Engström Erica, required up to 22% more inspiratory work than a continuous flow CPAP system despite most sensitive trigger settings [2].

To minimize this problem, the manufacturers of ventilators introduced a new technique of augmenting spontaneous inspiration called inspiratory pressure support (IPS) or assisted spontaneous breathing (ASB). A small IPS is already provided without activation of this mode in some ventilators (Servo C) [3]. IPS or ASB reduce the work of inspiration and eliminate most of the additional inspiratory work required by the machine. However, in contrast to the continuous flow system an isovolemic trigger effort is still necessary (see also chapter by L. Brochard and F. Lemaire in this book).

Recently, demand valve IMV/CPAP systems (Servo C, EV-A, Bennett 7200) have reached a high technological standard allowing spontaneous breathing with a minimum of added work required [2]. Moreover a new continuous flow system ("flow by", Puritan Bennett) has become commercially available. This is advantageous because the required trigger effort is further reduced (Fig. 1).

On the other hand flow-by cannot be used simultaneously with the IPS option. The combination of flow-by and IPS would theoretically eliminate all work required due to resistances external to the patient including the inspiratory work necessary to overcome the resistance of the endotracheal tube (Fig. 2). IMV and IPS/ASB relieve the patient from a certain fraction of the required ventilation, thus providing partial ventilatory support (PVS) in contrast to full ventilatory support (FVS) as in controlled mechanical ventilation [4].

Conventional assisted mechanical ventilation (AMV) in which each spontaneous breath initiates a mechanical breath can also be considered to provide partial ventilatory support. These various techniques of mechanical ventilatory assistance can be put in a simple order (Table 1).

DEMANDFLOW (III)

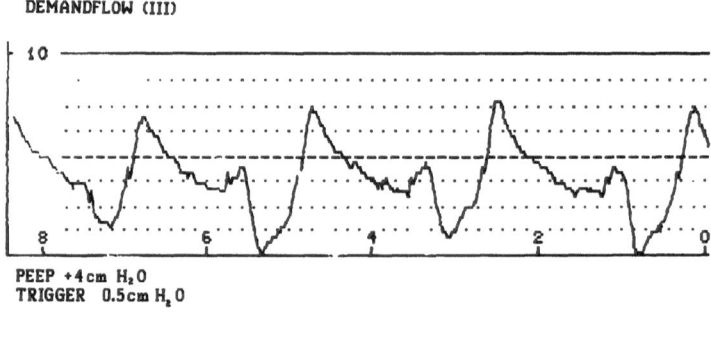

PEEP +4cm H₂0
TRIGGER 0.5cm H₂0

FLOW BY

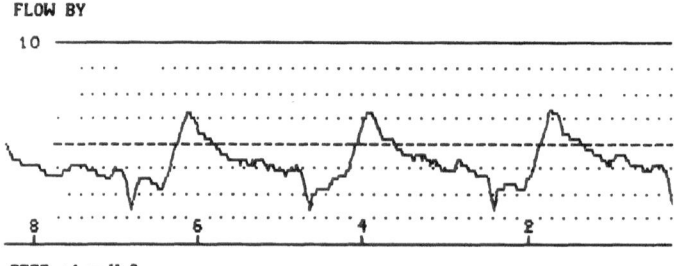

PEEP +4 cm H₂0
BASISFLOW 20 LpM
FLOWSENSIBILITAET 1 LpM

Fig. 1. Airway pressure (vertical axis: cmH₂O, horizontal axis: sec) during spontaneous breathing with demand-valve system without pressure support (top) and with the flow-by option (bottom) (ventilator Puritan Bennett 7200).
Negative inspiratory pressure swings were reduced with flow-by, indicating that either inspiratory flow conditions are improved or the added inspiratory work due to the resistance of the circuit is reduced

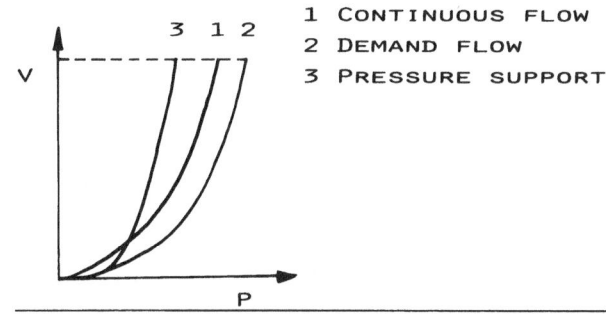

Fig. 2. Schematic pressure volume relationship representing the work of inspiration (V = tidal volume, P = transpulmonary pressure).
The work of inspiration is equivalent to the area encircled by the vertical axis, the pressure volume curves (1–3) and the horizontal dotted line. It is increased with the demand-flow (or -valve) (2) if compared with the continuous flow system (1). With inspiratory pressure support (IPS) (3) the required work of inspiration is decreased. The left shift of the pressure volume curve indicate that the patient can breathe as if the compliance was improved. However, IPS does not eliminate the required work in the beginning of inspiration (trigger effort). From this graph it appears that the combination of continuous flow plus IPS would most efficiently reduce the required work of inspiration

Table 1. Types of mechanical ventilatory assistance

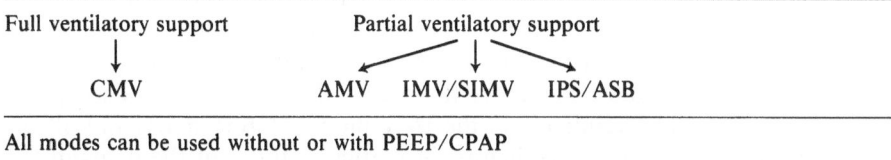

All modes can be used without or with PEEP/CPAP

Table 2. Advantages and disadvantages of MV

Advantages:	Disadvantages:
– Spontaneous breathing possible without deterioration of blood gases [5, 6]	– Risk of ineffective, energy consuming spontaneous breathing
– Reduced need to suppress spontaneous breathing	– Possible occurrence of inspiratory muscle fatigue
– Reduced dead space with spontaneous breaths [7]	– Permanent weaning conditions
– Possible gradual transition from high to low mean intrathoracic pressures	– Increased level of attention required by nurses and doctors
– Cardiocirculatory and renal function less compromized than with CMV [5–7]	– Possible worsening of LV failure by spontaneous breathing
	– Complicated technology

Advantages and Disadvantages of IMV

Some of the important potential advantages and disadvantages of IMV are listed in Table 2. During recent years pro's and con's of IMV have been discussed in much detail sometimes in a very critical manner [4, 8, 9]. Theoretically one would expect that the reduced intrathoracic pressure associated with spontaneous breathing minimizes the potentially adverse effects of controlled positive pressure ventilation in particular if PEEP is used. In fact, some of the listed advantages have been substantiated by appropriate studies, e.g. the benficial effect of IMV on renal function when compared to CMV at identical levels of PEEP. However, this was studied only during short periods of a few hours [5, 6]. Whether long term use of IMV leads to less water retention than CMV remains unknown.

It was hoped that IMV would eliminate at least in part the negative influence of CMV on ventilation-perfusion-ratio (VA/Q). Recent clinical studies using the six inert-gases elimination technique did not show a consistent improvement of VA/Q during IMV if compared to CMV (Radermacher, personal communication).

Today IMV is widely used despite the fact that its beneficial effect on organ function, on the course and duration of acute respiratory failure and on the outcome has not been well substantiated. This high degree of acceptance may be explained by obvious practical advantages of IMV simplifying the management of patients on ventilators. In the author's opinion the most relevant advantage of IMV is that the majority of patients can be permitted to breathe spontaneously while being mechanically ventilated without deterioration in blood gases. Because most patients in acute respiratory failure (except if the respiratory center is depressed) have the inevitable desire to breathe, there is a tendency to systematically set mechanical ventilator in the IMV mode. Unfortunately not all presently available mechanical ventilators, in particular those of the demand valve type, can cope with the extreme breathing patterns of some critically ill patients.

Figure 3 shows an example where the inspiratory flow created by the patient exceeds the inspiratory flow delivered during a mechanical breath. This problem is recognized by the sharp drop of inspiratory airway pressure at the beginning of the positive pressure wave representing the mechanical breath. According to studies by Schlobohm et al. [10] and Quan et al. [11] such negative airway pressure swings may be detrimental to pulmonary function. Hence, the precondition for a successful use of a "IMV for all" concept requires mechanical ventilators providing constant positive airway pressures at the PEEP level during expiration as well as during inspiration despite excessive flow demands by the patient. In the mentioned example (Fig. 3) the problem was solved by increasing the inspiratory peak flow from 30 to 45 l/min and by changing the inspiratory flow pattern for the mandatory breath from a square to a decelerating flow wave providing the patient with the peak flow at the beginning of inspiration.

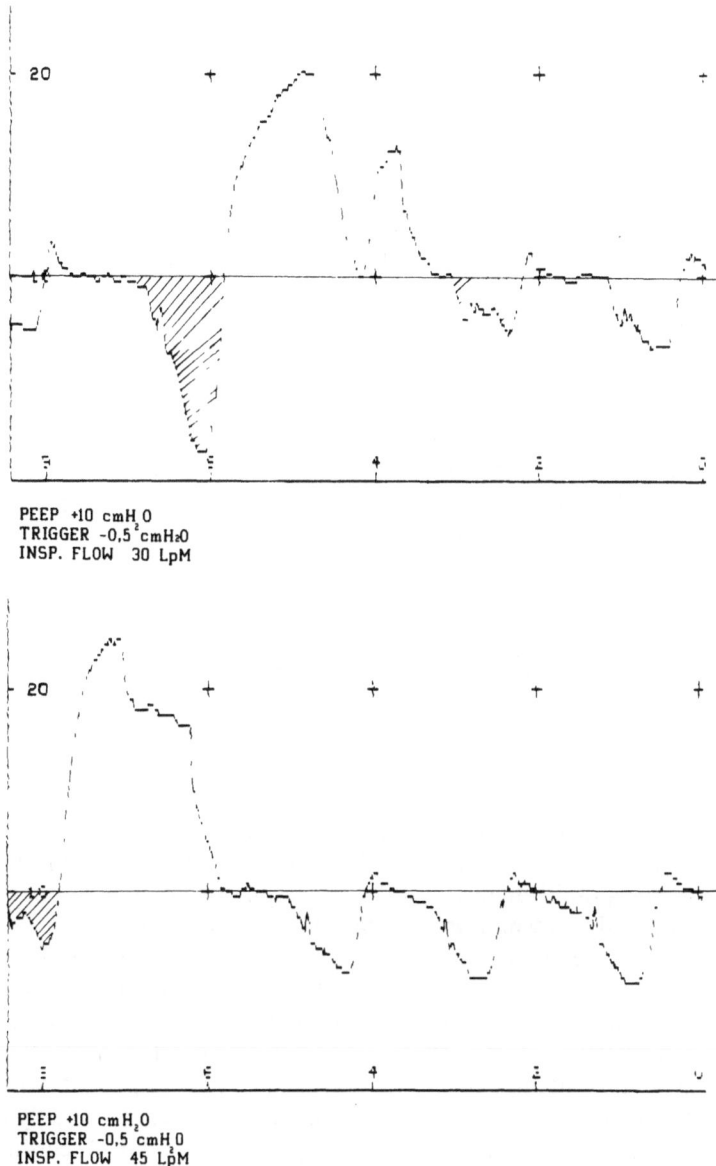

PEEP +10 cmH₂0
TRIGGER -0,5 cmH₂0
INSP. FLOW 30 LpM

PEEP +10 cmH₂0
TRIGGER -0,5 cmH₂0
INSP. FLOW 45 LpM

Fig. 3. Airway pressure during IMV (Puritan Bennett 7200), (vertical axis: cm H₂O, horizontal axis: sec). The large shaded area in the top panel represents inadequate flow delivered by the ventilator. This was improved (below) by rising the inspiratory flow set on the machine. (For further explanation see text)

IMV versus IPS/ASB

Both IMV and IPS provide partial ventilatory support. IMV intersperses volume-assisted breaths with non-assisted breaths. Conventional assisted mechanical ventilation also provides partial ventilatory support. However, according to

Marini et al. [12] AMV may be associated with an unexpected high work of breathing, a problem which may also occur with assisted breaths during SIMV.

In IPS or ASB each breath is augmented with an additional flow according to the flow demand of the patient up to a certain preselected pressure limit. In contrast to SIMV, IPS is associated with improved respiratory function parameters e.g. respiratory rate [13]. It reduces the mechanical inspiratory work of each breath and the patient inhales as if the compliance was increased [2, 14]. Moreover, IPS improves the efficacy of spontaneous breathing as judged by increased PaO_2, reduced $PaCO_2$, respiratory rate and pressure time index of the diaphragm [15]. Kanak et al. [16] found a marked reduction of oxygen consumption with the change from SIMV to IPS in a patient with chronic ostructive lung disease. These results indicate that IPS might provide physiologically more appropriate respiratory support than SIMV.

Until the role of IPS is further established by clinical studies, it is recommended to use 2-4 cm H_2O IPS in combination with SIMV (so far the only possibility with demand valve systems), to relieve the patient from most of the work required to overcome external resistances.

IMV and Inspiratory Muscle Fatigue

Under conditions of partial ventilatory support patients are always in a weaning situation. Hence, if the level of ventilatory support is insufficient to the ability of the patients to breathe spontaneously there is the inherent risk of developing inspiratory muscle fatigue. The classical clinical symptoms of an unsuccessful weaning trial are identical with those indicating inspiratory muscle fatigue, e.g. dyspnea, rapid shallow ventilation, respiratory muscle discoordination (abdominal paradox, respiratory alternans) and acidosis [17, 18].

Other possibilities to assess inspiratory muscle fatigue during partial ventilatory support has been described [19, 20]. Taylor et al. [18] used the trigger mechanism of a demand valve device (Ventilator Bear I) to measure tracheal occlusion pressure, which is the negative pressure created during the first 0.1 sec of an inspiratory attempt against an occluded airway. In patients with inspiratory muscle fatigue, the respiratory neuromuscular drive is abnormally high leading to an increase in the tracheal occlusion pressure [21-23]. Accordingly partial ventilatory support e.g. the number of mechanical breaths should be increased if signs of inspiratory muscle fatigue occur.

The early recognition of dyspnea and inspiratory muscle fatigue during partial ventilatory support relies on frequent careful assessment of the clinical status by nurses and doctors. Except for the surveillance of the respiratory rate automatic monitors are of little help.

The risk of developing inspiratory muscle fatigue is increased in patients with low or inadequate blood flow to the diaphragm, e.g. in low cardiac output [24]. Consequently, IMV should not be used under these circumstances. In severe shock, controlled mechanical ventilation is mandatory, at least in part to avoid respiratory muscle fatigue and failure.

One of the unresolved problems in respiratory care is whether weaning should be carried out continuously utilizing IMV and/or IPS or discontinuously interspersing T-piece or CPAP trials with phases of controlled mechanical ventilation. Anecdotal observations suggest that patients with underlying chronic lung disease (COPD) or muscle diseases benefit from phases of mechanical ventilation with complete rest. Unfortunately, inspiratory muscle fatigue has been studied mostly in COPD patients. In patients with acute respiratory failure undergoing partial ventilatory support its role needs still to be defined by appropriate clinical studies.

References

1. Downs JB, Klein EF, Desautels D, Modell JH, Kirby RR (1973) Intermittent mandatory ventilation: a new approach to weaning patients from mechanical ventilators. Chest 64:331–335
2. Samodelov LF, Falke K (1988) Total inspiratory work with modern demand valve devices compared to continuous flow CPAP. (submitted)
3. Falke KJ, Samodelov LF (1986) Inspiratory work of breathing with CPAP-systems. In: Update on Intensive Care and Emergency Medicine, vol 1. Springer, Berlin Heidelberg New York London Paris Tokyo, pp 96–100
4. Shapiro BA (1984) The IMV controversy: Full vs partial ventilatory support. In: JL Vincent (ed) Update in Intensive Care and Emergency Medicine, Springer, Berlin Heidelberg New York Tokyo, pp 36–38
5. Steinhoff H, Falke KJ, Schwarzhoff W (1982) Enhanced renal function associated with intermittent mandatory ventilation in acute respiratory failure. Intensive Care Med 8:69–74
6. Steinhoff H, Kohlhoff RJ, Falke KJ (1984) Facilitation of excretory function and hemodynamics of the kidneys by intermittent mandatory ventilation. Intensive Care Med 10:59–64
7. Wolff G, Brunner JX, Gradel E (1986) Gas exchange during mechanical ventilation and spontaneous breathing. Intermittent mandatory ventilation after open heart surgery. Chest 90:11–17
8. Shapiro BA, Cane RD (1984) The IMV-AMV controversy: a plea for clarification and redirection. Crit Care Med 12:472–473
9. Weisman IM, Rinaldo JE, Rogers RM, Sanders MH (1983) Intermittent mandatory ventilation. Am Rev Respir Dis 127:641–647
10. Schlobohm RM, Falltrick RT, Quan SF, Katz JA (1981) Lung volumes, mechanics, and oxygenation during spontaneous positive-pressure ventilation: the advantage of CPAP over EPAP. Anesthesiology 55:416–422
11. Quan SF, Falltrick RT, Schlobohm RM (1981) Extubation from ambient or expiratory positive airway pressure in adults. Anesthesiology 55:53–56
12. Marini JJ, Capps JS, Culver BH (1985) The inspiratory work of breathing during assisted mechanical ventilation. Chest 87:612–618
13. MacIntyre NR (1986) Respiratory function during pressure support ventilation. Chest 89:677–683
14. Brochard L, Harf A, Lorino H, Lemaire F (1987) Decreases work of breathing and oxygen consumption during weaning from mechanical ventilation (MV). Am Rev Respir Dis 135:A51 (Abstract)
15. Brochard L, Pluskwa F, Lemaire F (1987) Improved efficacy of spontaneous breathing with inspiratory pressure support. Am Rev Respir Dis 136:411–415
16. Kanak R, Fahey PJ, Vanderwarf C (1985) Oxygen cost of breathing: Changes dependent upon mode of mechanical ventilation. Chest 87:126–127
17. Cohen CA, Zagelbaum G, Gross D, Roussos C, Macklem PT (1982) Clinical manifestations of inspiratory muscle fatigue. Am J Med 73:308–316

18. Tobin MJ, Perez W, Guenther SM, et al (1986) The pattern of breathing during succesful and unsuccessful trials of weaning from mechanical ventilation. Am Rev Respir Dis 134:1111–1118
19. Herrera M, Blasco J, Venegas J, Barba R, Doblas A, Marquez E (1985) Mouth occlusion pressure in acute respiratory failure. Intensive Care Med 11:134–139
20. Taylor RF, Marini JJ, Smith TC, Lamb VJ (1987) Bedside estimation of respiratory drive during machine assisted ventilation. Am Rev Respir Dis 135:A51
21. Whitelaw WS, Derenne JP, Milic-Emili J (1975) Occlusion pressure as a measure of respiratory center output in conscious man. Resp Physiol 23:181–199
22. Milic-Emili J, Whitelaw WA, Derenne J-P (1975) Occlusion pressure-a simple measure of the respiratory center's output. N Engl J Med 292:1029–30
23. Sassoon CSH, Te TT, Mahutte K, Light RW (1987) Am important indicator for successful weaning in patients with chronic obstructive pulmonary disease. Am Rev Respir Dis 135:107–113
24. Aubier M, Trippenbach T, Roussos C (1981) Respiratory muscle fatigue during cardiogenic shock. J Appl Physiol 51:499–508

Inspiratory Pressure Support

L. Brochard and F. Lemaire

Introduction

During controlled mechanical ventilation, spontaneous inspiratory activity is decreased or abolished during the following circumstances: administration of sedative drugs, respiratory muscle fatigue or excessive loading [1], hypocapnic hyperventilation or central nervous system disorders. In other cases, a spontaneous diaphragmatic activity may be present during ventilatory support. Several modes of ventilatory assistance have been developed to allow spontaneous breathing of the patient. The use of such modes has became widespread during difficult weaning from mechanical ventilation. In a more general point of view, putative advantages of partial ventilatory support can be summarized as follows:

1. minimal need for sedation;
2. optimized ventilator synchrony;
3. prevention of respiratory muscle atrophy;
4. potential training of the respiratory muscles.

However, no clear advantage has been shown during weaning from mechanical ventilation. In addition, the assistance provided to the respiratory muscles can be ineffective [2]. In contrast, inspiratory pressure support ventilation provides an efficacious physiological assistance to respiratory muscles, as shown, by several authors [3–5]. Although clinical applications of pressure support ventilation cannot be clearly defined yet it appears as a promising alternative to other partial ventilatory supports.

Main Characteristics

During inspiratory pressure support (IPS) ventilation a constant positive pressure is applied to the circuit throughout patient's spontaneous inspiration. The level of pressure can be adjusted (Fig. 1). Expiration remains passive and PEEP may be added as in other conventional respiratory modes. Thus, the respiratory frequency remains under the patient's control, while the tidal volume and the minute ventilation are the result of both the patient's demand and the assistance pressure level.

According to the set-up of the parameters, a total ventilation can range from a full spontaneous ventilation (if the IPS level is nil) to a near controlled ventilation (if the IPS level is high).

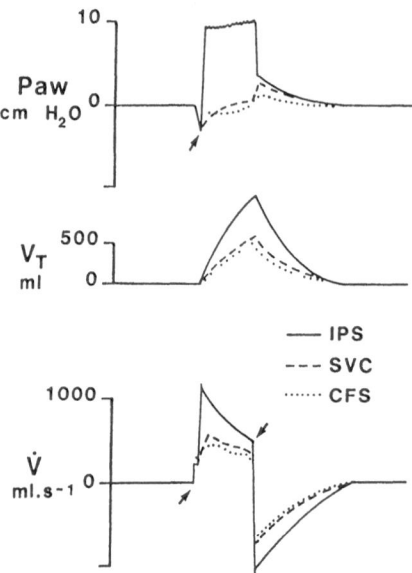

Fig. 1. Diagram of airway pressure (Paw), tidal volume (V_t) and flow ($\dot{V}$) during three modes of ventilatory assistance: inspiratory pressure support (IPS), spontaneous breathing through the Servo 900 C circuit (SVC) or through a continuous flow system (CFS). Opening of the demand valve is indicated with an arrow on the pressure trace. With IPS a plateau of pressure is produced during the entire inspiration (arrows on flow delineate pressure support time)

The way IPS work widly varies among the different systems available. Nevertheless, three events can be distinguished during a complete breath under IPS:

1. *The triggering* in response to a patient's inspiratory effort, most often detected by a pressure sensor.
2. *The inspiration:* at the onset of inspiration, the ventilator delivers a high inspiratory flow which decreases during inspiration. The servo regulation maintains the proper flow to reach the adequate pressure support level and maintains it constant until expiration. Whatever the IPS level, this always increases the patient's inspiratory flow in a way which remains under patient regulation. This characteristic differs strickingly from all the other ventilatory modes. For instance, during assist-control mode, any inspiratory effort leads to a reduction of the ventilator work. If the required flow becomes greater than the flow supplied by the ventilator, the patient exhausts his forces without any tidal volume increase.
3. *The expiration* which occurs either with the detection of a slight airways overpression (1–3 cm H_2O) over the IPS level or when the inspiratory flow drops under a given value (25% of the peak flow on the Servo 900C, Bear 5, EV-A). Generally, a time limit to inspiration is added to OPS regulation, which works mainly as a safety feature, whenever a leak in the circuit makes the two previous systems inoperative.

Physiological Aspects of Inspiratory Pressure Support Breathing

Breathing Pattern

During pressure support ventilation, tidal volume is higher and respiratory rate is lower than during spontaneous breathing [4, 5]. For increasing levels of IPS, tidal volume continues to increase and most often respiratory rate continues to decrease. For high levels of pressure (20 cm H_2O or more) inflation tends to occur more and more passively. Tidal volume then depends upon lung compliance and may reach excessive levels with potential risk of hyperinsufflations, generally followed by periods of apnea.

In patients unable to maintain normal arterial blood gas tensions during spontaneous breathing, pressure support ventilation allows improvement in gas exchange and normalization of $PaCO_2$ by increasing alveolar ventilation and decreasing oxygen consumption [5, 6].

Respiratory Muscles

Several means can be used to quantify respiratory muscle activity.

Oxygen consumption: the oxygen cost of breathing can be estimated as the difference between the $\dot{V}O_2$ measured during controlled mechanical ventilation (with all respiratory muscles relaxed) and the $\dot{V}O_2$ measured during spontaneous breathing [7]. Even though other determinants than respiratory muscle oxygen consumption may contribute to the oxygen cost of breathing, a good correlation was found with the inspiratory work of breathing [8, 9]. Several works have shown a reduced cost of breathing during pressure support by comparison to spontaneous breathing with or without a continuous positive airway pressure circuit. Increasing the level of pressure support results in a decreased oxygen cost of breathing. For instance from 0 to 20 cmH_2O, the cost of breathing has been shown to fall from 27 to 1% of total $\dot{V}O_2$ in patients experiencing difficult weaning [8].

Work of breathing: the inspiratory work of breathing can be measured as the area under an esophageal pressure versus tidal volume loop and the static P–V

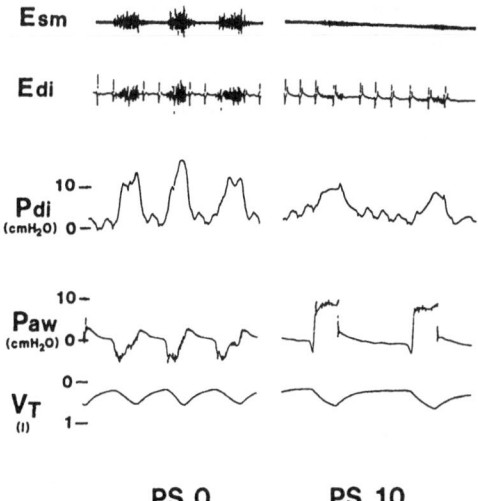

Fig. 2. Recordings of electrical activity of the sternocleidomastoid muscle (Esm) and of the diaphragm (Edi), trans-diaphragmatic pressure (Pdi), airway pressure (Paw) and tidal volume (V_t) for a patient without inspiratory pressure support (PS 0) and with pressure support of 10 cmH_2O (PS 10). Note the dramatic decrease in respiratory muscle activity, the increased tidal volume and the decreased respiratory rate during PS 10

curve of the chest wall. IPS decreases the work of breathing performed by the respiratory muscles [6]. When increasing levels of pressure support are used, the work of breathing is gradually diminished [6]. And the diaphragmatic activity is decreased [5]. In patients with low lung compliance and high respiratory resistance, IPS levels higher than 15 or 20 cmH_2O are sometimes necessary to significantly reduce this activity. In others patients, diaphragmatic activity may be dramatically decreased with 10 cmH_2O.

Diaphragmatic Fatigue

During unsuccessful weaning from mechanical ventilation, there is evidence that diaphragmatic fatigue is an important factor [8]. In such patients, IPS breathing can maintain spontaneous respiratory activity without fatigue [8].

Clinical Use

Advantages

IPS markedly increases the efficacy of spontaneous breathing while reducing the activity of the inspiratory muscles. The ventilator patient synchrony is good since the own patient respiratory rate is imposed and since each breath is efficiently assisted, allowing the patient to breathe spontaneously for sustained periods. Several authors reported that patients supported on IPS appeared comfortable. Monitoring of ventilation is extensively performed on ventilators offering the pressure support mode.

Inspiratory Pressure Support Level

A matter of difficulty with this mode of ventilatory assistance is to find the "optimum level" of pressure support for each patient. Indeed, an insufficient level may insufficiently assist respiratory muscles and result in fatigue, and an excessive level may be responsible for potentially deleterious hyperinsufflations. A way to set up this level is to give enough pressure to obtain a predetermined tidal volume.

The optimum level of JPS can also be defined as the lowest level maintaining diaphragmatic activity without fatigue [8]. The electrical muscular activity of the sternocleidomastoid muscle, considered as auxiliary inspiratory muscle is greater when the diaphragm is fatigued. The activation of this muscle is due to an increased demand for ventilation and is therefore minimal at the optimum pressure support level. Thus, monitoring pressure support ventilation could be done at the bedside by palpating the muscular activity of the sternomastoid, and by gradually decreasing IPS from high levels (30 cmH_2O for instance), until the phasic inspiratory activity of the sternomastoid appears to increase. Then a 5 cmH_2O higher level should be applied.

Clinical Use

To date there is no evidence that pressure support ventilation can shorten the weaning time or reduce complications related to mechanical ventilation. Thus, indications of pressure support cannot be clearly defined yet and are still a matter of personal choice. Pressure support ventilation is probably beneficial in difficult weaning from mechanical ventilation or as a ventilatory support without the need for sedation.

Need for sedation, total rest of the respiratory muscles or dramatic decrease of oxygen consumption should contraindicate the use of pressure support. In the same way, central neurologic disorders without efficacious ventilatory command does not allow the use of pressure support ventilation.

References

1. Rochester DF, Braun NMT, Laine S (1977) Diaphragmatic energy expenditure in chronic respiratory failure. The effect of assisted ventilation with body respirators. Am J Med 63:223–231
2. Marini JJ, Rodriguez RM, Lam V (1986) The inspiratory workload of patient initiated mechanical ventilation. Am Rev Respir Dis 134:902–909
3. Prakash O, Meij S (1985) Cardiopulmonary response to inspiratory pressure support during spontaneous ventilation versus conventional ventilation. Chest 88:403–408
4. MacIntyre NR (1986) Respiratory function during pressure support ventilation. Chest 89:677–683
5. Brochard L, Pluskwa F, Lemaire F (1987) Improved efficacy of spontaneous breathing with inspiratory pressure support. Am Rev Respir Dis 136:411–416
6. Brochard L, Harf A, Lorino H, Lemaire F (1987) Pressure support decreases work of breathing and oxygen consumption during weaning from mechanical ventilation. Am Rev Respir Dis 135:A51 (Abstract)
7. Fields S, Kelly SM, Macklem PT (1982) The oxygen cost of breathing in patients with cardiorespiratory disease. Am Rev Respir Dis 126:9–13
8. Brochard L, Harf A, Lorino H, Lemaire F (1987) Optimum level of pressure support in patients with unsuccessful weaning from mechanical ventilation. Am Rev Respir Dis 135:A51 (Abstract)
9. McGregor M, Blcklake M (1961) The relationship of oxygen cost of breathing to respiratory mechanical work and respiratory force. J Clin Invest 40:971–980

Airway Pressure Release Ventilation

J. Räsänen and J. B. Downs

Introduction

Patients with acute lung injury present with a spectrum of respiratory failure ranging from mild arterial hypoxemia with intact pulmonary mechanics to severe intrapulmonary shunting of blood and overt ventilatory insufficiency. Of the three components of respiratory therapy – continuous positive airway pressure (CPAP), oxygen supplementation, and positive pressure mechanical ventilation – only CPAP can be expected to reverse any of the pathophysiologic alterations causing the symptoms of hypoxemia and increased respiratory work [1, 2]. Mild acute lung injury can be treated successfully using relatively low levels of CPAP to correct hypoxemia and to improve derangement in ventilatory mechanics, adding oxygen supplementation as necessary. Mechanical ventilatory assistance rarely is indicated in mild cases. More severe cases of acute lung injury require higher levels of CPAP to decrease respiratory work, but once optimum CPAP is applied, the patient still may be able to breathe spontaneously without difficulty. In severe cases of acute lung injury, however, ventilatory failure often is present, even with optimum CPAP therapy, and mechanical ventilatory assistance must be initiated.

Administration of positive pressure mechanical ventilatory support reverses the physiologic respiratory variations in airway and intrathoracic pressure, inviting potential complications and therapeutic compromise [3]. High airway and intrathoracic pressure during positive pressure breaths limits the use of CPAP and, consequently, prevents optimization of gas exchange and the mechanics of spontaneous breathing. Increased spontaneous respiratory work and impaired matching of ventilation and perfusion diminish the efficiency of ventilation, so that the amount of mechanical ventilatory assistance required ultimately is larger than the extent of the patient's ventilatory failure would indicate [4, 5]. Despite careful adjustment of the ventilator, mean intrathoracic pressure is elevated by positive pressure ventilation with resultant cardiovascular compromise in normo- or hypovolemic patients. Periodic alveolar hypertension may cause barotrauma in compliant areas of the lung, may impair healing of the lung, and may even cause additional damage in the diseased alveoli. Attempts to unload excess respiratory work with positive pressure ventilation frequently creates serious problems, a fact that has sustained an intensive search for better ventilatory support techniques for the last decade.

Airway Pressure Release Ventilation

Airway pressure release ventilation (APRV) is a new respiratory support modality designed to augment alveolar ventilation as an adjunct to CPAP therapy [6]. A CPAP circuit can be modified to deliver APRV by including a pressure release valve that allows rapid transient release of circuit pressure from CPAP to a lower level (Fig. 1). As the release valve opens, and the circuit pressure falls, gas exits the lungs and lung volume decreases below functional residual capacity. When CPAP is re-established, the lungs are reinflated with fresh gas to the previous volume. Tidal volume of the APRV breath depends on lung compliance, airway resistance, the gradient of pressure release, and the pressure release time. The patient's spontaneous respiration is unimpeded throughout the APRV cycle. The intrathoracic pressure pattern during APRV resembles that recorded during spontaneous breathing with CPAP (Fig. 2).

Appropriate CPAP therapy is essential in the use of APRV. Optimization of CPAP assures minimum impairment in pulmonary gas exchange, maximum lung compliance, and the highest possible tidal volume for a given APRV pressure release gradient. Appropriate CPAP therapy also allows spontaneous breathing with minimum respiratory work between mechanical respiratory cycles. When

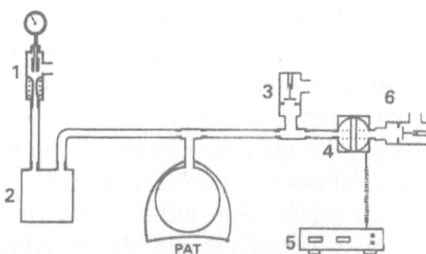

Fig. 1. The APRV circuit. An oxygen-powered venturi flow generator (*1*) creates a high flow of gas that traverses a humidifier (*2*) and exits through a threshold resistor valve (*3*) creating CPAP when the pressure release valve (*4*) is open. When the timer (*5*) opens the pressure release valve, airway pressure and lung volume decrease abruptly to a level determined by a second threshold resistor valve (*6*). When the pressure release valve closes, CPAP and lung volume are re-established. PAT = patient

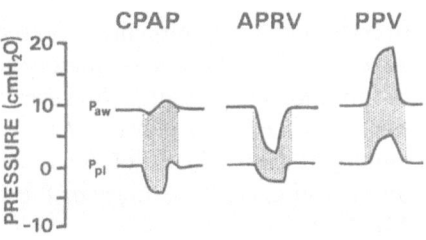

Fig. 2. Changes in airway (P_{aw}) and intrathoracic (P_{pl}) pressure during spontaneous breathing with CPAP, during APRV and during PPV. Transpulmonary pressure differential (shaded area) is directly related to lung volume

APRV breaths are added to CPAP, mean airway and intrathoracic pressure decreases, and peak airway pressure remains equal to the level of CPAP. Therefore, initiation of mechanical ventilation using APRV should neither depress cardiovascular performance nor subject the patient to high airway pressure and the risk of barotrauma.

The pressure release time must be sufficiently long to allow adequate emptying of the lungs, yet sufficiently short not to compromise the efficacy of ventilatory augmentation, or CPAP therapy. A pressure release time of 1.5 sec has been used successfully in all previously published studies.

Documentation of APRV

Experimental and clinical investigations have shown that alveolar ventilation and arterial oxygenation can be maintained effectively using APRV [7-9]. No significant differences in oxygenation or ventilation have been observed between APRV and conventional positive pressure ventilation (PPV) in experimental animals with normal lung function. However, in dogs with oleic acid induced lung injury, Stock et al. found that the use of APRV resulted in significantly lower arterial blood carbon dioxide tension and higher arterial blood oxygen tension compared to PPV, when the two ventilatory modalities were administered using a similar mean airway pressure, tidal volume, and ventilator rate [7]. These results indicate that the airway pressure pattern of APRV may favor a more uniform distribution of ventilation than PPV in injured lungs. Räsänen et al. compared spontaneous breathing, APRV, and PPV using a similar level of CPAP in dogs with oleic acid induced lung injury, and found that ventilatory failure and arterial desaturation that existed during spontaneous breathing could be effectively corrected by either APRV or PPV [8].

Peak airway pressure during APRV is 30-75% of that during PPV [7-9]. The extent of peak airway pressure reduction achieved with APRV depends on whether APRV and PPV have been adjusted to a similar mean airway pressure or to a similar level of CPAP. In a recently published case report, Väisänen et al. described a patient, in whom weaning from mechanical ventilation and removal of the endotracheal tube was successfully accomplished by APRV delivered by a mask-CPAP circuit [10]. Since airway pressure during APRV never exceeds the CPAP level, APRV may be administered with a mask.

Mean intrathoracic pressure is the major determinant of the circulatory effects of any ventilatory modality. Therefore, hemodynamic effects of APRV, compared to other types of ventilatory support, depend on the corresponding levels of intrathoracic pressure. Not surprisingly, no differences in circulatory function have been observed between APRV and PPV in experimental studies that have employed similar levels of mean airway pressure, regardless of the presence or absence of acute lung injury or the volume status of the experimental animal [7, 11].

However, APRV originally was designed to be used as an adjunct to CPAP therapy. When APRV and PPV are added to existing CPAP therapy, the hemodynamic advantages of APRV become obvious. A recent experimental investigation in dogs with induced lung injury revealed that ventilation could be controlled using APRV, with no depression of stroke volume, cardiac output, and tissue oxygen delivery compared to spontaneous breathing with CPAP [8]. When PPV is used in a similar fashion, stroke volume decreased by 42%, oxygen delivery diminished by 32% and oxygen utilization coefficient increased by 33%. Such depression in circulatory performance during PPV also is commonly seen in clinical practice, and it frequently cannot be avoided. Instead, it must be compensated for by lowering CPAP to a suboptimal level, by infusing large amounts of fluid to augment central blood volume, or by using inotropic agents to increase left ventricular contractility. All of these measures are potentially harmful to the patient and complicate therapy considerably. If APRV is available, they may be unnecessary.

Clinical application of APRV is under intensive investigation. Garner et al. compared APRV and PPV in patients with mild acute lung injury following cardiac operations and cardiopulmonary bypass [9]. APRV provided effective ventilation and oxygenation for all patients in the study. Mean airway pressures during APRV and PPV were similar in this study, and no hemodynamic differences were observed between the two ventilatory modalities. Peak airway pressure, however, was greatly reduced during APRV. The patients were weaned successfully from ventilatory support using APRV, and no complications were reported.

Effectiveness of APRV in the treatment of moderate to severe acute lung injury currently is being evaluated in a multicenter study involving seven institutions in three countries. The initial results of this investigation will be presented in the Eighth International Symposium on Intensive Care and Emergency Medicine.

References

1. Kirby RR, Downs JB, Civetta JM, et al (1975) High level positive end-expiratory pressure (PEEP) in acute respiratory insufficiency. Chest 67:156–163
2. Katz JA, Marks JD (1985) Inspiratory work with and without continuous positive airway pressure in patients with acute respiratory failure. Anesthesiology 63:598–607
3. Montgomery AB, Stager MA, Carrico CJ, Hudson LD (1985) Causes of mortality in patient with the adult respiratory distress syndrome. Am Rev Respir Dis 132:485–489
4. Froese AB, Bryan AC (1974) Effects of anesthesia and paralysis on diaphragmatic mechanics in man. Anesthesiology 41:242–255
5. Wolff G, Brunner JX, Grädel E (1986) Gas exchange during mechanical ventilation and spontaneous breathing. Chest 89:11–17
6. Downs JB, Stock MC (1987) Airway pressure release ventilation: A new concept in ventilatory support. Crit Care Med 15:459–461
7. Stock MC, Downs JB, Frolicher DA (1987) Airway pressure release ventilation. Crit Care Med 15:462–466
8. Räsänen J, Downs JB, Stock MC. Cardiovascular effects of conventional positive pressure ventilation and airway pressure release ventilation. Chest (In press)
9. Garner W, Downs JB, Stock MC, Räsänen J. Airway pressure release ventilation (APRV) (Submitted for publication)
10. Väisänen IT, Nikki P, Tahvanainen J. Airway pressure release ventilation by mask – A case report. Crit Care Med (In Press)
11. Halpern P, Downs JB, Räsänen J. Hemodynamic effects of airway pressure release ventilation and positive pressure ventilation in hypovolemic dogs (Submitted for publication)

Independent Lung Ventilation

R. Scherer and U. Hartenauer

Pathophysiology

Acute respiratory failure (ARF) following shock, trauma, major surgery or sepsis still has a very high mortality, between 50 and 60% [1]. ARF is the pathophysiological endpoint of a progressive deterioration of pulmonary alveolar ventilation to capillary perfusion relationship (V/Q), impeding gas exchange and leading to hypoxemia and high intrapulmonary shunt (Q_s/Q_t). Dysfunction of lung mechanics is caused by decreased transpulmonary compliance (CTP) and functional residual capacity (FRC). Major reductions in FRC as seen in patients suffering massive trauma, sepsis or following major surgery [2] may promote airway closure and alveolar collapse, i.e. perfusion of non-ventilated areas. Anatomic distribution of these areas of "true" shunt can be diffuse or asymmetric. V/Q mismatching is further increased by non uniform distribution of pulmonary blood flow because gravitational forces increase perfusion in the dependent parts of the lung [3]. Ordinarily, hypoxic pulmonary vasoconstriction in non-ventilated areas of a diseased lung has a tendency to shift perfusion to better ventilated areas of the lung. However, in areas of the lung with pneumonitis [4], contusion or in sepsis, local vasodilation and the hyperdynamic cardiovascular response tend to overcome the vasoconstrictive response. Thus, increased perfusion of dependent lung segments with low V/Q ratios results in a large shunt and hypoxemia.

It is well documented that ARF with decreased FRC and hypoxemia responds well to application of volume-controlled ventilation with positive end-expiratory pressure (PEEP) [1]. The premise of PEEP ventilation is based of equal and homogeneous distribution of both airway resistance and compliance characteristics of the lungs. However, cases have been reported, where PEEP therapy did not improve gas exchange and, in some cases, had a deleterious effect [5, 6].

Some of the cases involved unilateral or asymmetrical diseases such as unilateral aspiration, atelectasis or bronchopleural fistula. If one lung is much stiffer than the other one ventilation will be preferentially directed to the more compliant lung. The result is over distension of the more compliant lung, with transmission of the pressures to the distended normal alveolar capillary beds. This increased capillary resistance diverts pulmonary blood flow toward the less-compliant lung which has a low V/Q ratio [6] so that gas exchange worsens [5]. However, the increase of V/Q mismatch induced by PEEP can occur not only in asymmetrical lung disease, but also in bilateral ARF when there is a marked disparity in disease severity between lung segments. Therefore, PEEP application to prevent small airway closure and alveolar collapse also results in overdistension of more compliant areas of the lung and blood flow diversion towards areas of the lung with a low V/Q ratio [5, 7].

In order to improve distribution of ventilation to perfusion in asymmetrical lung disease it has been suggested to place the patient in the lateral position [8] with the healthier lung in dependent position to increase PaO_2 [9, 10]. The explanation is that the more compliant dependent lung will be better perfused by gravity and that the less-compliant lung receives a smaller blood flow.

As prolonged nursing of ARF patients in the lateral decubitus position is very difficult, positional maneuvers are usually temporary. Independent lung ventilation (ILV) has been proposed to better match ventilation to perfusion in patients with unilateral asymmetrical lung disease. Separating the right and left lung by an appropriate endobronchial tube offers the opportunity to ventilate both lungs by selecting independently tidal volume, frequency and airway pressure (PEEP). The pressure generated secondary to the volume delivery varies inversely with the compliance characteristics of the two lungs, i.e. the lower the compliance, the higher the pressure required. Consequently overdistension or alveolar collapse can be avoided during mechanical breath [12]. Significant differences in compliance between the two lungs have therefore become a major indication to ventilate each lung separately [11], (Fig. 1).

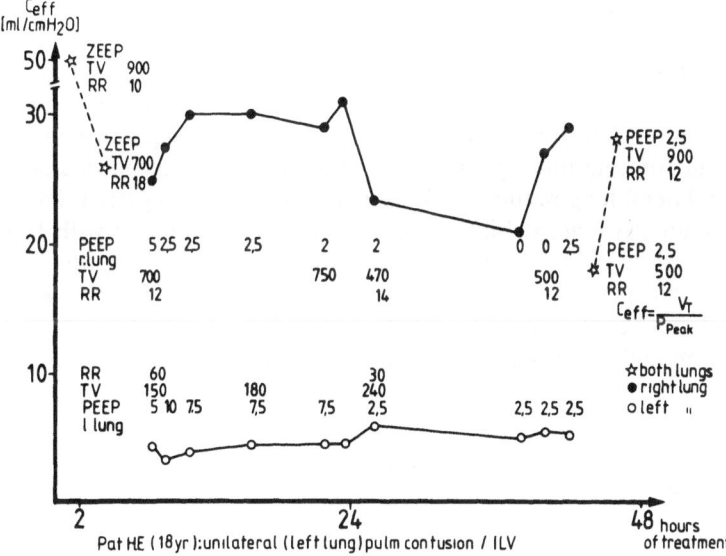

Fig. 1. Total lung compliance and individual compliances of the right and left lung in a patient with contusion of the left lung. (From [26], with permission)

Indication of Independent Lung Ventilation

While the clinical use of ILV has become possible due to the commercially availability of double-lumen endobronchial tubes suitable for this technique [13], no clear and easily applied guidelines have been established for initiating and qualifying the need for ILV [14]. The spectrum of indications where ILV has been used successfully in clinical practice is given in Table 1.

In the presence of a broncho-pleural fistula the indication for ILV depends upon the opening pressure of the fistula and the magnitude of the air-leak. A chest X-ray demonstrating asymmetric lung disease like contusion, atelectasis, pneumonia, aspiration pneumonitis or unilateral edema is a very helpful criterion for initiation of ILV. However, asymmetry of a lung lesion can be radiologically inapparent at its onset but can become apparent with unilateral overexpansion after PEEP is initiated. Primary radiological evidence of a unilateral lung lesion is not a necessary prerequisite to consider therapy with ILV; a firm criterion for ILV is the demonstration of redistribution of pulmonary blood flow and increase in shunt induced by PEEP: qualitative (serial bedside pulmonary angiogram via pulmonary arterial catheter [6]) as well as quantitative (lung scans [5, 27]) or inert gas [13] methods have been used for studies of V/Q distribution in conjunction with physiological measurements showing increase in shunt. Unfortunately, while valuable, these methods are cumbersome, expensive and often require the transport of the critically ill patient to a specialized laboratory. Furthermore, these techniques cannot be repeated frequently to allow fine tuning of ILV therapy.

A computer-based pulmonary evaluation technique for quantifying static and dynamic compliance changes by the delineation of flow, pressure and volume relationships has been presented [14]. This technique provides quantitative criteria for determining when ILV should be started, particularly in patients with bilateral lung pathology. Recently, it has been suggested that even patients with acute asymmetric bilateral lung disease may improve with ILV and differential PEEP in the lateral position [7, 13, 27]. However, initiation of ILV in these particular patients needs great deal of clinical intuition. The influence of conventional ventilation with PEEP in combination with lateral position on oxygenation and shunt may be a simple and effective maneuver to assess the physiolog-

Table 1. Indications of independent lung ventilation

	References
Unilateral lung contusion	[11, 12, 14, 15, 26]
Unilateral aspiration	[11, 23, 26]
Unilateral lung edema	[11, 25]
Refractory unilateral atelectasis	[18, 19, 23, 24]
Unilateral or lobar pneumonia	[15, 19, 21, 23]
Bronchopleural fistula	[11, 16, 18, 26]
Postpulmonary or esophageal surgery	[6, 17, 23, 26]
Acute asymmetric bilateral lung disease	[7, 11, 13]

ical consequences of asymmetric pulmonary involvement in radiologically diffuse bilateral process.

Techniques of Independent Lung Ventilation

The Endobronchial Tube

The modified left-sided Robertshaw double-lumen endobronchial tube ("Broncho-cath" National Catheter) made from transparent polyvinylchloride with radiopaque markers and low pressure, high volume cuffs is the most common endobronchial tube for ILV. A double-lumen tracheostomy tube for long term use has recently been presented [28]. Insertion of the "Broncho-cath" has been described extensively elsewhere [29]. Although insertion and positioning are usually easy, bronchoscopic guidance is recommended to prevent malpositioning [30, 31]. A safe method to secure the tube to the patient is essential. Correct tube position and cuff seal should be checked after each suctioning and change in patient position. Specifically, due to the narrow lumina, suctioning of the airway can be difficult. A double-lumen tube can cause considerable patient discomfort by virtue of its position in the trachea which may require the judicious use of sedative or narcotic drugs. While there are at least two reports of bronchial rupture associated with "low-pressure" cuffed tubes [32, 33], we have experienced no problems with over 400 "Broncho-cath" tubes used in anethesia and intensive care in the last 8 years.

Choice of Respirators and Ventilatory Modes

A variety of breathing circuits, single ventilators and ventilators in tandem have been used to deliver ILV. In earlier reports using single ventilator set-ups with double breathing circuits [20, 21, 34], PEEP was adjusted upward on the less compliant lung and inspiration to the "better" lung was retarded until volume between the two sides were equal. With growing experience most investigators have used two ventilator systems [6, 7, 12–14, 18, 23, 25–27]. Some suggest that synchronization of the two ventilators is not necessary [35]. Others used alternating ventilation, when one lung is ventilated 180 degrees out of phase with the other [36, 37]. Compared with synchronous ventilation, alternating ventilation can cause a decrease in airway pressure and may have a positive effect on total lung compliance and pulmonary vascular resistance in animal experiments; no report has used alternating ventilation in humans.

The distribution of the tidal volume between the two lungs and the application of different PEEP levels on each lung is by far a more important issue in ILV than the use of one or two ventilators, synchronized or not. The methods employed for partitioning the tidal volume, gas flow and airway pressure between the two lungs have varied between the reports. Most studies aimed to an even distribution of tidal volume between the two lungs [6, 20, 21, 34]. This strategy is supported by the experimental evidence [38] that arterial oxygenation was better

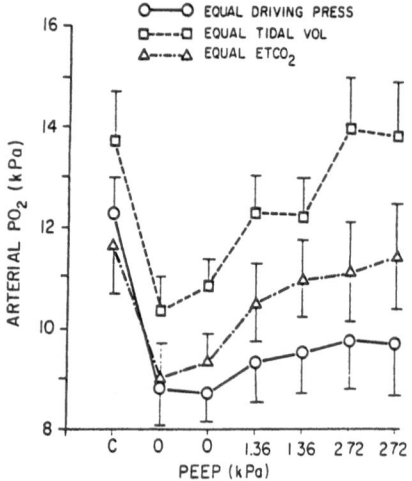

Fig. 2. Comparison of PaO_2 between three methods of differential lung ventilation tidal volume allocation at two levels of unilateral PEEP (mean ± SEM). ($ETCO_2$ = end tidal CO_2 fraction). (From [39], with permission)

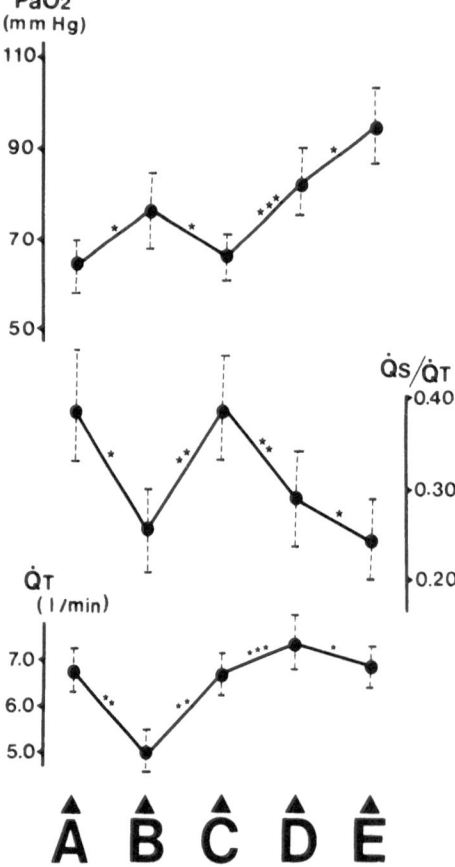

Fig. 3. Cardiac output (Q_T), venous admixture ($\dot{Q}_S/\dot{Q}_T$), and arterial oxygen tension (PaO_2) from 11 patients in acute respiratory failure, illustrating the effects of the different ventilator settings: *A*) conventional ventilation with PEEP in the supine posture; *B*) conventional ventilation with general PEEP in the supine posture; *C*) conventional ventilation with PEEP in the lateral decubital posture; *D*) differential ventilation with even tidal volume distribution and PEEP in the lateral decubital posture; *E*) differential ventilation with even tidal volume distribution and selective PEEP to the dependent lung in the lateral decubital posture. (From [7], with permission)
Mean value ± SEM; * p < 0,005; ** p < 0,001; *** p > 0,001

with even distribution of tidal volume than with ventilator settings resulting in equal end-tidal CO_2 and airway pressure (Fig. 2).

It has been suggested that in acute asymmetrical bilateral lung pathology matching of ventilation and perfusion in each lung can be improved by application of differential ventilation with selective PEEP in the lateral position [7, 13, 39], to increase perfusion to the dependent lung and increase ventilation to the non-dependent lung. ILV with selective PEEP to the dependent lung, and simultaneously increases ventilation to the hyperperfused dependent lung, thereby improving V/Q matching and PaO_2 without a concomitant deleterious effect on the cardiac output [7] (Fig. 3).

ILV has also been used successfully in the management of bronchopleural fistula [11, 16, 18, 19]. The lung with the bronchopleural fistula may not be ventilated at all but lung inflation can be maintained with a CPAP level just below the critical opening pressure of the fistula. The contralateral normal lung is ventilated with or without PEEP. An alternative of ILV for these cases is selective PEEP with high frequency positive pressure ventilation plus CPAP contralaterally [22, 40].

Monitoring of Independent Lung Ventilation

Monitoring of ILV should include V_T distribution between the two lungs, static compliance of each lung as well as airway resistance. In addition, the examination of pressure-volume curves is a relatively simple bedside method to evaluate the compliance of each lung and determine the minimal opening pressure of collapsed alveoli [14]. The pressure-volume curve obtained during conventional ventilation of both lungs may show two distinct slopes as a sign of asymmetrical lung disease. A trial of ILV and examination of individual pressure-volume curves of each lung is then indicated. A variety of other measurements can be obtained, such as FRC, V_D/V_T and CO_2 production [35, 38], but these are not mandatory for succesfull initiation of ILV therapy. The effects of ILV on oxygenation and hemodynamics are monitored by standard methods.

Conclusions

A variety of case reports have shown the usefulness of ILV to improve oxygenation in unilateral pneumonia, pulmonary edema, pulmonary hermorrhage, aspiration pneumonitis and lung contusion, to maintain alveolar ventilation in patients with bronchopleural fistula and to reexpand atelectatic lungs [6, 7, 11-27, 39, 40]. ILV should also be considered in bilateral, diffuse lung damage. In combination with the lateral decubitus position ILV may provide a level of oxygenation not attainable by conventional modes of therapy. The physiological and clinical justification of the use of ILV is well established, the necessary technology to initiate and apply ILV is available. Therefore, ILV is a valuable, safe and effective therapy and a true enrichment of our methods of ventilatory therapy.

References

1. Rinaldo JE, Rogers RM (1982) Adult respiratory distress syndrome. N Engl J Med 306:902–912
2. Katz JA, Ozanne GM, Zin SE, Fairley HB (1981) Time course and mechanism of lung-volume increase with PEEP in acute pulmonary failure. Anesthesiology 54:9–16
3. West JB (1977) Blood flow. In: West JB (ed) Regional differences in the lung. Academic Press, New-York, pp 85–165
4. Light RB, Mink SN, Wood LDH (1981) Pathophysiology of gas exchange and pulmonary perfusion in pneumococcal lobar pneumonia in dogs. J Appl Physiol 50:524–530
5. Kanarek DJ, Shannon DC (1979) Adverse effects of positive end-expiratory pressure on pulmonary perfusion and oxygenation. Am Rev Respir Dis 112:457–459
6. Carlon GC, Kahn R, Howland WS (1978) Acute life-threatening ventilation perfusion inequality: an indication for independent lung ventilation. Crit Care Med 6:380–383
7. Baehrendtz S, Hedenstierna G (1984) Differential ventilation and selective positive end-expiratory pressure: effects on patients with acute bilateral lung disease. Anesthesiology 61:511–517
8. Fishman A (1981) Down with the good lung. N Engl J Med 9:537
9. Zack MB, Pontoppidan H, Kazemi H (1974) The effect of lateral positions on gas exchange in pulmonary disease. Am Rev Respir Dis 110:49–55
10. Ramolina C, Khan AU, Santiago TV (1981) Positional hypoxemia in unilateral disease. N Engl J Med 9:523–527
11. Carlon GC, Ray C, Klein R, Goldiner PL, Miodownik S (1978) Criteria for selective positive and expiratory pressure and independent synchronized ventilation of each lung. Chest 74:501–507
12. Geiger K (1983) Differential lung ventilation. In: Geiger K (ed) European Advances in Intensive Care. Int Anaesthesiol Clin 21:83–96
13. Baehrendtz S, Bindslev L, Hedenstierna G, Santesson J (1983) Selective PEEP in acute bilateral lung disease: effect on patients in the lateral lung posture. Acta Anaesthesiol Scand 27:311–317
14. Siegel JH, Stoklosa JC, Borg U, et al (1985) Quantification of asymmetric lung pathophysiology as a guide to the use of simultaneous independent lung ventilation in posttraumatic and septic ARDS. Am Surg 202:425–439
15. Hurst JM, DeHaven B, Branson RD (1985) Comparison of conventional mechanical ventilation and synchronous independent lung ventilation in the treatment of unilateral lung injury. J Trauma 25:766–770
16. Rafferty TD, Palma J, Motoyama EK, Schachter N, Giarcia M (1980) Management of a bronchopleural fistula with differential lung ventilation and PEEP. Respiratory Care 25:654–657
17. Neidhardt A (1984) Prevention of early respiratory complications in esophageal surgery by ventilation of the independent lung. Cah Anaesthesiol 32:613–616
18. Schulte am Esch J, Keiser R, Horstmann R (1982) Zur Indikation des endobronchialen Doppellumentubus in der Intensivbehandlung einseitiger Lungenkomplikationen. Anaesthesist 31:400–407
19. Venus B, Pratap KS, OP 'Tholt T (1980) Treatment of unilateral pulmonary insufficiency by selective administration of CPAP through a double-lumen tube. Anesthesiology 52:74–77
20. Rivara D, Bourgain JL, Rieuf P, Harf A, Lemaire F (1979) Differential ventilation in unilateral lung disease: effects on respiratory mechanics and gas exchange. Intensive Care Med 5:189–191
21. Powner DJ, Eross B, Grenvik A (1977) Differential ventilation with PEEP in the treatment of unilateral pneumonia. Crit Care Med 5:170–172
22. Miranda DR, Stoutenbeck C, Kingma L (1981) Differential lung ventilation with HFPPV. Intensive Care Med 7:139–141
23. Hillman KM, Barber JD (1980) Asynchronous independent lung ventilation (AILV). Crit Care Med 8:390–395
24. Glass DD, Tonnesen AS, Gabel JC, Arens JF (1976) Therapy of unilateral pulmonary insufficiency with a double-lumen endotracheal tube. Crit Care Med 4:323–326

25. Scherer R, Reinhold P, Buchholz B (1983) Einseitiges Lungenödem nach Thoraxtrauma: Eine Indikation zur seitendifferenten Beatmung. Anästh Intensivther Notfallmed 18:65–67

26. Hartenauer U (1981) Seitengetrennte Beatmung. In: Lawin P, Wendt M (eds) Das Thoraxtrauma. Bibliomed., Melsungen, pp 207–216

27. Hedenstierna G, Baehrendtz S, Klingstedt C, Santesson J, Sönderborg B, Dahlborn M, Bindslev L (1984) Ventilation and Perfusion of each lung during differential ventilation with selective PEEP. Anesthesiology 61:369–376

28. Rommelsheim K (1985) A new double-lumen tracheostomy tube for long-terme use. Anaesth Intensivther Notfallmed 20:342–344

29. Benumof JL (1983) Physiology of the open chest and one-lung ventilation. In: Kaplan JA (ed) Thoracic Anesthesia. Churchill Livingstone, New York, pp 287–296

30. Benumof JL (1986) Fiberoptic bronchoscopy and double-lumen tube position. Anesthesiology 65:117–119

31. Brodsky JB, Skulman MS, Mark JBD (1985) Malpositioning of left-sided double-lumen endotracheal tubes. Anesthesiology 62:233–235

32. Burton NA, Fall S, Lyons T, et al (1983) Rupture of the left main-stem bronchus with a polyvinyl-chloride double-lumen tube. Chest 83:929

33. Wagner DL, Gammage GW, Wong MC (1985) Tracheal rupture following the insertion of a disposable double-lumen endotracheal tube

34. Cavanilles JM, Garrigosa F, Prieto C, et al (1979) A selective ventilation distribution circuit. Intensive Care Med 5:95–98

35. East TD, Pace NL, Westenskow DR (1983) Synchronous versus asynchronous differential lung ventilation with PEEP after unilateral acid aspiration in the dog. Crit Care Med 11:441–444

36. Muneyki M, Konishi K, Horiguchi R, et al (1983) Effects of alternating lung ventilation on cardiopulmonary function in dogs. Anesthesiology 58:353–356

37. Reinhold P (1986) Alternierende seitengetrennte Lungenbeatmung. Thieme Copytek

38. East TD, Pace L, Westenskow OR, Lund K (1983) Differential lung ventilation with unilateral PEEP following unilateral hydrochloric acid aspiration in the dog. Acta Anaesthesiol Scand 27:356–360

39. Hedenstierna G, Baehrendtz S, Frostell C, Mebius C (1984) Differential ventilation in acute respiratory failure Indications and outcome. Bull Eur Physiopathol Respir 21:281–285

40. Crimi G et al (1986) Clinical applications of independent lung ventilation with unilateral high-frequency jet ventilation. Intensive Care Med 12:90–94

High Frequency Ventilation

N. Mutz, M. Baum, and H. Benzer

Historical Review

The need to maintain adequate gas exchange in patients with respiratory insufficiency led already in the early beginning of the 20th century to the development of certain methods which can be apostrophized as the basis of the today techniques of the so called "High Frequency Ventilation" (HFV). It was Volhard in 1908 [1], who reported successful oxygenation in dogs without any movement of the lungs only by adjusting bias flow of oxygen across the upper airways. However, continuously increasing hypercarbia was the limiting factor of this method. Activation of CO_2 elimination leading to normocarbia was the goal of Draper and Whitehead [2] in 1944, calling this advanced method "Diffusion Respiration". However, assisted by a stream of air, guided additionally into the airways, CO_2 elimination could be improved in animal experiment [2]. Because of rapid development of "Intermittent Positive Pressure Ventilation" (IPPV) there was no clinical need for further pursuing of this methods. Thus, it lasted about 3 decades until new impulses reactivated the idea to ensure gas exchange without excessive lung movement due to periodical gas displacement ("bulk flow") [3, 4].

Classification of HFV-systems and Their Terminology

Different HFV systems have been described. All have a common feature, namely ventilatory frequencies at least four times higher than that of normal spontaneous breathing [5]. However, clinical application and interaction with the lungs may vary with different types of HFV ventilators. In the following an attempt for a HFV classification is made.

Set-Up of Different HF Ventilation (Fig. 1)

High Frequency Positive Pressure Ventilation (HFPPV) [6]: In a Y-piece attached to the proximal end of an endotracheal tube gas enters the system during inspiration in the side stream. At the same time a pneumatic valve on the top of the Y-piece is closed. For expiration gas flow is interrupted and the valve opens.

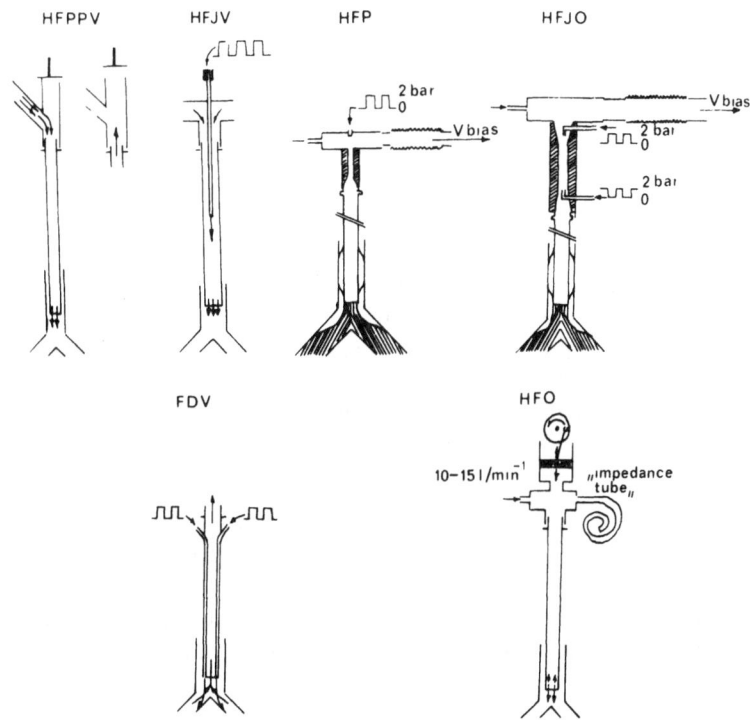

Fig. 1. Set-up of different types of high frequency ventilators

High Frequency Jet Ventilation (HFJV) [4]: A catheter is inserted into a common endotracheal tube. High pressure impulses of breathing gas are supplied to this catheter and discharged as a jet at its tip. The diameter of the jet increases with the distance from the tip. Once it has widened enough to reach the wall of the endotracheal tube the system acts similar to an injector. Gas is entrained from the upstream, side and bulk flow impulses are leaving the distal end of the tube.

High Frequency Pulsation (HFP) [7]: High pressure impulses of breathing gas are fed into a nozzle on top of a T-piece attached to the endotracheal tube. The jet discharges into a Venturi throat which is part of the T-piece. In contrast to HFJV bulk flow impulses are already present in the proximal part of the endotracheal tube. In addition, a bias flow of gas is used to cover the entrainment.

High Frequency Jet Oscillation (HFJO) [8]: Two sources of high pressure impulses of breathing gas 180 degrees out of phase are supplied to a pair of nozzles implemented into a T-piece. Again a Venturi throat is placed in between the nozzles. The nozzle directed towards the lungs acts as injector whereas the other one is used as an ejector. Thus positive and negative pressure impulses are applied to the lungs. Again a bias flow system is necessary to cover the entrainment.

High Frequency Oscillation (HFO) [9]: A motor driven piston pump with the desired stroke volume is connected to a 4-way patient adapter on top of an endotracheal tube. An oscillatory flow is directed towards the lungs. Breathing gas enters the system from a high impedance gas source. To avoid extensive losses of oscillatory volume the bias flow must leave the system via an impedance tube.

Forced Diffusion Ventilation (FDV) [10]: Two sources of high pressure impulses of breathing gas are supplied to pressure lines implemented into the wall of an endotracheal tube. Two jets enter the lungs at the tip of the tube approximately 2 cm above the carina. Under this condition the jets remain focused even when they get in contact with the bronchial wall and breathing gas can penetrate a large number of airway generations. Exhaled gas can leave the lungs through the main lumen of the endotracheal tube.

Frequency Ranges of Different Types of HFV-Ventilators

Figure 2 gives the frequency range achievable under clinical conditions in adult patients. For all HFV-systems except HFO the maximal frequency is limited by

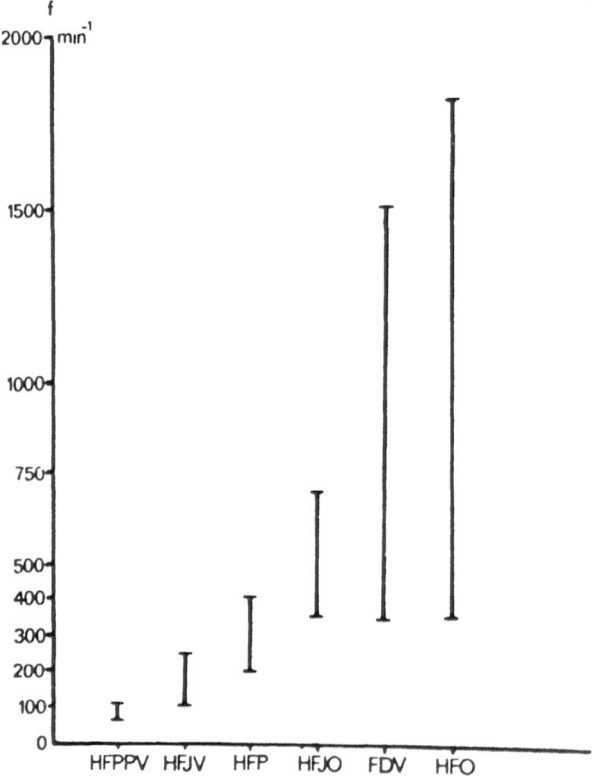

Fig. 2. Frequency range of different modes of HFV

poor CO_2 elimination and depends on the metabolic rate and the mechanical property of the patient's lungs.

Tidal Volume Ranges of Different Types of HFV-Ventilators

Figure 3 depicts the volume ranges necessary to ventilate adult patients under clinical conditions. Although tidal volume decreases with high frequencies, minute ventilation is increasing. Due to the totally different gas transport mechanism, FDV does not fit into this correlation.

Classification According to Volume Constancy

There are two reactions of HFV ventilators when frequency is varied with all other settings remaining unchanged.

Ventilators with constant minute volume: HFPPV, HFV, HFJV, HFJO, FDV

All gas driven systems act in this way because a present gasflow is supplied to the lungs independently of the frequency of the interrupting mechanism.

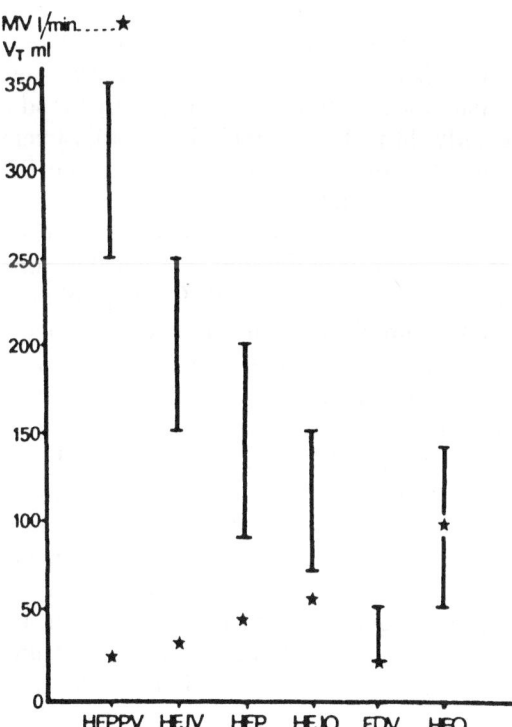

Fig. 3. Tidal volume range and average minute ventilation (*) of different modes of HFV in adult patients

Ventilators with constant stroke volume: HFO

The adjusted stroke volume is applied to the lungs and thus minute volume is a function of frequency.

Classification According to Mode of Exhalation

Exhalation by natural lung recoil: HFPPV, HFJV, HFP

The ventilator only supports inspiration by positive pressure impulses. Expiratory volume is governed by the time constancy of the lung recoil and by mean alveolar pressure.

Exhalation by an active mechanism supporting expiratory flow: HFO, HFJO, FDV.

The support of exhalation can be achieved either by applying a suction phase (HFO, HFJO) or by a scavenge process as initiated during FDV. Mean alveolar pressure does not influence expiratory volumes.

Although this classification is incomplete, it helps to understand the different results reported from experiences with HFV.

Clinical and Technical Problems Associated with Different Types of HFV-Ventilators

Using conventional ventilators, one can rely on certain ventilatory parameters applied to the lungs regardless of their mechanical properties. The effect of the settings on the lungs can be followed by monitoring the airway pressure, expiratory volume etc. These features are often not available in HFV, so that setting is often based on trials and checked by blood gas analysis and chest X-ray. Particularly difficult with HFV is the adjustment of mean airway pressure and its relevance for lung volume. In HFJV and FDV pressures are not measurable at the proximal end of the endotracheal tube, but usually by an extra pressure line at tracheal level. All other types allow pressure monitoring at the patient adapter. However, it is questionable whether this reflects the pressure in peripheral airways which is responsible for lung volume. Due to the peak flow rates most of the pressure drop occurs along the resistive elements such as endotracheal tube and large airways. Thus peak pressure and end-expiratory pressure are meaningless for lung inflation, particularly at frequencies above 200/min, when inspiration and expiration becomes short compared to the time constancy of the lungs. In mechanical lung models with rigid bronchial systems we observed a good correlation between mean airway pressure, measured at the endotracheal tube, and the mean alveolar pressure. This may be quite different in natural lungs, where secondary movements of the bronchial wall can create large differences between inspiratory and expiratory airway resistance.

High frequency ventilators only supporting inspiration (HFPPV, HFJV, HFP) by principle produce positive airway pressures. Fig. 4 demonstrates the influence of the I/E ratio on the magnitude of this mean pressure during HFP at a rate of 300/min. I/E ratio was increased from 1/3 to 1/2 to 1/1. All other settings were

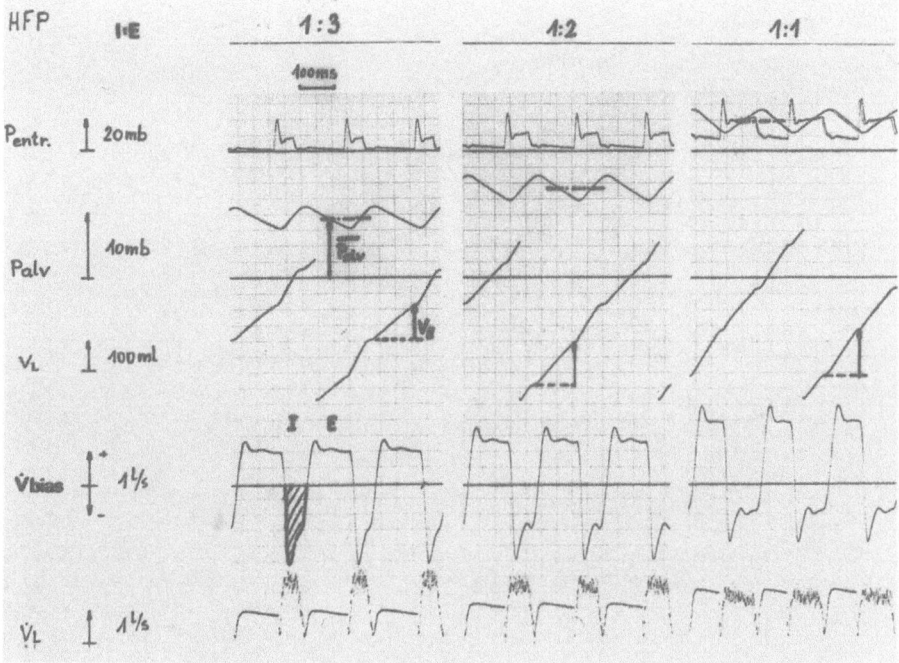

Fig. 4. Pressure flow conditions during HFP recorded at a lung model
P_{entr}: pressure in the entrance section of the endotracheal tube; P_{alv}: pressure in terminal structures of the lung model; VL: volume displaced to the lungs; $\dot{V}E$: expired volume; $\dot{V}bias$: bias flow measured in the expiratory limb of the patient adapter; $\dot{V}_L$: hot wire tracing of the total flow entering and leaving the lung model

kept constant. The baseline of the positive pressure pulses measured in the entrance section of the endotracheal tube shows a slight elevation from step to step. The end-expiratory pressure at 1/1 is in the range of 4 mb. However, the mean alveolar pressure (Palv.) in the compliance section of the lung model increases from 9 to 14 to 25 mb (dotted lines). Thus lung inflation is much higher than indicated by the end-expiratory pressure. With this type of HFV lung volume is mainly adjusted by the I/E ratio. Frequency is only a factor of second order as long as it is not increased above 500–600/min [11].

High frequency ventilators with an active support of expiration (HFO, HFJP, FDV) do not necessarily create positive mean pressures with HFJO (Fig. 5). Expiration is supported by a negative pressure pulse which is identical to the inspiration pulse. Under this condition mean alveolar pressure remains about zero, regardless of frequency and driving pressure. In this system as well as in FDV, lung volume has to be adjusted by an additional device similar to a PEEP valve and does not interfere with other ventilator settings. In HFO a similar effect can be achieved by variation of bias flow.

The second unknown factor in most of the high frequency ventilators is the tidal volume applied to the patient. Only in HFPPV and in FDV tidal or minute volume can be monitored by collecting expiratory volume. Although the ad-

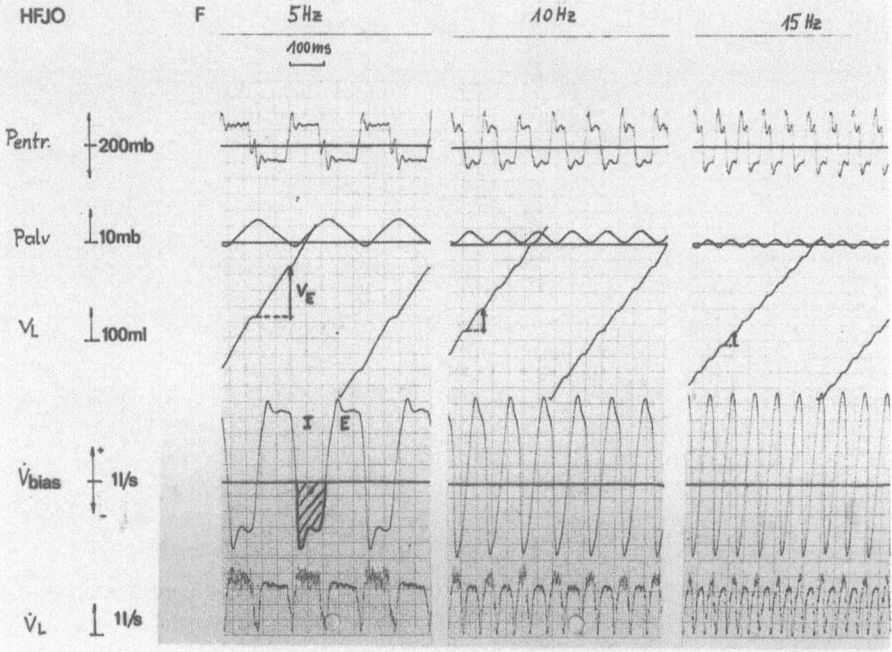

Fig. 5. Pressure flow conditions during HFJO recorded at the lung model

justed displacement of the pump in HFO is well defined, the volume portion transmitted to the patient is reduced due to losses into the bias flow system and into the compressible volume between pump and patient.

In all systems using an injector (HFJV, HFP, HFJO) tidal volume is a function of driving pressure, I/E ratio and frequency (VE in Figures 4 and 5). However, the most important factor influencing tidal volume is the geometry of the injector (nozzle diameter, diameter of endotracheal tube or Venturi throat and jet entry position (HFJV). The injector geometry further determines the reaction of lung impedance and tidal volume. A badly matched geometry will result in excessive tidal volume losses with increasing airway resistance. Thus the often used driving pressure as a measure for ventilation is not valid under these circumstances. A further attribute of an injector is its ability to entrain gas. The amount of gas entrained is governed by the same factors that are determining tidal volume. With a properly matched geometry more than 60% of the tidal volume comes from the entrainment (shaded area of Vbias in Figures 4 and 5). This can be used to reduce total gas consumption of the ventilator which is sometimes a limiting factor for the use of HFV in case of low line pressures (below 4 bar). On the other hand the entrained gas must have the same FiO_2 as the driving gas. This must be covered by the bias flow system. To handle the high peak flows on entrained gas with justifiable bias flow of 20 l/min, a reservoir tube has to be added at the expiratory limb of the patient adapter (HFP, HFJO in Fig. 1). This reservoir tube causes a certain amount of rebreathing, because part of the entrained gas has now expiratory quality.

A main problem is given by the still unsolved humidification of breathing gas in HFV. The driving gas for the jets and for the Venturi pump is still dry. Humidification of a high pressure gas is rather complex because water vapor of high temperature and high pressure has to be added to the driving gas. The dosage of the water vapor is critical for an excess will lead to condensation in the pressure line. Thus from a technical point of view a sufficient humidifier can be even more costly than the ventilator itself.

One of the most important points in HFV are safety mechanism. Since breathing gas enters the system from the high pressure source, obstruction of the expiratory way or malfunction of the switching mechanisms bears the potential risk of lung rupture. At the usual fresh gas rates of 0.5-1 l/sec. dangerous levels of pressure and volume can be reached within 3-6 seconds. A high frequency ventilator for clinical use must therefore have fast responding, automatic switch-off features. The pressure signal can be either taken from the patient adaptor (HFPPV, HFP, HFJO, HFO) or from a separate pressure line at the distal end of the endotracheal tube (HFJV, FDV). A further possibility is to use the jet line during expiration for pressure monitoring purposes.

FDV is an example that a lack of patients safety can limit the clinical use of a high frequency ventilator. As already mentioned the unique flow pattern of FDV, which allows a continuous wash-out of CO_2 can only be reached with a gas entry position close to the carina. As soon as the endotracheal tube is removed to more than 2 cm above carina, CO_2 elimination becomes poor and as a result a rapid increase in $PaCO_2$ occurs [10, 12]. Except for intraoperative use the clinical application of FDV over longer periods was hardly possible due to this source of complications.

Further Developments of HFV

In the last years a number of modifications of the original HFV-systems has taken place, resulting in a large number of different apparatus. Further expression of the euphoria during that "High Frequency Ventilation – Boom" was the variety of clinical indications for HFV. Using HFV in severely lung-injured patients suffering from bronchopleural fistulae these techniques were applied to nearly all areas of artificial ventilation (intraoperatively, postoperatively, respiratory therapy etc.) [13-15]. An increasing number of publications focused on HFV as a "universal method" of respiratory treatment.

Disapointment was later aroused because of serious incidents when using HFV-techniques [16, 17]. Inadequate humidification, poor safety (difficult monitoring), confusion about respirator settings, inability to maintain gas exchange in extremely damaged lungs (ARDS-patients) as well as the improvement of "conventional" respirators and the development of new ventilatory techniques led to limited further enthusiastic application of HFV.

Therefore, apart from some very specialized indications such as various pediatric lung disorders, massive bronchopleural fistulae, some particular weaning maneuvers and distinct surgical procedures like surgery of the larynx and upper airways [18, 21], HFV seemed left as an established tool within mechanical ventilation in clinical practice.

However the fascinating idea to achieve adequate gas exchange without extensive lung movement ("Immobilization of the diseased lung – Quiet Lungs") gave new impulses for further research on the field of HFV. Particularly attractive in presence of massive lung damage is to ensure respiration in the so-called "equilibrium value" (= minimized surfactant loss) [22].

Today, research of the "second wave" of HFV focuses on the following areas:

1. Improvement of physiologic as well as pathophysiologic knowledge, e.g. gas distribution modalities, mucociliary clearance, lung fluid balance, behavior of surfactant, interactions with the heart and the circulatory system etc.;
2. Improvement of understanding of the operational characteristics of the ventilators themselves;
3. Clarification of the rationale for ventilator settings during FDV based on the pathophysiology of specific disease states;
4. Development of a special monitoring providing rapid recognizion of system dysfunction;
5. Development of automatically effective security equipments (to prevent barotrauma);
6. Development of effective humidification systems especially for long-term ventilation in ICU-patients;
7. Critical searching for new special indications and their practicability, such as airway surgery, flexible bronchoscopy and specific application modalities in severe lung damage;
8. Development of new methods to assess the influence therapeutic of decisions on the actual course of lung injury and repair.
9. Development of strategies to teach effective respirator adjustments.

Future Aspects

Clarifying physiological and technical mysteries and unsolved problems, the proper place of HFV in acute respiratory failure will delineated with much more objectivity. This will lead to more realistic therapeutic decisions applying HFV at a definite course of lung disorder.

Several actions for improving ventilator's safety and selecting special modes of HFV may prevent uncertainty especially in severely lung-injured patients. Hopefully, clear guidelines will be given for the adjustment of the respirator, based on pathophysiologic mechanisms.

References

1. Volhard F (1908) Über künstliche Beatmung durch Ventilation der Trachea und eine einfache Vorrichtung zur rhythmischen künstlichen Atmung. Münch Med Wschr 55(5)
2. Draper WB, Whitehead RW (1944) Diffusion respiration in the dog anesthesized by pentobarbital sodium. Anesthesiology 5:262
3. Lunkenheimer PP, Rafflenbeul W, Keller H, Frank I, Dickhut HH, Fuhrmann C (1972) Application of transtracheal pressure oscillations as a modification of "diffusion respiration". Br J Anesth 44:627
4. Klain M, Smith RB (1977) High Frequency percutaneous transtracheal jet ventilation. Crit Care Med 5(6):280
5. Froese AB (1984) High Frequency Ventilation: a critical assessment. In: "State of the art", Society of Critical Care Medicine, (ed) WC. Shoemaker, Fullteron, California
6. Sjöstrand UH, Bunegin L, Smith RB, Babinski MF (1983) Development and clinical application of High Frequency Ventilation. In: PA Scheck, UH Sjöstrand (eds) Perspectives in High Frequency Ventilation. Nijhoff Publishers, Boston, p 12
7. Benzer H, Baum M, Duma St, Geyer A, Mutz N (1983) Peri- and postoperative aplication of various types of High Frequency Ventilation (HFV). In: Perspectives in High Frequency Ventilation. Nijhoff Publishers, Boston, p 240
8. Baum M, Benzer H, Golschmied W, Mutz N (1983) Pressure Flow pattern and gas transport using various types of High Frequency Ventilation. In: Perspectives in High Frequency Ventilation, Nijhoff Publishers, Boston, p 51
9. Bohn CJ, Miyasaka K, Marchak BE, Thompson WK, Froese AP (1980) Ventilation by high frequency oscillation. J Appl Physiol, Respir Env Ex Physiol 48:710–716
10. Baum M, Benzer H, Geyer A, Haider W, Mutz N (1980) Forcierte Diffusionsventilation (FDV) Anaesthesist 29:586–591
11. Fletcher PR (1983) Alveolar pressures during High Frequency Ventilation. In: Perspectives in High Frequency Ventilation. Nijhoff Publishers, Boston, p 92
12. Mutz N (1984) Hochfrequenzbeatmung. Entwicklung neuer Beatmungssysteme – experimentelle und klinische Ergebnisse. Wien Klin Wschr 96. Jhg. Suppl 146
13. Crawford MR, Rehder K (1983) High frequency small volume ventilation (HFV) in anesthetized man. Anesthesiology 59 (3):503
14. Dedhia HV (1981) Hemodynamic effect of high frequency ventilation in open heart surgery. Crit Care Med 9:158
15. Kalla R, Wald M, Klain M (1981) Weaninig of ventilator dependent patients by high frequency jet ventilation. Crit Care Med 9:162
16. Chang JL, Meeuwis H, Belyaert A, Babinski M, Petruscak J (1978) Severe abdominal distension following jet ventilation during general anaesthesia. Anesthesiology 49:216
17. Mette PJ (1980) Avoiding complications during jet ventilation. Anesthesiology 52:451
18. Babinski MF, Sierra OG, Smith RB, Leano E, Chavez A, Castellanos P (1985) Clinical Application of Continuous Flow Apneic Ventilation. Acta Anaesth Scand 29:750–752
19. Boynton BP, Mannino FL, Davis RF, Kopotic RJ, Friedrichsen G (1984) Combined high-frequency oscillatory ventilation and intermittent mandatory ventilation in critically ill neonates. J Pediatrics 105:297–302
20. Mutz N, Baum M, Benzer H, Koller W, Moritz E, Pauser G (1984) Intraoperative application of high-frequency ventilation. Crit Care Med 12:800–802
21. Rontal E, Rontal M, Wenokur ME, Southfield MI (1985) Jet insufflation anaesthesia for endolaryngeal laser surgery: a review of 318 consecutive cases. Laryngoscope 95:990–992
22. Benzer H, Coraim F, Mutz N, Geyer A, Pauser G (1979) Probleme der "Respiratorischen" Beatmung bei der Schocklunge. In: Mayrhofer-Krammel O (Hrsg) Akutes Progressives Lungenversagen. (Intensivmedizin, Notfallmedizin, Anaesthesiologie Bd 16, S 263)

Neonatal Extra-Corporeal Membrane Oxygenation (ECMO)

J. C. Mercier, F. Laborde, and F. Beaufils

Introduction

Extracorporeal membrane oxygenation (ECMO) has been successfully used to treat acute respiratory failure (ARF) in over 1000 neonates since Dr. Bartlett's pioneering efforts and his first survivor in 1975 [1]. The key component of ECMO is the ability of oxygen transport across a semi-permeable membrane. The cardiopulmonary bypass concept was developed in the early 1950s. Devices at that time were bubble or disk oxygenators with a direct oxygen-blood interface, resulting in marked hemolysis after a few hours of bypass, precluding their use for long-term problems. With the development of the first membrane oxygenator by Clowes et al. [2] in 1956, prolonged cardiopulmonary bypass became feasible.

Advancement in techniques and research occurred in the 1960s and 1970s. During this period, a nine-collaborative study was organized by the National Heart, Lung and Blood Institute to study ECMO therapy in adults with ARF [3]. Unfortunately, survival was not improved (9.5% in ECMO patients vs 8.3% in the controls). However, this study suffered serveral clues: 1) the patients pulmonary diseases were very heterogenous; 2) a 10% survival prediction was the entry criteria and pathological changes in the lung were probably irreversible; 3) intensive ventilator support was continued which probably perpetuated lung damage [4, 5]. The ECMO experience in children was similar to that in the adult, with many of the same problems [6, 7]. However, during this important period, the critical concept emerged that ECMO was not only technically feasible but might potentially reverse pulmonary failure in patients in whom irreversible fibrosis of the lung had not yet occurred.

Unfortunately, the early neonatal experience was not either conclusive, since the first newborn population chosen for ECMO was the premature infant with hyaline membrane disease (HMD) who developed significant intra-cranial hemorrhage secondary to systemic heparinization, with a high mortality [8–10]. It was not until Bartlett pioneered the treatment of full-term and near-term newborns with ARF [11, 12] that ECMO entered its successful period. This preliminary results have been confirmed by other works [13–17] from now more than 36 centers with present-day survival rates of over 90% in newborns selected on a predicted mortality of 80% mainly from historical retrospective studies (Table 1). The single randomized study was published by Bartlett et al. in 1985 [18]. A very peculiar "play-the-winner" statistic method was applied because of this group's very positive experience and ethical considerations. There was a single control

Table 1. Data from the ECMO Central Registry summarizing the total infant population treated with ECMO (through August 1987)

	No. of Patients	Survival (%)
Meconium aspiration syndrome	424	89.9
Hyaline membrane disease	140	75.7
Congenital diaphragmatic hernia	150	62.0
Sepsis	84	73.8
Persistent pulmonary hypertension	134	85.1
Pneumothorax	4	75.0
Cardiac	14	50.0
Other	26	80.8
Total	978	80.7

case who died and 11 ECMO patients who all survived. However, the results were criticized because of the unusual but correct statistical methodology [19]. A new double-arm randomized study is at the moment conducted by Dr. Bartlett's group in Ann Arbor comparing conventional treatment and ECMO on a 50% and a 80% predicted mortality.

Patient Population and Criteria for ECMO

Currently, the appropriate patient population for ECMO therapy is the full-term or near-term (35 to 40 weeks gestation) who fail "maximal medical therapy" including appropriate ventilatory and pharmacological support and who, by institutional criteria, has 80% risks of mortality [20, 21].

A congenital heart disease must be first excluded, using two-dimensional echocardiography and in difficult cases angiography (most centers have experienced difficulties to rule out total abnormal pulmonary venous return). Second, since systemic heparinization is required, infants with any major bleeding disorder, including severe intracranial hemorrhage must be excluded. Thirdly, the infant's lung disease must be potentially reversible within a 1 to 2-weeks period. Therefore, infants having been severely mechanically ventilated for more than one week should be excluded, since the likelihood of severe bronchopulmonary dysplasia (BPD) which cannot be reversed by ECMO is high. Finally, infants not having an expected good quality of life must be excluded, such as those with highly suspected karyotypic abnormalities.

Most candidates fort ECMO have, as an underlying process, persistent pulmonary hypertension of the neonate (PPHN), which results in right-to-left shunting through the foramen ovale and the ductus arteriosus [22]. This condition is a common pathway in the majority of severe neonatal ARF such as meconium aspiration, sepsis, HMD, idiopathic PPHN, and congenital diaphragmatic hernia. When these diseases are very severe, the use of ECMO therapy for some days would be logical if the various systems eventually implicated in the pulmonary vasomotricity (catecholamines, prostanoids) are disturbed only for a few days [23]. The medical treatment of PPHN includes apropriate ventilatory and pharmacological support [24]. Hyperventilation is still the cornerstone of this treatment. Its aim is to obtain respiratory alkalosis with a $PaCO_2$ under a critical value between 20 and 25 Torr (value of the continuous monitoring of PCO_2 using transcutaneous PCO_2 ($tcPCO_2$)) and a pH above a critical value of 7.5 to 7.6 to reduce pulmonary hypertension, reverse the right-to-left shunt, and improve systemic oxygenation continuously monitored by transcutaneous PO_2 ($tcPO_2$) or pulse oximeter [25]. In order to obtain effective hyperventilation, leaks around the endotracheal tube should be avoided using tubes of appropriate size, conventional continuous-flow time-cycled ventilators should not be used at unconventional rates [26] but volume-cycled ventilators, and sometimes high-frequency ventilation trials may be tested [27]. Analgesia and muscle relaxants may help mechanical ventilation and prevent occurrence of pulmonary arterial vasospasms in response to pain or tracheal suction [28]. Sodium bicarbonate drips may facilitate alkalinization, provided CO_2 is adequately eliminated through the lungs. Vasodilators try to decrease pulmonary hypertension, although none is specific of the pulmonary vascular bed [29]. Tolazolin has been extensively used but several adverse effects have been described including deleterious systemic hypertension, mainly because its pharmacology was not taken into account [30]. Finally catecholamines such as dopamine or dobutamine try to overcome the induced systemic hypotension as well as to support the overload right ventricle [25].

Congenital diaphragmatic hernia (CDH) raise two additional questions: 1) is urgent surgical repair of the diaphragmatic defect still mandatory? 2) does any criteria exist to indicate definite pulmonary hypoplasia which is incompatible with extra-uterine life? For the majority of the authors, primary surgical repair of the diaphragm should be done as early as possible and is mandatory before ECMO is considered [31]. However, on the basis that diaphragmatic repair was not followed by immediate pulmonary expansion and that the latter could be obtained by efficient digestive decompression using both gastric suction and gastrografin enema, some groups have tried not to operate before a few days, allowing better pre-operative stabilization [32]. Moreover, it seems that the predictive indices of mortality developed by Bohn et al. [33, 34] are not modified by surgical repair. Thus, our therapeutic protocol as in some other European centers is first to stabilize the patient for a few hours up to a few days. In addition, this therapeutic approach would have the advantage of avoiding the bleeding complications during ECMO which represent the major cause of death of CDH treated with ECMO. In fact, 40 bleeding complications with 30 deaths occurred in the 93 first infants with CDH treated with ECMO [35].

Nevertheles, in case of congenital diaphragmatic hernia, the main question still concerns the underlying pulmonary hypoplasia. The earlier in the intra-uterine life the diaphragmatic hernia has occurred, the larger the defect is (requiring the use of a prosthetic plaque), the earlier and the more severe the signs of respiratory distress are, the more severe the pulmonary hypoplasia would be. Some indices have been related to survival. Raphaely and Downes [36] found a significant difference in $AaDO_2$ gradient between survivors (260 Torr) and non-survivors (614 Torr). However, this study was undertaken before the agressive medical treatment of PPHN using hyperventilation. Bohn et al. [33] suggested another index based on the relationship between $PaCO_2$ and a marker of mechanical ventilation intensity (Respiratory Rate x Mean Airway Pressure), two hours after surgery. All their patients who sat outside of the "survival triangle" finally died. Likely, in a new study, Bohn et al. [34] showed that this index could predict mortality either before or after surgery. In other words, surgical diaphragmatic repair did not influence the underlying pulmonary hypoplasia. In fact, trials of high-frequency ventilation were unsuccessful in 14 of the 16 nonsurvivors. Moreover, in 5 such patients in which the pre-operative as well as the postoperative indices were indicative of death there was strong evidence of pulmonary hypoplasia, although only mild signs of pulmonary artery muscular hypertrophy were found. Therefore, in an infant having congenital diaphragmatic hernia associated with some degree of pulmonary hypoplasia, respiratory support using ECMO for a few days, long enough to wait for the heal of the PPHN "profile", is still questionable, although 7 out of 12 such patients having apparently the same mortality indices as Bohn's finally survived after ECMO therapy (Heaton et al. 18th annual meeting of the American Pediatric Surgical Association, Hilton Head Island, SC, May 6–9, 1987).

Thus, when every possibility of "maximal medical treatment" has been found unsuccessful, ECMO therapy may salvage infants with severe ARF. Most centers have practically adopted indices indicative of 80% mortality, such as either a $AaDO_2$ gradient ≥ 610 Torr for 8 consecutive hours [37] or ≥ 605 Torr and peak inspiratory pressure > 38 cm H_2O for more than 4 hours [38] or the Oxygenation Index (OI) [39]. The various indices are listed in Table 2. However, for such infants, other alternative may exist such as High-Frequency oscillatory ventila-

Table 2. ECMO Criteria

Patients must meet **all** of the following criteria:
1. Weight greater than 2 kilograms
2. No suspected karyotypic anomalies
3. No congenital heart disease (Two-dimensional echocardiography)
4. No intracranial hemorrhage (Head ultrasound)
5. No severe coagulopathy
6. Failure of "maximal medical therapy" (100% oxygen, no tracheal leaks, appropriate hyperventilation, systemic arterial support, vasodilator trials)
7. Reversible lung disease within 1 to 2 weeks (no more than 7 days of mechanical ventilation)
8. **Plus** one of the following:
   - $P(A-a)O_2$[a] ≥ 610 Torr for 8 hours (80% mortality)
   - $P(A-a)O_2$[a] ≥ 605 Torr and PIP[b] ≥ 38 cm H_2O for 4 hours (84% mortality)
   - Oxygenation Index (O.I.) = Paw (cm H_2O) × FiO_2 (%) / post-ductal PaO_2 (Torr)
   - – if O.I. ≥ 25 for 5 subsequent values: 50% mortality
   - – if O.I. ≥ 40 for 5 subsequent values: 80% mortality

[a] $P(A-a)O_2 = $ (Barometric pressure (mmHg) $- 47$ mmHg) $\cdot FiO_2$ (should be I.O.) $- PaO_2 - PaCO_2$
[b] $PIP = $ Peak inspiratory pressure (cmH_2O)

tion (HFOV). In fact, both methods are not exclusive but complementary. Thus, Cornish et al. [40] treated 16 infants having ECMO criteria: one was put directly on ECMO, 15 underwent a HFOV trial; 7 were successfully treated but 8 ECMO were later treated with ECMO.

ECMO Equipment

The accepted ECMO procedure in neonates is venoarterial. The main reason is the need to support gas exchange as well as the impaired cardiac function secondary to right ventricular pressure overload. This technique needs however definite surgical ligation of major vessels, usually the right carotid artery and the internal jugular vein. No early or late deleterious adverse effects attributable to this has been definitely proved so far, mainly because effective cerebral perfusion is maintained through the Willis circle by the left vessels as well as the vertebral arteries.

A veno-venous alternative has been suggested and tested in several cases [41, 42]. This technique usually needs surgical cutdown of the right internal jugular vein and of a femoral vein. However, initiating veno-venous bypass required more surgical time because two incisions and dissections are required. The pump output usually needs to be 40% higher on veno-venous (requiring larger canulas) than on veno-arteria bypass to obtain appropriate systemic oxygenation. The veno-venous bypass does not support the failing right ventricle as efficiently as the veno-arterial bypass, and had to be converted in veno-arterial bypass in 7 of 15 cases [13]. Finally, after ECMO, there was a significant amount of early (groin infections) as well as late complications (enlarged leg).

There is no standard "ECMO" machine. The system has been designed from cardiopulmonary bypass equipment. The oxygenator must be a model using a silicone membrane (Sci-Med 0.8 m^2, Sci-Med Life Systems Inc., Minneapolis, MN). In fact, the column oxygenators become porous and leak significant amounts of serum after 24 to 48 hours of function, and are therefore inappropriate for a run which may last for 8 to 10 days. Other essential components are: a tubing pack individually designed for each institution; a 50 ml venous silicone reservoir bag (Sci-Med); a system which monitors venous return and alarms if there is a significant drop (this is not commercially available); a roller head occlusion pump; a 45 ml-heat exchanger (Sci-Med) with a heating unit; an oxygen flow (0.1 L/min) and CO_2 flow (0.01 L/min)meters.

ECMO Procedure [43]

Preparation of the Bypass Circuit

The first step in the ECMO procedure is the preparation of the bypass circuit. All the parts: tubing, venous reservoir, membrane oxygenator, heat exchanger, pigtail connections, and two-way stopcocks are unpacked then assembled with aseptic conditions. All stopcocks are turned off but one, next to the oxygenator. Then a tubing is connected between the CO_2 source and the priming bag through a filter. The CO_2 gas flow (1 L/min) is turned on for 5 minutes in order to remove all the air in the circuit. This is followed by vacuum application. Then, a crystalloid solution is introduced through the priming bag to fill the system. While the pump runs the flow at 200–250 ml/min, special care is taken to remove bubbles from all parts including the oxygenator. To decrease platelet adhesion, 200 ml of 20 or 25% albumin is added to the circuit, which is then primed with 2 units of unwashed packed red cells. The pH is adjusted in adding 10 to 15 ml of sodium bicarbonate. The red cell/albumin prime is allowed to circulate through the circuit with room air added to the membrane for a few minutes. Blood gases are obtained to ensure normal acid-base status.

Cannulation

While the ECMO circuit is set up, the surgical team starts the cannulation procedure, at the bedside in the ICU. Anesthesia insured by Fentanyl (10 to 15 µg/kg) and supplemented with local anesthesia (0.5% xylocaine) to the surgical site. Often the baby was already paralyzed with pancuronium or vecuronium (0.1 mg/kg). A 2 cm-long vertical incision is performed over the right sternomastoid muscle, starting at 1 cm above the calvicula. During dissection, meticulous hemostasis is necessary using electrocautery, since the baby will be systematically heparinized. The internal jugular vein and the carotid artery are exposed. Heparin is given intravenously as a 150 U/kg bolus. The artery is clamped then opened up and the intima carefully sewed with 6–0 silk, in order to prevent intimal dissection during the cannulation procedure. The arterial catheter (8 to 10 F) is advanced to the aortic arch. The venous catheter should be the largest possible (10 to 14 F) and have several side holes in order to allowed left venous return through the innominate vein, when its tip is advanced to the low right atrium. Surgical and hemostatic glue is placed on the wound. The catheter placement is checked by X-ray then the wound is closed.

Starting ECMO

The ECMO circuit (Fig. 1) is carfully connected to the cannulas to ensure that no air has been introduced into the system, while the priming is still running through the bridge. Bypass is started by removing first the arterial clamp, second clamping the bridge, third removing the venous clamp. The bypass flow is increased slowly by 50-ml increments as the ventilator is decreased. During all the procedure, care is taken to the infant's arterial pressure, and its transcutaneous O_2/CO_2 which should be maintained within physiological values. In order to obtain adequate systemic blood gases, bypass flows should be as high as 300 to 500 ml/min or 70 to 80% of the normal cardiac output which is estimated to be 150–200 ml/kg, and easily measured using pulsed-Doppler echocardiography [44]. This allowed to reduce the ventilator settings to: FiO_2 0.21, rate 10 to 15

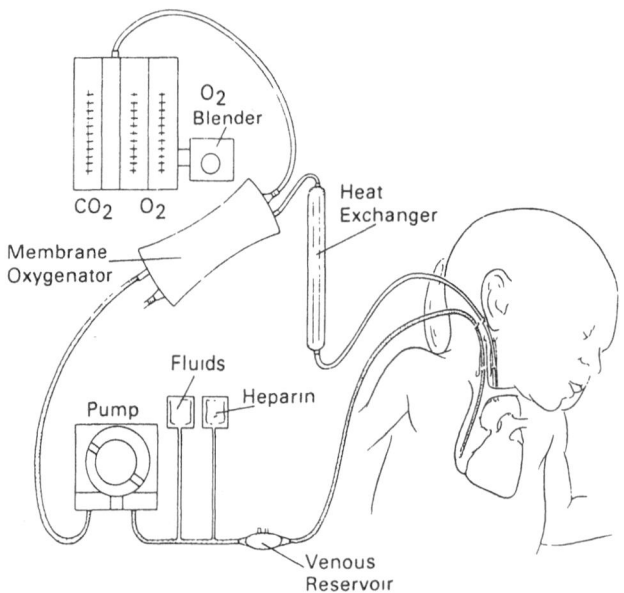

Fig. 1. The arteriovenous ECMO circuit

breaths min, inspiratory time (TI) 0.5 second, peak inspiratory pressure (PIP) 15, and positive end-expiratory pressure (PEEP) 5 cm H_2O.

Routine Management on ECMO

The amount of oxygen delivered to the patient on ECMO is related to the gas transfer characteristics of the membrane lung. As in the human lung, oxygen transfer across the membrane depends on the flow rate and the degree of the blood's oxyhemoglobin desaturation entering the membrane lung: O_2 delivery = Flow x O_2 content. Therefore, to increase oxygenation, one must increase the percent of cardiac output going through the membrane lung. The usual size for a newborn is 0.8 m^2. The Sci-Med membrane will transfer 60 to 70 ml of O_2/m^2. Gas flow across the membrane is usually kept between 1 and 2 L/min. Caution must be taken not to increase gas flow higher than 2.4 L/min (for the 0.8 m^2 membrane) since gasous bubbles may appear in the blood and induce air embolism. Because of the large oxygen gradient across the membrane, oxygen transfer is not affected by changes in gas flow.

Since CO_2 is much more diffusible than oxygen, the CO_2 gradient across the membrane lung is small, provided there is no fluid accumulation on the gasous side of the membrane. Therefore, CO_2 is efficiently removed, and often some low stream of CO_2 (0.01–0.04 L/min) must be added in order to maintain the infant's $PaCO_2$ in the range of 35 to 45 Torr. Thus, CO_2 levels may be altered by two methods: 1) changing the sweep-gas flow: if the gas flow is increased, more CO_2 will be removed and vice-versa; 2) changing the CO_2 amount entering the oxygenator.

The infant's blood gases should be measured every hour. However, the use of non-invasive devices such as transcutaneous oxygen saturation with a pulse oximeter (which works only if a pulse pressure is maintained) or transcutaneous PO_2/PCO_2 may decrease the number of blood gas samplings. Likewise, the continuous measurement of venous oxygen saturation is very helpful for adjusting the necessary bypass flow. Normal post-pump blood gases should range from pH 7.35 to 7.45, PCO_2 35 to 40 Torr, and PO_2 350 to 400 Torr. Since veno-arterial ECMO provides cardiac and pulmonary support, inotropic drugs such as dopamine and vasodilators such as tolazoline may be discontinued. Muscle relaxants are also unnecessary. The infant is allowed to awaken and breathe spontaneously. Respiratory care is continued but limited to vibration and suctioning, the cannulas restricting the changes in the infant's position.

The infant must have enough circulating blood volume to obtain adequate blood flow rates. A practical way of assessing the neccessary blood volume is to look at the bypass flow which makes the infant's pulsatile arterial contour to flatten. It means, in fact, that bypass flow is too high in comparison to the infant's own cardiac output. Blood losses are often large: blood sampling, wound drainage ... and careful and complete intake and output should be done hourly. Volume replacement (packed red blood cells if the hematocrit is less than 45% and if not 10 or 20% albumin) must be given however slowly in order ro avoid a sudden increase in blood volume with subsequent sudden increase in the pulmonary blood flow and hypoxemia. Fluid intakes must be in the normal range (90–150 ml/kg/d), trying to keep the infant on the "dry" side. Urinary output is usually high (2–4 ml/kg/min) in response to improved oxygenation. However, over 90% of the infants will develop a left-to-right shunt through the patent ductus arteriosus (PDA) on day 2 to 3 and will be treated with more severe fluid restriction (< 100 ml/kg/d). Electrolyte needs are slightly less for Na^+ (1–2 mMol/kg/d), and increased for K^+ (4–5 mMol/kg/d) and Ca^{++} (50–70 mg/kg/d). Total parenteral nutrition should supply at least 90 kcal/kg/d of a balanced intralipid, sugar, and protein solution.

Systemic anticoagulation must be maintained during the ECMO course. The most practical test is the activated clotting time (ACT). It is measured as needed, every 30 to 60 minutes, on blood sampled before the venous reservoir. Measurements are made at the bedside using a Hemochron (International Technidyne Corp, Edison, NJ) or Actester (Kendall McGaw Inc, Santa Ana, CA). ACTs should to maintained between 220 and 260 seconds. This requires a constant heparin drip of 20 to 70 U/kg/h which must arrive at the venous reservoir level but after the sampling port. Platelets are sequestered at the membrane lung level, and frequent platelet transfusions are needed to keep the platelet counts above $60000/mm^3$. All platelet transfusions must be given after the membrane lung to decrease membrane platelet adherence. Head ultrasonography must be done daily to detect intracranial hemorrhage.

Special care must be taken to aseptic procedures, specially at the levels of samplings and injections. Blood cultures are taken daily. One must be aware that vancomycin reacts with heparin.

Weaning from ECMO

For the first 1 to 2 days, bypass flow should be kept at 70 to 80% of the infant's cardiac output, in order to maintain the infant's PaO_2 between 60 to 80 Torr. As the infant's lungs improve, the PaO_2 increases above this level and the bypass flow may be slowly decreased by 10 to 20 ml/min-steps, gradually diminishing the amount of cardiac output bypassed. When the ECMO flows are decreased to 30% of the cardiac output, the FiO_2 delivered to the ventilator is increased to 0.30 to accommodate the increased pulmonary blood flow. The weaning process continues until the bypass flow reaches 40 to 50 ml/min (around 10% of cardiac output), whereas PaO_2 are well maintained in the normal range. Once these "idling" flows are reached, no further changes are made for 8 to 12 hours to ensure that the infant's condition is sufficiently stable before decannulation.

The chest X-ray is characterized by a pattern of diffuse atelectasis ("white lungs"), for the first days. Then, the lung fields clear up a few hours before the infant could be weaned off. This radiological sequence parallels to the dynamic lung compliance (CL) measurements [45]. As the lungs heal, surfactant-associated protein concentrations in lung lavage increases [46], CL improves, and a value of 0.8 ml/cm H_2O or greater predict successful decannulation.

Decannulation

After a successful idling period, the infant is ready to be taken off ECMO. The decannulation procedure is similar to cannulation, although it can usually be scheduled at a more convenient time. The infant is paralyzed with a short-action muscle relaxant such as vecuronium (0.1 mg/kg) and sedated with fentanyl (5μg/kg). The neonatologist monitors vital signs and makes appropriate ventilatory changes as needed. Ventilator settings are increased to FiO_2 30 to 40, rate 40 to 45 breath/min. Tl 6 second, PIP 18 to 20 cm H_2O. It is important to avoid air embolus when removing the venous cannula using the respiratory hold of the ventilator. Both the internal jugular vein and carotid artery are ligated.

The infant is allowed to breathe spontaneously shortly after decannulation. The average time to extubation in most institutions is 24 hours, followed by oxygen therapy for 5 to 7 days. Platelets must be monitored closely because severe thrombocytopenia post-ECMO is common. Few infants have BPD; most of them were placed on ECMO after more than 6 days of ventilator therapy.

ECMO Complications

Bleeding

Most complications of ECMO therapy are related to the use of heparin and its sytemic effects. Bleeding from the neck operative site is usually small, but if it exceeds 5 to 6 ml per hour the site should be explored. However, the most frequent finding is generalized oozing from surrounding tissues, which can usually be stopped by applying surgical glue or packing with gelfoam soaked in topical thrombin. Congenital diaphragmatic hernia repaire may have significant bleeding and if not brought under control may require early removal from ECMO support [35]. The frequency of stump bleeding may justify the new concept of delayed diaphragmatic repair. Other bleeding complications have included: pulmonary hemorrhage, nose bleeding, umbilical site bleeding, and chest tube bleeding. All of these should be treated with low ACTs, higher flows and higher platelet counts than usual.

Nevertheless, the most common cause of death is severe intracranial hemorrhage (ICH) [13, 17]. Its incidence greatly depends upon the gestational age. Thus, among the first 100 infants treated by Bartlett et al. [13] ICH occured in 17 out of 19 (89%) having less than 35 weeks of gestation and only in 12 out of 81 (15%) having more than 35 weeks. Moreover, more appropriate criteria for ECMO therapy may explain the decrease in its incidence. Thus, during Phase I (1973-1982) in which ECMO was used when all other therapy has failed, ICH incidence was 38% (17/50); during Phase II (1982-1984) in which ECMO was applied as a prospective controlled randomized study following high mortality risk criteria, ICH incidence was 13% (4/30); finally, during Phase III (1984-1986) in which ECMO was applied for all patients if mortality risk was 80% or greater, ICH incidence was only 10% (2/20). The pre-ECMO events are important for ICH incidence, and an ultrtasound scanogram should be systematically obtained before ECMO. Systemic heparinization places these infants at risk for such complications and thus heparin therapy must be monitored closely. If the bleed is limited, ECMO may be continued but the heparin dose is lowered to decrease ACTs to 200 to 210 seconds while ECMO flows are increased to 80% of cardiac output to decrease the risks of clot formation in the circuit. Meanwhile, platelets are maintained at greater than 80000 to 100000/mm^3. Massive ICH justifies to discontinue ECMO and reinitiating maximum ventilatory assistance.

Other neurological complications than ICH may intervene during ECMO, such as seizures. Seizures occurred in 25% of the infants [13, 17], and are often easily controlled with anticonvulsant therapy. Their pathophysiology remains speculative, probably not linked to carotid artery ligation. However, they seem to be associated with some developmental delay [47].

Patent Ductus Arteriosus

More than 90% of infants on their second or third day on ECMO will developed a left-to-right shunt through the patent ductus arteriosus (PDA). This is manifested by persistence of white lungs on X-ray, decreasing CL, and the need to increase ECMO flows to maintain a normal PaO$_2$. The best diagnostic tools are probably at the moment a combination of pulsed-Doppler and contrast echocardiography. Severe fluid restriction and diuretics over several days will permit closing of most patent ductus arteriosus. Indomethacin use is discouraged because it may dramatically increase bleeding risks. Surgical ligation may be necessary but is unusual.

Acute Renal Insufficiency

Acute renal insufficiency seems unusual, involving 10 of 100 patients in Bartlett et al's study [13]. This is presumably due to acute tubular necrosis. Its treatment is now simplified by the use of an hemofilter (Minifilter, Amicon, Danvers, MA) hooded between the pump and the venous reservoir bag. However, special care must be taken to restrict the ultrafiltrate in order to prevent rapid and severe dehydration.

Technical Failures

Technical failures such as breakage of the lung membrane, rupture of the race-way, dysfunction of the heat exchanger, disconnection of tubings ... are not unu-sual, if one considers the 31% rate reported by Bartlett et al. [13]. However, all these adverse events were not directly associated with mortality. This fact em-phasizes the need of a highly trained ECMO team.

Inability to Wean from ECMO

Inability to wean from the ECMO circuit can be due to a number of causes including undiagnosed cardiac disease such as total abnormal pulmonary ve-nous return (TAVPR), significant patent ductus arteriosus, hypoplastic lungs. A mechanical problem should be considered: insufficient occlusion of the pump head. However, the most common cause is undiagnosed TAVPR. Most infants require ECMO for 5 days. So, if the flows cannot be reduced to 60% of cardiac output by day 5, cardiac re-evaluation and cardiac catheterization must be con-sidered. The diagnosis of hypoplastic lungs is more common in congenital diaphragmatic hernia than in other pulmonary diseases.

Outcome and Follow-up

The overall results of neonatal ECMO are very impressive, if one considers the overall results of the ECMO Central Registry Report (Table 1). Up to August 1987, 978 infants have been treated with ECMO in 36 centers, including 3 Eu-ropean centers with an overall survival of 80.7% (data due to the courtesy of Dr. Bartlett and Dr. Toomasian). These results are remarkable, if one considers that the majority of these infants have been selected on the basis of an 80% mortality risks.

However, because of the severity of the primary disease and the possibility of late complications, a critical evaluation of the long-term follow-up is mandatory. Although the permanent ligation of two major neck vessels did not appear to be associated with early morbidity, it was necessary to evaluate the potential late sequellae. Towne et al. [48] studied 18 children ranging from 4 to 11 years of age. The evaluation of carotid arteries output using continuous Doppler exhibited:

1) a minimal flow in the right carotid artery due to retrograde flow coming from the right external carotid artery; 2) a compensatory flow in the left carotid artery. Moreover, the evoked potentials were found diminished on the right side but without any clinical significance.

Likewise, the long-term follow-up studies are extremely encouraging. Kirkpatrick et al. [46] examined at 1 year of age 6 survivors out of 8 newborns treated with ECMO: five were normal, and one was delayed. However, she suffered a cardiopulmonary arrest due to presumed air embolization at decannulation. Towne et al. [45] followed up 18 of 24 survivors out of 47 newborns treated by Dr. Bartlett: thirteen were normals and five were delayed: one required shunting for hydrocephalus and one had a defect that lateralized to the right hemisphere. Andrews et al. [49] evaluated the long-term results of the newborns treated by Dr. Bartlett in Ann Arbor, MI: 7 out of 14 (50%) survivors were totally normal with 1 to 3-year follow-up but 10 out of 14 (71%) were mentally normal. Glass et al. [50] systematically examined the newborns treated at the National Children's in Washington, DC: out of 120 neonates treated with ECMO within 2 years and a half, 85% survived; 42 out of 46 were more than 1 year follow-up; 62% were normal both for motor and mental Bailey scores, 18% were "suspect" (1 of 2 scores lower than 90), and 20% delayed (both scores lower than 90) but only 10% significantly delayed. The latter were precisely those who suffered birth asphyxia.

However, these optimistic results should be tempered by the neuro-imaging (ultrasound during ECMO and CT scan prior to discharge) results on the 84 survivors of the first 100 patients: major ICH (grade > II, intraparenchymal or cerebellar hemorrhage) in 6 (7%), 3 of whom required shunts; minor ICH (subependymal or petecchial hemorrhage) in 16 (19%); non-hemorrhagic intracranial abnormalities in 10 (12%): atrophy = 5, hypodensities = 3, periventricular leukomalacia = 1, partial thrombosis of the sagittal sinus = 1, i.e. altogether 38% of abnormalities [51]. Likewise, 34 survivors in Ann Arbor were longitudinally reviewed. Ten infants had a CT scan: 4 were diffusely abnormal, 1 had bilateral focal lesions, and all three unifocal lesions were right-sided [52]. Our single case with CDH suffered also right-sided cortical hypoperfusion using single positron emitting tomography [53].

On the other hand, the incidence of bronchopulmonary dysplasia was markedly low in this high-risk population. Bartlett et al. [13] experienced only 8 (3 will ultimately die) out of 72 (11%). Miller et al. [17] had 13 out of 84 (15%) infants with low oxygen-dependence ($FiO_2 < 30$) and 7 for longer than 1 month.

Future Developments

ECMO therapy is still in its infancy. The equipment used will probably dramatically change in the next few years. One of the most expected breakthrough is the development of a circuit totally heparin-bonded, obviating the need for systemic heparinization [54, 55]. The recent development of a new technique which

covalently bonds by end-point attachment the active sites of heparin will probably definitely solve this problem.

If ECMO is proved to improve not only survival but also to reduce the morbidity of infants with ARF selected on the basis of only 50% mortality risks,
ECMO would be applied earlier on less sick newborns. In these conditions, a
less effective circuit such as venovenous bypass would be appropriate for pulmonary as well as cardiovascular support. The lower bypass flow would allow
the use of smaller cannula which might be inserted percutaneously. Similarly, a
double-lumen single venous canula might be employed [56]. Moreover, if the
lung may be proved to be safely ventilated with higher setting, the necessary
ECMO flow would be lower and the system will greatly approach the CO_2 removal system successfully applied in the adults by Gattinoni [57].

Costs of ECMO

Health costs have become one of the major limits for medicine and particularly
intensive care medicine. ECMO has been evaluated also from this point of
view. Pearson and Short [58] compared the costs of the 25 first newborns treated
with ECMO from June 1984 to June 1985 to those of 34 matched control newborns treated with conventional treatment:

1. survival was 80.8% in the ECMO group vs 28.6% in the control group ($p \leqslant$
   0.05);
2. average length of stay in the hospital was 21 days in the ECMO group vs 37
   days in the control group ($p \leqslant 0.05$);
3. total average charges per patient were respectively \$ 91,804 and \$ 93,524
   ($p = NS$), i.e. the costs per patient were similar;
4. however, when only survivors of both groups were compared, average length
   of stay was much shorter for ECMO (25 days) than for conventional treatment (76 days) ($p < 0.001$) as well as average charges per patient \$ 98,320 vs \$
   173,282 ($p \leqslant 0.001$). Therefore, the necessary financial investment for ECMO
   has been positive for the Society.

Conclusion

The use of ECMO has been undoubtedly successful in a large number of full-
term or near-term infants with severe acute respiratory failure. The mortality of
these patients has been dramatically reduced (roughly 80% survival vs 20% with
conbentional medical treatment). However, the morbidity of such treated disease processes appears to be acceptable, provided a careful selection of the patients as well as a highly trained ECMO team.

In fact, ECMO is very labor-intensive and requires a well-organized team including neonatologists or intensivists, cardiovascular surgeons, perfusionists,
technical specialists, and trained nursing staff on the supervision of a full-time
coordinator. Likewise, the cardiology and radiology services, pharmacy, blood

bank, and almost all support systems are affected. It is why ECMO could not be unorganized. ECMO programs should be regionalized and restricted to large mainly University Hospitals. In Europe, such a program as every other expensive and labor-intensive programs should be discussed at both national health and medical organization levels. The latter has partially justified the foundation of the European Society of Pediatric Intensive Care. This is in our opinion the single way to contribute to the development of a successful ECMO program.

Finally, with improvement in the technique and the hope in a next future of totally nonthrombogenic systems, ECMO may soon become available to a much larger population of infants who presently die of their respiratory disease or survive with a severe bronchopulmonary dysplasia.

Acknowledgments: We would like to warmly thank Dr. R. H. Bartlett, Dr. B. L. Short, Dr. Arensman, and Dr. A. M. Salzberg for their strong support and their fraternal advices.

References

1. Bartlett RH, Gassaniga AB, Jeffreis MR, et al (1976) Extracorporeal membrane oxygenation cardiopulmonary support in infancy. Trans Am Soc Artif Int Organs 22:80-93
2. Clowes GHA, Hopkins AL, Neville WE (1976) An artificial lung dependent upon diffusion of oxygen and carbon dioxide through plastic membranes. J Thorac Cardiovasc Surg 32:630-637
3. Zapol WM, Snider MT, Hill DJ, et al (1979) Extracorporeal membrane oxygenation in severe acute respiratory failure: A randomized study. JAMA 242:2193-2196
4. Gille JP, Bagniewski AM (1976) Ten years of use of extracorporeal membrane oxygenation (ECMO) in the treatment of acute respiratory insufficiency (ARI). Trans Am Soc Artif Intern Organs 22:102-108
5. Pratt PC, Vollmer RT, Shelburne JD, et al (1979) Pulmonary morphology in a multihospital collaborative extracorporeal membrane oxygenation project. Am J Pathol 95:191-208
6. Bartlett RH, Gazzaniga AB, Fong SW, et al (1973) Extracorporeal membrane oxygenator support for cardiopulmonary failure. Experience in 28 cases. J Thorac Cardiovasc Surg 66:214-218
7. Redmond CR, Graves ED, Falterman KW, et al (1987) Extracorporeal membrane oxygenation for respiratory and cardiac failure in infants and children. J Thorac Cardiovasc Surg 93:199-204
8. Callaghan JC, Cardoza D, Boracchia B (1962) Study of prepulmonary bypass in the development of an artificial placenta for prematurity and respiratory distress of the newborn. J Thorac Cardiovasc Surg 44:600-604
9. Rashkind WJ, Freedman A, Klein D, et al (1965) Evolution of a disposable plastic low volume, pumpless oxygenator as a lung substitute. J Pediatr 66:94-102
10. White JJ, Andrews HG, Risenberg H, et al (1971) Prolonged respiratory support in newborn infants with a membrane oxygenator. Surgery 70:288-296
11. Bartlett RH, Andrews AF, Toomasian JM, et al (1982) Extracorporeal membrane oxygenation for newborn respiratory failure: Forty-five cases. Surgery 92:425-433
12. Bartlett RH, Gazzaniga AB, Huxtabie RH, et al (1979) Extracorporeal membrane oxygenation (ECMO) in neonatal respiratory failure: Technical considerations. Trans Am Soc Artif Intern Organs 25:173-175
13. Bartlett RH, Toomasian JM, Roloff DW, et al (1986) Extracorporeal membrane oxygenation (ECMO) in neonatal respiratory failure: 100 cases. Ann Surg 204:236-244
14. Trento A, Griffith BP, Hardesty RL (1986) Extracorporeal membrane oxygenation experience at the University of Pittsburg. Ann Thorac Surg 42:56-59

15. Loe WA, Graves ED, Oschner JL, et al (1985) Extracorporeal membrane oxygenation for newborn respiratory failure. J Pediatr Surg 20:684–688
16. Weber TR, Plennington DG, Connors R, et al (1986) Extracorporeal membrane oxygenation for newborn respiratory failure. Ann Thorac Surg 42:529–535
17. Miller MK, Short BL, Glass P, et al (1987) Outcome of 100 infants with extracorporeal membrane oxygenation (ECMO). Pediatr Res 21:369A (Abstr)
18. Bartlett RH, Roloff DW, Cornell RG, et al. (1985) Extracorporeal circulatory support in neonatal respiratory failure: A prospective randomized study. Pediatrics 76:479–487
19. Paneth N, Wallenstein S (1985) Extracorporeal membrane oxygenation and the play the winner rule. Pediatrics 76:622–623
20. Andrews AF, Roloff DW, Bartlett RH (1984) Use of extracorporeal membrane oxygenation in persistent pulmonary hypertension of the newborn. Clin Perinatol 11:729–735
21. Short BL, Pearson GD (1986) Neonatal extracorporeal membrane oxygenation: A review. J Intens Care Med 1:48–54
22. Gersony WM (1984) Neonatal pulmonary hypertension: Pathophysiology, classification, and etiology. Clin Perinatol 11:517–524
23. Stolar CJH, Dillon PW, Stalcup SA (1985) Extracorporeal membrane oxygenation and congenital diaphragmatic hernia: Modification of the pulmonary vasoactive profile. J Pediatr Surg 20:681–683
24. Fow WW, Duara S (1983) Persistent pulmonary hypertension in the neonate: Diagnosis and management. J Pediatr 103:505–514
25. Drummond WH, Gregory GA, Heyman MA, et al (1981) The independent effects of hyperventilation, tolazoline and dopamine on infants with persistent pulmonary hypertension. J Pediatr 98:603–609
26. Boros SJ, Ring DR, Mammel MC, et al (1984) Using conventional infant ventilators at unconventional rates. Pediatrics 74:497–492
27. Wetzel RC, Gisia FR (1987) High frequency ventilation. Pediatr Clin N Am 34:15–38
28. Vacanti JP, Crone RK, Murphy JD, et al (1984) The pulmonary hemodynamic response to perioperative anesthesia in the treatment of high-risk infants with congenital diaphragmatic hernia. J Pediatr Surg 19:672–679
29. Drummond WH, Lock JE (1984) Neonatal "pulmonary vasodilator" drugs. Pharmacol Ther 7:1–20
30. Ward RM (1984) Pharmacology of tolazoline. Clin Perinatol 11:703–713
31. Hardesty RL, Griffith BP, Debski RF, et al (1981) Extracorporeal membrane oxygenation: Successful treatment of persistent fetal circulation following repair of congenital diaphragmatic hernia. J Thorac Cardiovasc Surg 81:556–563
32. Cartlidge PHT, Mann NP, Kapila L (1986) Preoperative stabilisation in congenital diaphragmatic hernia. Arch Dis Child 61:1226–1228
33. Bohn DJ, James I, Filler RM, et al (1984) The relathionship between $PaCO_2$ and ventilation parameters in predicting survival in congenital diaphragmatic hernia. J Pediatr Surg 19:666–671
34. Bohn, D, Tamura M, Perrin D, et al (1987) Ventilatory predictors of pulmonary hypoplasia in congenital diaphragmatic hernia, confirmed by morphologic assessment. J Pediatr 111:423–431
35. Langham MR, Krummel TM, Greenfield LJ, et al (1987) Extracorporeal membrane oxygenation following repair of congenital diaphragmatic hernia. Ann Thorac Surg 44:247
36. Raphaely RC, Downes JJ Jr (1973) Congenital diaphragmatic hernia: Prediction of survival. J Pediatr Surg 8:815–823
37. Krummel TM, Greenfield LG, Krikpatrick BV, et al (1984) The early evaluation of survivors after extracorporeal membrane oxygenation for neonatal respiratory failure. J Pediatr Surg 19:585–590
38. Beck R, Anderson KD, Pearson GD, et al (1986) Criteria for extracorporeal membrane oxygenation in a population of infants with persistent pulmonary hypertension of the newborn. J Pediatr Surg 21:297–302
39. Ortiz RM, Cilley RE, Bartlett RH (1987) Extracorporeal membrane oxygenation in pediatric respiratory failure. Pediatr Clin N Am 34:39–46

40. Cornish JD, Gertsmann DR, Clark RH, et al (1987) Extracorporeal membrane oxygenation and high frequency oscillatory ventilation: Potential therapeutic relationship. Crit Care Med (in press)

41. Andrews AF, Klein MD, Toomasian JM, et al (1983) Venovenous extracorporeal membrane oxygenation in neonates with respiratory failure J Pediatr Surg 18:339–346

42. Klein MD, Andrews AF, Wesley JR, et al (1985) Venovenous perfusion in 02–CEC for newborn respiratory insufficiency. A clinical comparison with venoarterial perfusion. Ann Surg 201:520–526

43. Toomasian JM, Chapman RA, Bartlett RH (eds) (1987) Extracorporeal membrane oxygenation. Technical specialist manual, 8th edition. The University of Michigan, Ann Arbor

44. Tibballs J, Mercier JC, Trang TTH, et al (1986) Mesure du débit cardiaque par Doppler pulsé chez l'enfant Réan, Soins Intens, Méd Urg 2:231 (Abstr)

45. Lotze A, Short BL, Taylor GA (1987) Lung compliance as a measure of lung function in newborns with respiratory failure requiring extracorporeal membrane oxygenation. Crit Care Med 15:226–229

46. Lotze A, Short BL, Whitsett JA (1987) Surfactant-associated protein (SAP) concentrations in lung lavage fluid in infants requiring extracorporeal membrane oxygenation (ECMO) Pediatr Res 21:458A (Abstr)

47. Conry JA, Miller MK, Glass P, et al (1987) Neonatal seizures and EEG in infants following extracorporeal membrane oxygenation (ECMO). Pediatr Res 21:490A (Abstr)

48. Towne BH, Lott IT, Hicks DA, et al (1985) Long-term follow-up of infants and children treated with extracorporeal membrane oxygenation (ECMO): A preliminary report. J Pediatr Surg 20:410–414

49. Andrews AF, Nixon CA, Cilley RE, et al (1986) One- to three-year outcome for 14 neonatal survivors of extracorporeal membrane oxygenation. Pediatrics 78:692–698

50. Glass P, Miller MK, Short BL (1987) Extracorporeal membrane oxygenation (ECMO): Outcome at 1 year of age. Pediatr Res 21:395A (Abstr)

51. Miller MK, Glass P, Taylor GA, et al (1987) Neuroimaging of ECMO patients. Pediatr Res 21:494A (Abstr)

52. Shumacher RE, Barks JDE, Johnston MV, et al (1987) Right-sided brain lesions in infants following carotid ligation for extracorporeal membrane oxygenation. Pediatr Res 21:375A (Abstr)

53. Mercier JC, Laborde F, Aigrain Y, et al (1986) Oxygénation extra-corporelle: un cas de hernie diaphragmatique congénitale traité avec succès. Réan, Soins Intens, Méd Urg 2:261 (Abstr)

54. Risohk HV, Calabrese D, Sanematsu L, et al (1984) Bound and circulating heparin in an ECMO system: Thrombogenicity versus functionality. Trans Am Soc Artif Intern Organs 30:636–643

55. Toomasian JM, Zwischenberger JB, Okam AD, et al (1984) The use of bound heparin in prolonged extracorporeal membrane oxygenation. Trans Am Soc Artif Intern Organs 30:133–136

56. Zwischenberger JB, Toomasian JM, Drake K, et al (1985) Total respiratory support with single cannula venovenous ECMO: double lumen continuous flow vs single lumen tidal flow. Trans Am Soc Artif Intern Organs 31:610–615

57. Gattinoni L, Pesenti A, Masheroni D, et al (1986) Low frequency positive-pressure ventilation with extracorporeal CO_2 removal in severe acute respiratory failure. JAMA 256:881–886

58. Pearson GD, Short BL (1987) An economical analysis of extracorporeal membrane oxygenation. J Intens Care Med 2:116–120